Body Structures & Functions

10th Edition

Ann Senisi Scott

Elizabeth Fong

THOMSON

DELMAR LEARNING   Australia   Canada   Mexico   Singapore   Spain   United Kingdom   United States

THOMSON

DELMAR LEARNING

Body Structures & Functions, 10th edition
by Ann Senisi Scott and Elizabeth Fong

Executive Director, Health Care Business Unit
William Brottmiller

Executive Editor
Cathy L. Esperti

Acquisitions Editor
Sherry Gomoll

Developmental Editor
Darcy M. Scelsi

Editorial Assistant
Jennifer Conklin

Executive Marketing Manager
Dawn F. Gerrain

Channel Manager
Jennifer McAvey

Project Editor
Shelley Esposito

Production Editor
John Mickelbank

Art and Design Coordinator
Robert Plante

For permission to use material from this text or product contact us by
Tel   (800) 730-2214
Fax   (800) 730-2215
www.thomsonrights.com

Library of Congress Cataloging-in-Publication Data

Scott, Ann Senisi, 1935–
   Body structures & functions.—10th ed. / Ann Senisi Scott, Elizabeth Fong.
      p. cm.
   ISBN 1-40180-995-2
   1. Human physiology. 2. Human anatomy. I. Title: Body structures and functions. II. Fong, Elizabeth. III. Title.

QP34.5 .F66 2004
612—dc21

2004031519

NOTICE TO THE READER

Publisher does not warrant or guarantee any of the products described herein or perform any independent analysis in connection with any of the product information contained herein. Publisher does not assume, and expressly disclaims, any obligation to obtain and include information other than that provided to it by the manufacturer.

The reader is expressly warned to consider and adopt all safety precautions that might be indicated by the activities herein and to avoid all potential hazards. By following the instructions contained herein, the reader willingly assumes all risks in connection with such instructions.

The Publisher makes no representation or warranties of any kind, including but not limited to, the warranties of fitness for particular purpose or merchantability, nor are any such representations implied with respect to the material set forth herein, and the publisher takes no responsibility with respect to such material. The publisher shall not be liable for any special, consequential, or exemplary damages resulting, in whole or part, from the readers' use of, or reliance upon, this material.

CONTENTS

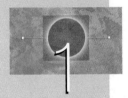

INTRODUCTION TO THE STRUCTURAL UNITS / 1

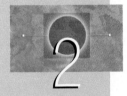

CHEMISTRY OF LIVING THINGS / 12

CELLS / 28

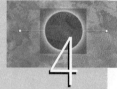
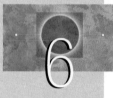
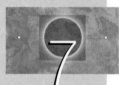
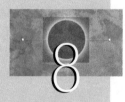

PERIPHERAL AND AUTONOMIC NERVOUS SYSTEM / 159

SPECIAL SENSES / 172

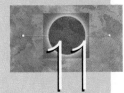

ENDOCRINE SYSTEM / 196

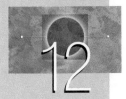

BLOOD / 222

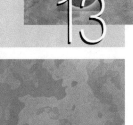

HEART / 240

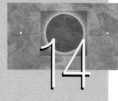

CIRCULATION AND BLOOD VESSELS / 265

THE LYMPHATIC SYSTEM AND IMMUNITY / 288

INFECTION CONTROL AND STANDARD PRECAUTIONS / 307

RESPIRATORY SYSTEM / 326

DIGESTIVE SYSTEM / 349

PREFACE

INTRODUCTION

The tenth edition of *Body Structures & Functions* has been revised to reflect the many changes that are occurring in today's health science and medical fields. The multi-skilled health practitioner (MSHP) of today must know the structure and function of each body system as well as the common diseases. All diseases and disorders content is integrated within each chapter as appropriate.

SPECIAL FEATURES

- Delmar's Anatomy and Physiology CD-ROM accompanies each text. Organized by body system, separate quiz and tutorial modes allow students to master key concepts.

- Effects of Aging boxes have been integrated within the chapters to highlight the changes that are associated with the body systems as we age.

- Medical Terminology review has been added to each chapter to acquaint the reader with common medical suffixes and prefixes and how they work to form medical terms.

- Case Studies have been added to promote a real-world view of medical careers and to hone critical thinking skills.

- Lab Activities have been added to incorporate an element of interactivity to the content, further enhancing comprehension.

- The art program has been revamped with new illustrations and gross anatomy images to enhance visual learners and add to the real-world appeal.

MAJOR CHANGES TO THE TENTH EDITION

- Chapter 3: Cells—revised discussion of mitosis and meiosis for ease of understanding, and new discussion of stem cell research

- Chapter 15: The Lymphatic System and Immunity—increased discussion of autoimmunity, updated discussion of AIDS/HIV infection, and updated immunization schedule

- Chapter 16: Infection Control and Standard Precautions—new chapter presents an overview of infection and the body's defense mechanisms and presents content on maintaining health and safety in the health care work environment

- Chapter 17: Respiratory System—added discussion on asbestosis and anthrax

- Chapter 19: Nutrition—updated discussion on the new adequate intakes and upper tolerable limits that are replacing the Recommended Dietary Allowances, updated discussion on the revised Dietary Guidelines for Americans, and new discussion on body mass index and basal metabolic rate

- Chapter 21: Reproductive System—updated and expanded discussion on infertility treatments and new tables on fetal development

MEDICAL HIGHLIGHTS

- Medical Imaging
- Stem Cell Research
- Genetic Engineering and Cloning
- Arthroscopy and Microdiskectomy
- Acupuncture
- Massage Therapy
- West Nile Virus
- Connection Between Nerves and Muscles
- Limbic System
- Cumulative Trauma Disorders
- Eye Strain and Computers
- Headaches
- Lasers
- Sunshine Disorder
- Diabetes
- Uses for Newborn's Umbilical or Cord Blood
- Treatment for Sickle Cell Anemia
- Triglycerides and Cholesterol Levels
- Pacemakers, Defibrillators, and Heart-Assistive Devices
- White Coat Hypertension
- Development in AIDS Research

- Bioterrorism
- Emphysema and Asthma
- Sleep Apnea
- Swallowable Imaging Capsule
- Body Mass Index
- Foods that Heal
- Kidney Stone Removal
- Fertility Tests
- Treatment for Cancer
- Gene Therapy

CAREER PROFILES

- Radiologic Technologists
- Physicians
- Physical Therapist and Physical Therapy Assistants
- Sports Medicine/Athletic Trainer
- Chiropractor
- Electroneuro Diagnostic Technician/EEG Technician
- Audiologists, Optometrists, and Dispensing Opticians
- Medical Assistant
- Clinical Laboratory Technician/Medical Laboratory Technician and Clinical Laboratory Technologists/Medical Technologist
- Emergency Medical Technicians and Paramedics
- Cardiovascular Technologists and Technicians/EKG Technicians
- Registered Nurses (RNs) and Nurse Practitioners
- Nurses Aides and Psychiatric Aides, Licensed Practical Nurses
- Dentists, Dental Hygienists, Dental Assistants, and Dental Laboratory Technicians
- Dietitians and Nutritionists
- Renal Dialysis Technician

SUPPLEMENTS

Student Workbook—includes activities that focus on applied academics through a variety of practical application exercises including multiple choice, fill-in-the-blank, matching, labeling, and word puzzles, basic skill problems, application of theory to practice, plus a Surf-the-Net feature.

Instructor's Manual—is completely revamped to make this an invaluable tool for the instructor. Instructional strategies and resources have been added to aid the instructor in preparation for class work. Quizzes, case studies, and lab activities have been added to provide the instructor with additional class materials.

Online Companion—has additional resources available online in support of the text for both students and instructors. A PowerPoint presentation will be available correlating to each chapter. Additional activities and web links can also be accessed online. Visit www.delmarlearning.com/companions to access this resource.

ABOUT THE AUTHOR

Ann Senisi Scott is the author of the tenth edition of *Body Structures & Functions*. Ann was previously the Coordinator of Health Occupations and Practical Nursing at Nassau Tech Board of Cooperative Education Services, Westbury, New York. As the Health Occupations Coordinator, she worked to establish a career ladder program from health care worker to practical nurse. Before becoming the administrator of these programs, she taught Practical Nursing for over 12 years.

ACKNOWLEDGMENTS

A special thanks to my husband, Wayne Scott, my personal reviewer, and my children, Vincent, Margaret, Carolyn, Daniel, Michael, Kenneth, Leslie, and Scotty, along with their spouses. Special appreciation for research work done by Alycia Markoff Senisi. I also want to say "thank you" to my students who made teaching a wonderful experience.

REVIEWERS

We are particularly grateful to the reviewers who continue to be a valuable resource in guiding this book as it evolves. Their insights, comments, suggestions, and attention to detail were very important in guiding the development of this textbook.

Lisa M. Carrigan, RN
Applied Technology Center
Rock Hill, South Carolina

Judy B. Conlin, RN
Florida Department of Education
Tallahassee, Florida

Kathleen Park, M. Ed, MT (ASCP), EMSC
Lamar State College
Orange, Texas

Janet L. Bailey, BS, MT (ASCP), M.Ed, EMT-B
Plano Senior High School
Plano, Texas

Beverly Fenley, RN, BSN, M.Ed
The Academy of Irving Independent School District
Irving, Texas

Ann Marie Trzasko, RN, BAN, MSA
Career Prep Center
Sterling Heights, Michigan

HOW TO STUDY USING BODY STRUCTURES & FUNCTIONS

Preview the text before attempting to study the material covered in the individual chapters. By reviewing each section of this textbook, you will better understand its organization and purpose. Reading comprehension and long-term memory levels improve dramatically when you take the time to review the text and learn how it can help you learn.

To get the most from this course, take an active role in your learning by integrating your senses to increase your retention. You may want to:

- *Visually* highlight important material.

- *Read* critically—turn headings, subheadings, and sentences into questions.

- *Recite* important material aloud to stimulate your auditory memory.

- *Draw* your own illustrations of anatomy or function processes and check them for accuracy.

- *Answer* (in writing or verbally) the review questions at the end of the chapter.

- Review the content on the Anatomy and Physiology CD-ROM that accompanies the textbook.

Each time you encounter a new chapter, preview it first to understand its overall structure. Review the **Objectives** presented at the beginning of each chapter to easily identify the key facts *before* you read the chapter. These objectives are also useful to review *after* you have completed a chapter. After reading a chapter, test yourself to see whether you can answer each objective. If you cannot, you will know exactly which areas to study again. The **Key Words** are listed at the beginning of each chapter, are highlighted in *red* (at first usage) within the chapter, and are also defined in the glossary.

Read the **main headings**, **subheadings**, and first sentence of each paragraph—these elements serve as the outline for the whole chapter. Be careful not to overlook the **illustrations**, **photographs**, and **tables** to help you comprehend the difficult material.

Career Profiles provide descriptions of many health professions in today's dynamic health and medical environment. These profiles describe the role of each professional, and may even provide you with insight into possible future career paths.

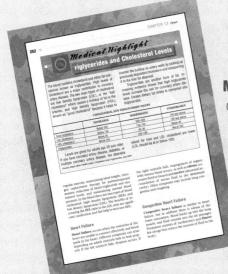

Medical Highlights provide information on technology, innovations, discoveries, and bioethical issues in research and medicine. These topics are based on current information obtained from research on various medical websites.

Review Questions will help you measure whether you have mastered the material that you have covered. Questions in a variety of formats are presented to reinforce important information within each chapter. Also integrated here and in the workbook are applied academic activities for math, spelling, communication, and legal-ethical issues.

The **Glossary of Terms** provides you with a concise definition for all the *key words* in the textbook. The **Index** serves as an alphabetical listing of topics, terms, concepts, and important names for easy reference. Note that figure page numbers are listed in **boldface** in the index.

PROLOGUE

Much of the early study of gross anatomy and physiology comes from Aristotle, a Greek philosopher. Aristotle believed that every organ had a specific function and that function is based upon the organ's structure. Most of Aristotle's ideas were based upon the dissection of plants and animals. He never dissected a human body.

In the third century BC, Herophilus founded the first school of anatomy and encouraged the dissection of the human body. He is credited with demonstrating the brain as being the center of the nervous system. It was a Greek physician, Galen, however, who is credited with the creation of the first standard medical text expanding upon Aristotle's ideas. Galen was the first to discover many muscles and the first to find the value in monitoring an individual's pulse. Galen never performed human dissections and many of his theories were later proven wrong.

The first medical schools were founded in the Middle Ages, however, instructors at this time were hesitant to question the theories and beliefs founded by the early Greeks such as Aristotle and Galen. As a result, very few ideas or discoveries were made in the medical field in the Middle Ages.

During the Renaissance, however, interest in anatomy was renewed due in part to the work of artist Leonardo da Vinci who studied the form and function of the human body. It was during this period in history that the first systematic study of the structure of the human body was made. Many of these early scientists were hindered in their pursuit of knowledge of the human body because it was believed by many that human dissections were immoral and illegal. For example, Andreas Vesalius, a founder of modern anatomy, was sentenced to death because of his anatomical dissections of humans.

In the seventeenth century, the invention of the microscope aided in new anatomical discoveries and research. Scientists could now see structures that were invisible to the naked eye. Robert Hooke's investigation of cork under the microscope was the foundation of the theory that the cell is the basic unit of life. This theory was later proved and expanded upon by other scientists in the eighteenth century as technological advances continued to improve.

Advances in technology have continued into today and new anatomical and physiological discoveries are still being made. With the mapping of the Human Genome, completed in 2003, the complete genetic code has been documented. It is hoped that this knowledge will enable discoveries into disease processes and the development of cures for many of the diseases that continue to plague our society.

At the end of each chapter within this book, use the internet to research early discoveries related to that body system and the scientists that made those discoveries.

Chapter 1

INTRODUCTION TO THE STRUCTURAL UNITS

Key Words

abdominal cavity
abdominopelvic
   cavity
anabolism
anatomical
   position
anatomy
anterior
biology
buccal cavity
catabolism
caudal
comparative
   anatomy
coronal (frontal)
   plane
cranial
cranial cavity
cytology
deep
dermatology
developmental
   anatomy

distal
dorsal
dorsal cavity
embryology
endocrinology
epigastric
external
gross anatomy
histology
homeostasis
hypogastric
inferior
internal
lateral
life function
medial
metabolism
microscopic
   anatomy
midsagittal plane
morphology
nasal cavity

neurology
oral cavity
orbital cavity
organs
organ system
pelvic cavity
physiology
planes
posterior
proximal
sagittal plane
section
spinal cavity
superficial
superior
systematic
   anatomy
thoracic cavity
tissues
transverse
umbilical
ventral

ANATOMY AND PHYSIOLOGY

Anatomy and physiology are branches of a much larger science called **biology.** Biology is the study of all forms of life. Biology studies microscopic one-celled organisms, multicelled organisms, plants, animals, and humans.

Anatomy studies the shape and structure of an organism's body and the relationship of one body part to another. The word *anatomy* comes from the Greek, *ana,* meaning "apart", and *temuein,* "to cut"; thus, the acquisition of knowledge on human anatomy comes basically from dissection. However, one cannot fully appreciate and understand anatomy without the study of its sister science, **physiology.** Physiology studies the function of each body part and how the functions of the various body parts coordinate to form a complete living organism.

Branches of Anatomy

Anatomy is subdivided into many branches based on the investigative techniques used, the type of knowledge desired, or the parts of the body under study.

1. **Gross anatomy.** Gross anatomy is the study of large and easily observable structures on an organism. This is done through dissection and visible inspection with the naked eye. In it the different body parts and regions are studied with regard to their general shape, external features, and main divisions. The study of shape is called **morphology.**

2. **Microscopic anatomy.** With the invention and perfection of the microscope, the knowledge of gross anatomy can be extended down to the microscopic level. Microscopic anatomy is subdivided into two branches. One branch is **cytology,** which is the study of the structure, function, and development of cells that comprise the different body parts. For example, cytology can study the heart cells or the nerve cells comprising the brain. The other subdivision is **histology,** which studies the tissues and organs that make up the entire body of an organism.

3. **Developmental anatomy.** Developmental anatomy studies the growth and development of an organism during its lifetime. More specif-

ically, **embryology** studies the formation of an organism from the fertilized egg to birth.

4. **Comparative anatomy.** Humans are one of many animals found in the animal kingdom. The different body parts and organs of humans can be studied with regard to similarities and differences to other animals in the animal kingdom.

5. **Systematic anatomy.** Systematic anatomy is the study of the structure and function of various organs or parts that comprise a particular organ system. Depending on the particular organ system under study, a specific term is applied, for example:

   a. **Dermatology**—study of the integumentary system (skin, hair, and nails)

   b. **Endocrinology**—study of the endocrine or hormonal system

   c. **Neurology**—study of the nervous system

ANATOMIC TERMINOLOGY

In the study of anatomy and physiology, special words are used to describe the specific location of a structure or organ, or the relative position of one body part to another.

The following terms are used to describe the human body as it is standing in the **anatomical position,** Figure 1-1. A human being in such a position is standing erect, with face forward, arms at the side, and palms forward.

Terms Referring to Location or Position and Direction

- See Figures 1-1 and 1-2.

- **Anterior** or **ventral** means "front" or "in front of." For example, the knees are located on the anterior surface of the human body. A ventral hernia may protrude from the front or belly of the abdomen.

- **Posterior** or **dorsal** means "back" or "in back of." For example, human shoulder blades are found on the posterior surface of the body. The dorsal aspect of the foot is the back or sole of the foot.

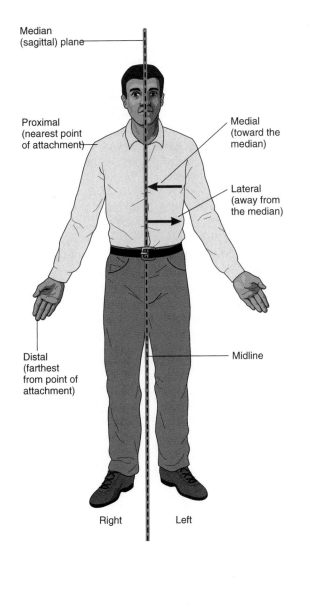

Figure 1-1 *Anatomical terms are used to describe body division parts*

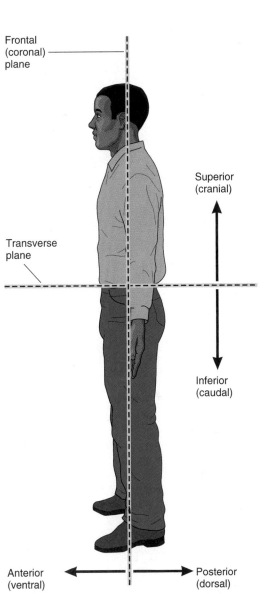

Figure 1-2 *Imaginary lines, or places, separate body structures*

- **Cranial** and **caudal** refer to direction: Cranial means "skull or head end" of the body; caudal means "tail end." For example a blow to the skull may increase cranial pressure and cause headaches. Caudal anesthesia is injected in the lower spine.

- **Superior** and **inferior**—superior means "upper" or "above another"; inferior refers to "lower" or "below another." For example, the heart and lungs are situated superior to the diaphragm, while the intestines are inferior to it.

- **Medial** and **lateral**—medial signifies "toward the midline or median plane of the body"; while lateral means "away", or toward the side of the body." For example, the nose is medial to the eyes and the ears are lateral to the nose.

- **Proximal** and **distal**—proximal means "toward the point of attachment to the body, or toward the trunk of the body"; distal means "away from the point of attachment or origin, or farthest from the trunk."

For example, the hand is proximal to the wrist; the elbow is distal to the shoulder. Note: these two words are used primarily to describe the appendages or extremities.

■ **Superficial** or **external** and **deep** or **internal**—superficial implies "on or near the surface of the body." For example, a superficial wound involves an injury to the outer skin. A deep injury involves damage to an internal organ such as the stomach. The terms *external* and *internal* are specifically used to refer to body cavities and hollow organs.

Terms Referring to Body Planes and Sections

Planes are imaginary anatomical dividing lines which are useful in separating body structures, Figures 1-1 and 1-2. A **section** is a cut made through the body in the direction of a certain plane.

The **sagittal plane** divides the body into right and left parts. If the plane started in the middle of the skull and proceeded down, bisecting the sternum and the vertebral column, the body would be divided equally into right and left halves. This would be known as the **midsagittal plane.**

A **coronal (frontal) plane** is a vertical cut at right angles to the sagittal plane, dividing the body into anterior and posterior portions. The term *coronal* comes from the coronal suture which runs perpendicular (at a right angle) to the sagittal suture. A **transverse** or cross section is a horizontal cut that divides the body into upper and lower parts.

Terms Referring to Cavities of the Body

The organs that comprise most of the body systems are located in four cavities: cranial, spinal, thoracic, and abdominopelvic, Figure 1-3. The cranial and spinal cavities are within a larger region known as the dorsal (posterior) cavity. The thoracic and abdominopelvic cavities are found in the ventral (anterior) cavity.

The **dorsal cavity** contains the brain and spinal cord: The brain is in the **cranial cavity** and the spinal cord is in the **spinal cavity** (see Figure 1-3). The diaphragm divides the ventral

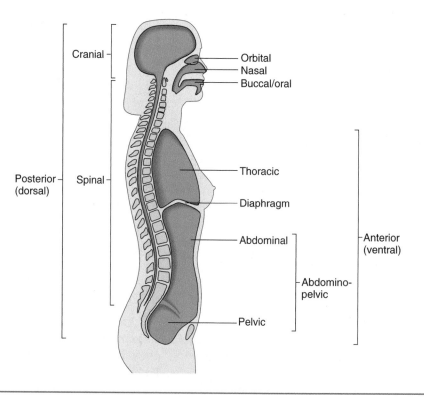

Figure 1-3 *Cavities of the body*

cavity into two parts: the upper thoracic and lower abdominopelvic cavities.

The central area of the thoracic cavity is called the mediastinum. It lies between the lungs and extends from the sternum (breast bone) to the vertebrae of the back. The esophagus, bronchi, lungs, trachea, thymus gland, and heart are located in the thoracic cavity. The heart itself is contained within a smaller cavity, called the pericardial cavity.

The **thoracic cavity** is further subdivided into two pleural cavities: The left lung is in the left cavity, the right lung is in the right cavity. Each lung is covered with a thin membrane called the pleura.

The **abdominopelvic cavity** is actually one large cavity with no separation between the abdomen and pelvis. To avoid confusion, this cavity is usually referred to separately as the abdominal cavity and the pelvic cavity. The **abdominal cavity** contains the stomach, liver, gallbladder, pancreas, spleen, small intestine, appendix, and part of the large intestine. The kidneys are close to but behind the abdominal cavity. The urinary bladder, reproductive organs, rectum, remainder of the large intestine, and appendix are in the **pelvic cavity.**

Terms Referring to Regions in the Abdominopelvic Cavity

To locate the abdominal and pelvic organs more easily, anatomists have subdivided the abdominopelvic cavity into nine regions, Figure 1-4.

The nine regions are located in the upper, middle, and lower parts of the abdomen:

- Upper or **epigastric** region is located just below the sternum (breast bone), and the right hypochondriac and the left hypochondriac regions are located below the ribs.

- Middle or **umbilical** area is located around the navel or umbilicus, and the right lumbar region and the left lumbar region extend from anterior to posterior. (A person will complain of back pain or lumbar sprain.)

- Lower or **hypogastric** region may also be referred to as the pubic area; the left iliac and right iliac may also be called the left inguinal and right inguinal areas.

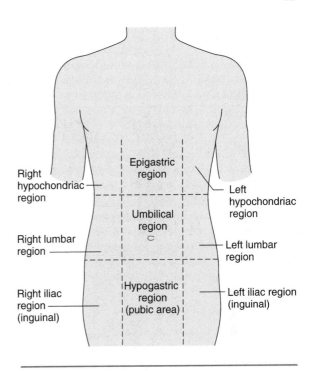

Figure 1-4   *Nine regions of the abdominal area*

Smaller Cavities

In addition to the cranial cavity, the skull also contains several smaller cavities. The eyes, eyeball muscles, optic nerves, and lacrimal (tear) ducts are within the **orbital cavity.** The **nasal cavity** contains the parts that form the nose. The **oral** or **buccal cavity** encloses the teeth and tongue.

LIFE FUNCTIONS

When we examine humans, plants, one-celled organisms, or multicelled organisms, we recognize that all of them have one thing in common: They are alive.

All living organisms are capable of carrying on life functions. **Life functions** are a series of highly organized and related activities which allow living organisms to live, grow, and maintain themselves.

These vital life functions include movement, ingestion, digestion, transport, respiration, synthesis, assimilation, growth, secretion, excretion, regulation (sensitivity), and reproduction, see Table 1-1.

Table 1-1 *Review of the Life Functions and Body Systems*

LIFE FUNCTIONS/ BODY SYSTEMS	DEFINITION
Movement / Muscle System	The ability of the whole organism—or a part of it—to move
Ingestion / Digestive System	The process by which an organism takes in food
Digestion / Digestive System	The breakdown of complex food molecules into simpler food molecules
Transport / Circulatory System	The movement of necessary substances to, into, and around cells, and of cellular products and wastes out of and away from cells
Respiration / Respiratory System	The burning or oxidation of food molecules in a cell to release energy, water, and carbon dioxide
Synthesis / Digestive System	The combination of simple molecules into more complex molecules to help an organism build new tissue
Assimilation / Digestive System	The transformation of digested food molecules into living tissue for growth and self-repair
Growth / Skeletal System	The enlargement of an organism due to synthesis and assimilation, resulting in an increase in the number and size of its cells
Secretion / Endocrine System	The formation and release of hormones from a cell or structure
Excretion / Urinary System	The removal of metabolic waste products from an organism
Regulation (sensitivity) / Nervous System	The ability of an organism to respond to its environment so as to maintain a balanced state (homeostasis)
Reproduction / Reproductive System	The ability of an organism to produce offspring with similar characteristics (This is *essential* for species survival as opposed to individual survival.)

HUMAN DEVELOPMENT

During our lifetime, the body carries on numerous life functions that keep us alive and active. Living depends on the constant release of energy in every cell of the body. Powered by the energy that is released from food, the cells are able to maintain their own living condition and, thus, the life of human beings.

A complex life form like a human being consists of over 50 trillion cells. Early in human development, certain groups of cells become highly specialized for specific functions, such as movement or growth.

Special cells—grouped according to function, shape, size, and structure—are called **tissues.** Tissues, in turn, form larger functional and structural units known as **organs.** For example, human skin is an organ of epithelial, connective, muscular, and nervous tissue. In much the same way, kidneys consist of highly specialized connective and epithelial tissue.

The organs of the human body do not operate independently. They function interdependently with one another to form a live, functioning organism. Some organs are grouped together because more than one is needed to perform a function. Such a grouping is called an **organ system.** One example is the digestive system composed of the teeth, esophagus, stomach, small intestine, and large intestine. In this textbook you will study the various body systems and the organs that comprise these systems.

BODY PROCESSES

The functional activities of cells that result in growth, repair, energy release, use of food, and secretions are combined under the heading of **metabolism.** Metabolism consists of two processes that are opposite to each other: anabolism and catabolism. **Anabolism** is the building up of complex materials from simpler ones such as food and oxygen. **Catabolism** is the breaking down and changing of complex substances into simpler ones, with a release of energy and carbon dioxide. The sum of all the chemical reactions within a cell is therefore called metabolism.

The proper function and maintenance of the human body depends on numerous activities. The body must constantly respond to changes in the environment by exchanging substances between its surroundings and its cells. Maintaining the body's cellular environment and function helps to ensure regular body functions. Thus, optimum cell functioning requires a stable cellular environ-ment (within very narrow limits of acidity, nutri-ents, oxygen, temperature, and fluid balance).

The maintenance of such (optimal) internal environmental conditions is known as **home-ostasis.** Human survival depends on mainte-nance or restoration of homeostasis.

Medical Terminology

-al	pertaining to
ana	apart
-tom	cutting
-y	process of
ana/tom/y	process of cutting apart; study of body parts by dissection
-ology	study of
bio	life
bio/logy	study of life
physio	nature
physi/ology	study of nature or natural
ante	in front of
anter/ior	in the front
poster	behind
poster/ior	in back of
super	above
super/ior	above a part
infer	below
infer/ior	below a part
al	pertaining to
caud	tail
caud/al	pertaining to the tail
crani	skull
crani/al	pertaining to the skull
dist	distant
dist/al	pertaining to a distant part
dors	back
dors/al	pertaining to the back
later	side
later/al	pertaining to the side
medi	middle
med/ial	pertaining to the middle
proxim	near
proxim/al	pertaining to nearness or close
ventr	belly, front side
ventr/al	pertaining to the belly or front side

REVIEW QUESTIONS

Select the letter of the choice that best completes the statement.

1. Anatomy is the study of:
   a. the structure of a body part
   b. the structure and function of a body part
   c. the function of a body part
   d. the formation of a body part

2. The study of the function of cells is called:
   a. anatomy
   b. physiology
   c. histology
   d. cytology

3. The anatomical position is described as:
   a. body erect, arms at the side, palms forward
   b. body supine, arms at the side, palms forward
   c. body erect, arms at the side, palms backward
   d. body supine, arms at the side, palms backward

4. A plane that divides the body into right and left parts is:
   a. transverse plane
   b. coronal plane
   c. sagittal plane
   d. frontal plane

5. If a wound occurred near the surface of the skin, it would be:
   a. deep
   b. superficial
   c. medial
   d. lateral

6. The heart is described as superior to the diaphragm because it is:
   a. in back of the diaphragm
   b. in front of the diaphragm
   c. above the diaphragm
   d. below the diaphragm

7. The brain and the spinal cavity are located in the:
   a. ventral cavity
   b. spinal cavity
   c. cranial cavity
   d. dorsal cavity

8. The epigastric region of the abdominal area is located:
   a. just above the sternum
   b. in the umbilical area
   c. just below the sternum
   d. in the pelvic area

9. The sum of the chemical reactions in a cell is known as:
    a. homeostasis
    b. metabolism
    c. anabolism
    d. catabolism

10. The formation and release of hormones from a cell or structure is called:
    a. digestion
    b. excretion
    c. synthesis
    d. secretion

MATCHING

Match each term in Column I with its correct description in Column II.

Column I	Column II
_____ **1.** catabolism	a. balanced cellular environment
_____ **2.** pelvic cavity	b. constructive chemical processes which use food to build complex materials of the body
_____ **3.** pericardial cavity	
_____ **4.** anabolism	c. useful breakdown of food materials resulting in the release of energy
_____ **5.** abdominal cavity	
_____ **6.** diaphragm	d. contained within the oral cavity
_____ **7.** homeostasis	e. cavity in which the reproductive organs, urinary bladder, and lower part of large intestine are located
_____ **8.** tissue	
_____ **9.** kidneys	f. cavity in which the stomach, liver, gallbladder, pancreas, spleen, appendix, cecum, and colon are located
_____ **10.** teeth and tongue	
_____ **11.** cranial cavity	g. cavity containing the heart
_____ **12.** organ system	h. a group of cells which together perform a particular job
	i. portion of the dorsal cavity containing the brain
	j. divides the ventral cavity into two regions
	k. structure located behind the abdominal cavity
	l. organs grouped together because they have a related function
	m. an activity that a living thing performs to help it live and grow

APPLYING THEORY TO PRACTICE

1. In each of the following examples, choose the term that correctly describes the human body according to anatomical position.
    a. In the anatomical position, the palms are forward or backward.
    b. The liver is superior or inferior to the diaphragm.

    c. The hand is proximal or distal to the elbow.

    d. The sole of the foot is on the anterior or posterior part of the body.

    e. Cranial refers to the head or tail end of the body.

    f. The coronal plane divides the body into front and back or right and left sections.

    g. The arms are located on the medial or lateral side of the body.

    h. The transverse plane divides the body into superior and inferior or anterior and posterior parts.

2. Describe the following to a physician using the correct anatomical term.

    a. The location of an appendectomy scar

    b. A wound that is on the front of the leg

    c. The end of the spine

    d. A pain near the breast bone

3. Think about what your body does within a 24-hour period and name the life functions that take place.

CASE STUDY

An EMT responds to a call for a fall out of a tree. Upon arrival, the EMT sees a young boy lying at the bottom of the tree; his right arm is visibly deformed. The EMT suspects the arm may be broken.

1. Describe the anatomical terms the EMT will use to describe the injury to the ER doctor.

2. What life function will be affected by the fall?

3. The boy is right handed; describe other life functions that may be affected by his injury.

Lab Activity

1-1

Anatomical Directions

■ *Objective:* To properly use directional terms to reference anatomical regions

■ *Materials needed:* pencil, paper

Step 1: You may work individually or with a lab partner. Each student will assume the anatomical position. Is it comfortable? Record your response on paper.

Step 2: Ask your lab partner if he or she is comfortable in the anatomical position. Record your partner's response on paper.

Step 3: State the reason why you think this position is comfortable or uncomfortable. Write your response on paper.

Step 4: The student will locate his or her own anterior, posterior, lateral, medial, superior, and inferior body surface, and then repeat the step on his or her partner.

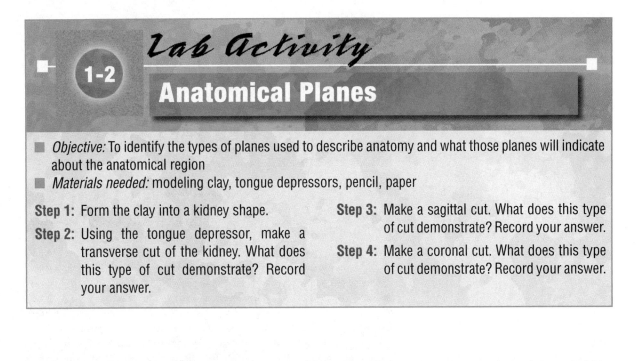

Lab Activity 1-2
Anatomical Planes

■ *Objective:* To identify the types of planes used to describe anatomy and what those planes will indicate about the anatomical region

■ *Materials needed:* modeling clay, tongue depressors, pencil, paper

Step 1: Form the clay into a kidney shape.

Step 2: Using the tongue depressor, make a transverse cut of the kidney. What does this type of cut demonstrate? Record your answer.

Step 3: Make a sagittal cut. What does this type of cut demonstrate? Record your answer.

Step 4: Make a coronal cut. What does this type of cut demonstrate? Record your answer.

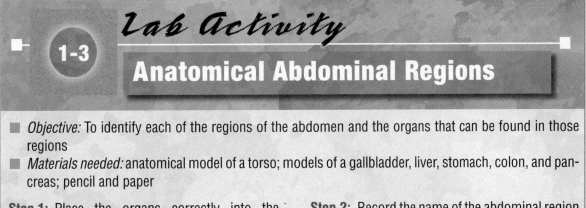

Lab Activity 1-3
Anatomical Abdominal Regions

■ *Objective:* To identify each of the regions of the abdomen and the organs that can be found in those regions

■ *Materials needed:* anatomical model of a torso; models of a gallbladder, liver, stomach, colon, and pancreas; pencil and paper

Step 1: Place the organs correctly into the anatomical model.

Step 2: Record the name of the abdominal region in which each of the organs is located.

Chapter 2

CHEMISTRY OF LIVING THINGS

Key Words

acid	element	multicellular
alkali	energy	neutralization
amino acid	enzyme	nucleic acid
atom	extracellular fluid	organic catalyst
base	fat (triglyceride)	organic compound
biochemistry	glycogen	phospholipid
buffer	hydroxide	pH scale
carbohydrate	intracellular fluid	polysaccharide
chemistry	ion	potential energy
cholesterol	ionize	protein
coenzyme	isotopes	radioactive
compound	kinetic energy	ribonucleic acid
deoxyribonucleic	lipid	(RNA)
acid (DNA)	matter	salt
disaccharide	molecule	steroid
electrolytes	monosaccharide	unicellular

To be an effective health care professional, an individual must have a thorough understanding of the normal and abnormal functioning of the human body and a knowledge of basic chemistry and biochemistry.

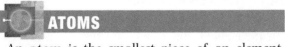

CHEMISTRY

Chemistry is the study of the structure of matter and the composition of substances, their properties, and their chemical reactions. Many chemical reactions occur in the human body. These reactions can range from the digestion of a piece of meat in the stomach and formation of urine in the kidneys, to the manufacture of proteins in a microscopic human cell. Ultimately, the chemical reactions necessary to sustain life occur in the cells. Thus, the study of the chemical reactions of living things is called **biochemistry.**

MATTER AND ENERGY

Matter is anything that has weight (mass) and occupies space. Matter exists in the forms of solid, liquid, and gas. An example in our bodies of solid matter is bone; liquid matter is blood; gas is oxygen.

Matter is neither created nor destroyed, but it can change form through physical or chemical means. A physical change occurs when we chew a piece of food and it breaks up into smaller pieces. A chemical change occurs when the food is acted on by various chemicals in the body to change its composition. For example, imagine a piece of toast that becomes molecules of fat and glucose to be used by the body for energy.

Energy is the ability to do work or to put matter into motion. Energy exists in our body as **potential energy** or **kinetic energy.** Potential energy is energy stored in cells waiting to be released, whereas kinetic energy is work resulting in motion. Lying in bed is an example of potential energy; getting out of bed is an example of kinetic energy.

ATOMS

An **atom** is the smallest piece of an element. Atoms are invisible to the human eye, yet they surround us and are part of our human structure. Hydrogen is an example of an atom.

The normal atom is made up of subatomic particles: protons, neutrons, and electrons. Protons have a positive (+) electric charge; neutrons have no electric charge. Protons and neutrons make up the nucleus of the atom (which differs from the nucleus of the cell), Figure 2-1. Electrons have à negative (−) electric charge and are arranged around the nucleus in orbital zones or electron shells. Atoms usually have more than one electron shell. The arrangement of the subatomic particles is how the atoms of one element differ from atoms of another element; the structure of the hydrogen atom is different from the structure of the oxygen atom.

The number of protons of an atom is equal to the number of electrons; atoms are electrically neutral—neither negative nor positive. An atom can share or combine an electron with another atom to form a chemical bond. If one atom gives up an electron to another atom to form this bond, it will now have more protons than electrons and will have a positive charge.

Atoms of a specific element that have the same number of protons but a different number of neutrons are called **isotopes.** All isotopes of a specific element have the same number of electrons.

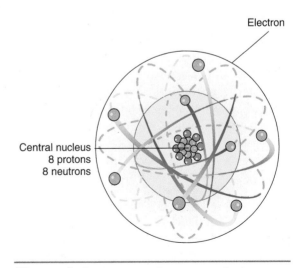

Figure 2-1 *Structure of an atom. Eight protons and eight neutrons are tightly bound in the central nucleus, around which the eight electrons revolve*

Certain isotopes are called **radioactive** isotopes, because they are unstable and may decay (come apart). As they decay they give off (emit) energy in the form of radiation which can be picked up by a detector. The detector not only detects the emission from a radioactive isotope but, with the aid of a computer, also forms the image of its distribution within the body. Radioactive isotopes can be used to study structure and function of particular tissue. In addition, strong radiation from certain isotopes may destroy body tissue. This radiation is useful in the treatment of cancer and other diseases.

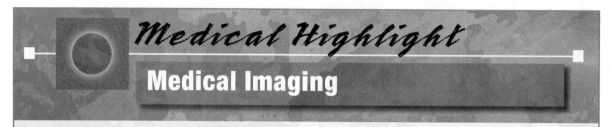

Medical Highlight
Medical Imaging

Nuclear medicine uses radionuclides (also known as radioisotopes) to scan the body. It can be used to identify abnormal and normal body structures that are unable to be seen by x-ray.

CAT or CT scan combines x-ray emission with nuclear medicine to look inside the body. The images produced are cross-sectional, patterned much like slices of bread. By taking a series of such images, a CAT scan creates a multidimension view of the body. The main feature of the equipment is a large "ring." The patient passes through the ring while the x-ray tube rotates 360 degrees around the patient and takes pictures. After taking many pictures, the computer has enough information to combine segments of the pictures and create views of the internal organs. These views are projected onto a television screen. Still photos are taken to record significant findings. CAT scans have all but eliminated exploratory surgery. They are most useful in evaluating brain and abdominal findings.

Positron emission tomography (PET) scan is a procedure in which the patient is given an injection of a short-lived radionuclide and then positioned in the PET scanner. The radionuclides are absorbed by active brain cells and high-energy gamma rays are released as a result. A computer analyzes these rays and produces a color picture of the brain's biochemical activity. The patient must remain alert for this test. Blindfolds and earplugs may be used to reduce external stimuli to the brain. The patient is also asked questions or told to recite, to see how the brain activity changes for reasoning and remembering. PET scans are most useful to diagnose the effects of stroke, some aspects of Alzheimer's disease, epilepsy, and mental illness.

Sonography or ultrasound imaging uses high-frequency sound waves for diagnostic purposes. Ultrasound is completely noninvasive and uses no radiation. To date, no harmful effects on living tissue have been noted. Sound waves are sent into the body tissues by a small transducer, which also receives returning sound echoes as they are deflected off various internal structures. The returning sound waves are converted into electric signals that are fed into a computer. The computer transforms the signals into scans or graphs which are used to construct visual images of the body. This is the imaging choice for obstetrics to visualize the fetal embryo and placenta. It is useful to examine the pelvic and abdominal areas. The Doppler method is a variation of sonography in which returning sound waves are transformed into audible sounds that can be detected by earphones. The Doppler method measures blood flow by moving the transducer along the path of a blood vessel. Data can be obtained concerning the velocity of flow in the area over which the transducer moves.

Magnetic resonance imaging (MRI) uses a magnetic field and radio frequency waves to

continues

continued

produce cross-section images of the body. The patient is inserted into a chamber built within a huge magnet. A new open MRI is actually open on all four sides, so the patient is not placed inside a chamber. The magnetic field causes the atomic ions in the tissue to align in a parallel fashion. Radio waves are sent into the patient and the aligned ions pick up this energy and change their orientation. When the radio waves are turned off, the ions revert to the lined fashion produced by the magnetic field. These changes in the energy field are sensed and translated by a computer into a visual image. MRI is a good diagnostic tool for degenerative disease such as multiple sclerosis. Caution

must be used, however, as strong magnetic fields may damage pacemakers and metal prostheses such as hips and knees. Patients must remove all hair clips, jewelry, and watches when receiving an MRI.

Health care workers must be aware of the anxiety people feel when they see the CAT scan and closed MRI machines. Patient education is critical. Patients may feel a sense of claustrophobia (a pathological fear of confinement) when placed inside the chamber. Patients must also be told that when they are inside the chamber, the "clicking" noises they hear are normal. No one may be in the room with them during the test, but a technician will always be within voice contact.

ELEMENTS

Atoms that are alike combine to form the next stage of matter, which is an **element.** An element is a substance that can neither be created nor destroyed by ordinary means. Elements can exist in more than one phase in our bodies. Our bones are solid and contain the element calcium. The air we take into our lungs contains the element oxygen, which is a gas. Our cells are bathed in fluids that contain the elements of hydrogen and oxygen. When these two elements unite, they form water.

There are 92 elements found naturally in our world; additional elements have been manmade by scientists. Each of the elements is represented by a chemical symbol or an abbreviation. Table 2-1 shows a sampling of elements and their chemical symbols.

Table 2-1 *Some Sample Elements and Their Symbols*

ELEMENT	SYMBOL
Calcium	Ca
Carbon	C
Chlorine	Cl
Hydrogen	H
Iodine	I
Iron	Fe
Magnesium	Mg
Nitrogen	N
Oxygen	O
Phosphorus	P
Potassium	K
Sodium	Na
Zinc	Zn

COMPOUNDS

Various elements can combine in a definite proportion by weight to form **compounds.** A compound has different characteristics or properties depending on its elements. For example, the compound water (H_2O) is made of two parts hydrogen and one part oxygen. Separately, hydrogen and oxygen are gaseous elements, but when combined to form water, the resulting compound is a liquid. Common table salt is a compound made from the two elements sodium (Na) and chlorine (Cl), chemically called sodium chloride (NaCl). Separately, sodium is a metallic element. It is light, silver-white, and shiny when freshly cut, but rapidly becomes dull and gray when exposed to air. Chlorine, on the other hand, is an irritating, greenish-yellow poisonous gas with a suffocating odor. However, the chemical combination of both sodium and chlorine results in sodium chloride, which is a crystalline powder that can be dissolved in water.

Just as elements are represented by symbols, compounds are represented by something called a formula. A formula shows the types of elements present and the proportion of each element present by weight. Some common formulas are H_2O (water), NaCl (common table salt), HCl (hydrogen chloride or hydrochloric acid), $NaHCO_3$ (sodium bicarbonate or baking powder), NaOH (sodium hydroxide or lye), $C_6H_{12}O_6$ (glucose or grape sugar), $C_{12}H_{22}O_{11}$ (sucrose or common table sugar), CO_2 (carbon dioxide), and CO (carbon monoxide).

A living organism, whether it is a **unicellular** (one celled) microbe or a **multicellular** animal or plant, can be compared with a chemical factory. Most living organisms will take the 20 essential elements and change them into needed compounds for the maintenance of the organism. In many living organisms, the elements carbon, hydrogen, and oxygen are united to form **organic compounds** (compounds found in living things containing the element carbon).

Molecules

The smallest unit of a compound that still has the properties of the compound and the capability to lead its own stable and independent existence is called a **molecule.** For example, the common compound water can be broken down into smaller and smaller droplets. The absolutely smallest unit is a molecule of water, H_2O.

IONS AND ELECTROLYTES

In addition to combining to form elements, atoms can share or combine their electrons with other atoms to form chemical bonds. If one atom gives up an electron to another atom to form a bond, it will have more protons than electrons and will have a positive (+) charge. The atom that took the extra electron will now have more electrons than protons and thus have a negative (−) charge. Such a positively or negatively charged particle is called an **ion.** The attraction between the opposite charges produces an ionic bond.

When compounds are in solution and act as if they have broken into individual pieces (ions), the elements of the compound are **electrolytes.** For example, a salt solution consists of sodium (Na^+) ions with a positive charge and chlorine (Cl^-) ions with a negative charge.

In the cells and tissue fluids of the body, ions make it possible for materials to be altered, broken down, and recombined to form new substances or compounds. Electrolytes are responsible for the acidity or alkalinity of solutions and can conduct an electrical charge. The ability to record electric charges within the tissue is invaluable for diagnostic tools such as an electrocardiogram, which measures the electrical conduction of the heart.

TYPES OF COMPOUNDS

The various elements can combine to form a great number of compounds. All known compounds, whether natural or synthetic, can be classified into two groups: inorganic compounds and organic compounds.

Inorganic Compounds

Inorganic compounds are made of molecules that do not contain the element carbon (C). A few exceptions are carbon dioxide (CO_2) and calcium carbonate ($CaCO_3$). Water is an inorganic compound. It comprises between 55% and 65% of human body weight. Water is the most important inorganic compound to living organisms.

Organic Compounds

Organic compounds are found in living things and the products they make. These compounds always contain the element carbon, combined with hydrogen and other elements. Carbons have the ability to combine with other elements to form a large number of organic compounds. There are more than a million known organic compounds. Their molecules are comparatively large and complex. By comparison, inorganic molecules are much smaller. The four main groups of organic compounds are carbohydrates, lipids, proteins, and nucleic acids.

Career Profile
Radiologic Technologists

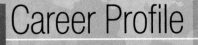

Medical uses of radiation go far beyond the diagnosis of broken bones by x-ray. Radiation is used to produce images of the interior of the body and to treat cancer. The term "diagnostic imaging" not only Involves x-ray technique but also ultrasound and MRI scans.

Radiographers produce x-ray films for use in diagnosing disease. They prepare the patients for procedures by explaining the process, positioning the patient, preventing unnecessary radiation exposure, and taking the picture. Experienced radiographers may also perform more complex imaging tests such as fluoroscopy, operate CT scanners, and use MRI machines.

Radiation therapy technologists prepare cancer patients for treatment and administer prescribed doses of ionizing radiation to specific body parts. They check for radiation side effects.

Sonographers project nonionizing, high-frequency sound waves into specific areas of the patient's body; the equipment then collects the reflected echoes to form an image.

Education for these positions is offered in hospitals, colleges, and vocation-technical institutes. Course of study includes class and clinical practice. The Joint Review Committee on Education in Radiologic Technology accredits most formal training programs in this field. Specialty areas in radiology include MRI technology, nuclear medicine technology, diagnostic technology, ultrasound technology, and mammography technology. Most specialty areas require additional education and certification. The job outlook in this field is expected to grow faster than average.

CARBOHYDRATES

All **carbohydrates** are compounds of the elements carbon (C), hydrogen (H), and oxygen (O). These compounds have twice as many hydrogen as oxygen and carbon atoms. Carbohydrates are divided into three groups: the monosaccharides, disaccharides, and polysaccharides.

Monosaccharides

Monosaccharides (from the Greek words *mono*, meaning "one," and *sakcharon*, meaning "sugar") are sugars that cannot be broken down any further. Hence, they are also called single or simple sugars. The types of monosaccharide sugars are glucose, fructose, galactose, ribose, and deoxyribose.

Glucose is an important sugar. It is the main source of energy in cells. Glucose, sometimes referred to as blood sugar, is carried by the bloodstream to individual cells, and is stored in the form of **glycogen** in the liver and muscle cells. Glucose combines with oxygen in a chemical reaction called oxidation that produces energy.

Fructose is the sweetest of the monosaccharides and is found in fruit and honey. Deoxyribose sugar is found in **deoxyribonucleic acid (DNA)** and ribose sugar is found in **ribonucleic acid (RNA).**

Disaccharides

A **disaccharide** is known as a double sugar, because it is formed from two monosaccharide

MONOSACCHARIDE + MONOSACCHARIDE − H_2O (DEHYDRATION SYNTHESIS)	FORMS	DISACCHARIDE
Glucose + Fructose − H_2O	→	Sucrose
Glucose + Glucose − H_2O	→	Maltose
Glucose + Galactose − H_2O	→	Lactose

Table 2-2 *The Monosaccharide Composition of Sucrose, Maltose, and Lactose*

molecules by a chemical reaction called dehydration synthesis. This reaction involves the synthesis of a large molecule from small ones by the loss of a molecule of water. Table 2-2 illustrates the process of dehydration synthesis.

The opposite reaction to dehydration synthesis is hydrolysis. In this reaction, a large molecule is broken down into smaller molecules by the addition of water. Examples of disaccharides are sucrose (table sugar), maltose (malt sugar), and lactose (milk sugar).

Disaccharides must be broken down by the process of digestion (hydrolysis) to monosaccharides to be absorbed and used by the body.

Polysaccharides

A large number of carbohydrates found in or made by living organisms and microbes are **polysaccharides.** These are large, complex molecules of hundreds to thousands of glucose molecules bonded together in one long chainlike molecule. Examples of polysaccharides are starch, cellulose, and glycogen. Under the proper conditions, polysaccharides can be broken down into disaccharides and then finally into monosaccharides. Starch is a polysaccharide found in grain products and root vegetables such as potatoes. Cellulose is the main structural component of plant tissue.

LIPIDS

Lipids are molecules containing the elements carbon, hydrogen, and oxygen. Lipids are different from carbohydrates because they have proportionately much less oxygen in relation to hydrogen. Examples of lipids are fats, phospholipids, and steroids.

Characteristics of Lipids

Everywhere you look today you see the words "no fat," yet lipids or fats are essential to health. Lipids are an important source of stored energy. They make up the essential steroid hormones and help to insulate our bodies. It is when the intake of lipids in the form of fat becomes excessive that a health problem may occur.

Fats consist of glycerol and fatty acids. Fats also may be known as **triglycerides.** This type of lipid is the most abundant in the body.

Phospholipids contain carbon, hydrogen, oxygen, and phosphorus. This type of lipid may be found in the cell membranes, the brain, and the nervous tissue.

Steroids are lipids that contain **cholesterol.** Cholesterol is essential in the structure of the semipermeable membrane of the cell. It is necessary in the manufacture of vitamin D and in the production of male and female hormones. Cholesterol is needed to make the adrenal hormone cortisol. In certain people, however, cholesterol can accumulate in the arteries, becoming a problem. The most common food sources of cholesterol are meat, eggs, and cheese. Yet, even without these food sources, the liver will still manufacture cholesterol.

PROTEINS

Proteins are organic compounds containing the elements carbon, hydrogen, oxygen, and nitrogen and, most times, phosphorus and sulfur. Proteins are among the most diverse and essential organic compounds found in all living organisms. They are found in every part of a living cell; they are also an important part of the outer protein coat of all viruses. Proteins also serve as binding and structural components of all living things. For example,

Table 2-3 *Nine Essential Amino Acids*

ESSENTIAL AMINO ACIDS	SYMBOL
Histidine	His
Isoleucine	Ileu
Leucine	Leu
Lysine	Lys
Methionine	Met
Phenylalanine	Phe
Threonine	Trp
Tryptophan	Try
Valine	Val

large amounts of protein are found in fingernails, hair, cartilage, ligaments, tendons, and muscle.

The small molecular units that make up the very large protein molecules are called **amino acids.** There are 22 different amino acids that can be combined in any number and sequence to make up the various kinds of proteins.

Table 2-3 gives a list of the nine essential amino acids. Essential amino acids must be ingested because they cannot be made by the body.

Large protein molecules are constructed from any number and sequence of these amino acids. The number of amino acids in any given protein molecule can number from 300 to several thousand. Therefore, the structure of proteins is quite complicated.

Enzymes

Enzymes are specialized protein molecules found in all living cells. They help to control the various chemical reactions occurring in a cell, so each reaction occurs at just the right moment and at the right speed. Enzymes help provide energy for the cell, assist in the making of new cell parts, and control almost every process in a cell. Because enzymes are capable of such activity, they are known as **organic catalysts.** An enzyme or organic catalyst affects the rate or speed of a chemical reaction without itself being changed. Enzymes can also be used over and over again. An enzyme molecule is highly specific in its action. Enzymes are made up of all protein or part protein (apoenzyme) attached to a nonprotein part (**coenzyme**).

The name of an enzyme usually ends in -*ase*.

NUCLEIC ACIDS

Nucleic acids are important organic compounds containing the elements carbon, oxygen, hydrogen, nitrogen, and phosphorus. The two major types of nucleic acids are deoxyribonucleic acid (DNA) and ribonucleic acid (RNA).

Structure of Nucleic Acids

Nucleic acids are the largest known organic molecules. They are made from thousands of smaller, repeating subunits called nucleotides. A nucleotide is a complex molecule composed of three different molecular groups. Figure 2-2 shows a typical nucleotide. Group 1 is a phosphate or phosphoric acid group, H_3PO_4; group 2 represents a five-carbon sugar. Depending on the nucleotide, the sugar could be either a ribose or a deoxyribose sugar. Group 3 represents a nitrogenous base. The two groups of nitrogenous bases are the purines and the pyrimidines. The purines are either adenine (A) or guanine (G); the pyrimidines are cytosine (C) and thymine (T).

DNA Structure and Function

DNA is involved in the process of heredity. The nucleus of every human cell contains 46 (23 pairs of) chromosomes, creating a long coiled molecule of DNA. The chromosomes contain about 100,000 genes. This genetic information tells a cell what structure it will possess and what function it will have. The DNA molecule passes on this genetic information from one generation to the next.

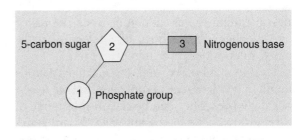

Figure 2-2   *Structure of a typical nucleotide*

DNA is a double-stranded molecule referred to as a double helix. This structure resembles a twisted ladder. The sides of the ladder are formed by alternating bands of a sugar (deoxyribose) unit and a phosphate unit. The rungs of the ladder are formed by the nitrogenous bases which always pair in specific ways: thymine (T) pairs with adenine (A), and cytosine (C) pairs with guanine (G), Figure 2-3.

DNA structures are unique for each person and so are usable as a means of identification. Because all cells contain DNA, a very small amount can identify anyone.

RNA Structure and Function

The RNA nucleotide consists of a phosphate group, the ribose sugar, and any one of the following nitrogenous bases: adenine, cytosine, guanine, and uracil instead of thymine. The RNA molecule is single stranded, whereas the DNA molecule is double stranded.

The three different types of RNA in a cell are the messenger RNA (m-RNA), the transfer RNA (t-RNA), and the ribosomal RNA (r-RNA). Messenger RNA carries the instructions for protein synthesis from the DNA molecule located in the nucleus of a cell into the cytoplasm. The m-RNA molecule carries the code for protein synthesis from the DNA in the nucleus to the ribosomes in the cytoplasm. The transfer RNA molecule picks up amino acid molecules in the cytoplasm and transfers them to the ribosomes where they combine to form proteins. The ribosomal RNA helps in the attachment of the m-RNA to the ribosome. Table 2-4 shows the basic differences between the DNA molecule and the RNA molecule.

ACIDS, BASES, AND SALTS

Before ending the discussion of basic chemistry and biochemistry, a brief discussion of acids, bases, salts, and pH is essential.

Many inorganic and organic compounds found in living organisms are ones that we use in our daily lives. They can be classified into one of three groups: acids, bases, and salts. We are familiar with the sour taste of citrus fruits (grapefruits,

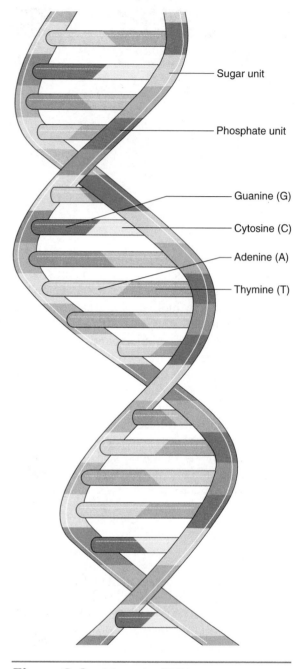

Figure 2-3 *Schematic of DNA*

lemons, and limes) and vinegar. The sour taste is due to the presence of compounds called acids. What characteristics do acids have to set them apart from the bases and salts?

Table 2-4 *Differences Between DNA and RNA Molecules*

TYPE OF NUCLEIC ACID	TYPE OF SUGAR PRESENT	TYPES OF BASES PRESENT	PHOSPHATE GROUP	LOCATION	NUMBER OF STRANDS PRESENT
DNA	Deoxyribose	A, T, G, C	Same as RNA	Cell nucleus, chromosomes	2
RNA	Ribose	A, U, G, C	Same as DNA	Cytoplasm, nucleoli, ribosomes	1

Table 2-5 *Names, Formulas, and Locations or Uses of Common Acids*

NAME OF ACID	FORMULA	WHERE FOUND OR USAGE
Acetic acid	CH_3COOH	Found in vinegar
Boric acid	H_3BO_3	Weak eyewash
Carbonic acid	H_2CO_3	Found in carbonated beverages
Hydrochloric acid	HCl	Found in stomach
Nitric acid	HNO_3	Industrial oxidizing acid
Sulfuric acid	H_2SO_4	Found in batteries and industrial mineral acid

Acids

An **acid** is a substance that, when dissolved in water, will **ionize** into positively charged hydrogen ions (H^+) and negatively charged ions of some other element. (Basically, an acid is a substance that yields hydrogen ions (H^+) in solution.) For example, hydrogen chloride (HCl) in pure form is a gas. But when bubbled into water, it becomes hydrochloric acid. How does this happen? Simply. In a water solution, hydrogen chloride ionizes into one hydrogen ion and one negatively charged chloride ion.

$HCl + H_2O \longrightarrow H^+ + Cl^-$

Hydrogen ⟶ Hydrogen + Chloride
chloride in   ion   ion
solution

It is the presence of the hydrogen ions that gives hydrochloric acid its acidity and sour taste. (However, one should *not* taste any substance to identify it as an acid. There are other more reliable and safer methods for identification.) A substance can be tested for its acidity through the use of specially treated paper called litmus. In the presence of an acid, blue litmus paper turns red. Table 2-5 names some common acids, their formulas, and where they are found or how they are used.

Bases

A **base** or **alkali** is a substance that, when dissolved in water, ionizes into negatively charged **hydroxide** (OH^-) ions and positively charged ions of a metal. For example, sodium hydroxide (NaOH) ionizes into one sodium ion (Na^+) and one hydroxide ion (OH^-). The reaction can be shown as follows:

$NaOH \longrightarrow Na^+ + OH^-$

Sodium ⟶ Sodium + Hydroxide
hydroxide   ion   ion
in solution

Bases have a bitter taste and feel slippery between the fingers. They turn red litmus paper blue. Table 2-6 names some common bases, their formulas, and location or use.

Neutralization and Salts

When an acid and a base are combined, they form a salt and water. This type of reaction is called a **neutralization,** or exchange reaction. In a neutralization reaction, hydrogen ions (H^+) from the acid and hydroxide ions (OH^-) from the base join to form water. At the same time, the negative ions

Table 2-6 *Names, Formulas, and Locations or Uses of Common Bases*

NAME OF BASE	FORMULA	WHERE FOUND OR USAGE
Ammonium hydroxide	NH_4OH	Household liquid cleaners
Magnesium hydroxide	$Mg(OH)_2$	Milk of magnesia
Potassium hydroxide	KOH	Caustic potash
Sodium hydroxide	$NaOH$	Lye

Hydrochloric acid   +   Sodium hydroxide ⟶ Sodium chloride (salt)   +   Water

HCL   +   NaOH   ⟶   NaCL   + H_2O

Figure 2-4   *Neutralization or exchange reaction*

of the acid combine with the positive ions of the base to form the compound **salt.** For example, hydrochloric acid and sodium hydroxide combine to form sodium chloride and water. The hydrogen ions from the acid unite with the hydroxide ions from the base to form water. The sodium ions (Na^+) combine with the chloride ions (Cl^-) to form sodium chloride (NaCl). When the water evaporates, solid salt remains. The neutralization reaction is shown in Figure 2-4.

 PH SCALE

pH is a measure of the acidity or alkalinity (basicity) of a solution. Special pH meters determine the hydrogen or hydroxide ion concentration of a solution on a scale called the **pH scale.** The pH scale, which is used to measure the acidity or alkalinity of a solution, ranges from 0 to 14. A pH of 7 indicates that a particular solution has the same number of hydrogen ions as hydroxide ions. This is a neutral pH, and distilled water is neutral with a pH value of 7.0. Any pH value between 0 and 6.9 indicates an acidic solution. The lower the pH number, the stronger the acid or higher hydrogen ion concentration. Any pH value between 7.1 and 14.0 means a solution is basic or alkaline. Thus, the greater the number above 7.0, the stronger the base or greater hydroxide ion concentration. Figure 2-5 shows the pH values of some common acids, bases, and human body fluids. It also shows the color changes that occur on a pH strip.

Homeostasis

As shown in Figure 2-5, living cells and the fluids they produce are usually neither strongly acidic nor strongly alkaline. These fluids, in fact, are nearly neutral. For instance, human tears have a pH of 7.3 and human blood a range of 7.35 to 7.45.

For living cells to function optimally, their biochemical reactions must maintain homeostasis. In humans and other living organisms, the maintenance of a balanced pH is achieved through a compound called a **buffer.** Sodium bicarbonate ($NaHCO_3$) acts as a buffer in many living organisms. Buffers help a living organism to maintain a constant pH value, which contributes to the homeostasis or balanced state within all living things.

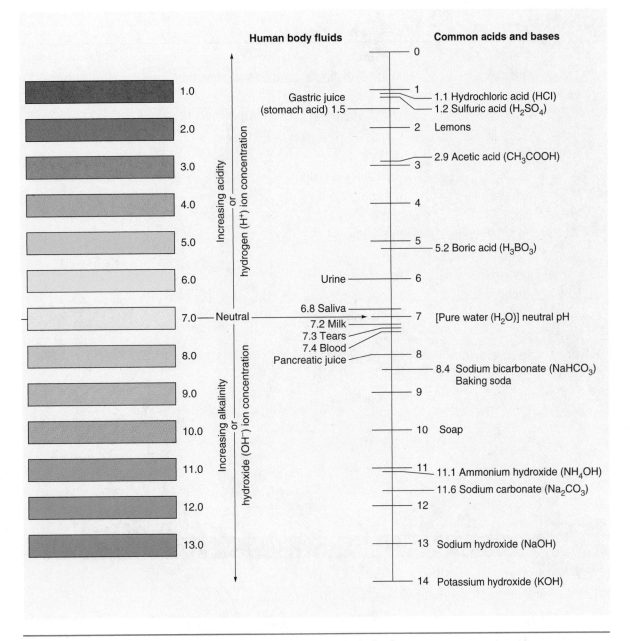

Figure 2-5 *pH values of common acids, bases, and human body fluids*

It is important that the fluid within the cell (**intracellular fluid**) and the fluid surrounding the cell (**extracellular fluid**) maintain the proper chemical balance for the cell to function. A state of homeostasis is required for the body to function at an optimum level of health. If a control system like the acid-base or electrolyte balance is not maintained, cells and tissue will become damaged. A moderate dysfunction causes illness; a severe dysfunction causes death.

Medical Terminology

chem	chemical
chemistry	study of chemical composition of matter
di	two
-saccharide	sugar containing carbon, hydrogen, and oxygen
disaccharide	contains two sugars
extra	outside
-cellular	pertaining to cell(s)
extra/cellular	outside the cell
intra	inside
intra/cellular	inside the cell
mono	one
mono/saccharide	has one sugar
multi	many
multi/cellular	many cells
poly	many
poly/saccharide	has many sugars
uni	one
uni/cellular	one celled

REVIEW QUESTIONS

Select the letter of the choice that best completes the statement.

1. A substance that has weight and occupies space is called:
   a. kinetic energy
   b. catalyst
   c. matter
   d. potential energy

2. Walking is an example of:
   a. catalyst
   b. kinetic energy
   c. matter
   d. potential energy

3. Water is classified as a(n):
   a. atom
   b. element
   c. mineral
   d. compound

4. A monosaccharide sugar is:
   a. sucrose
   b. cellulose
   c. maltose
   d. glucose

5. Sugar stored in the liver and muscle cells for energy is called:
   a. glucose
   b. glycogen
   c. fructose
   d. ribose

6. A chemical reaction in the cell is affected by:
   a. enzymes
   b. organic compounds
   c. nucleic acids
   d. energy

7. The strongest acid is found in the stomach. It is:
   a. sulfuric
   b. acetic
   c. hydrochloric
   d. nitric

8. The compound with a pH of 8.4 is alkaline and is:
   a. milk of magnesia
   b. baking soda
   c. ammonia
   d. lye

9. When proper amounts of an acid and base are combined, the products formed are a salt and:
   a. gas
   b. water
   c. another base
   d. another acid

10. The name given to the atomic particle found outside the nucleus of an atom is:
   a. proton
   b. neutron
   c. electron
   d. ion

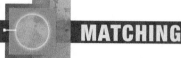

MATCHING

Match each term in Column I with its correct description in Column II.

Column I		Column II
_____	**1.** glucose	a. fluid within the cell
_____	**2.** electrolyte	b. double sugar
_____	**3.** intracellular	c. triglycerides
_____	**4.** disaccharides	d. chromosomes
_____	**5.** HCL	e. conducts an electrical charge in a solution
_____	**6.** steroid	f. blood sugar
_____	**7.** energy	g. positively or negatively charged particle of an atom
_____	**8.** ion	h. ability to do work
_____	**9.** DNA	i. cholesterol
_____	**10.** fats	j. found in the stomach

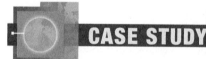

APPLYING THEORY TO PRACTICE

1. Read the label on a loaf of bread and state why the bread can be advertised as "no cholesterol."

2. Compare the fat content in one slice of pizza, a fast-food quarter pound hamburger, a serving of ice cream, and a serving of yogurt.

3. Should DNA identification be required at birth? Have a panel discussion on the ethics of DNA testing as part of a pre-employment physical.

CASE STUDY

Patricia Savon is 34 years old. She has come to the clinic because of a general feeling of weakness and some difficulty in walking. She also has had problems with her vision. When you bring Patricia to the examining room, she asks you to leave the door open because she is afraid of being shut inside.

  The doctor does a physical examination on Patricia and orders some diagnostic tests. A possible diagnosis for Patricia is multiple sclerosis.

1. The fear that Patricia experiences is known as _____.

2. Understanding Patricia's fears, what type of nuclear imaging test will be ordered for her?

3. Patricia wants to know how nuclear imaging works; she is afraid of radiation. Explain to her how imaging devices work.

4. What additional instructions and information can you give Patricia regarding the test?

5. Are there other imaging tests that could be ordered for Patricia?

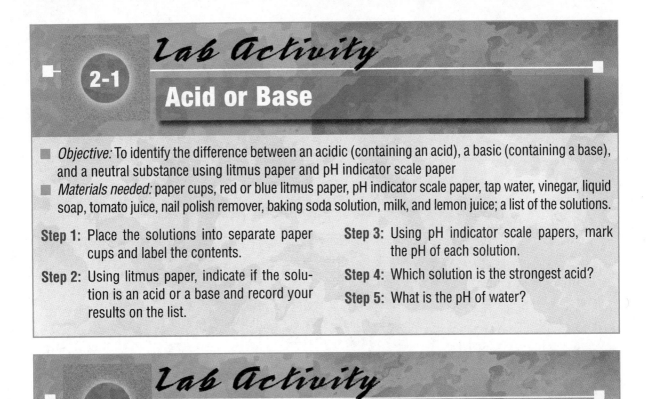

Lab Activity 2-1

Acid or Base

■ *Objective:* To identify the difference between an acidic (containing an acid), a basic (containing a base), and a neutral substance using litmus paper and pH indicator scale paper

■ *Materials needed:* paper cups, red or blue litmus paper, pH indicator scale paper, tap water, vinegar, liquid soap, tomato juice, nail polish remover, baking soda solution, milk, and lemon juice; a list of the solutions.

Step 1: Place the solutions into separate paper cups and label the contents.

Step 2: Using litmus paper, indicate if the solution is an acid or a base and record your results on the list.

Step 3: Using pH indicator scale papers, mark the pH of each solution.

Step 4: Which solution is the strongest acid?

Step 5: What is the pH of water?

Lab Activity 2-2

Effects of Antacid on an Acidic Stomach

■ *Objective:* To determine the effectiveness of various antacid preparations or household remedies on an acidic stomach; the stomach under normal conditions has a pH of about 7

■ *Materials needed:* vinegar, water, paper cups, Tums, Rolaids, Pepcid AC, Alka-Seltzer, baking soda solution, pH indicator paper, and paper on which to record your results

Step 1: Mix 1 oz of vinegar with 8 oz of water to make a solution to represent an acidic stomach.

Step 2: Use pH indicator papers to test the pH of the acidic stomach preparation. Record your result.

Step 3: Place approximately 1.5 oz of the acidic stomach solution into each of five different paper cups.

Step 4: Add one type of antacid preparation or 1 tablespoon of the baking soda solution to separate cups of the acidic stomach solution.

Step 5: After adding antacid preparation, does the solution fizz? What is occurring?

Record your results.

Step 6: After the tablets and baking soda solutions have dissolved, retest each of the solutions with pH indicator paper to measure any changes in the pH of the solution. Record your results.

Step 7: Did the antacid preparation raise the pH of the acidic stomach solution?

Step 8: Which preparation was most effective as an antacid?

Step 9: Obtain the prices of the various antacids. Which preparation is most cost effective (least expensive to produce the desired result)?

Step 10: Record your results for steps 7, 8, and 9.

Chapter 3

CELLS

Key Words

active transport
adenosine
   triphosphate
   (ATP)
anaphase
benign
cell
cell membrane
centriole
centrosome
chromatid
chromatin
chromosome
cloning
cytoplasm
cytoskeleton
diffusion
endoplasmic
   reticulum
   (smooth and
   rough)

equilibrium
filtration
genetic
   engineering
Golgi apparatus
hypertonic
   solution
hypotonic solution
interphase
isotonic solution
lysosome
meiosis
metaphase
metastasis
mitochondria
mitosis
neoplasm
nuclear membrane
nucleolus
nucleoplasm
nucleus

organelle
osmosis
osmotic pressure
passive transport
perioxisome
phagocytosis
phase
pinocytic vesicle
pinocytosis
prophase
protein synthesis
replication
ribosome
selective
   permeable
   membrane
solutes
telophase
tumor
vacuole
wart (papilloma)

When a field of grass is seen from a distance, it resembles a solid green carpet. Closer observation, however, shows that it is not a solid mass but is made up of countless separate blades of grass. So it is with the body of a plant or animal; it seems to be a single entity, but when any portion is examined under a microscope it is found to be made up of many small, discrete parts. These tiny parts, or units, are called **cells.** (*Note:* These units were first discovered in the 1600s by Robert Hook. When examining a piece of cork under a crude microscope, the units reminded him of a monk's room, which was called a cell). All living things—whether plant or animal, unicellular or multicellular, large or small—are composed of cells. A cell is microscopic in size. *The cell is the basic unit of structure and function of all living things.*

Because cells are microscopic, a special unit of measurement is used to determine their size. This is the micrometer (μm), or micron (μ). It is used to describe both the size of cells and their cellular components, Table 3-1.

To better understand the structure of a cell, let us compare a living entity—such as a human being—to a house. The many individual cells of this living organism are comparable to the many rooms of a house. Just as each room is bounded by four walls, a floor, and a ceiling, a cell is bounded by a specialized cell membrane with many openings. Cells, like rooms, come in a variety of shapes and sizes. Every kind of room or cell has its own unique function. A house can be made up of a single room or many. In much the same fashion, a living thing can be made up of only one cell (unicellular), or many cells (multicellular).

Basic and *typical* are terms used to identify structures common to most living cells, Figure 3-1.

Table 3-1 *Units of Length in the Metric System*	
1 meter = 39.37 inches	
1 centimeter (cm) = 1/100 or 0.01 meter	
1 millimeter (mm) = 1/1000 or 0.001 meter	
1 micrometer (μm) or micron (μ) = 1/1,000,000 or 0.000001 meter	
1 nanometer (nm) = 1/1,000,000,000 or 0.000000001 meter	
1 angstrom (Å) = 1/10,000,000,000 or 0.0000000001 meter	

CELL MEMBRANE

Every cell is surrounded by a **cell membrane.** It is sometimes called a plasma membrane. The cell membrane separates the cell from its external environment and from the neighboring cells. It also regulates the passage or transport of certain molecules into and out of the cell, while preventing the passage of others. This is why the cell membrane is often called a selective semipermeable membrane. The cell membrane consists of protein and lipid (fatty substance) molecules arranged in a double layer.

NUCLEUS

The **nucleus** is the most important organelle (Little Body) within the cell. It has two vital functions: to control the activities of the cell and to facilitate cell division. This spherical organelle is usually located in or near the center of the cell. Various dyes or stains, such as iodine, can be used to make the nucleus stand out. The nucleus stains vividly because it contains deoxyribonucleic acid (DNA) and protein. Surrounding the nucleus is a membrane called the nuclear membrane.

The DNA and protein are arranged in a loose and diffuse state called **chromatin.** When the cell is ready to divide, the chromatin condenses to form short, rodlike structures called **chromosomes.** There is a specific number of chromosomes in the nucleus for each species. The number of chromosomes for the human being is 46.

When a cell reaches a certain size, it may divide to form two new cells. The nucleus divides first by a process called mitosis. It is only during the process of mitosis that the chromosomes can be seen.

Chromosomes are important because they store the hereditary material DNA, which is passed on from one generation of cells to the next.

Nuclear Membrane

The nucleus of a cell is contained within a **nuclear membrane,** or nuclear envelope. This membrane is a double-layered structure that has openings (pores) at regular intervals. Materials can pass through these openings from either the nucleus to the cytoplasm (the material found between the

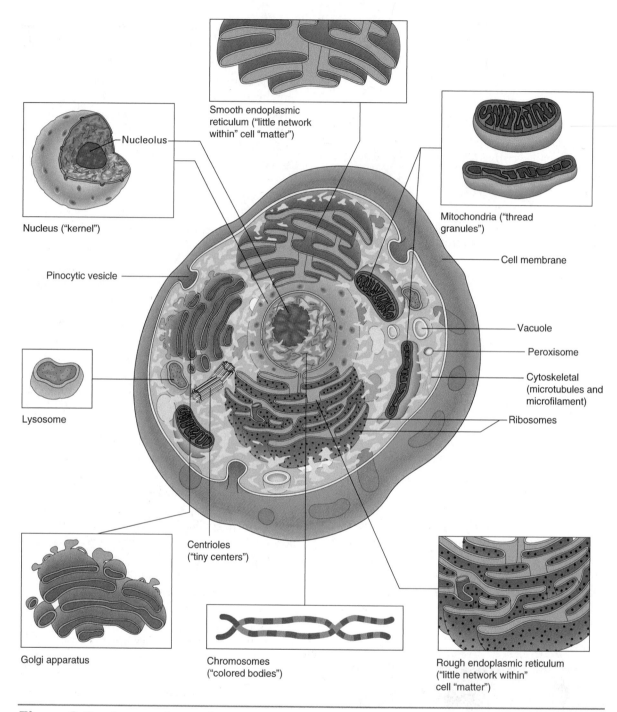

Smooth endoplasmic reticulum ("little network within" cell "matter")

Nucleolus

Nucleus ("kernel")

Pinocytic vesicle

Lysosome

Mitochondria ("thread granules")

Cell membrane

Vacuole

Peroxisome

Cytoskeletal (microtubules and microfilament)

Ribosomes

Golgi apparatus

Centrioles ("tiny centers")

Chromosomes ("colored bodies")

Rough endoplasmic reticulum ("little network within" cell "matter")

Figure 3-1 *Structure of a typical animal cell*

nucleus and the cell membrane) or the cytoplasm to the nucleus. The outer layer of the nuclear membrane is continuous with the endoplasmic reticulum of the cytoplasm and may have small round projections on it called ribosomes.

Nucleoplasm

Nucleoplasm is a clear, semifluid medium that fills the spaces around the chromatin and the nucleoli within the nucleus.

Nucleolus and the Ribosomes

Within the nucleus are one or more nucleoli (plural of nucleolus). Each **nucleolus** is a small round body, Figure 3-1. It contains **ribosomes** composed of ribonucleic acid and protein. The ribosomes can pass from the nucleus through the nuclear pores into the cytoplasm. There the ribosomes aid in protein synthesis. They may exist freely in the cytoplasm, be in clusters called polyribosomes, or be attached to the walls of the endoplasmic reticulum.

CYTOPLASM

Cytoplasm is a sticky, semifluid material found between the nucleus and the cell membrane. Chemical analysis of the cytoplasm shows that it consists of proteins, lipids, carbohydrates, minerals, salts, and water (70% to 90%). Each of these substances other than water varies greatly from one cell to the next and from one organism to the next. The cytoplasm is the background for all chemical reactions that take place in a cell, such as protein synthesis and cellular respiration. Molecules are transported about the cell by the circular motion of the cytoplasm. Embedded in the cytoplasm are **organelles,** or cell structures that help a cell to function. Table 3-2, summarizes the organelles and their functions.

Centrosome and Centrioles

The **centrioles** are two cylindrical organelles found near the nucleus in a tiny round body called the **centrosome.** The centrioles are perpendicular to each other. Figure 3-1 shows two centrioles near the nucleus. During mitosis, or cell division, the two centrioles separate from each other. In the process of separation, thin cytoplasmic spindle fibers form between the two centrioles. This structure is called a spindle-fiber apparatus. The spindle fibers attach themselves to individual chromosomes to help in the equal distribution of these chromosomes to two daughter cells.

Endoplasmic Reticulum

Crisscrossing the cellular cytoplasm is a fine network of tubular structures called the **endoplas-**

Table 3-2 *Functions of Cell Organelles*

ORGANELLE	FUNCTION
Cell membrane	Regulates transport of substances into and out of the cell.
Cytoplasm	Provides an organized watery environment in which life functions take place by the activities of the organelles contained in the cytoplasm.
Nucleus	Serves as the "brain" for the control of the cell's metabolic activities and cell division.
Nuclear membrane	Regulates transport of substances into and out of the nucleus.
Nucleoplasm	A clear, semifluid medium that fills the spaces around the chromatin and the nucleoli.
Nucleolus	Functions as a reservoir for RNA.
Ribosomes	Serve as sites for protein synthesis.
Endoplasmic reticulum	Provides passages through which transport of substances occurs in cytoplasm.
Mitochondria	Serves as sites of cellular respiration and energy production; stores ATP.
Golgi apparatus	Manufactures carbohydrates and packages secretions for discharge from the cell.
Lysosomes	Serve as centers for cellular digestion.
Peroxisome	Enzymes oxidize cell substances.
Centrosome and centrioles	Contains two centrioles that are functional during animal cell division.
Cytoskeleton	Forms internal framework.

mic reticulum (reticulum means "network"). Some of this endoplasmic reticulum connects the nuclear membrane to the cell membrane; thus, it serves as a channel for the transport of materials in and out of the nucleus. Sometimes the endoplasmic reticulum will accumulate large masses of proteins and act as a storage area.

The two types of endoplasmic reticulum are **rough** and **smooth.** Rough endoplasmic reticulum has ribosomes studding the outer membrane. The ribosomes are the sites for protein synthesis in the cell. The smooth endoplasmic reticulum has a role in cholesterol synthesis, fat metabolism, and detoxification of drugs.

Mitochondria

Most of the cell's energy comes from spherical or rod-shaped organelles called **mitochondria** (singular, mitochondrion; *mito* means "thread," *chondrion* means "granule"). These mitochondria vary in shape and number. There can be as few as one in each cell or more than a thousand. Cells that need the most energy have the greatest number of mitochondria. Because they supply the cell's energy, mitochondria are also known as the "power-houses" of the cell.

The mitochondria have a double-membraned structure which contains enzymes. These enzymes help to break down carbohydrates, fats, and protein molecules into energy to be stored in the cell as **adenosine triphosphate** (ATP). All living cells need ATP for their activities.

Golgi Apparatus

The **Golgi apparatus** is also called Golgi bodies or the Golgi complex. It is an arrangement of layers of membranes resembling a stack of pancakes. Scientists believe that this organelle synthesizes carbohydrates and combines them with protein molecules as they pass through the Golgi apparatus. In this way, the Golgi apparatus stores and packages secretions for discharge from the cell. These organelles are abundant in the cells of gastric glands, salivary glands, and pancreatic glands.

Lysosomes

Lysosomes are oval or spherical bodies in the cellular cytoplasm. They contain powerful digestive enzymes that digest protein molecules. The lysosome thus helps to digest old, wornout cells, bacteria, and foreign matter. If a lysosome should rupture, as sometimes happens, the lysosome will start digesting the cell's proteins, causing it to die. For this reason lysosomes are also known as "suicide bags."

Perioxisomes

Membranous sacs that contain oxidase enzymes are called **perioxisomes.** These enzymes help to digest fats and detoxify harmful substances.

Cytoskeleton

Cytoskeleton is the internal framework of the cell which consists of microtubules, intermediate filaments, and microfilaments. The filaments provide support for the cells; the microtubules are thought to aid in movement of substances through cytoplasm.

Pinocytic Vesicles

Large molecules such as protein and lipids, which cannot pass through the cell membrane, will enter a cell by way of the pinocytic vesicles. The **pinocytic vesicles** form when the cell membrane folds inward to create a pocket. The edges of the pocket then close and pinch away from the cell membrane, forming a bubble or **vacuole** in the cytoplasm. This process by which a cell forms pinocytic vesicles to take in large molecules is called pinocytosis or "cell drinking."

CELLULAR METABOLISM

For cells to maintain their structure and function, chemical reactions must occur inside the cell. These chemical reactions require energy most commonly from a molecule called ATP (adenosine triphosphate). ATP is created from the decomposition of organic molecules from the carbohydrates, proteins, and fats we eat. Calories released from the decomposition of food are used to synthesize ATP. ATP is then available to be used for maintenance of cellular structure and function.

CELL DIVISION

Cells divide for two purposes: meiosis and mitosis. The process of **meiosis** involves reproduction. The process of **mitosis** involves growth or maintenance of cells in the human body.

Meiosis

Meiosis is the process of cell division of the sex cell or gamete. During meiosis, the ovum from the female and the spermatozoa from the male *reduce* their respective chromosomes by half, from 46 to 23. When fertilization (the union of the ovum and the spermatozoa) occurs, the two sex cells combine to form a simple cell called the zygote, with the full set of 46 chromosomes, 23 from each parent, Figure 3-2.

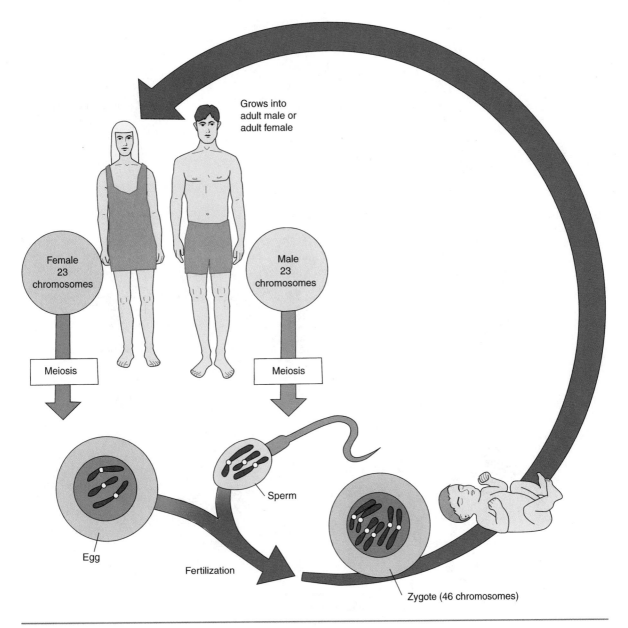

Figure 3-2 *The process of meiosis*

Mitosis

Cell division is divided into two distinct processes; the first stage is the division of the nucleus and the second stage is the division of the cytoplasm.

Mitosis essentially is an orderly series of steps by which the DNA in the nucleus of the cell is equally distributed to two daughter, or identical, nuclei. During the process, the nuclear material is distributed to each of the two new nuclei. This is followed by the division of the cytoplasm into two approximately equal parts through the formation of a new membrane between the two nuclei.

All cells do not reproduce at the same rate. Blood-forming cells in the bone marrow, cells of the skin, and cells of the intestinal tract reproduce continuously. Muscle cells only reproduce every few years.

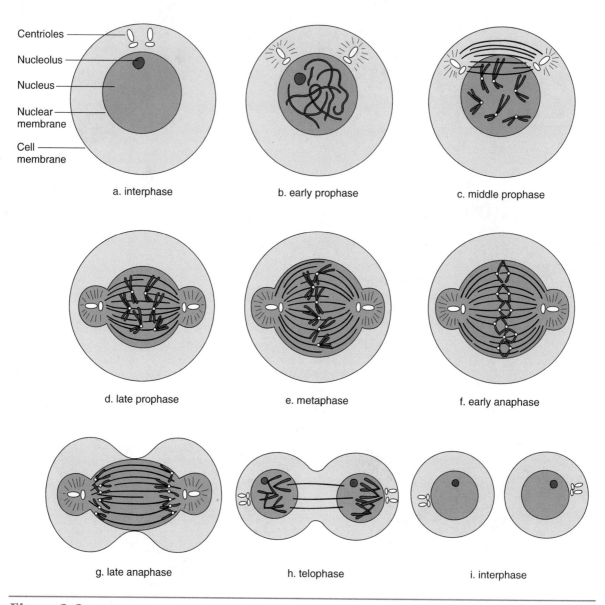

Figure 3-3 The five phases of mitosis: interphase, prophase, metaphase, anaphase, and telophase

Mitosis in a Typical Animal Cell

Mitosis is a smooth, continuing process. For ease and convenience of study, however, five stages, or **phases,** have been identified by the cell biologist. These five phases are discussed subsequently with accompanying diagrams, Figure 3-3. The normal human somatic cell contains 46 chromosomes in the nucleus, which is equal to 23 pairs of chromosomes. This particular chromosome number (46) is called the diploid number of chromosomes. The illustration of a cell in interphase is a repre-

sentative animal cell with a diploid number of 46 chromosomes. This cell will help to illustrate the process of mitosis. (Refer to Figure 3-3 for phases 1 through 5.)

Phase 1—Interphase (Resting Stage). In the **interphase** or "resting" stage, an animal cell undergoes *all* metabolic cellular activities to help in the maintenance of cell homeostasis. The term *resting* refers only to the fact that the cell is not undergoing the visible steps of mitosis yet. Interphase occurs between nuclear divisions. During early interphase, an exact duplicate of each nuclear chromosome is made. This process is called **replication.** Replication is the duplication of the molecules of DNA within a chromosome.

At the start of mitosis, each chromosome has already replicated. Each strand of the replicated chromosome is called a **chromatid.** The two chromatid strands are joined by a small structure called the centromere. During interphase, two centrioles located near the periphery of the nucleus are quite visible. The two centrioles are found in an area called the centrosome. They also replicate during interphase in preparation for the next cell division.

Phase 2—Prophase. During **prophase,** the two pairs of centrioles start to separate toward the opposite ends or poles of the cell. As the two pairs of centrioles migrate, an array of cytoplasmic microtubules forms between them.

There are changes in the nucleus as well. The nuclear membrane starts to dissolve and the nucleolus disappears. The DNA in the chromosomes becomes more highly coiled or condensed and forms very deeply staining, rodlike structures.

Phase 3—Metaphase. During **metaphase,** the nuclear membrane has dissolved completely. The chromatid pairs arrange themselves in a single file, one chromatid pair per spindle fiber between the two centrioles. The area where the chromatid pairs align is called the equatorial plate.

Phase 4—Anaphase. During **anaphase,** the chromatid pairs separate and are pulled by the shortening spindle fibers toward the centrioles. The two chromatids of each replicated chromosome are now fully separated.

Phase 5—Telophase. During **telophase,** the chromosomes migrate to the opposite poles of the cell. There they start to uncoil to become loosely arranged chromatin granules. The nuclear membrane and the nucleolus reappear to help reestablish the nucleus as a definite organelle again.

When cytoplasmic division is finished, two new daughter cells are formed.

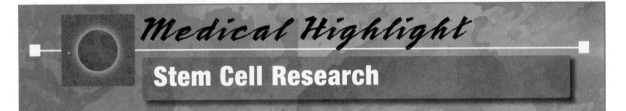

Stem Cell Research

The development of stem cell lines deserves close scientific examination, evaluation of the promises for new therapies and prevention strategies, and open discussion of the ethical issues.

Stem cells have the ability to divide for indefinite periods in culture and give rise to a wide range of specialized cells. Human development begins when a sperm fertilizes an egg and creates a single cell that has the potential to form an entire organism. This fertilized egg is referred to as totipotent, meaning that its potential is total. In the first hours after fertilization, this cell divides into identical cells; any one of these cells, if placed into a woman's uterus, has the potential to develop into a fetus. About 4 days after fertilization and after several cycles of cell division, these cells begin to specialize and form a hollow sphere of cells called a blastocyst. The blastocyst has an outer layer of cells, and inside the hollow sphere is a cluster of cells called the inner cell mass. The outer layer of cells will form the placenta and other tissues needed to support fetal development, but these cells do not become part of the fetus. The inner cell mass cells are called pluripotent, and are capable of giving rise to all tissues of the organism.

The pluripotent stem cells undergo specialization into stem cells, which are committed to give rise to cells of a particular function. These more specialized cells are called multipotent. Multipotent cells may be found in adults and children.

continues

continued

They can be found in some types of adult tissue, as stem cells are needed to replenish human cells that normally wear out. The difficulty in using adult stem cells is they have not been isolated for all tissues of the body and are often present in only minute quantities.

At present, human pluripotent stem cells are developed from two sources. One source is stem cells isolated directly from the inner cell mass of human embryos at the blastocyst stage. These embryo cells come from in vitro fertilization clinics. The clinics provide excess cells used for infertility treatment. The second source is isolated stem cells from fetal tissue obtained from terminated pregnancies. Donors must provide informed consent in both cases.

POTENTIAL APPLICATIONS OF PLURIPOTENT STEM CELLS

Pluripotent stem cells could help us to understand the complex events that occur during human development. A primary goal of this work could be the identification of factors involved in the cellular decision-making process that helps in cell specialization. Some of our most serious medical conditions, such as cancer and birth defects, are due to abnormal cell specialization and cell division.

The most far-reaching potential application of stem cells is the generation of cells and tissue that could be used for so-called cell therapies. Stem cells stimulated to develop into specialized cells offer the possibility of renewable sources of replacement cells to treat a myriad of diseases and injuries, including Parkinson's disease, Alzheimer's disease, spinal cord injury, stroke, and burns. Every realm of medicine may be touched by this innovation.

Much controversy has developed over ethical issues involved in stem cell research. The main reason for the debate over the use of stem cells is these cells can come from an embryo. For many people, an embryo is a living human and thus destroying an embryo for any reason is morally unacceptable.

The National Institute of Health (NIH) on August 23, 2000, announced that stem cell research is eligible for federal funding. The NIH has established strict guidelines regarding the source of the stem cells, informed consent, and access to information about the experiments.

Source: Stem Cells: A Primer, National Institute of Health, May 2000. Website: http://nih.gov/NEWS/STEMCELL/primer.htm

PROTEIN SYNTHESIS

Cells produce proteins such as albumin or globulin, which are essential to life, through a process called **protein synthesis.** Within each cell, the DNA determines the kinds of proteins that are produced. The blueprint for each individual kind of protein is contained within a specific gene which resides in the DNA chain.

MOVEMENT OF MATERIALS ACROSS CELL MEMBRANES

The cell membrane controls passage of substances into and out of the cell. The fluid within the cell and the fluid outside the cell must maintain a proper balance to maintain homeostasis. This is important because a cell must be able to acquire materials from its surrounding medium, after which it either secretes synthesized substances or excretes wastes. The physical processes that control the passage of materials through the cell membrane are diffusion, osmosis, filtration, active transport, phagocytosis, and pinocytosis. Diffusion, osmosis, and filtration are examples of **passive transport,** which means they do not need energy to function. Active transport, phagocytosis, and pinocytosis are active processes that require an energy source.

Diffusion

Diffusion is a physical process whereby molecules of gases, liquids, or solid particles spread or scatter themselves evenly through a medium. When solid particles are dissolved within a fluid, they are known

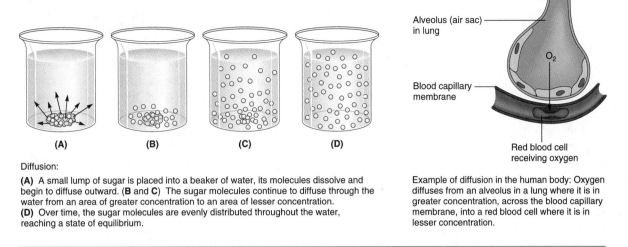

(A)   (B)   (C)   (D)

Diffusion:

(A) A small lump of sugar is placed into a beaker of water, its molecules dissolve and begin to diffuse outward. (**B** and **C**) The sugar molecules continue to diffuse through the water from an area of greater concentration to an area of lesser concentration.
(D) Over time, the sugar molecules are evenly distributed throughout the water, reaching a state of equilibrium.

Alveolus (air sac) in lung

O₂

Blood capillary membrane

Red blood cell receiving oxygen

Example of diffusion in the human body: Oxygen diffuses from an alveolus in a lung where it is in greater concentration, across the blood capillary membrane, into a red blood cell where it is in lesser concentration.

Figure 3-4   *The process of diffusion: The sugar molecules eventually reach a state of equilibrium.*

as **solutes.** Diffusion also applies to a slightly different process, where solutes and water pass across a membrane to distribute themselves evenly throughout the two fluids, which remain separated by the membrane. Generally, *molecules move from an area where they are greatly concentrated to an area where they are less concentrated.* The molecules will eventually distribute themselves evenly within the space available; when this happens, the molecules are said to be in a state of **equilibrium,** Figure 3-4.

The three common states of matter are gases, liquids, and solids. Molecules will diffuse more quickly in gases and more slowly in solids. Diffusion occurs due to the heat energy of molecules. As a result of this, molecules are always in constant motion, except at absolute zero ($-273°C$). In all cases, the movement of molecules increases with an increase in temperature.

A few familiar examples of the rates of diffusion may be helpful. For instance, if a person thoroughly saturates a wad of cotton with ammonia and places it in a far corner of a room, the entire room will soon smell of ammonia. Air currents quickly carry the ammonia fumes throughout the room. Another test for diffusion is to place a pair of dye crystals on the bottom of a water-filled beaker. Eventually the crystals will uniformly permeate and color the water. This diffusion process will take quite a while, especially if no one stirs, shakes, or heats the beaker. In still another test, a dye crystal placed on an ice cube moves even more

slowly through the ice. Diffusion of the dye can be accelerated by melting the ice.

The diffusion rate of molecules in the various media (gas, liquid, and solid) depends on the distances between each molecule and how freely they can move. In a gas, molecules can move more freely and quickly; within a liquid, molecules are more tightly held together. In a solid substance, molecular movement is highly restricted and thus very slow.

Diffusion plays a vital role in permitting molecules to enter and leave a cell in maintenance of homeostasis. Oxygen diffuses from the bloodstream, where it dwells in greater concentration. From the bloodstream, the oxygen enters the fluid surrounding a cell, then into the cell itself, where it is far less concentrated. In this manner, the flow of blood through the lungs and bloodstream provides a continuous supply of oxygen to the cells. Once oxygen has entered a cell, it is utilized in metabolic activities.

Osmosis

Osmosis is the diffusion of water or any other *solvent* molecule through a selective permeable membrane (e.g., the cell membrane). A **selective permeable membrane** is any membrane through which some solutes can diffuse, but others cannot.

Sausage casing is a selective permeable membrane which can be used to substitute for a cell membrane. A solution of salt, sucrose (table sugar), and gelatin is placed into the sausage casing. This mixture is then suspended into a beaker filled with distilled water, Figure 3-5. The sausage casing is permeable to water and salt, but not to gelatin and sucrose. Thus, only the water and salt molecules can pass through the casing. Eventually more salt molecules will move out of the mixture through the casing, because of the low concentration of salt molecules in the distilled water than in the casing. At the same time, more water molecules move through the casing, into the mixture.

The volume of water increases inside the casing, causing it to expand because of the entry of water molecules. When the number of water molecules entering the casing is equal to the number exiting, an equilibrium has been achieved: The casing will expand no further.

The pressure exerted by the water molecules within the casing at equilibrium is called **osmotic pressure.**

Osmosis is the movement of water molecules across a semipermeable membrane from an area of higher concentration of a solution to an area of lesser concentration of a solution to maintain homeostasis. The key word is *solute,* the amount of concentration of a dissolved substance.

In the human body this is well illustrated by a red blood cell in blood plasma, Figure 3-6. If a red blood cell is put into blood plasma, which has the same number of sodium particles as a red blood cell, the osmotic pressures of the red blood cell and that of the plasma are the same, representing an **isotonic solution.**

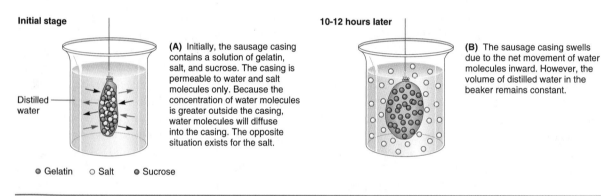

Initial stage

Distilled water

(A) Initially, the sausage casing contains a solution of gelatin, salt, and sucrose. The casing is permeable to water and salt molecules only. Because the concentration of water molecules is greater outside the casing, water molecules will diffuse into the casing. The opposite situation exists for the salt.

10-12 hours later

(B) The sausage casing swells due to the net movement of water molecules inward. However, the volume of distilled water in the beaker remains constant.

● Gelatin ○ Salt ● Sucrose

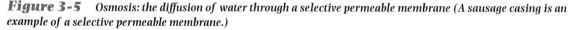

Figure 3-5   *Osmosis: the diffusion of water through a selective permeable membrane (A sausage casing is an example of a selective permeable membrane.)*

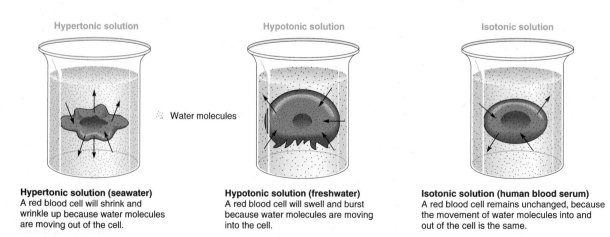

Hypertonic solution

Hypotonic solution

Isotonic solution

Water molecules

Hypertonic solution (seawater)
A red blood cell will shrink and wrinkle up because water molecules are moving out of the cell.

Hypotonic solution (freshwater)
A red blood cell will swell and burst because water molecules are moving into the cell.

Isotonic solution (human blood serum)
A red blood cell remains unchanged, because the movement of water molecules into and out of the cell is the same.

Figure 3-6   *Movement of water molecules in solutions of different osmotic pressure*

If a red blood cell is put into freshwater, which has less sodium particles than the red blood cell, water will rush into the red blood cell. The freshwater represents a **hypotonic solution.**

If a red blood cell is put into seawater, which has more sodium particles than the red blood cell, water will leave the red blood cell to dilute the seawater. The seawater represents a **hypertonic solution.**

The health care worker must know which type of solutions are used in health care. When a physician orders intravenous fluids, the patient's condition will determine what type of solution is ordered. Most intravenous fluids are isotonic solutions. Hypertonic solution is used for patients with edema; hypotonic solutions are used for patients with dehydration.

Filtration

Filtration is the movement of solutes and water across a semipermeable membrane. This results from some mechanical force, such as blood pressure or gravity. The solutes and water move from an area of higher pressure to an area of lower pressure to maintain homeostasis. The size of the membrane pores determines which molecules are to be filtered. Thus, filtration allows for the separation of large and small molecules. Such filtration takes place in the kidneys. The process allows larger protein molecules to remain within the body and smaller molecules to be excreted as waste, Figure 3-7.

Active Transport

Active transport is a process whereby molecules move across the cell membrane from an area of lower concentration against a concentration gradient, to an area of higher concentration. This process requires the high-energy chemical compound adenosine triphosphate (ATP). ATP runs the cell's machinery. The food we eat (a form of chemical energy) must be transformed into another form of chemical energy that allows cells to maintain, repair, and reproduce. The ATP is supplied by cell metabolism.

How does active transport work? One theory suggests that a molecule is picked up from the outside of the cell membrane and brought inside by a carrier molecule. Both molecule and

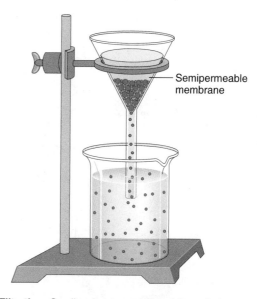

Filtration: Small molecules are filtered through the semipermeable membrane, while the large molecules remain in the funnel.

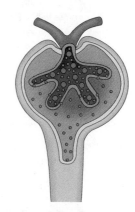

Example of filtration in the human body: Glomerulus of kidney, large particles such as red blood cells and proteins remain in the blood, and small molecules such as urea and water are excreted as a metabolic excretory product—urine.

Figure 3-7 *Filtration: a passive transport process*

carrier are bound together, forming a temporary carrier-molecule complex. This carrier-molecule complex shuttles across the cell membrane; the molecule is released at the inner surface of the membrane, from where it enters the cytoplasm. At this point, the carrier acquires energy at the inner surface of the cell membrane. Then it returns to the outer surface of the cell membrane to pick up another molecule for transport. Accordingly, the carrier can also convey molecules in the opposite direction, from the inside to the outside, Figure 3-8.

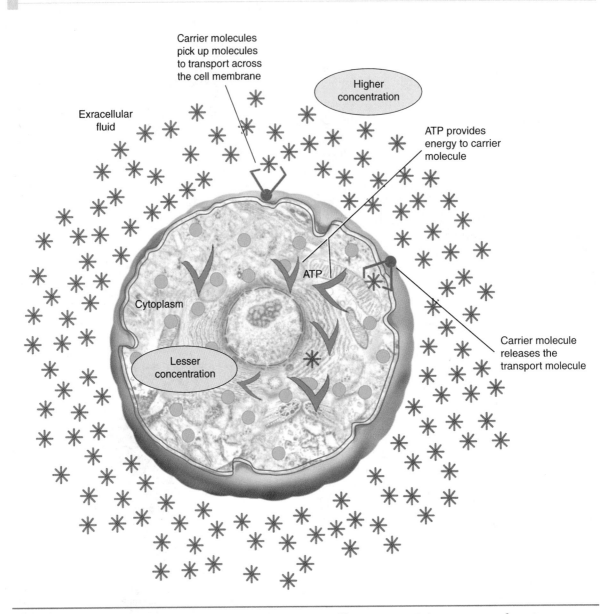

Carrier molecules
pick up molecules
to transport across
the cell membrane

Higher
concentration

Exracellular
fluid

ATP provides
energy to carrier
molecule

ATP

Cytoplasm

Carrier molecule
releases the
transport molecule

Lesser
concentration

Figure 3-8 *The active transport of molecules from an area of lesser concentration to an area of greater concentration, according to one theoretical model*

Phagocytosis

Phagocytosis, or "cell eating," is quite similar to pinocytosis, with an important difference. In pinocytosis, the substances engulfed by the cell membrane are in solution; however, in phagocytosis, the substances engulfed are within particles. Human white blood cells undergo phagocytosis. The particulate substance will be engulfed by an enfolding of the cell membrane to form a vacuole enclosing the material. When the material is com-pletely enclosed within the vacuole, digestive enzymes pour into the vacuole from the cytoplasm to destroy the entrapped substance.

Pinocytosis

As stated earlier, **pinocytosis,** or "cell drinking," involves the formation of pinocytic vesicles which engulf large molecules in solution. The cell then ingests the nutrient for its own use.

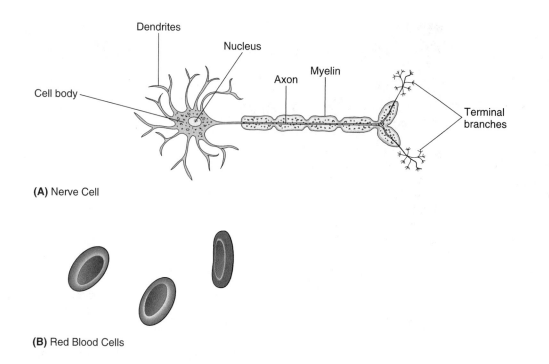

(A) Nerve Cell

(B) Red Blood Cells

Figure 3-9   *Specialized cells: nerve cells and red blood cells*

SPECIALIZATION

There are many kinds of cells of different shapes and sizes. Most of them have the characteristics shown in Figure 3-1, which is a generalized diagram of a basic cell. Some of the more specialized types, such as nerve cells and red blood cells, look very different, Figure 3-9.

Human beings are composed entirely of cells and the nonliving substances which cells build up around themselves. The interaction of the various parts of the cell within the cellular structure constitutes the life of the cell. These interactions result in the life activities, life processes, or life functions that were discussed in Chapter 1. In complex organisms, however, groups of cells become specialists in a particular function. Nerve cells, for example, have become specialized in response; red blood cells specialize in oxygen transport.

Specialized cells may lose the ability to perform some of the other functions, such as reproduction (cell division). Normally, when nerve cells are destroyed or damaged, others cannot be formed to replace them. Heart muscle cells no longer divide when they reach maturity. If a person has a heart attack, loss of heart muscle cells occurs, and the

Effects of Aging on Cells

Aging is a phase of normal development. It is estimated that an older person possesses 30% fewer cells than a younger adult (Eliopoulos), because of the slowing of cell division. Cells also change in their ability to perform specialized tasks. Cellular changes contribute to the fact that physiologic changes are universal and progressive. Aging is not a disease; however, the physiologic changes that occur may be predispositions to disease and illness.

Eliopoulis, C. (1995) Manual of Gerontological Nursing. St. Louis: Mosby

Medical Highlight

Genetic Engineering and Cloning

Genetic engineering is the ability to snip, rearrange, edit, or program DNA. The Human Genome Project (HGP) is an international 13-year effort started in 1990. Project goals are to discover the approximate 30,000 to 35,000 human genes (the human genome) and make them accessible for further biological study and to determine the complete sequence of the 3 billion DNA subunits (bases). Genes carry information for making all proteins required by all organisms.

In June 2000, scientists completed the first working draft of the human genome. With this information medical researchers will have the tools to:

- Improve diagnosis of disease
- Detect genetic predisposition to disease
- Devise novel therapeutic regimens based on new classes of drugs
- Design immunotherapy techniques
- Discover environmental conditions that may trigger disease
- Investigate the possibility of replacement of defective genes

Detailed genome maps have already helped researchers who seek genes associated with dozens of genetic conditions including inherited colon cancer, Alzheimer's disease, and familial breast cancer.

Cloning is an umbrella term used by scientists to describe duplication of biological material. The possibility of human cloning became a close reality in 1997 when Scottish scientists created the sheep named Dolly. She is the first fully grown mammal clone. To researchers at HGP, cloning refers to copying genes and other pieces of chromosomes to generate enough identical material for further study.

Dolly was cloned by taking the genetic material from the nucleus of an adult sheep's udder cell (donor) and fusing it with an egg whose nucleus, and thus its genetic material, had been removed. The fused cell developed into an embryo, which was implanted into a surrogate sheep. The embryo grew into a lamb, which was identical to the donor sheep. Scientists remain uncertain about whether changes in the cells used to obtain the nuclear material will lead to adverse effects on the cloned animal.

This breakthrough technology has a price: It is the question of who will govern experimentation and genetic engineering. American and international communities realize that humans should dictate future technology, not the opposite. Checks and balances must be developed and implemented to ensure that the studies and experiments pass strict ethical criteria.

Source: Human Genome Project Information http://www.orn/.gov/hgmis/project/benefits.html

---

cells are replaced by scar tissue. The heart then loses some of its ability to contract. Specialization also has resulted in an interdependence among cells—certain cells depend on other kinds of cells to aid them in carrying on the total life activities of the organism. In humans, this specialization and interdependence extends to the organs.

DISORDERS OF CELL STRUCTURE

Not all cell growth follows normal physical patterns. Cells may decrease in size, atrophy, usually due to aging or disease. Cells may also increase in size, hypertrophy; this is usually the result of an increase in workload. Cells can increase in number, called hyperplasia, which is related to hormonal stimulation. Cells also have the ability to change into another type of cell, called metaplasia; this may be a protective response to a stimulus, such as smoking. Dysplasia is the change to the size, shape, and organization of cells as a result of a stimulus. This type of cell alteration usually progresses to neoplasia. Neoplasia is the change in cell structure with an uncontrolled growth pattern. Cells can undergo abnormal growth that can range from simple swelling to complex cancerous growths. A variety of abnormalities can occur during cell growth. Some of these disorders are harmless, but others can cause serious illness or death.

Trauma or injury can also affect the structure of the cell. Hypoxia, a decreased blood flow to cellular structures, and anoxia, a lack of oxygen flow to cellular structures, most commonly caused death in cells. Bacterial toxins or viruses can also result in cell death.

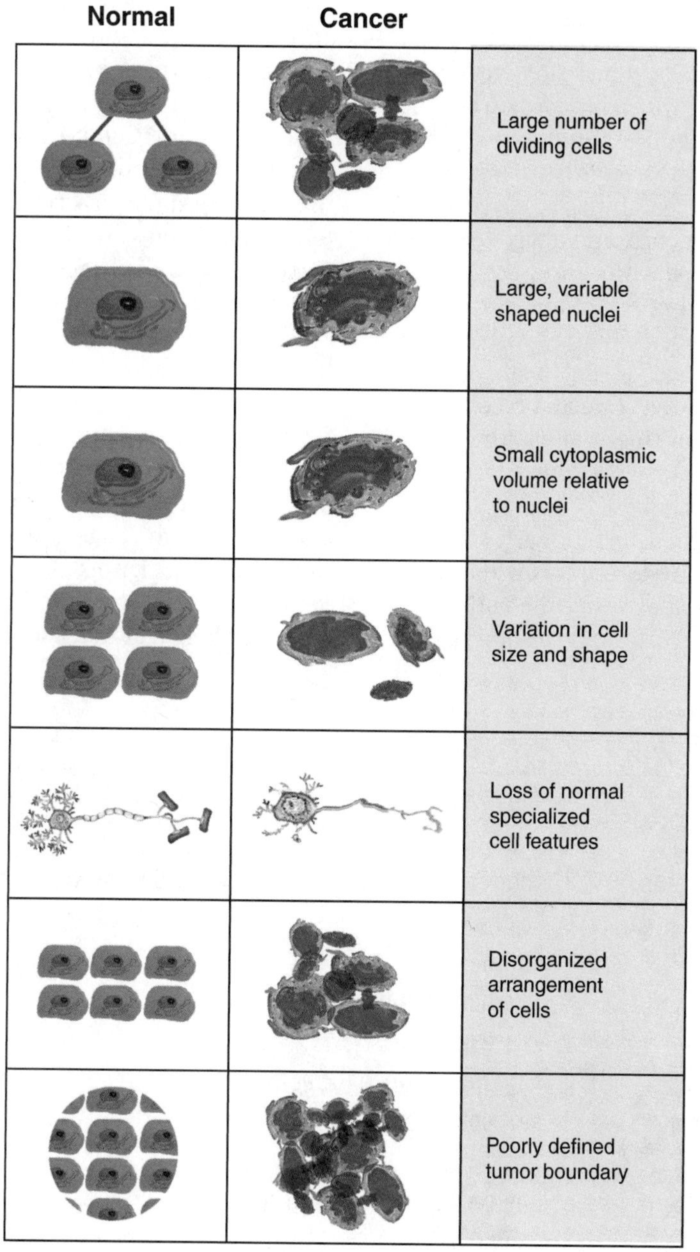

	Normal	Cancer
Large number of dividing cells		
Large, variable shaped nuclei		
Small cytoplasmic volume relative to nuclei		
Variation in cell size and shape		
Loss of normal specialized cell features		
Disorganized arrangement of cells		
Poorly defined tumor boundary		

Figure 3-10 *Comparison of normal cells to cancerous cells* (*Courtesy of National Cancer Society*)

Congenital defects (birth defects) alter cell structure. The majority of these defects are caused by an unknown factor. Other causes may include genetics, chromosomal alterations, and environmental factors.

Tumor

A **tumor** results when cell division does not occur in the usual pattern. If the pattern is interrupted by an abnormal and uncontrolled growth of cells, the result is a tumor, Figure 3-10. Tumors are also known as **neoplasms.** Tumors can be divided into two groups: benign and malignant.

A **benign** tumor is composed of cells confined to the local area. Benign tumors are given other names depending on their type or location (e.g., **wart** or **papilloma** is a type of tumor of the epithelial tissue). Most benign tumors can be surgically removed.

A malignant tumor is called cancer. Cancerous or malignant tumors continue to grow, crowding out healthy cells, interfering with body functions, and drawing nutrients away from the body tissues. These malignant tumors can spread to other parts of the body through a process called **metastasis.** Medical research has made remarkable advances in cancer care, and today well over half the people diagnosed with cancer are cured.

Any of the following symptoms may be an early indication of cancer: changes in bowel or bladder habits, sores that do not heal, obvious changes in a mole or wart, unusual bleeding or discharge, a new lump or thickening in the breast or elsewhere, difficulty in swallowing or frequent indigestion, a persistent cough, or hoarseness.

Diagnostic tests can detect the early stages of cancer. Some of these tests are x-ray, mammogram, sonagram, and biopsy. Give the patient information on procedures before any testing begins.

Cancer is classified by microscopic examination of the tumor cells removed during surgery. The tumor, node, and metastasis (TNM) system is the recommended classification by the American Joint Commission on Cancer. In the acronym TNM, T describes the size and extent of the main tumor, N describes if lymph nodes contain cancer cells and the number of nodes involved, and M describes if cancer has spread to other parts of the body.

Treatment of cancer depends on the type of tumor and where it is located. Treatment includes surgery, radiation, and use of drugs (chemotherapy). Other types of treatment include immunotherapy and laser treatment. Disadvantages of cancer treatment include toxic side effects from drugs and tissue damage caused by radiation. Scientists today are working to develop cancer treatments that are specific to the tumor to help eliminate such side effects.

Medical Terminology

chromo	colored
-some	body
chromo/some	colored body in the cell contains the DNA
cyto	cell
-skeleton	framework
cyto/skeleton	framework of the cell
hyper	excessive
-tonic	strength, concentration
hyper/tonic	excessive concentration
hypo	below normal
hypo/tonic	below normal concentration
iso	same as
iso/tonic	same concentration
mei	lessening or reduction
-o/sis	condition of
mei/osis	condition of lessening of chromosomes
meta	beyond or after
-stasis	controlling or stopping
metastasis	beyond control
neo	new
-plasm	growth

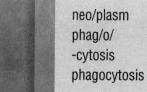	neo/plasm	new growth
	phag/o/	eat
	-cytosis	process of
	phagocytosis	process of cell eating

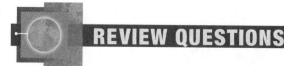

REVIEW QUESTIONS

Select the letter of the choice that best completes the statement.

1. Structures found in cytoplasm to help cells function are called:
   a. nucleolus
   b. organelles
   c. ribosomes
   d. vacuoles

2. Regulating transport of substances in and out of the cell is the:
   a. cell membrane
   b. nuclear membrane
   c. cytoplasm
   d. nucleus

3. A structure that digests worn out cells and bacteria is called:
   a. perioxisome
   b. ribosome
   c. lysosome
   d. mitochondria

4. The function of Golgi apparatus of the cell is:
   a. protein synthesis
   b. destroying bacteria
   c. digesting fats
   d. storing and packaging secretions

5. The internal framework of the cell is called:
   a. mitochondria
   b. cytoskeleton
   c. endoplasmic reticulum
   d. ribosomes

.6

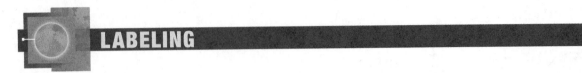

LABELING

Study the following diagram of a typical cell and name the labeled structures.

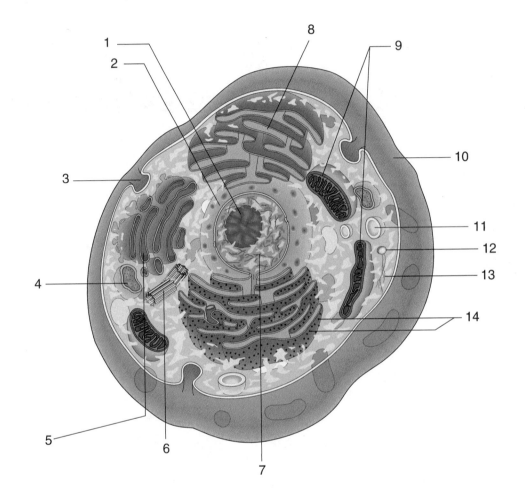

1. _____   8. _____

2. _____   9. _____

3. _____   10. _____

4. _____   11. _____

5. _____   12. _____

6. _____   13. _____

7. _____   14. _____

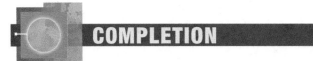

COMPLETION

Complete the following statements.

1. The powerhouse of the cell stores _____ and is called _____.

2. The rough endoplasmic reticulum is studded with _____ which serve as a site for _____ synthesis.

3. The perioxisomes contain _____ enzymes which help digest _____.

4. During the _____ stage of mitosis, the two pairs of centrioles start to move toward _____ end of the cell.

5. The _____ for each individual's kind of protein is contained within a specific _____ in the _____ chain.

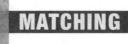

MATCHING

Match each term in Column I with its correct description in Column II.

Column I	Column II
_____ **1.** solute	a. cells confined to local area
_____ **2.** isotonic solution	b. has a higher concentration of Na than a red blood cell
_____ **3.** diffusion	c. needs ATP for energy
_____ **4.** phagocytosis	d. malignant tumor
_____ **5.** osmosis	e. solid particles dissolved within a fluid
_____ **6.** benign	f. cell reproduction
_____ **7.** hypertonic solution	g. molecules move from higher concentration to lower
_____ **8.** cancer	h. has same concentration of Na as the red blood cell
_____ **9.** mitosis	i. engulfs bacteria
_____**10.** active transport	j. diffusion of water molecules

APPLYING THEORY TO PRACTICE

1. The cell is a miniature of how the body works. Name the cellular structure responsible for each: digestion, respiration, energy, circulation, and the reproductive process.

2. Describe how the cell takes in nutrients and name at least three products that the cell manufactures.

3. You are working in an emergency care center. A person comes in dehydrated and the doctor orders a hypertonic solution. Explain why this solution is used instead of an isotonic solution.

4. You are asked to participate in an ethics discussion of the question "Should couples be required to undergo genetic screening before they are issued a marriage license?" State your opinion (yes/no) and list at least three positive and three negative arguments for this requirement.

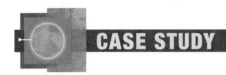

CASE STUDY

Jane Fitz, an LPN, admits Mrs. Smith, age 54, to Mercy Hospital. Mrs. Smith has had a persistent cough for 3 months and has lost 10 pounds over the past 6 weeks. Mrs. Smith has been a cigarette smoker for the past 30 years. The doctor orders a CT scan to determine if she has cancer of the lung.

1. Describe for Mrs. Smith the CT scan procedure.

2. Name the body system involved in lung cancer and describe the function of the system.

   The CT scan reveals a tumor of the lung and a biopsy (removal of tissue for examination) is scheduled.

3. Define cancer and the classification system that will be used to describe the tumor.

4. What actions can Jane Fitz take to reduce Mrs. Smith's anxiety?

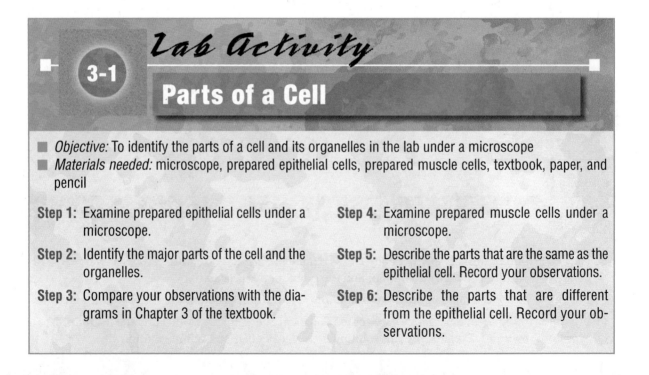

Lab Activity

3-1

Parts of a Cell

■ *Objective:* To identify the parts of a cell and its organelles in the lab under a microscope
■ *Materials needed:* microscope, prepared epithelial cells, prepared muscle cells, textbook, paper, and pencil

Step 1: Examine prepared epithelial cells under a microscope.

Step 2: Identify the major parts of the cell and the organelles.

Step 3: Compare your observations with the diagrams in Chapter 3 of the textbook.

Step 4: Examine prepared muscle cells under a microscope.

Step 5: Describe the parts that are the same as the epithelial cell. Record your observations.

Step 6: Describe the parts that are different from the epithelial cell. Record your observations.

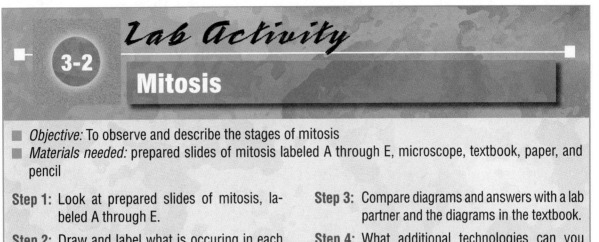

Lab Activity 3-2

Mitosis

- *Objective:* To observe and describe the stages of mitosis
- *Materials needed:* prepared slides of mitosis labeled A through E, microscope, textbook, paper, and pencil

Step 1: Look at prepared slides of mitosis, labeled A through E.

Step 2: Draw and label what is occuring in each slide labeled A through E.

Step 3: Compare diagrams and answers with a lab partner and the diagrams in the textbook.

Step 4: What additional technologies can you use to learn about and observe mitosis?

Lab Activity 3-3

Observation of Osmosis

- *Objective:* To observe and describe the process of osmosis
- *Equipment needed:* slices of potato, distilled water and 10% saline solution, saltshaker, and small glass containers or test tubes

Step 1: Place some distilled water and saline solution in separate containers and label.

Step 2: Mark the levels of the liquids in each container.

Step 3: Add a potato slice to each container and wait 30 minutes.

Step 4: Remove the potato slices and observe for differences.

Step 5: Observe the levels of liquids in each container.

Step 6: What has happened to the potato slices? To the liquid levels? Record your observations.

Step 7: Make two new containers with solutions and label (same as step 1).

Step 8: Mark the levels of liquid in each container.

Step 9: Take two new potato slices and salt each one with a saltshaker.

Step 10: Place salted potato slices in each container and wait 30 minutes.

Step 11: Remove the potato slices and observe for differences.

Step 12: What has happened to the potato slices? To the liquid levels? Record your observations.

Step 13: Explain what has occurred to cause the differences between step 6 and step 12.

TISSUES AND MEMBRANES

Key Words

adipose tissue	granulation	pleural membrane
aponeuroses	hyaline	primary repair
areolar tissue	intestinal mucosa	respiratory mucosa
bactericidal	ligament	scab
calcify	membrane	secondary repair
cardiac muscle	mucosa	serosa
cartilage	mucous membrane	serous fluid
cicatrix	muscle tissue	serous membrane
clean wound	nervous tissue	skeletal muscle
collagen	organ system	sutures
connective tissue	osseous	synovial
elastin	parietal membrane	membrane
epithelial tissue	pericardial	tendon
fasciae	membrane	tissue
gastric mucosa	peritoneal	visceral membrane
graft	membrane	

TISSUES

Multicellular organisms are composed of many different types of cells. Each of these cells performs a special function. These millions of cells are grouped according to their similarity in shape, size, structure, intercellular materials, and function. Cells so grouped are called **tissues.** There are four main types of tissue. (1) **Epithelial tissue** protects the body by covering internal and external surfaces. The cells of the epithelial tissue also produce secretions such as digestive juices. The epithelial tissue is named according to its structure. (2) **Connective tissue** supports and connects organs and tissue. (3) **Muscle tissue** contains cell material which has the ability to contract and move the body. (4) **Nervous tissue** contains cells that react to stimuli and conduct an impulse.

Specialization of cells can be seen in a study of the epithelial cells which make up epithelial tissue. Epithelial cells that cover the body's external and internal surfaces have a typical shape—either columnar, cubical, or platelike. This variation is necessary so the epithelial cells can fit together smoothly in order to line and protect the bodily surface. Muscle cells making up muscle tissue are long and spindlelike so they can contract.

Some tissues consist of both living cells and various nonliving substances which the cells build up around themselves. The variations, functions, and locations of each type are described in Table 4-1.

MEMBRANES

A **membrane** is formed by putting two thin layers of tissue together. The cells in the membrane may secrete a fluid. Membranes are classified as epithelial or connective.

Epithelial Membranes

Epithelial membranes are classified as either **mucous** or **serous membranes,** depending on the type of secretions produced, Figure 4-1.

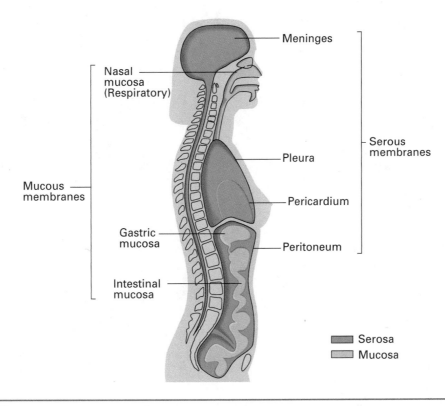

Meninges

Nasal mucosa (Respiratory)

Mucous membranes

Gastric mucosa

Intestinal mucosa

Pleura

Pericardium

Peritoneum

Serous membranes

Serosa
Mucosa

Figure 4-1　*Mucous and serous membranes*

Table 4-1 *Different Kinds of Human Tissue*

TYPE OF TISSUE	FUNCTION	CHARACTERISTICS AND LOCATION	MORPHOLOGY
I. EPITHELIAL	Cells form a continuous layer covering internal and external body surfaces, provide protection, produce secretions (digestive juices, hormones, perspiration), and regulate the passage of materials across themselves. **A. Covering and lining tissue** These cells can be stratified (layered), ciliated, or keratinized (hard, nonliving substance).		
		1. Squamous epithelial cells These are flat, irregularly shaped cells. They line the heart, blood and lymphatic vessels, body cavities, and alveoli (air sacs) of lungs. The outer layer of the skin consists of stratified and keratinized squamous epithelial cells. The stratified squamous epithelial cells on the outer skin layer protect the body against microbial invasion.	
		2. Cuboidal epithelial cells These cube-shaped cells line the kidney tubules and cover the ovaries and secretory parts of certain glands.	
		3. Columnar epithelial cells These cells are elongated, with the nucleus generally near the bottom and often ciliated on the outer surface. They line the ducts, digestive tract (especially the intestinal and stomach lining), parts of the respiratory tract, and glands.	

(continues)

Table 4-1 *(continued)*

TYPE OF TISSUE	FUNCTION	CHARACTERISTICS AND LOCATION	MORPHOLOGY
I. EPITHELIAL (continued)	**B. Glandular or secretory tissue** These cells are specialized to secrete materials such as digestive juices, hormones, milk, perspiration, and wax. They are columnar or cuboidal shaped.	**1. Endocrine gland cells** These cells form ductless glands which secrete their substances (hormones) directly into the bloodstream. For instance, the thyroid gland secretes thyroxin, and adrenal glands secrete adrenaline. **2. Exocrine gland cells** These cells secrete their substances into ducts. The mammary glands, sweat glands, and salivary glands are examples.	Duct (where secretions leave); Secretory cells; Exocrine (duct) gland cell e.g. sweat and mammary glands
II. CONNECTIVE	Cells whose intercellular secretions (matrix) support and connect the organs and tissues of the body. **A. Adipose tissue** This tissue stores lipid (fat), acts as filler tissue, cushions, supports, and insulates the body.	Connective tissue is found almost everywhere within the body: bones, cartilage, mucous membranes, muscles, nerves, skin, and all internal organs. Adipose tissue is a type of loose, connective tissue composed of saclike adipose cells; they are specialized for the storage of fat. Adipose cells are found throughout the body: in the subcutaneous skin layer, around the kidneys, within padding around joints, and in the marrow of long bones.	Cytoplasm; Collagen fibers; Nucleus; Vacuole (for fat storage)
	B. Areolar (loose) tissue This tissue surrounds various organs and supports both nerve cells and blood vessels which transport nutrient materials (to cells) and wastes (away from cells). Areolar tissue also (temporarily) stores glucose, salts, and water.	Areolar tissue is composed of a large, semifluid matrix, with many different types of cells and fibers embedded in it. These include fibroblasts (fibrocytes), plasma cells, macrophages, mast cells, and various white blood cells. The fibers are bundles of strong, flexible, white fibrous protein called **collagen**, and elastic single fibers of **elastin.** It is found in the epidermis of the skin and in the subcutaneous layer with adipose cells.	Mast cell; Reticular fibers; Collagen fibers; Fibroblast cell; Plasma cell; Elastic fiber; Matrix; Macrophage cell

(continues)

Table 4-1 (continued)

TYPE OF TISSUE	FUNCTION	CHARACTERISTICS AND LOCATION	MORPHOLOGY
II. CONNECTIVE (continued)	**C. Dense fibrous tissue** This tissue forms ligaments, tendons, and aponeuroses. **Ligaments** are strong, flexible bands (or cords) which hold bones firmly together at the joints. **Tendons** are white, glistening bands attaching skeletal muscles to the bones. **Aponeuroses** are flat, wide bands of tissue holding one muscle to another or to the periosteum (bone covering). **Fasciae** are fibrous connective tissue sheets that wrap around muscle bundles to hold them in place.	Dense fibrous tissue is also called white fibrous tissue, because .it is made from closely packed white collagen fibers. Fibrous tissue is flexible, but not elastic. This tissue has a poor blood supply and heals slowly	Closely packed collagen fibers — Fibroblast cell
	D. Supportive tissue **1. Osseous (bone) tissue** Comprises the skeleton of the body, which supports and protects underlying soft tissue parts and organs, and also serves as attachments for skeletal muscles.	This connective tissue's intercellular matrix is **calcified** by the deposition of mineral salts (like calcium carbonate and calcium phosphate). Calcification of bone imparts great strength. The entire skeleton is composed of bone tissue.	Bone lacunae — Bone cell — Cytoplasm — Nucleus
	2. Cartilage Provides firm but flexible support for the embryonic skeleton and part of the adult skeleton. **a. Hyaline** Forms the skeleton of the embryo.	Hyaline cartilage is found on articular bone surfaces, and also at the nose tip, bronchi, and bronchial tubes. Ribs are joined to the sternum (breastbone) by the costal cartilage. It is also found in the larynx and the rings in the trachea.	Cells (chondrocytes) — Matrix — Lacuna (space enclosing cells)
	b. Fibrocartilage A strong, flexible, supportive substance, found between bones and wherever great strength (and a degree of rigidity) is needed.	Fibrocartilage is located within intervertebral discs and pubic symphysis between the pubic bones.	Chondrocytes — Dense white fibers

(continues)

Table 4-1 *(continued)*

TYPE OF TISSUE	FUNCTION	CHARACTERISTICS AND LOCATION	MORPHOLOGY
II. CONNECTIVE (continued)	**D. Supportive tissue** (continued) **c. Elastic cartilage** The intercellular matrix is embedded with a network of elastic fibers and is firm but flexible.	Elastic cartilage is located inside the auditory ear tube, external ear, epiglottis, and larynx.	 Elastic fibers Chondrocyte Nucleus
	E. Vascular (liquid blood tissue) **1. Blood** Transports nutrient and oxygen molecules to cells, and metabolic wastes away from cells (can be considered as a liquid tissue). Contains cells that function in the body's defense and in blood clotting.	Blood consists of two major parts: a liquid called plasma, and a solid cellular portion known as blood cells (or corpuscles). The plasma suspends corpuscles, of which there are two major types: red blood cells (erythrocytes) and white blood cells (leukocytes). A third cellular component (actually a cell fragment) is platelets (thrombocytes). Blood circulates within the blood vessels (arteries, veins, and capillaries) and through the heart.	 Thrombocytes (platelets) Lymphocyte Basophil Erythrocytes Monocyte Neutrophil Eosinophil
	2. Lymph Transports tissue fluid, proteins, fats, and other materials from the tissues to the circulatory system. This occurs through a series of tubes called the lymphatic vessels.	Lymph fluid consists of water, glucose, protein, fats, and salt. The cellular components are lymphocytes and granulocytes. They flow in tubes called lymphatic vessels, which closely parallel the veins and bathe the tissue spaces between cells.	 Red blood cells White blood cell Lymph Blood capillary Cells Lymph capillary

(continues)

Table 4-1 *(continued)*

TYPE OF TISSUE	FUNCTION	CHARACTERISTICS AND LOCATION	MORPHOLOGY
III. MUSCLE	**A. Cardiac muscle** These cells help the heart contract in order to pump blood through and out of the heart.	Cardiac muscle is a striated (having a cross-banding pattern), involuntary (not under conscious control) muscle. It makes up the walls of the heart.	Centrally located nucleus — Striations — Branching of cell — Intercalated disc
	B. Skeletal (striated voluntary) muscle These muscles are attached to the movable parts of the skeleton. They are capable of rapid, powerful contractions and long states of partially sustained contractions, allowing for voluntary movement.	Skeletal muscle is striated (having transverse bands that run down the length of muscle fiber), voluntary because the muscle is under conscious control, and skeletal because these muscles attach to the skeleton (bones, tendons, and other muscles).	Nucleus Myofibrils
	C. Smooth (nonstriated involuntary) These provide for involuntary movement. Examples include the movement of materials along the digestive tract, and controlling the diameter of blood vessels and the pupil of the eyes.	Smooth muscle is nonstriated because it lacks the striations (bands) of skeletal muscles; its movement is involuntary. It makes up the walls of the digestive tract, genitourinary tract, respiratory tract, blood vessels, and lymphatic vessels.	Spindle-shaped cell — Cells separated from each other — Nucleus
IV. NERVE	**Neurons (nerve cells)** These cells have the ability to react to stimuli. **1. Irritability** Ability of nerve tissue to respond to environmental changes. **2. Conductivity** Ability to carry a nerve impulse (message).	Nerve tissue consists of neurons (nerve cells). Neurons have branches through which various parts of the body are connected and their activities coordinated. They are found in the brain, spinal cord, and nerves.	Axon Myelin Terminal branches Nucleus Dendrites Cell body

Mucous membranes. Mucous membranes line surfaces and spaces that lead to the outside of the body; they line the respiratory, digestive, reproductive, and urinary systems. The mucous membrane produces a substance called mucus which lubricates and protects the lining. For example, the mucus in the digestive tract protects the lining of the stomach and small intestines from the digestive juices. The term **mucosa** is used for the following specific mucous membranes (Figure 4-1).

- **Respiratory mucosa** lines the respiratory passages.

- **Gastric mucosa** lines the stomach.

- **Intestinal mucosa** lines the small and large intestines.

Serous membrane. The serous membrane is a double-walled membrane that produces a watery fluid and lines closed body cavities. The fluid produced is called **serous fluid.** The outer part of the membrane that lines the cavity is known as the **parietal membrane.** The part that covers the organs within is known as the **visceral membrane.** The fluid produced allows the organs within to move freely and prevents friction. The name **serosa** is given to the specific serous membranes, all beginning with the letter *p.* The serous membranes are as follows (Figure 4-1):

- **Pleural membrane** lines the thoracic or chest cavity and protects the lungs. The fluid is called pleural fluid.

- **Pericardial membrane** lines the heart cavity and protects the heart. The fluid is called pericardial fluid.

- **Peritoneal membrane** lines the abdominal cavity and protects the abdominal organs. The fluid is called peritoneal fluid.

Cutaneous membrane (skin). The cutaneous membrane is a specialized type of epithelial membrane. See Chapter 5 for a complete discussion.

Connective Membranes

Connective membranes consist of two layers of connective tissue. In this classification is the **synovial membrane,** which lines joint cavities. Synovial membranes secrete synovial fluid which prevents friction inside the joint cavity.

ORGANS AND SYSTEMS

An organ is a structure of several types of tissues grouped together to perform a single function. For instance, the stomach is an organ consisting of highly specialized vascular, connective, epithelial, muscular, and nerve tissues. These tissues function together to enable the stomach to perform digestion and absorption.

The skin that covers our bodies is no mere simple tissue, but a complex organ of connective, epithelial, muscular, and nervous tissue. These tissues enable the skin to protect the body and remove its wastes (water and inorganic salts).

The various organs of the human body do not function separately. Instead, they coordinate their activities to form a complete, functional organism. A group of organs that acts together to perform a specific, related function is called an **organ system,** Figure 4-2.

The digestive system has the special function of processing solid food into liquid for absorption into the bloodstream. This organ system includes the mouth, salivary glands, esophagus, stomach, small intestine, liver, pancreas, gallbladder, and large intestine. The circulatory system transports materials to and from cells. It consists of the heart, arteries, veins, capillaries, lymphatic vessels, and spleen.

The human body has 10 organ systems. Each is highly specialized to perform a specific function; together they coordinate their functions to form a whole, live, functioning organism.

The systems of the body are the skeletal, muscular, digestive, respiratory, circulatory, excretory, nervous, endocrine, reproductive, and integumentary systems. The functions and organs of each system are shown in Table 4-2.

DISEASE AND INJURY TO TISSUE

Tissue can be affected by infection or inflammation. Inflammation is a protective response to an injury or irritant. Inflammation will result in pain, swelling, redness, and loss of motion. Infection refers to the invasion of a microorganism causing disease. Infection usually results in inflammation.

Trauma resulting from an external force will cause tissue damage and injury. There is a wide variety of traumatic events that may occur

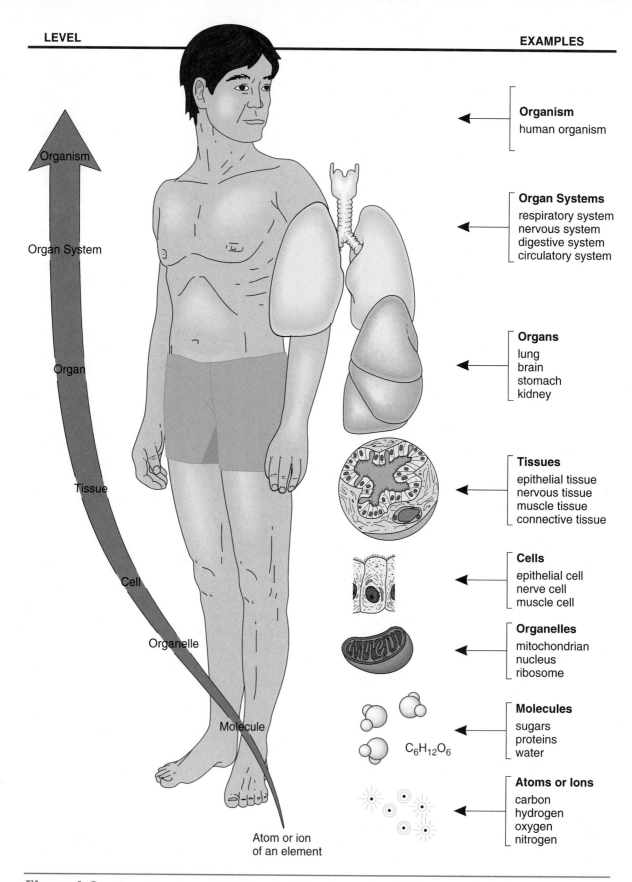

LEVEL   EXAMPLES

Organism

Organ System

Organ

Tissue

Cell

Organelle

Molecule

Atom or ion
of an element

Organism
human organism

Organ Systems
respiratory system
nervous system
digestive system
circulatory system

Organs
lung
brain
stomach
kidney

Tissues
epithelial tissue
nervous tissue
muscle tissue
connective tissue

Cells
epithelial cell
nerve cell
muscle cell

Organelles
mitochondrian
nucleus
ribosome

Molecules
sugars
proteins
water

$C_6H_{12}O_6$

Atoms or Ions
carbon
hydrogen
oxygen
nitrogen

Figure 4-2   *The various organs of the human body function together. The formation of the human organism progresses from simple to complex.*

Table 4-2 *The Ten Body Systems*

SYSTEM	SYSTEM FUNCTIONS	ORGANS
Skeletal	Gives shape to body; protects delicate parts of body; provides space for attaching muscles; is instrumental in forming blood; stores minerals.	Skull, spinal column, ribs and sternum, shoulder girdle, upper and lower extremities, pelvic girdle
Muscular	Determines posture; produces body heat; provides for movement.	Striated voluntary muscles—skeletal Striated involuntary muscles—cardiac Smooth muscles—nonstriated
Digestive	Prepares food for absorption and use by body cells through modification of chemical and physical states.	Mouth (salivary glands, teeth, tongue), pharynx, esophagus, stomach, intestines, liver, gallbladder, pancreas
Respiratory	Acquires oxygen; rids body of carbon dioxide.	Nose, pharynx, larynx, trachea, bronchi, lungs
Circulatory	Carries oxygen and nourishment to cells of body; carries waste from cells; provides body defense.	Heart, arteries, veins, capillaries, lymphatic vessels, lymph nodes, spleen
Excretory	Removes waste products of metabolism from body.	Skin, lungs, kidneys, bladder, ureters, urethra
Nervous	Communicates; controls body activity; coordinates body activity.	Brain, nerves, spinal cord, ganglia
Endocrine	Manufactures hormones to regulate organ activity.	Glands (ductless): pituitary, thyroid, parathyroid, pancreas, adrenal, gonads (ovaries, testes)
Reproductive	Reproduces human beings.	*Male* *Female* Testes Ovaries Scrotum Fallopian tubes Epididymis Uterus Vas deferens Vagina Seminal vesicles Bartholin's gland Ejaculatory duct External genitals (vulva) Prostate gland Breasts (mammary glands) Cowper's gland Penis Urethra
Integumentary	Helps regulate body temperature; establishes a barrier between the body and environment; eliminates waste; synthesizes vitamin D; contains receptors for temperature, pressure, and pain.	Epidermis, dermis, sweat glands, oil glands

but the most frequent cause of serious injury is motor vehicle collisions. Emergency management of trauma is necessary to prevent complications such as shock, hemorrhage, and infection.

Abnormal growth of cells can also alter tissue and cause tissue damage and trauma. These types of growth patterns were discussed in an earlier chapter.

Birth defects can also impair tissue. This can result from a change in structure or function of tissue at the chromosomal level or as a result of environmental factors.

DEGREE OF TISSUE REPAIR

Repair of damaged tissues occurs continually under the everyday activities of living.

Depending on the type and location of injury, some tissue is quickly repaired. Muscle tissue heals slowly and bone tissue repairs are slow because broken bone ends must be kept aligned and immobilized until the repair is done. Heart muscle tissue does not repair itself, and nerve cell bodies destroyed by infection or injury do not grow back.

PROCESS OF EPITHELIAL TISSUE REPAIR

There are two types of epithelial tissue repair. One is called **primary repair** and the other one is called **secondary repair.**

Primary Repair

Primary repair takes place in "clean" wounds. A **clean wound** is a cut or incision on the skin where infection is not present. In a simple skin injury, the deep layer of stratified squamous epithelium divides. The new stratified squamous epithelial cells "push" themselves upward toward the surface of the skin. The damage or wound is quickly and completely restored to normal. However, if the damage is over a larger area, then the underlying connective tissue cells and fibroblasts are also involved.

Primary Repair Over a Large Skin Area. If a large area of skin is damaged, fluid will escape from the broken capillaries. This capillary fluid dries and seals the wound, and the typical **scab** forms. Epithelial cells multiply at the edges of the scab and continue to grow over the damaged area until it is covered. If a great or deep area of skin is destroyed, skin **grafts** may be needed to help in wound healing.

Primary Repair of Deep Tissues. When damage occurs to deep tissues, the edges of the wound must be brought (sewn) together with **sutures.** For example, operative incisions or wounds have a tremendous amount of serous fluid that leaks out onto the wound. This helps to form a coagulation (clot) that seals the wound. The coagulum contains tissue fragments and white blood cells. In 24 to 36 hours, the epithelial cells lining the capillaries (endothelium) and fibroblasts of connective tissue are rapidly regenerating. The newly formed cells remain along the edges of the wound. On the third day following injury, new vascular tissue starts to form. These multiply across the wound along with connective tissue formation.

On the fourth or fifth day, fibroblast cells become very active in making new collagen fibers. In addition, capillaries grow and "reach" across the wound, holding the edges firmly together. Toward the end of the healing process, the collagenous fibers shorten, reducing scar tissue to a minimum.

Secondary Repair

During secondary repair, a process called **granulation** occurs in a large open wound with small or large tissue loss. The granulation process will form new vertically upstanding blood vessels. These new blood vessels are surrounded by young connective tissue and wandering cells of different types. Granulation causes the surface area to have a pebbly texture. Fibroblasts will be quite active in their production of new collagenous fibers. The activity of this repair causes the large open wound to eventually heal. As granulation occurs, a fluid also is secreted. This fluid has strong **bactericidal** (bacterial-destructing) properties, which helps reduce the risk of infection during wound healing.

As in any type of tissue repair, a certain amount of scar tissue will form. The amount of

VITAMIN	FUNCTION
Vitamin A	Aids in repair of epithelial tissue, especially the epithelial cells lining the respiratory tract.
Vitamin B (thiamine, nicotinic acid, and riboflavin)	Helps to promote the general well-being of the individual. Specifically helps to promote appetite, metabolism, vigor, and pain relief in some cases.
Vitamin C	Helps in the normal production of and maintenance of collagen fibers and other connective tissue substances.
Vitamin D	Needed for the normal absorption of calcium from the intestine. Possibly helps in the repair of bone fractures.
Vitamin K	Helps in the process of blood coagulation.
Vitamin E	Helps healing of tissues by acting as an antioxidant protector. It prevents important molecules and structures in the cell from reacting with oxygen. (When delicate components of living protoplasm are attacked by oxygen, they are literally "burnt.")

Table 4-3 *Vitamins Favorable to Tissue Repair*

Medical Terminology

adipos	fatty
-e	pertaining to
adipos/e	pertaining to fatty
bacteria	single cell microorganisms
-cidal	to kill or destroy
bacteri/cidal	to destroy rod-shaped microorganisms
cardi	heart
-ac	pertaining to
cardi/ac	pertaining to heart
muc	slime
-ous	pertaining to
mucous	pertaining to a slimy substance
pariet	wall
-al	pertaining to
pariet/al	pertaining to the wall of a body cavity
peri	around
peri/cardi/al	pertaining to around the heart
ser	watery
-ous	pertaining to
ser/ous	pertaining to a watery substance
viscer	guts or internal organs
viscer/al	pertaining to the internal organs

scar (**cicatrix**) tissue formed depends on the extent of tissue damage. Careful attention must be given to patients whose body or body parts are undergoing massive tissue repair (these include victims of burns). These areas *must* be kept in alignment and immobile at the beginning; however, later active movement should be encouraged so as new tissue forms, pulling from scar tissue will not occur. It is the role of the health care professional to help prevent or minimize excessive scar tissue formation that can lead to disfigurement.

A health care professional should also be mindful that proper nutrition plays an important part in healing. Newly growing tissues require lots of protein for repair; thus, the need for protein-rich foods is important.

Vitamins also play an essential role in wound repair. They help the patient develop resistance to infections. Table 4-3 lists vitamins that are needed in tissue repair.

REVIEW QUESTIONS

Select the letter of the choice that best completes the statement.

1. Cells that are alike in size, shape, and function are called:
   a. elements
   b. tissues
   c. organs
   d. systems

2. The type of tissue found on the outer layer of skin is called:
   a. squamous epithelial
   b. stratified epithelial
   c. ciliated epithelial
   d. columnar epithelial

3. Collagen is a strong, flexible protein found mainly in:
   a. adipose tissue
   b. cartilage tissue
   c. loose connective tissue
   d. bone tissue

4. Connective tissue structures that hold bones firmly together at joints are called:
   a. fascia
   b. tendons
   c. aponeuroses
   d. ligaments

5. The membrane that covers linings to the outside of the body is:
   a. cutaneous
   b. serous
   c. mucous
   d. synovial

6. The membrane that covers the lungs is called:
   a. parietal pleura
   b. visceral pleura
   c. parietal pericardial
   d. visceral pericardial

7. An inflammation of the lining of the abdominal cavity is called:
   a. pleurisy
   b. pericarditis
   c. peritonitis
   d. gastritis

8. The system that provides for movement of the body is the:
   a. skeletal
   b. nervous
   c. muscle
   d. circulatory

9. The type of repair that takes place in a clean wound is called:
   a. primary repair
   b. granulation
   c. secondary repair
   d. secretion of bactericidal fluid

10. The vitamin necessary to help as an antioxidant is:
   a. A
   b. D
   c. K
   d. E

COMPLETION

Complete the following statements.

1. The tissue that has the ability to react to stimuli is _____.

2. The gastric mucosa is the mucous membrane lining of the _____ _____.

3. The secretion that prevents the bones in a joint from rubbing together is _____ _____.

4. The lining that protects the lung is the _____ membrane.

5. In secondary tissue repair when there is a large open wound, the process of tissue repair is called _____.

APPLYING THEORY TO PRACTICE

1. Feel your skin. What type of tissue is it? Is this tissue the same as the lining in your mouth?

2. Explain how mucus affects the air we breathe or the food we eat.

3. Name the organ systems involved when you eat a slice of pizza.

4. You hear the expression, "I sprained a ligament" or "I pulled my tendon." Describe the type of tissue involved with each injury. Describe the function of a ligament and a tendon.

5. Imagine you have a friend with severe injuries, who is hungry. Describe the lunch you would prepare for this person. The menu should include the vitamins necessary for tissue repair and help in pain relief.

CASE STUDY

Anthony, age 5, fell on the school playground and scraped his knee. His mother comes to the school nurse's office. She is worried about infection and whether a big scar will form.

1. Explain to Anthony's mother what a clean wound is.

2. Describe to the mother what takes place in the healing process.

3. Explain to the mother about scarring.

4. Give the mother information on the role of vitamins in healing and developing resistance to other infections.

5. Anthony is worried he cannot run and play. What will you tell Anthony about his mobility?

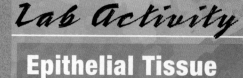

Lab Activity

4-1

Epithelial Tissue

■ *Objective:* To examine the structure of epithelial tissue and how the structure affects its function
■ *Materials needed:* slides of epithelial tissue: squamous, cuboidal, columnar, and glandular; microscope; paper and pencil

Step 1: Examine the prepared slides of the different types of epithelial tissue under a microscope. Record the observed differences.

Step 2: Draw a diagram of each type of epithelial tissue. Describe how the structure affects the function.

Step 3: Describe where each type of tissue is located in the body. Record your answers.

Step 4: What are the structural differences between the types of epithelial tissue? Record your conclusions.

Lab Activity

4-2

Connective Tissue

■ *Objective:* To examine connective tissue (the most common tissue type) and explain how it serves its general function to fasten, connect, support, and protect
■ *Materials needed:* labeled slides of connective tissue: adipose, areolar, dense fibrous, bone, cartilage, vascular (blood and lymph); unlabeled slides of connective tissue; microscope; pencil and paper

Step 1: Examine the prepared slides of the different types of connective tissue under the microscope.

Step 2: Describe what you see in each matrix of the tissue. Record your observations.

Step 3: List the categories of connective tissue.

Step 4: What is the difference between adipose tissue and bone tissue? Record your answers.

Step 5: With a lab partner, look at two types of connective tissue that are not labeled. Decide which types of connective tissue are shown on the slides. Record your opinion.

Chapter 5

INTEGUMENTARY SYSTEM

Key Words

acne vulgaris
alopecia
arrector pili
   muscle
athlete's foot
avascular
basal cell
   carcinoma
boils
cortex
cryosurgery
decubitus ulcer
dermatitis
dermis
eczema
epidermis
first degree burn
genital herpes

hair follicle
herpes
hyperthermia
hypothermia
impetigo
integumentary
   system
keratin
malignant
   melanoma
matrix
medulla
melanin
melanocytes
papillae
psoriasis
ringworm

root
rule of nines
sebaceous gland
sebum
second degree burn
shaft
shingles (herpes
   zoster)
skin cancer
squamous cell
   carcinoma
stratum corneum
stratum
   germinativum
sudoriferous gland
third degree burn
urticaria (hives)

The skin is our protective covering and is called the integument or **integumentary system** or cutaneous membrane. It is tough, pliable, and multifunctional.

FUNCTIONS OF THE SKIN

The skin has seven functions.

1. Skin is a covering for the underlying, deeper tissues, protecting them from dehydration, injury, and germ invasion.

2. Skin helps regulate body temperature by controlling the amount of heat loss. Evaporation of water from the skin, in the form of perspiration, helps rid the body of excess heat.

3. Skin helps to manufacture vitamin D. The ultraviolet light on the skin is necessary for the first stages of vitamin D formation.

4. Skin is the site of many nerve endings, Figure 5-1. A square inch of skin contains about 72 feet of nerves and hundreds of receptors.

5. Skin has tissues for the temporary storage of fat, glucose, water, and salts such as sodium chloride. Most of these substances are later absorbed by the blood and transported to other parts of the body.

6. Skin is designed to screen out harmful ultraviolet radiation contained in sunlight.

7. Skin has special properties to absorb certain drugs and other chemical substances. We can apply drugs for local application, as in the case of treating rashes; or we can apply medications that can be absorbed through the skin and have a general effect in the body. An example of this is Nitro-Bid paste, which is used to help dilate blood vessels in the treatment of angina pectoris (chest pain).

STRUCTURE OF THE SKIN

The skin consists of two basic layers.

1. The **epidermis** or outermost covering is made of epithelial cells with no blood vessels present (**avascular**).

2. The **dermis** or true skin is made of connective tissue and is vascular.

See Figure 5-2.

Epidermis

The epidermis consists of four distinct cell types and five layers. The thickness of the epidermis varies: It is thinnest on the eyelids and thickest on the palms of the hands and the soles of the feet. The surface layer (**stratum corneum**) consists of dead cells rich in keratin. **Keratin** is a protein that renders the skin dry and provides a waterproof covering, thus resisting evaporation and preventing excessive water loss. It also serves as a barrier against ultraviolet light, bacteria, abrasions, and some chemicals.

The epidermal cells are as follows:

a. Keratinocytes comprise most of the epidermis and produce the protein keratin.

b. Merkel cells are the sensory receptors for touch.

c. **Melanocytes** make the protein **melanin**, which protects the skin against the ultraviolet rays of the sun.

d. Langerhans cells (not the same as the islets of Langerhans in the pancreas) are macrophages which are effective in the defense of the skin against microorganisms.

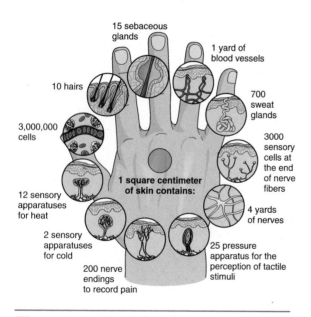

15 sebaceous glands

1 yard of blood vessels

10 hairs

700 sweat glands

3,000,000 cells

3000 sensory cells at the end of nerve fibers

1 square centimeter of skin contains:

12 sensory apparatuses for heat

4 yards of nerves

2 sensory apparatuses for cold

25 pressure apparatus for the perception of tactile stimuli

200 nerve endings to record pain

Figure 5-1   *The skin is well supplied with nerves.*

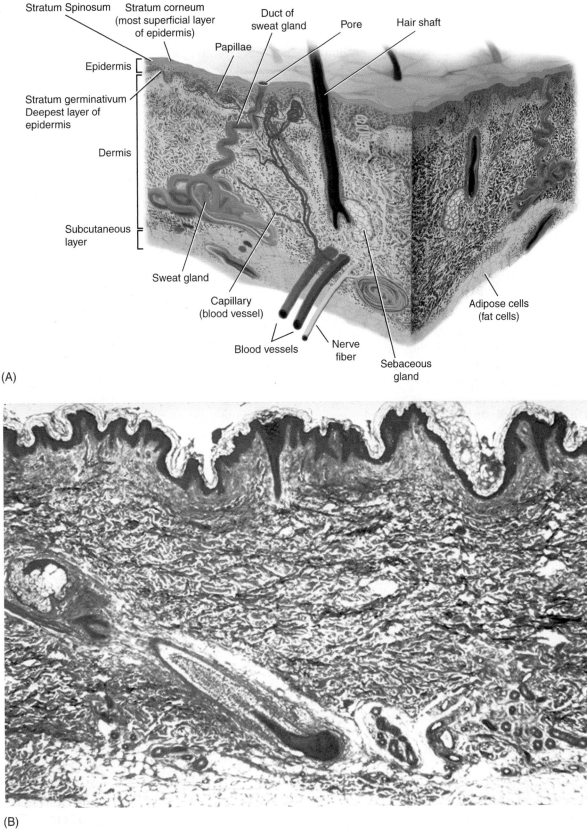

(A)

Stratum Spinosum

Stratum corneum
(most superficial layer
of epidermis)

Papillae

Duct of
sweat gland

Pore

Hair shaft

Epidermis

Stratum germinativum
Deepest layer of
epidermis

Dermis

Subcutaneous
layer

Sweat gland

Capillary
(blood vessel)

Blood vessels

Nerve
fiber

Sebaceous
gland

Adipose cells
(fat cells)

(B)

Figure 5-2 *A cross section of the skin* (B Courtesy of University of Wisconsin Medical School, Madison, WI.)

Following are the epidermal layers from the deepest to the most superficial.

1. The **stratum germinativum,** or stratum basale, undergoes continuous cell division; it is the deepest epidermal layer. It consists of a layer of cells that are mostly keratinocytes. They grow upward and become part of the more superficial layers, the stratum spinosum. Melanocytes and merkel cells are also found in the germinativum layer.

2. Stratum spinosum is 8 to 10 cell layers thick. Contained in this layer are melanocytes, keratinocytes, and Langerhans cells. Under a microscope the cells in this layer look prickly, and thus the name *spinosum,* meaning "little spine."

The stratum germinativum and stratum spinosum are adjacent to the dermis and thus contain the only epidermal cells that receive nourishment from the dermis. As the cells age, they are pushed upward by newly formed cells, away from the source of nourishment. They gradually die and their soft protoplasm becomes hard (keratinized).

3. The stratum granulosum is where the keratinization process begins and the cells begin to die.

4. The stratum lucidum is found only on the palms of the hand and the soles of the feet. The cells in this layer appear clear.

5. The stratum corneum is composed of dead, flat, scalelike keratinized cells, which slough off. This layer is also slightly acidic, which helps in the defense against harmful microorganisms.

Melanocytes produce two distinct classes of melanin: pheomelanin, which is red to yellow in color, and eumelanin, which is dark brown to black. People who have light skin generally have a greater proportion of pheomelanin in their skin than those who have dark skin. Both classes of melanin bind to a wide variety of compounds, including some drugs. Because of their affinity for melanin, some drugs make the skin burn more easily. In the elderly, melanin collects in spots, often called "aging" or "liver" spots.

Environment can also modify skin coloring. Exposure to sunlight may result in a temporary increase of eumelanin causing a darkened or tanned effect. Prolonged exposure to the ultraviolet rays of sunlight is dangerous because it may lead to the development of skin cancers.

As seen in Figure 5-2, the lower edge of the stratum germinativum is thrown into ridges. These ridges are known as the **papillae** of the skin. The papillae actually arise from the dermal layer of the skin and push into the stratum germinativum of the epidermis. In the skin of the fingers, soles of the feet, and the palms of the hands, these papillae are quite pronounced. So much so, in fact, that they raise the skin into permanent ridges. These ridges are so arranged that they provide maximum resistance to slipping when grasping and holding objects; thus, they are also referred to as friction ridges. The ridges on the inner surfaces of the fingers create individual and characteristic fingerprint patterns used in identification. Newborn infants are also footprinted for means of identity.

Dermis

The dermis, or corium, is the thicker, inner layer of the skin. It contains matted masses of connective tissue, collagen tissue bands, elastic fibers (through which pass numerous blood vessels), nerve endings, muscles, hair follicles, oil and sweat glands, and fat cells. The thickness of the dermis varies over different parts of the body. It is, for instance, thicker over the soles of the feet and the palms of the hand. The skin covering the shoulders and back is thinner than that over the palms, but thicker than the skin over the abdomen and thorax.

There are many nerve receptors of different types in the dermal layer. The sensory nerves end in nerve receptors which are sensitive to heat, cold, touch, pain, and pressure. The nerve endings vary in where they are located. The receptors for touch are closer to the epidermis so you can feel someone's touch. However, the pressure receptors are deeper in the dermal layer. This explains why you can sit for a long period before you feel uncomfortable. There are also nerve endings to sense pain located under the epidermis and around the hair follicles. These pain receptors are especially numerous on the lower arm, breast, and forehead.

Blood vessels in the dermis aid in the regulation of body temperature to maintain homeostasis. When external temperatures increase or decrease, blood vessels in the dermis dilate to bring more warmed blood flow to the surface of the body from deeper tissues. On a hot day the heat brought to the skin's surface can be lost through the process of radiation (transfer of heat from a warm body to a cooler environment), convection (air currents that pick up and transfer heat away from a warm surface), conduction (transfer of heat from a warm object to a cooler object it is in contact with), or evaporation (transfer of heat into body fluids which are then evaporated from the body surface). Heat loss through these means will cool the body. On a cold day this initial response aids in warming the body. In cold temperatures, however, this cannot be maintained for long periods of time. If the body is exposed to cold for an extended period of time the blood vessels will constrict to bring warmed blood closer to vital organs to warm and preserve them.

Subcutaneous or Hypodermal Layer

The subcutaneous or hypodermal layer lies under the dermis and sometimes is called superficial fascia. It is not a true part of the integumentary system. It consists of loose connective tissue and contains about one-half of the body's stored fat. The hypodermis layer attaches the integumentary system to the surface muscles underneath. Injections frequently given in this area are called hypodermic or subcutaneous.

APPENDAGES OF THE SKIN

The appendages of the skin include the hair, nails, sudoriferous (sweat) glands, and sebaceous (oil) glands and their ducts.

Hair

Hairs are distributed over most of the surface area of the body. They are missing from the palms of hands, soles of feet, glans penis, and inner surfaces of the vaginal labia.

The length, thickness, type, and color of hair vary with the different body parts and different races. The hairs of the eyelids, for example, are extremely short, whereas hair from the scalp can grow to a considerable length. Facial and pubic hair are quite thick.

A hair is composed of root shaft, the outer cuticle layer, the **cortex,** and the inner **medulla.** The cuticle consists of a single layer of flat, scale-like, keratinized cells that overlap each other. The cortex consists of elongated, keratinized, nonliving cells. Hair pigment is located in the cortex. In dark hair, the cortex contains pigment granules; as one ages, pigment granules are replaced with air, which looks gray or white.

The **root** is the part of the hair that is implanted in the skin. The **shaft** projects from the skin surface. The root is embedded in an inpocketing of the epidermis called the **hair follicle.** Hair varies from straight to curly. The shape of the hair follicle determines the curl of the hair. A round follicle makes straight hair, an oval follicle makes wavy hair, and a flat follicle makes curly hair. Toward the lower end of the hair follicle is a tuft of tissue called the papilla, which extends upward into the hair root. The papilla contains capillaries which nourish the hair follicle cells. This is important because the division of cells in the hair follicle gives rise to a new hair. There is a genetic predisposition in some males to a condition known as **alopecia** or baldness, which is a permanent hair loss. The normal hair is replaced by a very short hair which is transparent and for practical purposes invisible. Males typically experience more hair loss than women, and at a younger age. Treatment for baldness includes medications (topical and oral) and hair transplants.

Attached to each hair follicle on the side toward which it slopes is a smooth muscle called the **arrector pili muscle.** When the pili muscle is stimulated, as by a sudden chill, it contracts and causes the skin to pucker around the hair. It may be called "goosebumps" or "gooseflesh." When this occurs, a small amount of oil is produced, due to pressure on the sebaceous glands.

Nails

The nails are hard structures covering the dorsal surfaces of the last phalanges of the fingers and toes. They are slightly convex on their upper surfaces and concave on their lower surfaces. A nail is formed in the nail bed or **matrix,** Figure 5-3. Here the epidermal cells first appear as elongated cells. These then fuse together to form hard, keratinized plates. As long as a nail bed remains intact, a nail will always be formed. Occasionally, a nail is lost due to an injury or disease; however, if the nail bed is not damaged, a new nail will be produced.

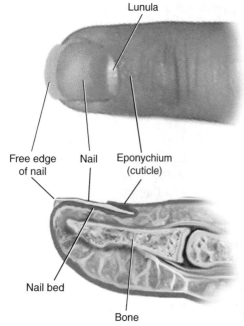

Lunula

Free edge of nail   Nail   Eponychium (cuticle)

Nail bed

Bone

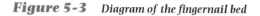

Figure 5-3 *Diagram of the fingernail bed*

Sweat Glands

While actual excretion is a minor function of the skin, certain wastes dissolved in perspiration are removed. Perspiration is 99% water with only small quantities of salt and organic materials (waste products). Sweat or **sudoriferous glands** are distributed over the entire skin surface. They are present in large numbers under the arms, and on the palms of the hands, soles of the feet, and forehead.

Sweat glands are tubular, with a coiled base and a tubelike duct that extends to form a pore in the skin, see Figure 5-2. Perspiration is excreted through the pores. Under the control of the nervous system, these glands may be activated by several factors including heat, pain, fever, and nervousness.

The amount of water lost through the skin is almost 500 ml a day, although this varies according to the type of exercise and the environmental temperature. In profuse sweating, a great deal of water may be lost; it is vital to replace the loss of water as soon as possible.

Ceruminous or wax glands are modifications of the sweat (sudoriferous) glands. These are found in the ear canals and produce ear wax.

Sebaceous Glands

The skin is protected by a thick, oily substance known as **sebum** secreted by the **sebaceous glands.** Sebum lubricates the skin, keeping it soft and pliable.

THE INTEGUMENT AND ITS RELATIONSHIP TO MICROORGANISMS

An intact skin surface is the best way the body can defend itself against pathogens (disease-producing, toxins), and water loss. If skin is especially dry, lotions or creams may prevent cracking.

Most of the skin surface is not a favorable place for microbial growth because it is too dry. Microbes live only on moist skin areas where they adhere to and grow on the surfaces of dead cells that compose the outer epidermal layer. The type of microbes found are of the Staphylococcus or Corynebacterium bacterial species. The other types are *fungi* and *yeasts.**

Most skin bacteria are associated with the hair follicles or sweat glands where nutrients are present and the moisture content is high. Underarm perspiration odor is caused by the interaction of bacteria on perspiration. This odor can be minimized or prevented either by decreasing perspiration with antiperspirants or killing the bacteria with deodorant soaps. Each hair follicle is associated with a sebaceous gland that secretes sebum. This lubricant fluid contains amino acids, lactic acid, lipids, salts, and urea. These are substances that can support microbial growth.

Handwashing

A health care worker must know that the number one way to prevent the spread of disease is by handwashing. The amount of time spent washing depends on the amount of contamination. The least amount of time is 10 to 30 seconds. If you are in contact with infectious material, the time should be from 2 to 4 minutes. If you are in contact with blood, infectious material, or any body secretions, first wash the hands, apply gloves before exposure, remove the gloves, and wash the hands again.

---

*Fungi are low forms of microscopic plant life lacking chlorophyll; may be filamentous (mold) or unicellular (yeast). Yeast is a microscopic, single-celled member of the fungi division.

Effects of Aging on The Integumentary System

The skin presents the most visible signs of aging. As one ages, the sebaceous glands secrete less lubrication and the outer layer of the skin becomes more fragile and dry. The elastin fibers shrink, becoming more rigid and leading to a loss of elasticity in the skin. Loss of subcutaneous fat results in lines, wrinkles, and sagging. The dermal vascular network decreases in its ability to respond to heat and cold. This predisposes an older person to hypothermia (condition in which body temperature drops below normal) and hyperthermia (condition in which body temperature rises above normal).

The melanocytes decrease, making the skin more sensitive to the ultraviolet rays of the sun. There may also be the appearance on the skin of small; cherry red bumps (cherry angiomas) which are benign skin tumors.

The physiological changes in the skin may affect a person's feelings of self-worth. This can be the most difficult part of aging in a society where youth translates into beauty.

REPRESENTATIVE DISORDERS OF THE SKIN

Acne vulgaris is a common and chronic disorder of the sebaceous glands. The sebaceous glands secrete excessive oil, or sebum, which is deposited at the openings of the glands. Eventually this oily deposit becomes hard, or keratinized, plugging up the opening. This prevents the escape of the oily secretions, and the area becomes filled with leukocytes (white blood cells). The leukocytes cause the accumulation of pus. Acne occurs most often during adolescence and is marked by blackheads, cysts, pimples, and scarring. Treatment may be topical medications that dry up oil and promote skin peeling. The physician may also order antibiotics if the skin becomes infected.

Athlete's foot is a contagious fungal infection. The fungus infects the superficial skin layer and leads to skin eruptions, Figure 5-4A. These eruptions are characterized by the formation of small blisters between the fingers and most often the toes. Accompanied by cracking and scaling, this condition is usually contracted in public baths or showers. Treatment involves thorough cleansing and drying of the affected area. In addition, special antifungal agents are administered and antifungal powders are applied liberally.

Dermatitis is an inflammation of the skin which may be nonspecific, Figure 5-4B. For example, some people may use a particular soap and develop contact dermatitis; the result is a rash. To treat contact dermatitis, remove the irritant that is causing the problem. Wash the area and apply topical ointments to reduce inflammation and itching. Another cause may be emotional; stress may cause a person's skin to become blotchy.

Eczema is an acute, or chronic, noncontagious inflammatory skin disease. The skin becomes dry, red, itchy, and scaly, Figure 5-4C. Various factors can lead to eczema. The most common type is atopic eczema, an allergic reaction that usually occurs in the first year of life. Eczema caused by ingested drugs is known as dermatitis medicamentosa. That caused by sunlight or artificial ultraviolet radiation is called dermatitis actinica. Treatment consists of removal or avoidance of the causative agent, as well as application of topical medications containing hydrocortisone. The medication, however, only helps to alleviate the symptoms.

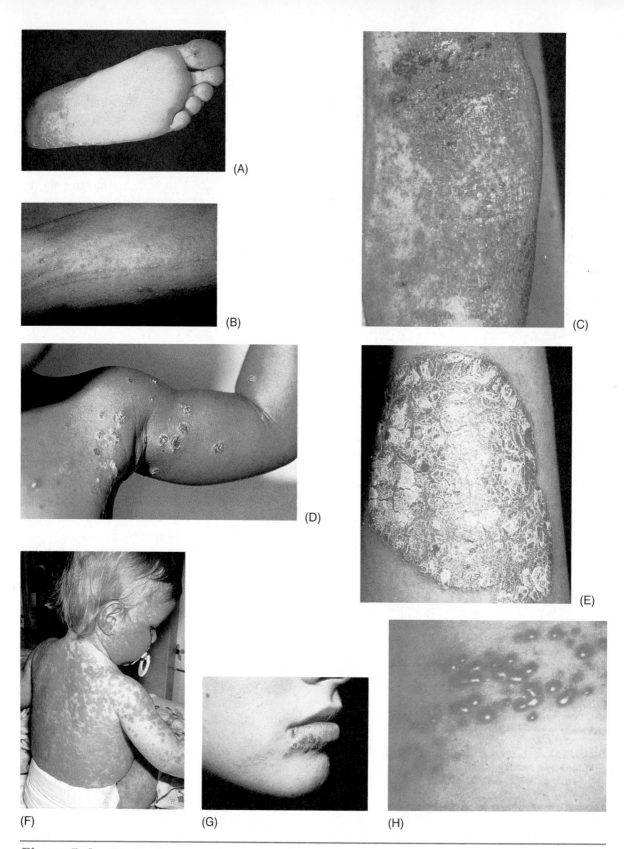

Figure 5-4 *Skin disorders: (A) athlete's foot; (B) allergic contact dermatitis; (C) eczema; (D) impetigo; (E) psoriasis; (F) urticaria or hives; (G) herpes simplex; and (H) shingles.* (A–C Courtesy of the Centers for Disease Control and Prevention; D–G Courtesy of Robert A. Silverman, M.D., Clinical Associate Professor, Department of Pediatrics, Georgetown University.)

Impetigo is an acute, inflammatory, and contagious skin disease seen in babies and young children. It is caused by the staphylococcus or streptococcus organism. This disorder is characterized by the appearance of vesicles that rupture and develop distinct yellow crusts, Figure 5-4D. Treatment is with a topical antibacterial cream and oral antibiotics.

Psoriasis is a chronic inflammatory skin disease characterized by the development of dry reddish patches which are covered with silvery-white scales. It affects the skin surface over the elbow's, knees, shins, scalp, and lower back, Figure 5-4E. The cause is unknown; onsets may be triggered by stress, trauma, or infection. Psoriasis has no definitive treatment at present; research is being done on many drugs for the treatment of this condition. Moisturizers help keep the skin soft and reduce scales and thus the pain of cracking skin.

Ringworm is a highly contagious fungal infection marked by raised, itchy, circular patches with crusts. It may occur upon the skin, scalp, and underneath the nails. Ringworm can be effectively treated with the drug griseofulvin.

Urticaria, or **hives,** is a skin condition recognized by the appearance of intensely itching wheals or welts. These welts have an elevated, usually white center, with a surrounding pink area. They appear in clusters distributed over the entire body surface, Figure 5-4F. The welts last 1 to 2 days. Urticaria is generally a response to an allergen, such as an ingested drug or foods like citrus fruits, chocolate, fish, eggs, shellfish, strawberries, and tomatoes. Complete avoidance and elimination of the causative factor(s) alleviate the problem.

Boils, or carbuncles, are painful. A boil is a bacterial infection of the hair follicles or sebaceous glands usually caused by the staphylococcus organism. If the boil becomes more extensive and is deeply embedded, it is called a carbuncle. Treatment requires antibiotics and excision and drainage of the affected area.

Herpes is a viral infection that is usually seen as a blister. The most common types are herpes simplex, genital herpes, and herpes zoster (shingles). Herpes simplex occurs around the mouth, and is known as a fever blister or cold sore, Figure 5-4G. It may be spread through oral contact.

Genital herpes is another form of the virus which may appear as a blister in the genital area. This virus is usually spread through sexual contact. Any type of herpes infection involves periods of remission and exacerbation (outbreak). Treatment is with acyclovir. A problem may arise when a woman becomes pregnant. If the woman has symptoms when the delivery date arrives, the baby may become infected when passing through the vaginal route for delivery. The physician must be told of a herpes condition to prevent infection of the newborn.

Shingles (herpes zoster) is a skin eruption due to a virus infection of the nerve endings. It is commonly seen on the chest or abdomen, accompanied by severe pain known as herpetic neuralgia, Figure 5-4H. The condition is especially serious in people who are elderly or debilitated. Treatment consists of medication for pain and itching and protecting the area.

SKIN CANCER

Skin cancer has been associated with exposure to ultraviolet light and scientists are cautioning people to limit their exposure to direct sunlight. Skin cancer is the most common type of cancer in people.

Basal cell carcinoma is the most common and least malignant type of skin cancer, usually occurring on the face. The abnormal cells start in the epidermis and extend to the dermis or subcutaneous layer. This cancer may be treated by surgical removal, radiation or cryosurgery. **Cryosurgery** is the destruction of tissue by freezing, using liquid nitrogen. Full recovery occurs in 99% of the cases.

Squamous cell carcinoma arises from the epidermis and occurs most often on the scalp and lower lip. This type grows rapidly and metastasizes to the lymph nodes. This cancer may be treated by surgical removal or radiation. Chances for recovery are good if found early.

Malignant melanoma occurs in pigmented cells of the skin called melanocytes. The cancer cells metastasize to other areas quickly. This

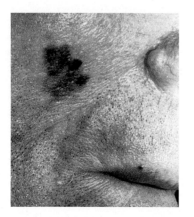

Figure 5-5 *Malignant melanoma (Courtesy of Robert A. Silverman, M.D., Clinical Associate Professor, Department of Pediatrics, Georgetown University.)*

type of tumor may appear as a brown or black irregular patch which occurs suddenly, Figure 5-5. A color or size change in a preexisting wart or mole may also indicate melanoma. Treatment is surgical removal of the melanoma and the surrounding area and chemotherapy.

BURNS

Burns are a traumatic injury as the result of radiation from the sun (sunburn), a heat lamp, or contact with boiling water, steam, fire, chemicals, or electricity. It is important to remind people that some medications cause increased sensitivity to sunlight. When the skin is burned, dehydration and infection may occur—either condition can be life threatening. The **rule of nines** measures the percent of the body burned: The body is divided into 11 areas and each area accounts for 9% of the total body surface. For example, the entire arm is 9%; the perineal area accounts for 1%.

Burns are usually referred to as first, second, or third degree, depending on the skin layers affected and the symptoms, Figure 5-6.

First degree burns involve only the epidermis. Symptoms are redness, swelling, and pain. Treatment consists of the application of cold water. Healing usually occurs within 1 week.

Second degree burns may involve the epidermis and dermis. Symptoms include pain,

swelling, redness, and blistering. The skin may also be exposed to infection. Treatment may include pain medication and dry sterile dressings applied to open skin areas. Healing generally occurs within 2 weeks.

Third degree burns involve complete destruction of the epidermis, dermis, and subcutaneous layers. Symptoms include loss of skin, eschar (blackened skin), yet possibly no pain. This may be a life-threatening situation, depending on the amount of skin damaged, and fluid and blood plasma lost. The person requires immediate hospitalization. Treatment consists of prevention of infection, contracture, and fluid replacement. Skin grafting is done as soon as possible.

SKIN LESIONS

The health care professional should be familiar with the different types of skin disorders or lesions. Sometimes skin lesions indicate only an outer skin disorder. Table 5-1 and Figure 5-7 describe the different types of skin lesions, their characteristics, and their dimensions.

Pressure Ulcer/Decubitus

Pressure ulcers, also known as **decubitus ulcers** or bedsores, are preventable and are a primary concern of health care workers. Decubitus ulcers occur when a person is constantly sitting or lying in the same position without shifting his or her weight. Any area of tissue that lies over a bone is much more likely to develop a decubitus ulcer. These areas include the spine, coccyx, hips, elbows, and heels. The constant pressure against the area causes a decrease in the blood supply there and thus the tissue begins to decay. These ulcers are classified in stages according to their severity.

■ Stage I involves surface reddening, but the skin is unbroken. Treatment is to alleviate the pressure.

■ Stage II is characterized by blistered areas that are either broken or unbroken; the surrounding area is red and irritated. Treatment is to protect and clean the area and alleviate the pressure.

■ Stage III presents with skin breaks through all layers of skin. It becomes a primary site

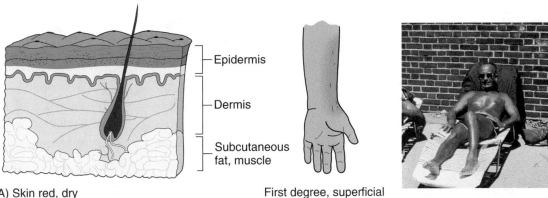

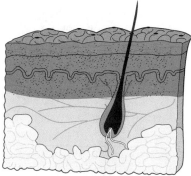

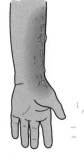

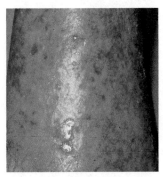

(A) Skin red, dry
First degree

First degree, superficial

(B) Blistered, skin moist, pink or red
Second degree

Second degree,
partial thickness

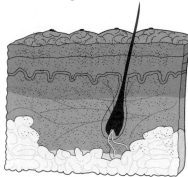

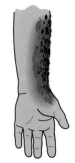

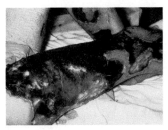

(C) Charring, skin black, brown, red
Third degree

Third degree, full thickness

Figure 5-6 *Burns are usually referred to as (A) first, (B) second, or (C) third degree.* (Photos courtesy of The Phoenix Society for Burn Survivors, Inc.)

for infection. Medical treatment is necessary to treat and prevent infection and promote healing.

- Stage IV ulcers have an ulcerated area that extends through skin and involves underlying muscles, tendons, and bones. This can produce a life-threatening situation. Treat-

ment is with surgical removal of necrotic (dead) or decayed area and antibiotics.

The best treatment for decubitus ulcers is prevention. Frequent turning and relief of pressure on bony prominences is essential. If the person is at home, family members must be educated on how to prevent the disorder.

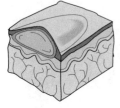

Bulla: (Large blister)
    Same as a vesicle only
    greater than 10 mm
Example:
    Contact dermatitis, large
    second degree burns,
    bulbous impetigo, pemphigus

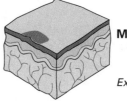

Macule:
    Localized changes in skin
    color of less than 1 cm
    in diameter
Example:
    Freckle

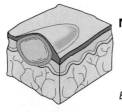

Nodules:
    Solid and elevated; however,
    they extend deeper than
    papules into the dermis or
    subcutaneous tissues, greater
    than 10 mm
Example:
    Lipoma, erythema, cyst, wart

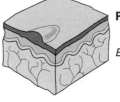

Papule:
    Solid, elevated lesion less
    than 1 cm in diameter
Example:
    Elevated nevi

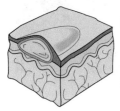

Pustule:
    Vesicles or bullae that
    become filled with pus,
    usually described as less
    than 0.5 cm in diameter
Example:
    Acne, impetigo, furuncles,
    carbuncles

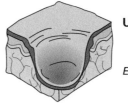

Ulcer:
    A depressed lesion of
    the epidermis and upper
    papillary layer of the dermis
Example:
    Stage 2 pressure ulcer

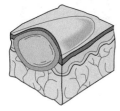

Tumor:
    The same as a nodule only
    greater than 2 cm

Example:
    Benign epidermal tumor
    basal cell carcinoma

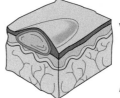

Vesicle: (Small blister)
    Accumulation of fluid between
    the upper layers of the skin;
    elevated mass containing
    serous fluid; less than 10 mm
Example:
    Herpes simplex, herpes
    zoster, chickenpox

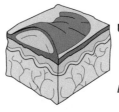

Urticaria, Hives:
    Localized edema in the
    epidermis causing irregular
    elevation that may be red
    or pale, may be itchy
Example:
    Insect bite, wheal

Figure 5-7   *Different types of skin lesions.*

Table 5-1 *Different Types of Skin Lesions, Their Characteristics, Sizes, and Examples of Each*

TYPE OF SKIN LESION	CHARACTERISTICS	SIZE	EXAMPLE(S)
Bulla (large blister)	Fluid-filled area	Greater than 10 mm across	A large blister Bleb-if it occurs in the lung
Macule	Flat area usually distinguished from its surrounding skin by its change in color	Smaller than 1 cm	• Freckle • Petechia
Nodule	Elevated solid area, deeper and firmer than a papule	Greater than 10 mm across	Wart
Papule	Elevated solid area	5 mm or less across	Elevated nevus
Pustule	Discrete, pus-filled raised area	Varying size	Acne
Ulcer	A deep loss of skin surface that may extend into the dermis that can bleed periodically and scar	Varies in size	• Venous stasis ulcer • Decubitus
Tumor	Solid abnormal mass of cells that may extend deep through cutaneous tissue	Larger than 1–2 cm	• Benign (harmless) epidermal tumor • Basal cell carcinoma (rarely metastasizing)
Vesicle Small blister	Fluid-filled raised area	10 mm or less across	• Chickenpox • Herpes simplex
Hives (wheal)	Itchy, temporarily elevated area with an irregular shape formed as a result of localized skin edema	Varies in size	• Hives • Insect bites

Medical Terminology

albin	white
-ism	abnormal condition of
albin/ism	abnormal condition of whiteness
alopec	baldness
-ia	abnormal condition of
alopec/ia	abnormal condition of baldness
a	without
vascul	little blood vessels
-ar	pertaining to
a/vascul/ar	being without little blood vessels
decubit	bedsore
-us	presence of
decubit/us	presence of bedsore, pressure sore
derma	skin
-titis	inflammation of
derma/titis	inflammation of the skin
epi	upon
epi/dermis	upon the skin; top layer of skin

hyper	above normal
thermia	heat
hyperthermia	above normal heat
hypo	below
hypo/-thermia	below normal heat
melan	black
-oma	tumor
melan/oma	tumor of blackness, usually malignant
papill	pimple
-a	presence of
papill/a	presence of pimple
sebac	grease or oil
-ous	pertaining to
sebac/e/ous	pertaining to oil glands
stratum	layer
corneum	horny
stratum corneum	horny layer of skin

Career Profile

Physicians

Physicians diagnose illnesses and prescribe and administer treatments for people suffering from illness and disease. Physicians examine patients, obtain medical histories, and order, perform, and interpret diagnostic tests. They counsel patients on hygiene, diet, and preventive health care.

Two types of physicians are the doctor of medicine (M.D.), and the doctor of osteopathy (D.O.). Both doctors may use all methods of treatment. Doctors of osteopathy place special emphasis on the body's musculoskeletal system and preventive and holistic medicine.

Some physicians are primary care physicians who practice general and family medicine. Some are specialists who are experts in their medical field such as dermatology, cardiology, or pediatrics.

Most physicians work long, irregular hours. Increasingly, they practice in groups or health care organizations. To become a physician requires 4 years of undergraduate study, 4 years of medical school, and 3 to 8 years of internship and residency depending on the specialization. Physicians must pass their medical boards to obtain a license to practice. Formal education and training requirements are among the longest of any occupation, but the earnings are among the highest.

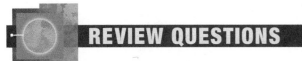

REVIEW QUESTIONS

Select the letter of the choice that best completes the statement.

1. The outmost layer of the skin is the:
   a. epidermis
   b. dermis
   c. hypodermis

2. The substance that serves best to keep our skin smooth and protected is:
   a. melanin
   b. keratin
   c. cortex

3. Nerve receptors are found in the:
   a. epidermis
   b. dermis
   c. hypodermis

4. Hair contains keratinized cells which are found in the:
   a. cuticle layer
   b. cortex
   c. medulla

5. The glands that secrete 99% water, small amounts of salt, and organic matter are called:
   a. endocrine glands
   b. sudoriferous glands
   c. sebaceous glands

COMPLETION

Complete the following statements.

1. Ulcers that occur because of a lack of blood supply to the area are known as _____ or _____.

2. A common and chronic disorder that occurs in the teen years is called _____ _____.

3. Inflammation of the skin is called _____.

4. Urticaria or hives is usually a reaction to an _____.

5. A chronic inflammatory disease characterized by silvery patches is known as _____.

6. A cold sore or fever blister is known as _____.

7. Painful viral infections of the nerve endings are called _____.

8. The most common type of cancer is _____ _____.

9. A skin cancer that occurs as a large brown or black patch is _____.

10. To determine the percent of the body burned, a health care worker may use a formula called the

_____ _____ _____.

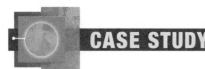

APPLYING THEORY TO PRACTICE

1. If you get a cut on your skin, what may be the result?

2. Doctors advise people to avoid overexposure to the sun. What is the reason for this warning? What measures can a person take to minimize overexposure to the sun? How effective are these measures?

3. The skin helps to regulate body temperature by evaporation of water from the skin. Why do you feel uncomfortable on a hot, humid day?

4. A person is brought to the emergency room with third degree burns, but is not complaining of pain. How is this possible?

5. The cosmetic industry sells many products that remove or prevent wrinkles. If this is true, why do people who use these creams still wrinkle as they age?

6. What are the effects of overexposure to the cold? What can be done to minimize these effects? How effective can these measures be?

CASE STUDY

Dan, age 38, owns a catering service. He is preparing a spaghetti dish for a catering order. While draining the spaghetti, he spills some of the water over his right hand and arm and burns both areas. He immediately runs his arm and hand under cold water, but he notices his right arm is starting to blister. A coworker drives him to the nearest hospital's emergency room. The ER physician says he has second degree burns of his right arm and first degree burns of his right hand.

1. Describe the appearance of Dan's right arm and right hand.

2. Did Dan experience pain in his arm or hand?

3. What layers of skin are involved with a first and second degree burn?

4. Describe how the physician treated the burn.

5. What other body functions may be affected because of the burn?

6. How long should it take for these areas to heal?

7. List safety precautions Dan should take to prevent future accidents.

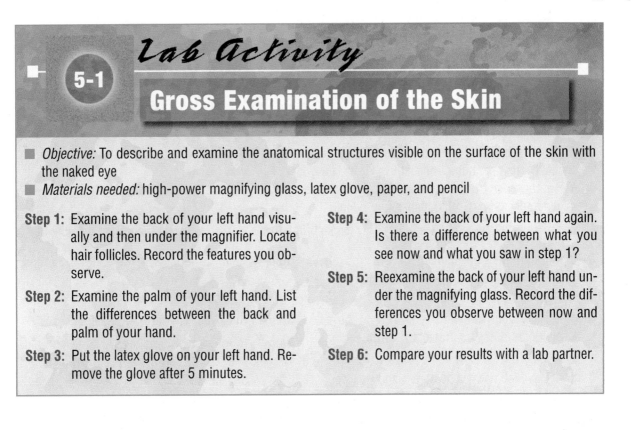

Lab Activity 5-1

Gross Examination of the Skin

■ *Objective:* To describe and examine the anatomical structures visible on the surface of the skin with the naked eye

■ *Materials needed:* high-power magnifying glass, latex glove, paper, and pencil

Step 1: Examine the back of your left hand visually and then under the magnifier. Locate hair follicles. Record the features you observe.

Step 2: Examine the palm of your left hand. List the differences between the back and palm of your hand.

Step 3: Put the latex glove on your left hand. Remove the glove after 5 minutes.

Step 4: Examine the back of your left hand again. Is there a difference between what you see now and what you saw in step 1?

Step 5: Reexamine the back of your left hand under the magnifying glass. Record the differences you observe between now and step 1.

Step 6: Compare your results with a lab partner.

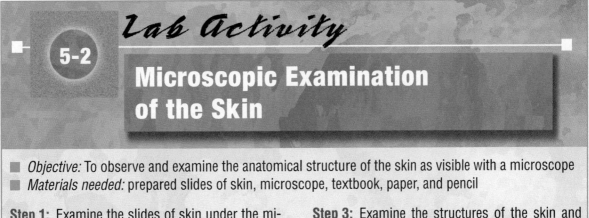

Lab Activity 5-2

Microscopic Examination of the Skin

■ *Objective:* To observe and examine the anatomical structure of the skin as visible with a microscope

■ *Materials needed:* prepared slides of skin, microscope, textbook, paper, and pencil

Step 1: Examine the slides of skin under the microscope.

Step 2: Examine the layers of the skin and compare with photos/drawings of skin in the textbook. Observe and record any differences you see.

Step 3: Examine the structures of the skin and compare with photos/drawings of skin in the textbook.

Step 4: Draw a diagram of what you see under the microscope. Label your diagram to identify layers and structures you observed.

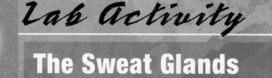

Lab Activity

The Sweat Glands

5-3

■ *Objective:* Observe the activity of the sweat glands with a lab partner. If you are allergic to iodine (or shellfish), do not attempt this lab

■ *Materials needed:* bond paper cut in 1-inch squares, tincture of iodine solution, adhesive tape, cotton-tipped applicators (Q-tips), paper, and pencil

*Note: Tincture of iodine is a poison. It may cause burns to the skin and it permanently stains clothing.

Step 1: Using the applicator, paint an area on your left forearm with iodine solution. Allow it to dry thoroughly.

Step 2: Have your lab partner securely tape a square of the bond paper over the iodine area. Leave in place for 20 minutes.

Step 3: Have lab partner do step 1 and you perform step 2 on your lab partner. Apply to the same area of the skin.

Step 4: After 20 minutes, remove the paper and tape; count the number of blue-black dots in the square of bond paper.

Step 5: Have your lab partner repeat step 4.

Step 6: Compare your results. Are the number of dots the same? What is the reason for the difference, if any? Record your observations.

Chapter 6

SKELETAL SYSTEM

Key Words

abduction
adduction
amphiarthroses
appendicular
  skeleton
arthritis
articular cartilage
atlas
axial skeleton
axis
ball-and-socket joint
bursa sacs
bursitis
calcaneus
carpal
cervical vertebrae
circumduction
clavicle
coccyx
diaphysis
diarthroses
dislocation
endosteum
epiphysis
ethmoid

extension
femur
fibula
flexion
fontanel
fracture
frontal
gliding joint
gout
hinge joint
humerus
hyoid
inferior concha
joint
kyphosis
lacrimal
lordosis
lumbar vertebrae
mandible
maxilla
medullary canal
metacarpal
metatarsal
nasal
occipital

ossification
osteoarthritis
osteoblast
osteoclast
osteocyte
osteomyelitis
osteoporosis
osteosarcoma
palatine
parietal
patella
periosteum
phalanges
pivot joint
pronation
radius
rheumatoid
  arthritis
rickets
rotation
sacrum
scapulae
scoliosis
skeletal system
  continues

Key Words continued

slipped (herniated) **disc**	**synarthroses**	**tibia**
sphenoid	**synovial cavity**	**true ribs**
spongy bone	**synovial fluid**	**ulna**
sprain	**synovial membrane**	**vomer**
supination	**tarsal**	**whiplash injury**
suture	**temporal**	**zygomatic**
	thoracic vertebrae	

If you have ever visited a beach, you may have seen a jellyfish floating lightly near the surface. The organs of the jellyfish are buoyed up by the water. If a wave should chance to deposit the jellyfish upon the beach, however, it would collapse into a disorganized mass of tissue, because the jellyfish has no supportive framework or skeleton. Fortunately, we humans do not suffer such a fate because we have a solid, bony skeleton to support body structures.

The **skeletal system** comprises the bony framework of the body. It consists of 206 individual bones in the adult. Some bones are hinged; others are fused to one another.

FUNCTIONS

The skeletal system has five specific functions:

1. It *supports* body structures and provides shape to the body.

2. It *protects* the soft and delicate internal organs. For example, the cranium protects the brain, the inner ear, and parts of the eye. The ribs and breastbone protect the heart and lungs; the vertebral column encases and protects the spinal cord.

3. It *allows movement and anchorage* of muscles. Muscles that are attached to the skeleton are called skeletal muscles. Upon contraction, these muscles exert a pull upon a bone and so move it. In this manner, bones play a vital part in body movement, serving as passively operated levers.

4. It *provides mineral storage.* Bones are a storage depot for minerals such as calcium and phosphorus. In case of inadequate nutrition, the body is able to draw upon these reserves. For example, if the blood calcium dips below normal, the bone releases the necessary amount of stored calcium into the bloodstream. When calcium levels exceed normal, calcium release from the skeletal system is inhibited. In this way the skeletal system helps to maintain blood calcium homeostasis.

5. It *is the site for hemopoiesis.* The red marrow of the bone is the site of blood cell formation. Red marrow is found in long bones, sternum, and ilia.

STRUCTURE AND FORMATION OF BONE

Bones consist of microscopic cells called **osteocytes** (from the Greek word *osteon,* meaning "bone"). An osteocyte is a mature bone cell. Bone is made up of 35% organic material, 65% inorganic mineral salts, and water.

The organic part derives from a protein called bone collagen, a fibrous material. Between these collagenous fibers is a jellylike material. The organic substances of bone give it a certain degree of flexibility. The inorganic portion of bone is made from mineral salts such as calcium phosphate, calcium carbonate, calcium fluoride, magnesium phosphate, sodium oxide, and sodium chloride. These minerals give bone its hardness and durability.

A bony skeleton can be compared with steel-reinforced concrete. The collagenous fibers may be compared with flexible steel supports, and mineral salts with concrete. When pressure is applied to a bone, the flexible organic material prevents bone damage, while the mineral elements resist crushing under pressure.

BONE FORMATION

The embryonic skeleton initially consists of collagenous protein fibers secreted by the osteoblasts (primitive embryonic cells). Later, during embryonic development, cartilage is deposited between the fibers. At this stage, the embryo's skeleton consists of collagenous protein fibers hyaline cartilage (a clear, tough, smooth, slippery material). During the eighth week of embryonic development, **ossification** begins. That is, mineral matter starts to replace previously formed cartilage, creating bone. Infant bones are very soft and pliable because of incomplete ossification at birth. A familiar example is the soft spot on a baby's head, the **fontanel.** The bone has not yet been formed there, although it will become hardened later. Ossification due to mineral deposits continues through childhood. As bones ossify, they become hard and more capable of bearing weight.

STRUCTURE OF LONG BONE

A typical long bone contains a shaft, or **diaphysis.** This is a hollow cylinder of hard, compact bone. It is what makes a long bone strong and hard yet light enough for movement. At each end (extreme) of the diaphysis is an **epiphysis,** Figures 6-1 A.

In the center of the shaft is the broad **medullary canal.** This is filled with yellow bone marrow, mostly made of fat cells. The marrow also contains many blood vessels and some cells which form white blood cells, called leukocytes. The yellow marrow functions as a fat storage center. The **endosteum** is the lining of the marrow canal that keeps the cavity intact.

The medullary canal is surrounded by compact or hard bone. Haversian canals branch into the compact bone. They carry blood vessels which nourish the osteocytes, or bone cells. Where less strength is needed in the bone, some of the hard bone is dissolved away leaving **spongy bone.**

The ends of the long bones contain the red marrow where some red blood cells called erythrocytes and some white blood cells are made. The outside of the bone is covered with the **periosteum,** a tough fibrous tissue which contains blood vessels, lymph vessels, and nerves. The periosteum is necessary for bone growth, repair, and nutrition.

Covering the epiphysis is a thin layer of cartilage known as the **articular cartilage.** This cartilage acts as a shock absorber between two bones that meet to form a joint.

GROWTH

Bones grow in length and ossify from the center of the diaphysis toward the epiphyseal extremities. Using a long bone by way of example, it will grow lengthwise in an area called the growth zone. Ossification occurs here, causing the bone to lengthen; this causes the epiphyses to grow away from the middle of the diaphysis. It is a sensible growth process, because it does not interfere with the articulation between two bones.

A bone increases its circumference by the addition of more bone to the outer surface of the diaphysis by osteoblasts. **Osteoblasts** are bone cells that deposit the new bone. As girth increases, bone material is being dissolved from the central part of the diaphysis. This forms an internal cavity called the marrow cavity, or medullary canal. The medullary canal gets larger as the diameter of the bone increases.

The dissolution of bone from the medullary canal results from the action of cells called osteoclasts. **Osteoclasts** are immense bone cells that secrete enzymes. These enzymes digest the bony material, splitting the bone minerals, calcium, and phosphorus and enabling them to be absorbed by the surrounding fluid. The medullary canal eventually fills with yellow marrow.

The length of a bone shaft continues to grow until all the epiphyseal cartilage is ossified. At this point, bone growth stops. This fact is helpful in determining further growth in a child. First, an x-ray of the child's wrists is taken. If some epiphyseal cartilage remains, there will be further growth. If there is no epiphyseal cartilage left, the child has reached his or her full stature (height).

The average growth in females continues to about 18 years; males grow to approximately 20 or 21 years. However, new bone growth can occur in a broken bone at any time. Bone cells near the site of a fracture become active, secreting large amounts of new bone within a relatively short time. Bone healing proceeds efficiently depending on age and health of the individual.

(B)

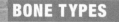

BONE TYPES

Bones are classified as one of four types on the basis of their shape, Figure 6-2. *Long* bones are found in both upper and lower arms and legs. The bones of the skull are examples of *flat* bones, as are the ribs. *Irregular* bones are represented by bones of the spinal column. The wrist and ankle bones are examples of *short* bones, which appear cubelike in shape.

   The bones in the hand are short, making flexible movement possible. The same is true of the irregular bones of the spinal column. The thigh bone is a long bone needed for support of the strong leg muscles and the weight of the body. The degree of movement at a joint is determined by bone shape and joint structure.

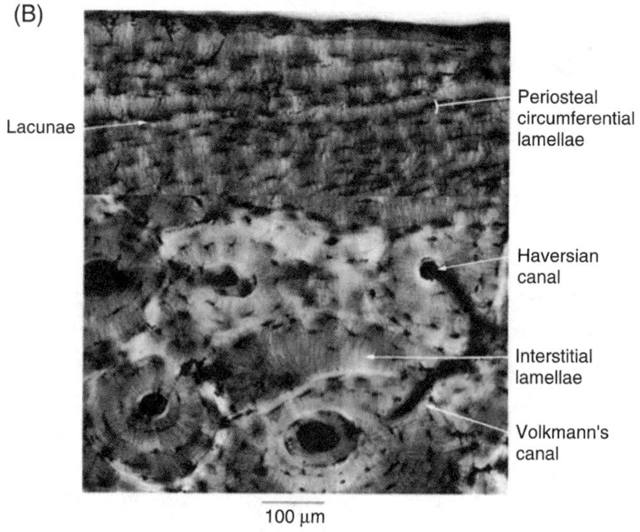

Lacunae

Periosteal circumferential lamellae

Haversian canal

Interstitial lamellae

Volkmann's canal

100 μm

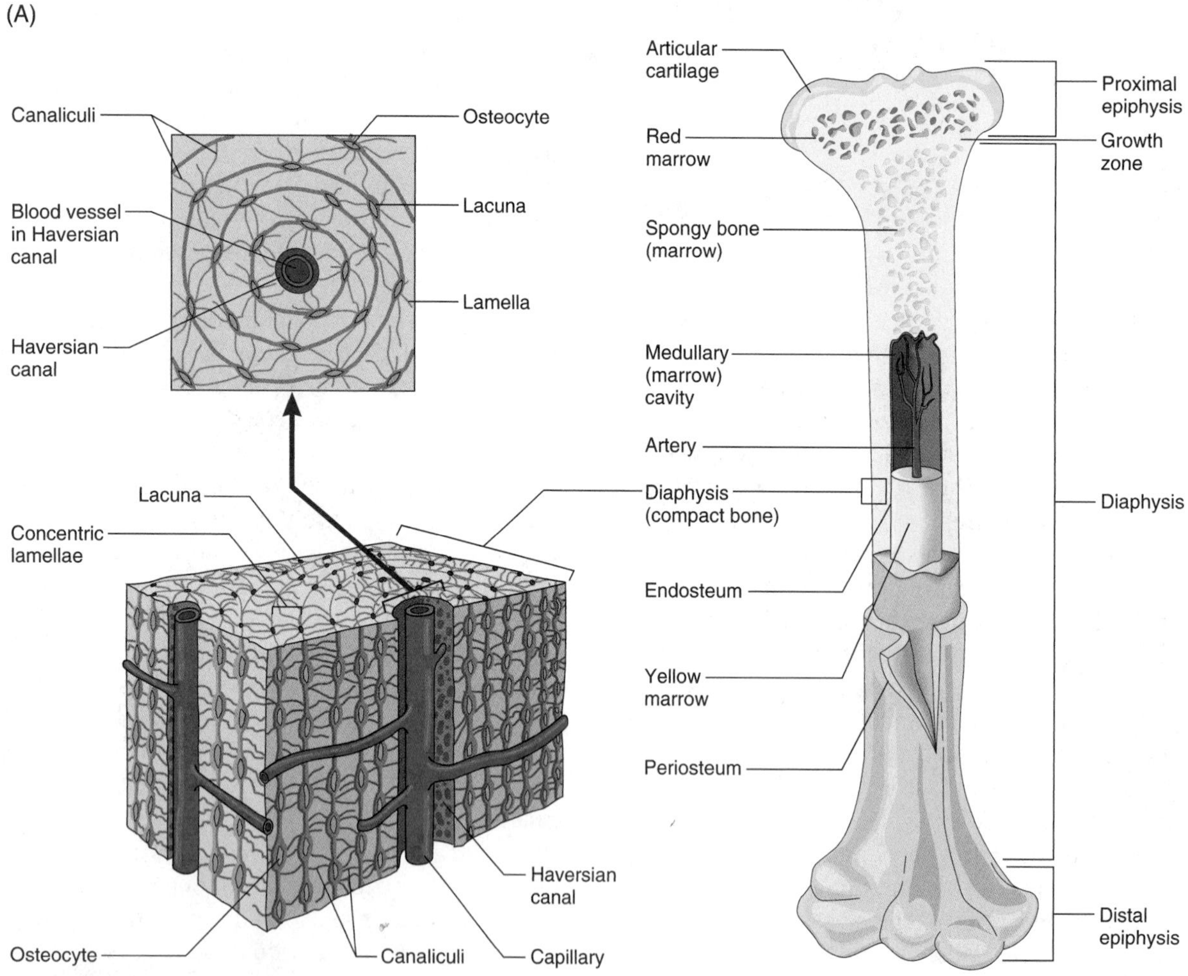

(A)

Canaliculi

Osteocyte

Blood vessel in Haversian canal

Lacuna

Haversian canal

Lamella

Lacuna

Concentric lamellae

Osteocyte

Canaliculi

Capillary

Haversian canal

Articular cartilage

Red marrow

Spongy bone (marrow)

Medullary (marrow) cavity

Artery

Diaphysis (compact bone)

Endosteum

Yellow marrow

Periosteum

Proximal epiphysis

Growth zone

Diaphysis

Distal epiphysis

Figure 6-1   *(A) Structure of a typical long bone; (B) cross section of bone*   (B is from Atlas of Microscopic Anatomy: A Functional Approach: Companion to Histology and Neuroanatomy, *by R. Bergman, A. Afifi, P. Heidger, 1999, www.vh.org/Providers/Textbooks/Microscopic Anatomy.html. Reprinted with permission.)*

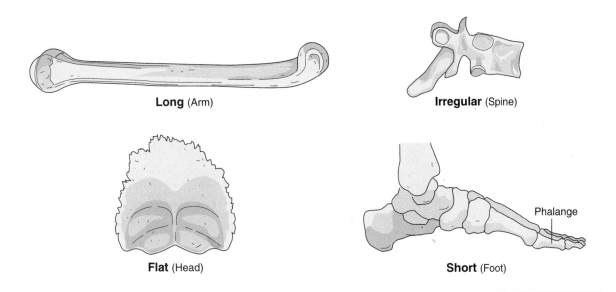

Long (Arm)

Irregular (Spine)

Flat (Head)

Short (Foot)

Phalange

Figure 6-2   *Bone shapes*

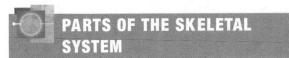

PARTS OF THE SKELETAL SYSTEM

The skeletal system consists of two main parts: the axial skeleton and the appendicular skeleton.

Axial Skeleton

The **axial skeleton** consists of the skull, spinal column, ribs, sternum (breastbone), and **hyoid** bone, Figure 6-3. The hyoid bone is a U-shaped bone in the neck, to which the tongue is attached (not seen in Figure 6-3).

Skull. The skull is the cranium and facial bones. The cranium houses and protects the delicate brain, while the facial bones guard and support the eyes, ears, nose, and mouth. Some of the facial bones, such as the nasal bones, are made of bone and cartilage. For example, the upper part of the nose (bridge) is bone, whereas the lower part is cartilage.

Cranial bones are thin and slightly curved. During infancy, these bones are held snugly together by an irregular band of connective tissue called a **suture.** As the child grows, this connective tissue ossifies and turns into hard bone. Thus, the cranium becomes a highly efficient, domed shield for the brain. The dome shape affords better protection than a flat surface, deflecting blows directed toward the head. However, it is not invulnerable and

a particularly hard blow may fracture the cranium. This can lead to a concussion. A traumatic injury to brain tissue may result, which may require surgery to relieve the pressure on the brain.

Collectively, there are 22 bones in the skull, Figure 6-4. The following 8 bones are in the cranium:

1 **frontal** forms the forehead.

2 **parietal** form the roof and sides of the skull.

2 **temporal** house the ears.

1 **occipital** forms the base of the skull and contains the foramen magnum.

1 **ethmoid** (located between the eyes) forms part of the nasal septum.

1 **sphenoid** (which resembles a bat) is considered the key bone of the skull; all other bones connect to it.

Following are the 14 facial bones.

5 **nasal** (2 are nasal bones that form the bridge of the nose [your glasses sit on this bone]; 1 is the **vomer** bone which forms the lower part, or midline, of the nasal septum; and 2 are **inferior concha** bones which make up the side walls of the nasal cavity).

2 **maxilla** make up the upper jaw.

2 **lacrimal** (in the inner aspect of the eyes) contain the tear ducts.

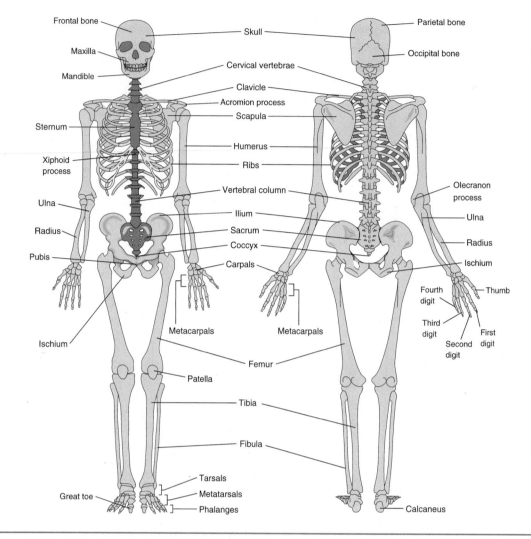

Figure 6-3   *The axial skeleton (blue) and the appendicular skeleton*

2 **zygomatic** form the prominence of the cheek.

2 **palatine** form the hard palate of the mouth.

1 **mandible** is the lower jaw and the only movable bone in the face.

The skull contains large spaces within the facial bones, referred to as paranasal sinuses. These sinuses are lined with mucous membranes. When a person suffers from a cold, flu, or hayfever, the membranes become inflamed and swollen, producing a copious amount of mucus. This may lead to sinus pain and a "stuffy" nasal sensation.

Spinal column/vertebra. The spine, or vertebral column, is strong and flexible. It supports the head and provides for the attachment of the ribs. The spine also encloses the spinal cord of the nervous system.

The spine consists of small bones called vertebrae which are separated from each other by pads of cartilage tissue called intervertebral disks, Figure 6-5. These disks serve as cushions between the vertebrae and act as shock absorbers. During our lifetime these disks become thinner, which accounts for the loss of height as we age.

The vertebral column is divided into five sections named according to the area of the body where they are located, see Figure 6-5A.

1. Cervical vertebrae (7) are located in the neck area. The **atlas,** Figure 6-5B, is the first

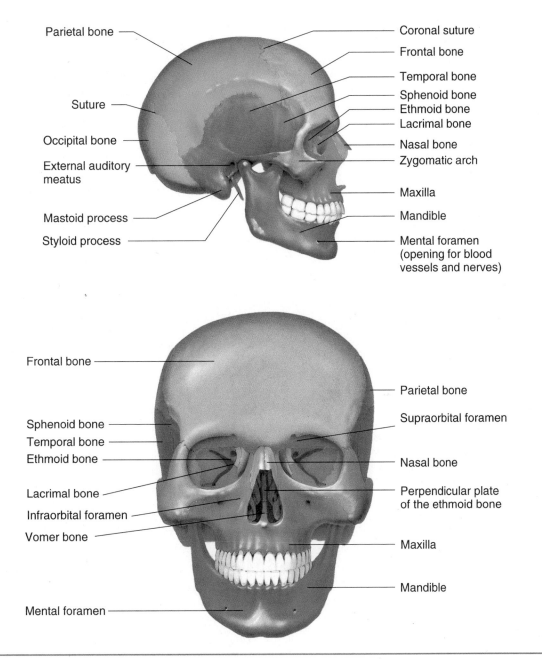

Figure 6-4 *Bones and sutures of the skull*

cervical vertebra that articulates, or is jointed, with the occipital bone of the skull. This permits us to nod our heads. On the **axis,** Figure 6-5C, the second cervical vertebra is the odontoid process which forms a pivot on which the atlas rotates; this permits us to turn our heads.

2. **Thoracic vertebrae** (12) are located in the chest area. They articulate with the ribs.

3. **Lumbar vertebrae** (5) are located in the back. They have large bodies that bear most of the body's weight.

4. **Sacrum** is a wedge-shaped bone formed by five fused bones. It forms the posterior pelvic girdle and serves as an articulation point for the hips.

5. **Coccyx** is also known as the tailbone. It is formed by four fused bones.

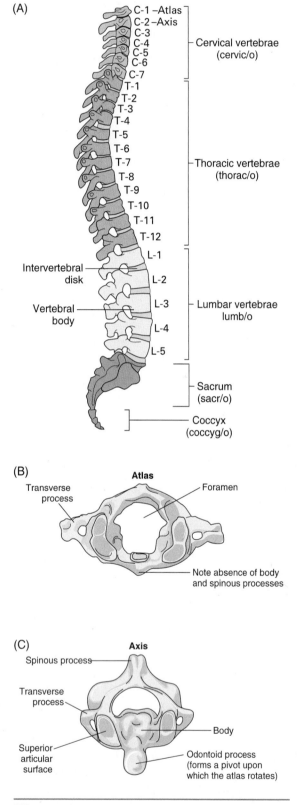

(A)

C-1 –Atlas
C-2 –Axis
C-3
C-4
C-5
C-6
C-7

Cervical vertebrae
(cervic/o)

T-1
T-2
T-3
T-4
T-5
T-6
T-7
T-8
T-9
T-10
T-11
T-12

Thoracic vertebrae
(thorac/o)

Intervertebral
disk

L-1
L-2
L-3
L-4
L-5

Lumbar vertebrae
lumb/o

Vertebral
body

Sacrum
(sacr/o)

Coccyx
(coccyg/o)

(B)

Atlas

Transverse
process

Foramen

Note absence of body
and spinous processes

(C)

Axis

Spinous process

Transverse
process

Superior
articular
surface

Body

Odontoid process
(forms a pivot upon
which the atlas rotates)

Figure 6-5 *(A) Lateral view of the spine; (B) view of the atlas; (C) view of the axis*

The spinal nerves enter and leave the spinal cord through the openings (foramen) between the vertebrae.

When you study a model of the human skeleton, note that the spine is curved instead of straight. A curved spine has more strength than a straight one would have. Before birth, the thoracic and sacral regions are convex curves. As the infant learns to hold up its head, the cervical region becomes concave. When the child learns to stand, the lumbar region also becomes concave. This completes the four curves of a normal, adult human spine.

A typical vertebra, as seen in Figure 6-6, contains three basic parts: body, foramen, and (several) processes. The large, solid part of the vertebra is known as the body; the central opening for the spinal cord is called the foramen. Above the foramen protrude two winglike bony structures called transverse processes. The roof of the foramen contains the spinous process (spine) and the articular processes.

Ribs and sternum. The thoracic area of the body is protected and supported by the thoracic vertebrae, ribs, and sternum.

The sternum (breastbone) is divided into three parts: the upper region (manubrium), the body, and a lower cartilaginous part called the xiphoid process. Attached to each side of the upper region of the sternum, by means of ligaments, are the two clavicles (collar bones).

Seven pairs of costal cartilages join 7 pairs of ribs directly to the sternum. These are known as **true ribs,** Figure 6-7. The human body contains 12 pairs of ribs. The first 7 pairs are true ribs. The next 3 pairs are false ribs, because their costal cartilages are attached to the seventh rib instead of directly to the sternum. Finally, the last 2 pairs of ribs, connected neither to the costal cartilages nor the sternum, are floating ribs.

The Appendicular Skeleton

The **appendicular skeleton** includes the upper extremities: shoulder girdles, arms, wrists, and hands; and the lower extremities: hip girdle, legs, ankles, and feet; refer to Figure 6-3. There are 126 bones in the appendicular skeleton.

Shoulder girdle. The shoulder girdle (also called pectoral girdle) consists of four bones: two curved

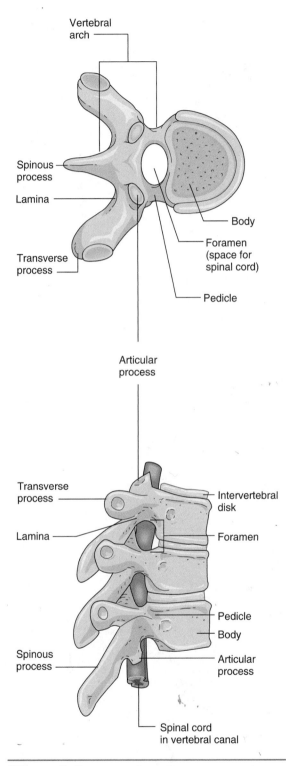

Figure 6-6 *A typical vertebra*

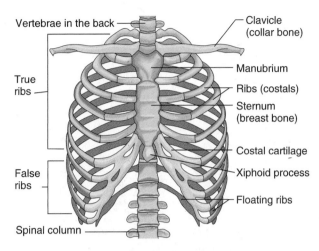

Figure 6-7 *Ribs and sternum*

clavicles (collar bones) and two triangular **scapulae** (shoulder bones); refer to Figure 6-3. On the skeleton, we observe two broad, flat triangular surfaces (scapulae) on the upper posterior surface. They permit the attachment of muscles that assist in arm movement and serve as a place of attachment for the arms. The two clavicles, attached at one end to the scapulae and at the other to the sternum, help to brace the shoulders and prevent excessive forward motion.

Arm. The bone structure of the arm consists of the humerus, radius, and ulna. The humerus is located in the upper arm and the radius and ulna are in the forearm.

The **humerus,** the only bone in the upper arm, is the second largest bone in the body. The upper end of the humerus has a smooth, round surface called the head, which articulates with the scapula. The upper humerus is attached to the scapula socket (glenoid fossa) by muscles and ligaments.

The forearm consists of two bones: the radius and the ulna. The **radius** is the bone running up the thumb side of the forearm. Its name derives from the fact that it can rotate around the ulna. This is an important characteristic, permitting the hand to rotate freely and with great flexibility. The **ulna,** by contrast, is far more limited. It is the largest bone in the forearm: At its upper end, it produces a projection called the olecranon process, forming the elbow, Figure 6-8. When you bang your elbow (the olecranon process) it is usually

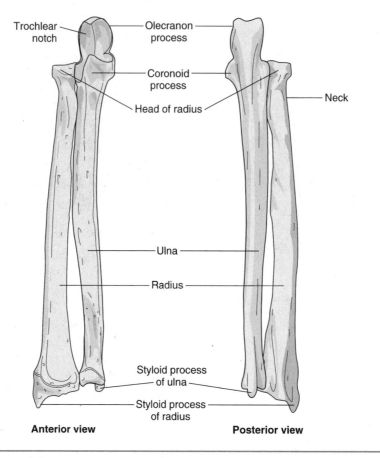

Anterior view   Posterior view

Figure 6-8   *Radius and ulna*

referred to as "hitting your funny bone." The olecranon process articulates with the humerus.

Hand. The human hand is a remarkable piece of
skeletal engineering and dexterity. It contains more
bones for its size than any other part of the body.
Collectively, the hand has 27 bones, Figure 6-9.

The wrist bone, or **carpals,** consists of eight
small bones arranged in two rows. They are held
together by ligaments which permit sufficient
movement to allow the wrist a great deal of mobility and flexion. There is only slight lateral (side)
movement of these carpal bones, however. Attached on the palm side of the hand are several
short muscles which supply mobility to the little
finger and thumb.

The hand consists of two parts: the palmer
surface with five **metacarpal** bones, and five fingers with 14 **phalanges** (singular, phalanx).
Each finger, except for the thumb, has three phalanges, whereas the thumb has two. There are

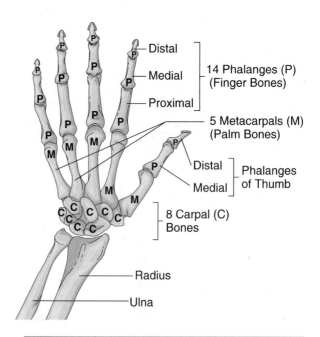

Figure 6-9   *The 27 bones of the left hand*

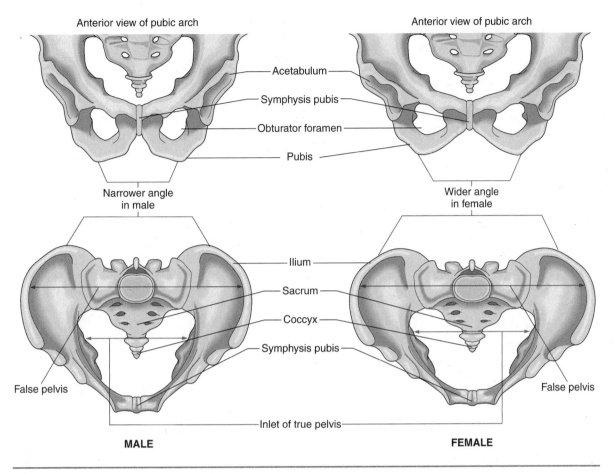

Anterior view of pubic arch

Anterior view of pubic arch

— Acetabulum —

— Symphysis pubis —

— Obturator foramen —

— Pubis —

Narrower angle
in male

Wider angle
in female

— Ilium —

— Sacrum —

— Coccyx —

— Symphysis pubis —

False pelvis

False pelvis

— Inlet of true pelvis —

MALE

FEMALE

Figure 6-10   *Comparison of the male and female pelvises*

hinge joints between each phalanx, allowing the fingers to be bent easily. The thumb is the most flexible finger because the end of the metacarpal bone is more rounded, and there are muscles attached to it from the hand itself. Thus, the thumb can be extended across the palm of the hand. Only humans and other primates possess such a digit, known as an opposable thumb.

Pelvic girdle. In youth, the pelvic girdle (innominate bones) consists of three bones. Found on either side of the midline of the body, the innominate bones include the ilium, ischium, and pubis. These bones eventually fuse with the sacrum to form a bowl-shaped structure called the pelvic girdle, Figure 6-10. Eventually these two sets of innominate bones form a joint with the bones in front, called the symphysis pubis, and with the sacrum in back, as the sacroiliac joint.

The pelvic girdle serves as an area of attachment for the bones and muscles of the leg. It also provides support for the viscera (soft organs) of the lower abdominal region. The obvious anatomical difference between the male and female pelvis is the female pelvis is much wider than that of the male. This is necessary for childbearing (pregnancy) and childbirth. In addition, the *pelvic inlet* is wider in the female, and the pelvic bones are lighter and smoother than those of the male.

Upper leg. The upper leg contains the longest and strongest bone in the body, the thigh bone or **femur.** The upper part of the femur has a smooth rounded head, Figure 6-11. It fits neatly into a cavity of the ilium known as the acetabulum, forming a ball-and-socket joint. The femur is an amazingly strong bone. A direct compressible force applied to the *top* of the femur of from 15,000 to 19,000 pounds per square inch is required to break it.

Lower leg. The lower leg consists of two bones: the **tibia** and the **fibula.** The tibia is the largest of

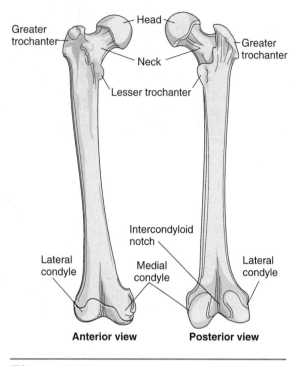

Greater trochanter

Head

Neck

Greater trochanter

Lesser trochanter

Intercondyloid notch

Lateral condyle

Medial condyle

Lateral condyle

Anterior view   **Posterior view**

Figure 6-11   *Anterior/posterior view of the femur*

the two lower leg bones. The **patella** (kneecap) is found in front of the knee joint. It is a flat, triangular, sesamoid bone; see Figure 6-3. The patella is formed in the tendons of the large muscle in front of the femur (quadriceps femoris). In females, it appears at around 2 or 3 years of age; in males, at about 6 years. The patella, attached to the tibia by a ligament, ossifies as early as puberty. Surrounding the patella are four bursae, which serve to cushion the knee joint.

Ankle. The ankle (tarsus) contains seven **tarsal** bones. These bones provide a connection between the foot and leg bones. The largest ankle bone is the heel bone or **calcaneus.** The tibia and fibula articulate with a broad tarsal bone called the talus. Ankle movement is a sliding motion, allowing the foot to extend and flex when walking.

Foot. The foot has five **metatarsal** bones which are somewhat comparable to the metacarpals of the hand; but the metatarsal and metacarpal bones are arranged to form two distinct arches, which are not found in the palm of the hand. One arch runs longitudinally from the calcaneus to the heads of the metatarsals: It is called the longitudi-

nal arch. The other, which lies perpendicular to the longitudinal arch in the metatarsal region, is known as the transverse arch. Strong ligaments and leg muscle tendons help to hold the foot bones in place to form those two arches. In turn, arches strengthen the foot and provide flexibility and springiness to the stride. In certain cases, these arches may "fall" due to weak foot ligaments and tendons. Then downward pressure by weight of the body slowly flattens them, causing fallen arches or flatfeet. Flatfeet cause a good deal of stress and strain on the foot muscles, leading to pain and fatigue. Factors that may lead to flatfeet include fatigue, overweight, poor posture, and shoes that do not fit properly.

The toes are similar in composition to the fingers. There are three phalanges in each, with the exception of the big toe which has only two. Because the big toe is not opposable like the thumb, it cannot be brought across the sole. There are a total of 14 phalanges in each foot, Figure 6-12.

Ligaments are fibrous bands that connect bones and cartilages and serve as support for muscles. Joints are also bound together by ligaments. Tendons are fibrous cords that connect muscles to bones.

JOINTS AND RELATED STRUCTURES

Joints, or articulations, are points of contact between two bones. They are classified into three main types according to their degree of movement: diarthroses (movable) joints, amphiarthroses (partially movable) joints, and synarthroses (immovable) joints, Figure 6-13.

Most of the joints in our body are **diarthroses.** They tend to have the same structure. These movable joints consist of three main parts: articular cartilage, a bursa (joint capsule), and a synovial (joint) cavity.

When two movable bones meet at a joint, their surfaces do not touch one another. The two articular (joint) surfaces are covered with a smooth, slippery cap of cartilage known as articular cartilage. As mentioned, this cartilage helps to absorb shocks and prevent friction between parts.

Enclosing two articular surfaces of the bone is a tough, fibrous connective tissue capsule called

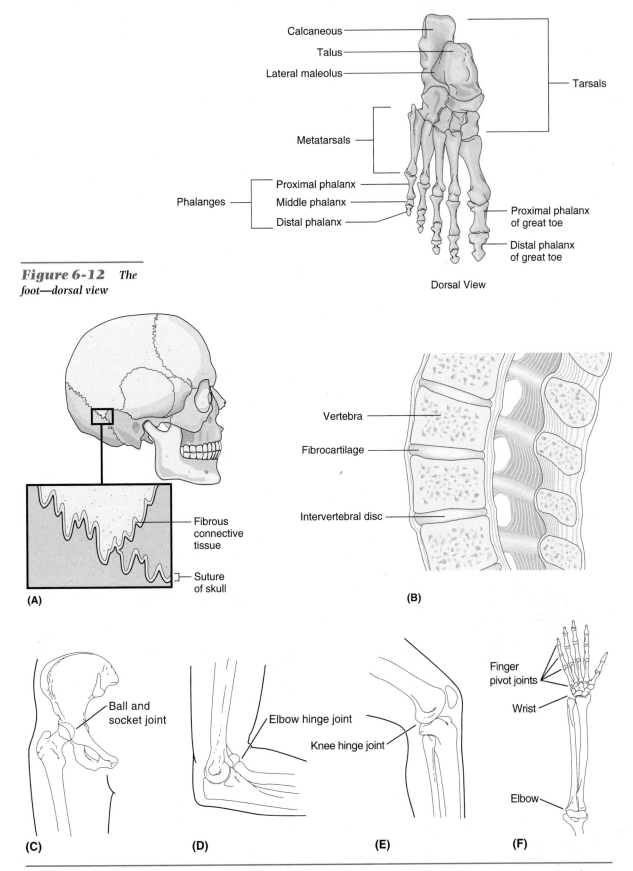

Figure 6-12 *The foot—dorsal view*

Calcaneous
Talus
Lateral maleolus
Tarsals
Metatarsals
Phalanges
Proximal phalanx
Middle phalanx
Distal phalanx
Proximal phalanx of great toe
Distal phalanx of great toe

Dorsal View

Fibrous connective tissue
Suture of skull

(A)

Vertebra
Fibrocartilage
Intervertebral disc

(B)

Ball and socket joint

(C)

Elbow hinge joint

(D)

Knee hinge joint

(E)

Finger pivot joints
Wrist
Elbow

(F)

Figure 6-13 *Types of joints: (A) a synarthrosis, an immovable fibrous joint (cranial bones); (B) an amphiarthrosis, a slightly movable cartilaginous joint (ribs or vertebra); (C–F) diarthroses, freely movable hinge or ball-and-socket joints*

an articular capsule. Lining the articular capsule is a **synovial membrane,** which secretes **synovial fluid** (a lubricating substance) into the **synovial cavity** (an area between the two articular cartilages). The synovial fluid reduces the friction of joint movement.

The clefts in connective tissue between muscles, tendons, ligaments, and bones contain **bursa sacs.** The synovial fluid secreted serves as a lubricant to prevent friction between a tendon and a bone. If this sac becomes irritated, injured, or inflamed, a condition known as **bursitis** develops. The synovial fluid can be aspirated (withdrawn) from the bursa sacs to examine for diagnostic purposes.

Diarthroses Joints

There are four types of diarthroses or moveable joints.

1. **Ball-and-socket joints** allow the greatest freedom of movement. Here, one bone has a ball-shaped head which nestles into a concave socket of the second bone. Our shoulders and hips have ball-and-socket joints.

2. **Hinge joints** move in one direction or plane, as in the knees, elbows, and outer joints of the fingers.

3. **Pivot joints** are those with an extension rotating in a second, arch-shaped bone. The radius and ulna (long bones of the forearm) are pivot joints. Another example is the joint between the atlas (first cervical vertebra in the neck) which supports the head, and the axis (second cervical vertebra) which allows the head to rotate.

4. **Gliding joints** are those in which nearly flat surfaces glide across each other, as in the vertebrae of the spine. These joints enable the torso to bend forward, backward, and sideways, as well as rotate.

Between each body of the vertebrae are fibrous disks. At the center of each fibrous disk is a pulpy, elastic material which loses its resiliency with increased usage and/or age. Disks can be compressed by sudden and forceful jolts to the spine. This may cause a disk to protrude from the vertebrae and impinge upon the spinal nerves resulting in extreme pain. Such a condition is known as a *herniated* or *slipped disk.*

Amphiarthroses Joints

Amphiarthroses are partially movable joints, with cartilage between their articular surfaces. Two examples are the attachment of the ribs to the spine and the symphysis pubis, which is the joint between the two pubic bones.

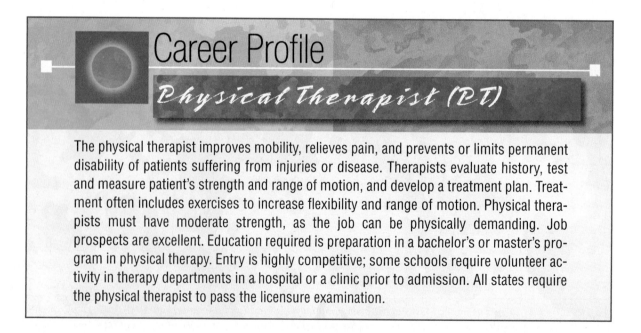

Career Profile
Physical Therapist (PT)

The physical therapist improves mobility, relieves pain, and prevents or limits permanent disability of patients suffering from injuries or disease. Therapists evaluate history, test and measure patient's strength and range of motion, and develop a treatment plan. Treatment often includes exercises to increase flexibility and range of motion. Physical therapists must have moderate strength, as the job can be physically demanding. Job prospects are excellent. Education required is preparation in a bachelor's or master's program in physical therapy. Entry is highly competitive; some schools require volunteer activity in therapy departments in a hospital or a clinic prior to admission. All states require the physical therapist to pass the licensure examination.

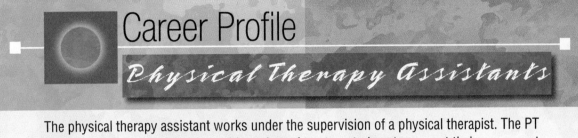

Career Profile
Physical Therapy Assistants

The physical therapy assistant works under the supervision of a physical therapist. The PT assistant instructs patients in a wide variety of treatment plans to prevent their permanent disability and help them resume activities of daily living. This occupation requires a moderate degree of strength because of its physical demands. Education requirement for the PT assistant is an associate degree from an accredited program for physical therapy assistants. Education requires a clinical component. At the present time, most states require licensure of certification. Job prospects are excellent because of the aging population.

Medical Highlight
Arthroscopy and Microdiskectomy

Arthroscopy is the examination into a joint using an arthroscope. The arthroscope is a small fiber optic viewing instrument made up of a tiny lens, light source, and video camera. Through an incision about 1/4 inch long, a physician may examine, diagnose, and treat injuries of joint areas. Most knee injuries are treated through arthroscopic technique.

Microdiskectomy is an operation to remove a prolapsed or damaged intervertebral disc through a tiny incision. The surgeon uses a bone plug to replace the damaged disc, which can either be a graft from the patient's hip bone or from a bone bank. Another option is to fill the space with coralline, which is obtained from sea coral. The patient may be out of bed the next day.

Synarthroses Joints

Synarthroses are immovable joints connected by tough, fibrous connective tissue. These joints are found in the adult cranium. The bones are fused together in a joint which forms a heavy protective cover for the brain. Such cranial joints are commonly called sutures.

TYPES OF MOTION

Joints can move in many directions, Figure 6-14. **Flexion** is the act of bringing two bones closer together, which decreases the angle between the two bones. **Extension** is the act of increasing the angle between two bones, which results in a

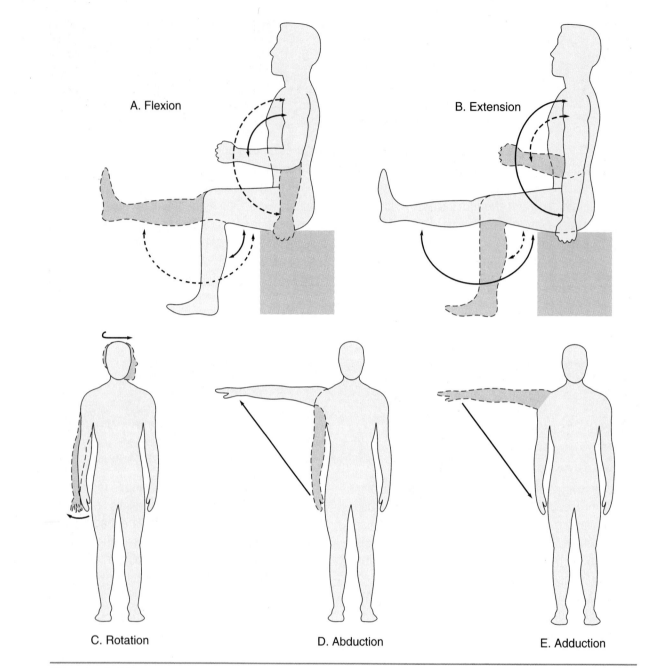

Figure 6-14 *Joint movements*

straightening motion. **Abduction** is the movement of an extremity away from the midline (an imaginary line that divides the body from head to toe). **Adduction** is movement toward the midline. **Circumduction** includes flexion, extension, abduction, and adduction.

A **rotation** movement allows a bone to move around one central axis. This type of pivot motion occurs when you turn your head from side to side (just say "no"). In **pronation,** the forearm turns the hand so the palm is downward or backward. In **supination,** the palm is forward or upward.

Effects of Aging on The Skeletal System

Around the age of 40, bone mass and density shift begin to decline. Women are more vulnerable to bone loss (osteoporosis) than men. Bone loss in women occurs especially in the decade following menopause.

The change in bones is gradual and is due to reabsorption of the interior matrix of the long and flat bones. The external surfaces of the bones begin to thicken. These changes are not directly observable, but are evident by alterations in position and stature. The intervertebral cartilage disks shrink, narrowing the space between disks, resulting in a loss of height. Posture also is affected; the center of balance is altered due to the shortening of the spinal column. Joints by the age of 70 reflect a lifetime of wear and tear. The joints become less mobile because the cartilage loses water and the joints fuse at the cartilage surface.

Hardening of ligaments, tendon, and joints leads to an increase in rigidity and a decrease in flexibility. Stiff, painful joints are due to the general wear and tear on the ligaments and synovial membrane. The discomfort and physically limiting changes will decrease the range of motion of the joints. The psychological fear of falling due to physical changes further adds to potential for inactivity and injury.

DISORDERS OF THE BONES AND JOINTS

The most common traumatic injury to a bone is a **fracture,** or break. When this occurs, there is swelling due to injury and bleeding tissues. The process of restoring bone is done through three main methods.

1. *Closed reduction*—the bony fragments are brought into alignment by manipulation, and a cast or splint is applied.

2. *Open reduction*—through surgical intervention, devices such as wires, metal plates, or screws are used to hold the bone in alignment and a cast or splint may be applied.

3. *Traction*—a pulling force is used to hold the bones in place (used for fractures of the long bone).

Following are the common types of fractures, Figure 6-15.

- *Greenstick* is the simplest type of fracture. The bone is partly bent, but it never completely separates. The break is similar to that of a young, sap-filled woodstick, where the fibers separate lengthwise when bent. Such fractures are common among children because their bones contain flexible cartilage.

- *Closed/simple* is when the bone is broken, but the broken ends do not pierce through the skin forming an external wound.

- *Open/compound* is the most serious type of fracture, where the broken bone ends pierce and protrude through the skin. This can cause infection of the bone and neighboring tissues.

- *Comminuted* is when the bone is splintered or broken into many pieces that can become embedded in the surrounding tissue.

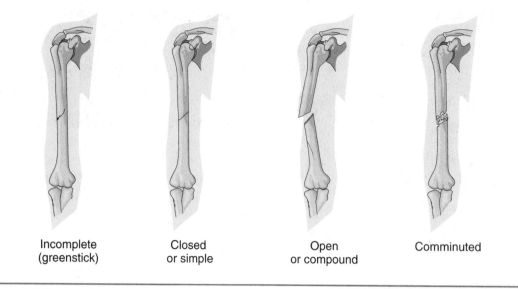

Incomplete
(greenstick)

Closed
or simple

Open
or compound

Comminuted

Figure 6-15   *Types of fractures*

Bone and Joint Injuries

A **dislocation** occurs when a bone is displaced from its proper position in a joint. This may result in the tearing and stretching of the ligaments. Reduction or return of the bone to its proper position is necessary, along with rest to allow the ligaments to heal.

A **sprain** is an injury to a joint caused by any sudden or unusual motion, such as "turning the ankle." The ligaments are either torn from their attachments to the bones or torn across, but the joint is not dislocated. A sprain is accompanied by rapid swelling and acute pain in the area and is treated with nonsteroidal anti-inflammatory drugs.

DISEASES OF THE BONES

Arthritis is an inflammatory condition of one or more joints, accompanied by pain and often by changes in bone position. There are at least 20 different types, the most common being rheumatoid arthritis and osteoarthritis, (Figure 6-16).

■ **Rheumatoid arthritis** is a chronic, autoimmune (when the body's immune system attacks the tissue) disease which affects the connective tissue and joints. There is acute inflammation of the connective tissue, thickening of the synovial membrane, and

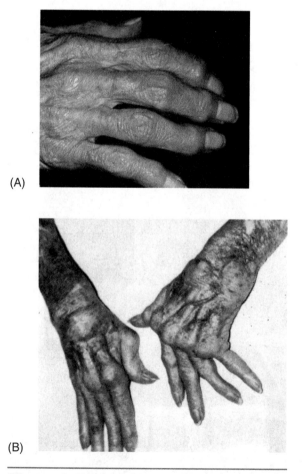

(A)

(B)

Figure 6-16   *Comparison of (A) osteoarthritis and (B) rheumatoid arthritis: hands and joints*

ankylosis (joints become fused) of joints. The joints are badly swollen and painful. The pain, in turn, causes muscle spasms which may lead to deformities in the joints. In addition, the cartilage that separates the joints will degenerate, and hard calcium fills the spaces. When the joints become stiff and immobile, muscles attached to these joints slowly atrophy (shrink in size). This disease affects approximately three times more women than men. Its cause is unknown.

- **Osteoarthritis** is known as degenerative joint disease. It occurs with aging; about 80% of all Americans are affected. In this disease the articular cartilage degenerates and a bony spur formation occurs at the joint. The joints may enlarge; there is pain and swelling, especially after activity.

At the present time there is no cure for arthritis, although there are many treatments to relieve pain and increase mobility. Treatment with nonsteroidal anti-inflammatory drugs may alleviate pain and reduce swelling. Glucosamine and chrondrotin sulfate substances found naturally in cartilage are available as over-the-counter dietary supplements; in some individuals they alleviate pain. A class of drugs called COX-2 inhibitors target the inflamed joints with less potential for harming the stomach than the nonsteroidal anti-inflammatory drugs. The most common are Vioxx and Celebrex. Hyaluronic acid is produced naturally in the body to lubricate cartilage in the joints. In osteoarthritis, the substance is broken down and lubrication is lost. Injection of this substance over a 3- to 5- week period helps lubricate the joint and alleviate pain. Some patients with rheumatoid arthritis get relief with injections of the drug Enbrel.

Acupuncture, nutrition supplements such as omega-3 fatty acids, and antioxidant vitamins A, C, and E may give temporary relief. Other treatments for arthritis include aromatherapy, copper bracelets, herbal preparations, and magnets. There are questions about the actual effectiveness of some of these alternative remedies. Currently, hip and knee replacement (arthroplasty) may be done for the affected joints.

Gout is a joint disorder characterized by an acute inflammation commonly affecting the big toe, although it may affect other joints as well. The pain and swelling is the body's response to the accumulation of uric acid crystals in the affected joint. Uric acid is formed by the breakdown of molecules called purines. Treatment is with nonsteroidal anti-inflammatory drugs.

Rickets is usually found in children and caused by a lack of vitamin D. Bones become soft, due to lack of calcification, causing such deformities as bowlegs and pigeon breast, (Figure 6-17). The disease may be prevented with sufficient quantities of calcium, vitamin D, and exposure to sunshine.

Slipped (herniated) disc is a condition where a cartilage disc (one of which is between each vertebra and acts as a shock absorber for the spine) ruptures or protrudes out of place and places pressure on the spinal nerve. This usually occurs in the lower back (lumbar-sacral) area. It may be treated by a chiropractor or with bed rest, traction, or surgery.

Whiplash injury is trauma to the cervical vertebra, usually the result of an automobile accident. The force generated by the car's abrupt change in speed or direction whips the head backward, putting tremendous strain on the cervical

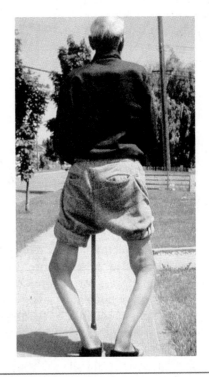

Figure 6-17 *Bowleggedness can result from rickets*

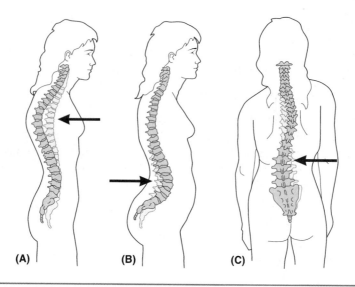

(A)   (B)   (C)

Figure 6-18 *Abnormal curvatures of the spine: (A) kyphosis, (B) lordosis, (C) scoliosis*

spine and neck muscles. Treatment depends on the extent of the injury.

Abnormal Curvatures of the Spine

Kyphosis (hunchback) is a humped curvature in the thoracic area of the spine, Figure 6-18A.

Lordosis (swayback) is an exaggerated inward curvature in the lumbar region of the spine just above the sacrum, Figure 6-18B.

Scoliosis is a side-to-side or lateral curvature of the spine, Figure 6-18C.

OTHER MEDICALLY RELATED DISORDERS

Osteoporosis is a disease that affects 25 million Americans—according to the National Osteoporosis Foundation, 80% are women. In osteoporosis, the mineral density of the bone is reduced from 65% to 35%. By age 55, the average postmenopausal woman has lost about 30% of her bone mass. This loss of bone mass leaves the bone thinner, porous, and susceptible to fracture, Figure 6-19. Ordinary x-rays do not detect osteoporosis until this 30% bone loss occurs. Symptoms may not be evident until a bone breaks in the wrist, hip, or spine. A bone mineral density scan measures the amount of calcium in the bone and can show

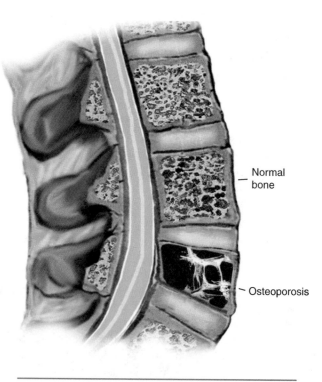

Normal bone

Osteoporosis

Figure 6-19 *Comparison of normal bone tissue to that of osteoporosis*

early signs of bone loss. Treatment is aimed at preventing or slowing the process. A person may take calcium supplements, increase calcium in the diet, and exercise. Postmenopausal women may take estrogen to help maintain bone mass.

Osteomyelitis is an infection which may involve all parts of the bone. It may result from injury or systemic infection and most commonly occurs in children between the ages of 5 and 14 years.

Osteosarcoma, or bone cancer, may occur in younger people. The most common site of affliction is just above the knee.

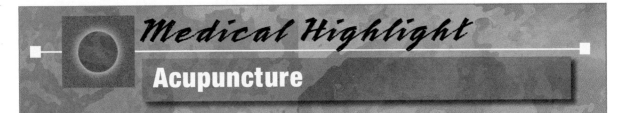

Medical Highlight
Acupuncture

Acupuncture is a form of traditional Chinese medicine that has been practiced for at least 2,500 years. Acupuncture has gained acceptance among some Western physicians as an alternative treatment for chronic pain and other medical conditions.

The Eastern philosophy behind acupuncture depends on a vital flow of life-force energy called qi ("chee"), which circulates along 12 major pathways called meridians. Along these meridians are several acupuncture points. It is believed that illness and pain cause a disruption, or traffic jam, in the normal flow of qi. Needles inserted into the acupuncture points unblock the flow of qi. The needles are hair thin and may be inserted in up to 20 local points, near the source of the pain. The needles are left in place for about 15 to 20 minutes. Once inserted, the needles may be moved or stimulated. Studies show this manipulation stimulates the release of the body's own pain-killing chemicals called endorphins. According to the National Institute of Health, acupuncture may be a reasonable pain management option for patients with osteoarthritis. Acupuncture is practiced by physicians who are members of the American Academy of Medical Acupuncture.

Source: *Mayo Clinical Medical Essay on Arthritis—2001*

Career Profile
Radiologic Technologists

Medical uses of radiation go far beyond the diagnosis of broken bones by x-ray. Radiation is used to produce images of the interior of the body and to treat cancer. The term "diagnostic imaging" not only involves x-ray technique but also includes ultrasound and magnetic resonance scans.

Radiographers produce x-ray films for use in diagnosing disease. They prepare the patients for procedures by explaining the process, positioning the patient, being certain to prevent unnecessary radiation exposure, and taking the picture. Experienced radiographers may perform more complex imaging tests such as fluoroscopy, operate computerized tomography scanners, and use magnetic resonance machines.

continues

continued

Radiation therapy technologists prepare cancer patients for treatment and administer prescribed doses of ionizing radiation to specific body parts. They check for radiation side effects.

Sonographers project nonionizing, high-frequency sound waves into specific areas of the patient's body; the equipment then collects the reflected echoes to form an image.

Education for these positions is offered in hospitals, colleges, and vocation-technical institutes. Course of study includes class and clinical practice. The Joint Review Committee on Education in Radiologic Technology accredits most formal training programs in this field. The job outlook in this field is growing faster than average.

Medical Terminology

ab	away from
duc	move
-tion	process
ab/duc/tion	process of moving away from
ad	to or toward
ad/duc/tion	process of moving toward
arthr	joint
-itis	inflammation
arthr/itis	inflammation of a joint
burs	small purselike sac
bursitis	inflammation of a small sac
carp	wrist
-al	pertaining to
carp/al	pertaining to the wrist
circum	around
circum/duc/tion	process of moving around
end	within
oste	bone
-um	presence of
end/oste/um	presence of lining within the bone
extens	straightening
-ion	process of
extens/ion	process of straightening
flex	bend
flex/ion	process of bending
kyph	humpback or hunchback
-osis	process of

kyph/osis	process of being hunchbacked
lord	bending backward, swayback
lord/osis	process of bending backward, inward curvature of the spine
meta	beyond
meta/carp/al	pertaining to beyond the wrist, bones of the palm of the hand
tars	ankle
meta/tars/al	pertaining to beyond the ankle bones of the sole of the foot
osteo/arthr/itis	inflammation of the joint
poro	pores in the bone
-sis	abnormal condition
osteo/poro/sis	abnormal condition of pores in the bone
peri	around
peri/oste/um	presence of lining around the bone
prona	placing face down
prona/tion	process of being face down
rheumat	painful changes in the joints
-oid	resembling
rheumat/oid	resembling painful changes in the joints
supina	placing on the back
supina/tion	process of placing on the back

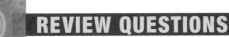

REVIEW QUESTIONS

Select the letter of the choice that best completes the statement.

1. Supination is one type of:
   a. extension
   b. abduction
   c. adduction
   d. rotation

2. The bones found in the skull are:
   a. irregular bones
   b. flat bones
   c. short bones
   d. long bones

3. The cranium protects the:
   a. lungs
   b. brain
   c. heart
   d. stomach

4. Pivot joints may be found in the:
   a. vertebral column
   b. skull
   c. wrist
   d. shoulder

5. Bones are a storage place for minerals such as:
   a. calcium and sodium
   b. calcium and potassium
   c. sodium and potassium
   d. calcium and phosphorous

6. The site of blood cell formation is:
   a. yellow marrow
   b. periosteum
   c. articular cartilage
   d. red marrow

7. Immovable joints are found in the:
   a. infant's skull
   b. adult cranium
   c. adult spinal column
   d. child's spinal column

8. Flexion means:
   a. bending
   b. rotating
   c. extending
   d. abduction

9. The degree of motion at a joint is determined by:
   a. the amount of synovial fluid
   b. the number of bursa
   c. the unusual amount of exercise
   d. bone shape and joint structure

10. The bone that forms the base of the skull is the:
   a. parietal
   b. temporal
   c. occipital
   d. frontal

11. The key bone of the skull is the:
   a. ethmoid
   b. frontal
   c. parietal
   d. sphenoid

12. The only moveable bone of the face is the:
   a. lacrimatic
   b. mandible
   c. maxilla
   d. palatine

13. The central opening on the vertebrae for passage of the spinal cord is the:
    a. transverse process
    b. intervertebral disc
    c. foramen
    d. spinous process

14. The shoulder girdle consists of two bones:
    a. radius and ulna
    b. clavicle and scapula
    c. tibia and fibula
    d. metatarsal and tarsal

15. The ribs attached directly to the sternum are called:
    a. floating
    b. true
    c. false
    d. humerus

16. The bone of the arm located on the thumb side is called:
    a. ulna
    b. radius
    c. humerus
    d. carpal

17. The bones of the wrist are called:
    a. tarsal
    b. metatarsals
    c. carpals
    d. metacarpals

18. The longest, strongest bone in the body is the:
    a. humerus
    b. tibia
    c. femur
    d. fibula

19. The heel bone is known as the:
    a. calcaneus
    b. patella
    c. fibula
    d. talus

20. An inflammation of the bone is known as:
    a. arthritis
    b. bursitis
    c. osteomyelitis
    d. osteoarthritis

LABELING

1. Label the parts of the skeleton.

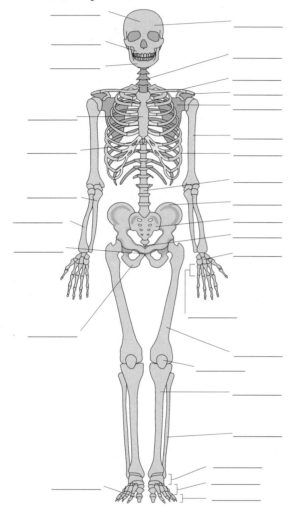

2. Label the parts of the long bone.

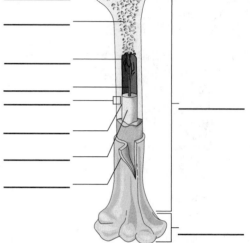

MATCHING

Match each term in Column I with its correct description in Column II.

Column I	Column II
_____ **1.** osteoarthritis	a. first cervical vertebra
_____ **2.** closed fracture	b. shock absorbers
_____ **3.** tendon	c. moveable joint
_____ **4.** endosteum	d. degeneration of articular cartilage

_____ **5.** bursa e. bone broken, skin intact
_____ **6.** epiphysis f. joint capsule
_____ **7.** periosteum g. fibrous cords that connect muscles to bone
_____ **8.** atlas h. lining of the marrow cavity
_____ **9.** intervertebral disc i. calcium and phosphorous
_____ **10.** diarthrosis joint j. end structure of long bone
                                         k. bone cells or osteocytes
                                         l. bone covering which contains blood vessels

APPLYING THEORY TO PRACTICE

1. What type of joint movement is used to shut off a light? What type is used to comb your hair?

2. When a skier breaks the long bone of his leg, what type of treatment will be used?

3. While running, you "turn your ankle." Name the bones involved. What is the best way to treat a sprain?

4. Your grandmother tells you her bones are stiff. Explain what causes this condition.

5. Your 70-year-old uncle, Mike, says, "I don't know what's happening to me. I used to be 5 feet 10 inches; now I'm only 5 feet 8 inches." Explain to your uncle why he is becoming shorter.

CASE STUDY

Your 80-year-old grandmother, Tess, while putting up dishes on a shelf, fell off a step stool and was unable to get up. She activated her medical lifeline and the emergency medical team arrived at the scene. They noticed her right leg was abducted and she was complaining of pain in her right leg and hip. Tess was taken to the emergency room where an x-ray revealed that the neck of her right femur was fractured. Further x-rays revealed a reduced bone mass in her right hip, femur, and vertebrae. Surgery was done to repair the hip. Your grandmother is now recuperating and having physical therapy treatment daily.

1. What organ and body system was affected by the injury?

2. Name the type of tissue involved and the cells responsible for healing.

3. The physician says she will do an open reduction to repair Tess's hip. Explain the process of an open reduction.

4. What disease condition did the x-ray of the vertebrae reveal?

5. What is the significance of your grandmother's age and gender?

6. What other body systems may be affected by the fall?

7. What will the role of the physical therapist be in your grandmother's rehabilitation?

8. Name the test that might have revealed the disease condition.

9. What measures can be taken to prevent osteoporosis?

10. What limitations will your grandmother have after her rehabilitation?

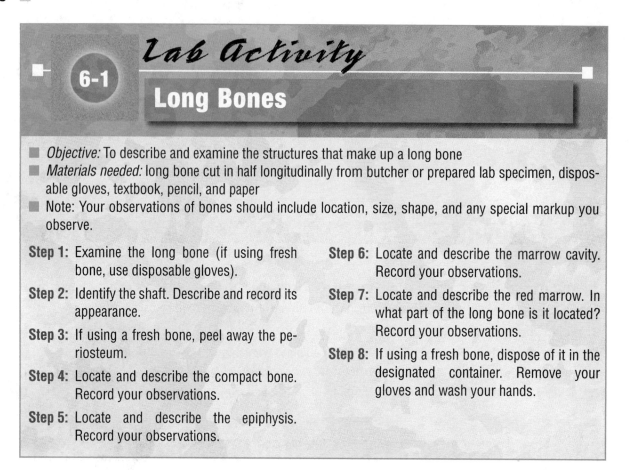

Lab Activity

6-1 Long Bones

- *Objective:* To describe and examine the structures that make up a long bone
- *Materials needed:* long bone cut in half longitudinally from butcher or prepared lab specimen, disposable gloves, textbook, pencil, and paper
- Note: Your observations of bones should include location, size, shape, and any special markup you observe.

Step 1: Examine the long bone (if using fresh bone, use disposable gloves).

Step 2: Identify the shaft. Describe and record its appearance.

Step 3: If using a fresh bone, peel away the periosteum.

Step 4: Locate and describe the compact bone. Record your observations.

Step 5: Locate and describe the epiphysis. Record your observations.

Step 6: Locate and describe the marrow cavity. Record your observations.

Step 7: Locate and describe the red marrow. In what part of the long bone is it located? Record your observations.

Step 8: If using a fresh bone, dispose of it in the designated container. Remove your gloves and wash your hands.

Lab Activity

6-2 Axial and Appendicular Skeleton

- *Objective:* To examine the size, shape, and location of the bones in the human skeleton
- *Materials needed:* articulated skeleton, textbook, paper, and pencil
- Note: Your observations of bones should include location, size, shape, and any special bone markings you observe.

Step 1: Locate and describe the bones of the cranium and facial bones. Record your observations.

Step 2: Locate and describe the bones of the rib cage. Note any differences. Record your observations.

Step 3: Locate the xiphoid process.

Step 4: Locate and describe the vertebrae. Compare your observation with the illustration in the textbook. Describe the types of vertebrae. Record your descriptions.

Step 5: Locate and describe the bones of the pectoral girdle. Record your observations.

continues

continued

Step 6: Locate the olecranon process. Record its location.

Step 7: Locate the radius and ulna bones. Which is the longer of the two bones? Record your answer.

Step 8: Count the bones located in a hand. Record your answer.

Step 9: Locate and describe the pelvic girdle. Record your observations.

Step 10: Find the acetabulum. What bone fits into this structure? Record your answer.

Step 11: Is the tibia longer or shorter than the fibula? What bone is called the shinbone? Record your answers.

Step 12: Locate the ankle bones. How many are in each foot? Record your answer.

Step 13: Locate and describe the structure of bones of the foot. Record your descriptions.

Step 14: Name three hinge joints that you can locate on the articulated skeleton. Record their names and location.

Step 15: Locate and describe two amphiarthroses joints. Record the location and features of this type of joint.

Chapter 7

MUSCULAR SYSTEM

Key Words

abdominal hernia
acetylcholine
action potential
antagonist
atrophy
belly
biceps
cardiac muscle
contractibility
deltoid
dilator muscle
elasticity
excitability
extensibility
fibromyalgia
flatfeet (talipes)
flexor
hernia
hiatal hernia

hypertrophy
inguinal hernia
insertion
intramuscular
irritability
isometric
isotonic
motor unit
muscle fatigue
muscle spasm
muscle tone
muscular dystrophy
myalgia
myasthenia gravis
neuromuscular
    junction
origin
physiotherapy

prime mover
rehabilitation
rotator cuff
    disease
sarcolemma
sarcoplasm
shin splints
skeletal muscle
smooth muscle
sphincter muscle
strain
strength
synergists
tennis elbow
tetanus
torticollis
triceps
vastus lateralis

The ability to move is an essential activity of the living human body which is made possible by the unique function of contractility in muscles. Muscles comprise a large part of the human body: Nearly half our body weight comes from muscle tissue. If you weigh 140 pounds, about 60 pounds of it comes from the muscles attached to your bones. Collectively, there are over 650 different muscles in the human body. Muscles are responsible for all body movement. They allow us to move from place to place, as well as perform involuntary functions such as the heart beating and our breathing. Muscles give our bodies form and shape; just think what you would look like if all your muscles "collapsed." Muscles are responsible for producing most of our body heat.

The muscle system has three main responsibilities.

1. Body movement
2. Body form and shape, to maintain posture
3. Body heat, to maintain body temperature

TYPES OF MUSCLES

Body movements are determined by one or more of the three principle types of muscles. They are skeletal, smooth, and cardiac muscle. These muscles are also described as striated, spindle shaped, and nonstriated because of the way their cells look under a microscope.

Skeletal muscles are attached to the bone of the skeleton. They are called striped or striated because they have cross bandings (striations) of alternating light and dark bands running perpendicular to the length of the muscle, Figure 7-1. Skeletal muscle is also called voluntary muscle, because it contains nerves under voluntary control. Skeletal muscle consists of bundles of muscle cells. Each cell is multinucleate (containing many nuclei). Each muscle cell is known as a muscle fiber. The cell membrane is **sarcolemma** and the cytoplasm is **sarcoplasm.**

The fleshy body parts are made of skeletal muscles. They provide movement to the limbs, but contract quickly, fatigue easily, and lack the ability to remain contracted for prolonged periods. Blinking the eye, talking, breathing, dancing, eating, and writing are all produced by the motion of these muscles. This chapter focuses on skeletal muscle.

Smooth (visceral) **muscle** cells are small and spindle-shaped. There is only one nucleus, located at the center of the cell. They are called smooth muscles because they are unmarked by any distinctive striations. Unattached to bones, they act slowly, do not tire easily, and can remain contracted for a long time, Figure 7-2.

Smooth muscles are not under conscious control; for this reason they are also called involuntary muscles. Their actions are controlled by the autonomic (automatic) nervous system. Smooth muscles are found in the walls of the internal

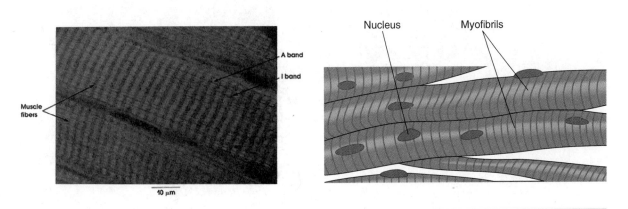

Figure 7-1 *Voluntary or striated (skeletal) muscle cells* (Photo is from Atlas of Microscopic Anatomy: A Functional Approach: Companion to Histology and Neuroanatomy, *by R. Bergman, A. Afifi, P. Heidger, 1999, www.vh.org/Providers/Textbooks/MicroscopicAnatomy.html. Reprinted with permission.)*

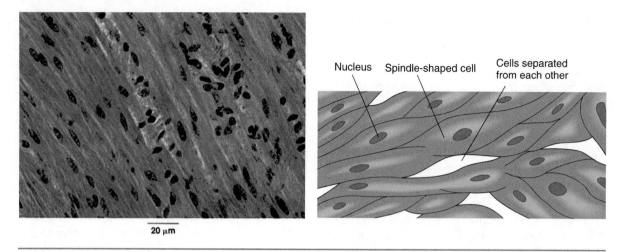

20 μm

Figure 7-2   *Involuntary or smooth muscle cells* (Photo is from Atlas of Microscopic Anatomy: A Functional Approach: Companion to Histology and Neuroanatomy, *by R. Bergman, A. Afifi, P. Heidger, 1999, www.vh.org/Providers/Textbooks/MicroscopicAnatomy.html. Reprinted with permission.)*

organs, including the stomach, intestines, uterus, and blood vessels. They help push food along the length of the alimentary canal, contract the uterus during labor and childbirth, and control the diameter of the blood vessels as the blood circulates throughout the body.

Cardiac muscle is found only in the heart. Cardiac muscle cells are striated and branched, and they are involuntary, Figure 7-3. Cardiac cells are joined in a continuous network without a sheath separation. The membranes of adjacent cells are fused at places called intercalated discs. A communication system at the fused area will not permit independent cell contraction. When one cell receives a signal to contract, all neighboring cells are stimulated and they contract together to produce the heart beat. When the heart beats normally, it holds a rhythm of about 72 beats per minute; however, the activity of various nerves leading to the heart can increase or decrease its rate. Cardiac muscle requires a continuous supply of oxygen to function. Should its oxygen supply be cut off for as little as 30 seconds, the cardiac muscle cells start to die.

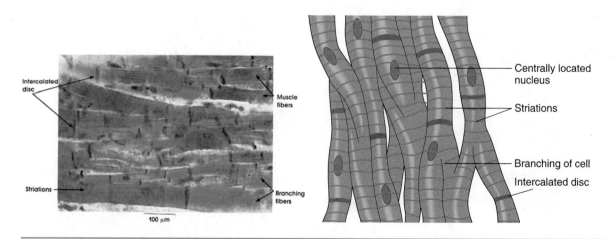

Figure 7-3   *Cardiac muscle cells* (Photo is from Atlas of Microscopic Anatomy: A Functional Approach: Companion to Histology and Neuroanatomy, *1999, by R. Bergman, A. Afifi, P. Heidger, www.vh.org/Providers/Textbooks/MicroscopicAnatomy.html. Reprinted with permission.)*

Table 7-1 *Characteristics of Major Muscle Types*

MUSCLE TYPE	LOCATION	STRUCTURE	FUNCTION
Skeletal muscle (striated voluntary)	Attached to the skelton and also located in the wall of the pharynx and esophagus.	A skeletal muscle fiber is long, cylindrical, multinucleated, and contains alternating light and dark striations. Nuclei located at edge of fiber.	Contractions occur voluntarily and may be rapid and forceful. Contractions stabilize the joints.
Smooth muscle (nonstriated, involuntary)	Located in the walls of tubular structures and hollow organs such as in the digestive tract, urinary bladder, and blood vessels.	A smooth muscle fiber is long and spindle shaped, with no striations.	Contractions occur involuntarily and are rhythmic and slow.
Cardiac (heart) muscle	Located in the heart.	Short, branching fibers with a centrally located nucleus; striations not distinct.	Contractions occur involuntarily and are rhythmic and automatic.

Sphincter, or dilator, muscles are special circular muscles in the openings between the esophagus and stomach, and the stomach and small intestine. They are also found in the walls of the anus, the urethra, and the mouth. They open and close to control the passage of substances.

Table 7-1 summarizes the characteristics of the three major muscle types.

CHARACTERISTICS OF MUSCLES

All muscles, whether they are skeletal, smooth, or cardiac, have four common characteristics. One is **contractibility,** a quality possessed by no other body tissue. When a muscle shortens or contracts, it reduces the distance between the parts of its contents, or the space it surrounds. The contraction of skeletal muscles that connect a pair of bones brings the attachment points closer together, thus causing the bone to move. When cardiac muscles contract, they reduce the area in the heart chambers, pumping blood from the heart into the blood vessels. Likewise, smooth muscles surround blood vessels and the intestines, causing the diameter of these tubes to decrease upon contraction.

Excitability or **irritability** is a characteristic of both muscle and nervous cells (neurons). It is the ability to respond to certain stimuli by producing electric signals called **action potentials** (impulses).

Extensibility is the ability to be stretched. When we bend our forearm, the muscles on the back of it are extended or stretched.

Muscles also exhibit **elasticity** (the ability to return to original length when relaxing). Collectively, these four characteristics of muscles—contractibility, excitability, extensibility, and elasticity—produce a veritable mechanical device capable of complex, intricate movements.

MUSCLE ATTACHMENTS AND FUNCTIONS

There are over 650 different muscles in the body. For any of these muscles to produce movement in any part of the body, it must be able to exert its force upon a movable object. Muscles must be attached to bones for leverage in order to have something to pull against. Muscles only pull, never push.

Muscles are attached to the bones of the skeleton by nonelastic cords called tendons. Bones are connected at joints. Skeletal muscles are attached to bones in such a way as to bridge these joints. When a skeletal muscle contracts, the bone to which it is attached will move.

Muscles are attached at both ends. Attachment may be to bones, cartilage, ligaments,

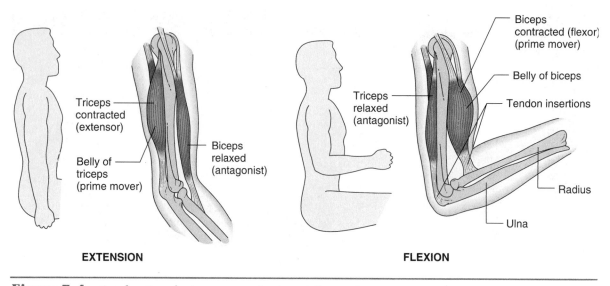

Figure 7-4 *Coordination of prime mover and antagonistic muscles*

tendons, skin, and sometimes to each other. The **origin** is the part of a skeletal muscle that is attached to a fixed structure or bone; it moves least during muscle contraction. The **insertion** is the other end, attached to a movable part; it is the part that moves most during a muscle contraction. The **belly** is the central body of the muscle, Figure 7-4.

The muscles of the body are arranged in pairs. One produces movement in a single direction called the **prime mover,** the other does so in the opposite direction called the **antagonist.** This arrangement of muscles with opposite actions is known as an antagonist pair.

By example, upper arm muscles are arranged in antagonist pairs, Figure 7-4. The muscle located on the front part of the upper arm is the **biceps.** One end of the biceps is attached to the scapula and humerus (its origin). When the biceps contract, these two bones remain stationary. The opposite end of the biceps is attached to the radius of the lower arm (its insertion); this bone moves upon contraction of the biceps.

The muscle on the back of the upper arm is the **triceps.** Try this simple demonstration: Bend your elbow. With your other hand, feel the contraction of the belly of the biceps. At the same time, stretch your fingers out (around the arm) to touch your triceps; it will be in a relaxed state. Now extend your forearm; feel the simultaneous contraction of the triceps and relaxation of the biceps. Now bend the forearm halfway and contract the biceps and triceps. They cannot move, because both sets of muscles are contracting at the same time. In some muscle activity, the role of prime mover and antagonist may be reversed. When you flex your arm, the biceps is the prime mover and the triceps is the antagonist. When you extend your arm, the triceps is the prime mover and the biceps is the antagonist.

Another group of muscles, called the **synergists,** help to steady a movement or stabilize joint activity.

SOURCES OF ENERGY AND HEAT

When muscles do their work, they not only move the body but also produce the heat which our bodies need. To get warm on a cold day, you jump up and down. Human beings usually maintain their body temperatures within a narrow range (98.6°F to 99.8°F). For muscles to contract and do their work, they need energy. The major source of this energy is adenosine triphosphate (ATP), a compound found in the muscle cell. To make ATP, the cell requires oxygen, glucose, and other material which is brought to the cell by the circulating blood. Extra glucose can be stored in the cell in the form of glycogen. When a muscle is stimulated, the ATP is released, thus producing the heat our bodies need and the energy the muscle needs to contract. During this process, lactic acid, which is a by-product of cell metabolism, builds up.

CONTRACTION OF SKELETAL MUSCLE

Movement of muscles occurs as a result of two major events: myoneural stimulation and contraction of muscle proteins. Skeletal muscles must be stimulated by nerve impulses to contract. A motor neuron (nerve cell) stimulates all of the skeletal muscles within a **motor unit.** A motor unit is a motor neuron plus all the muscle fibers it stimulates. The junction between the motor neuron's fiber (axon), which transmits the impulse, and the muscle cell's sarcolemma (muscle cell membrane) is the **neuromuscular junction.** The gap between the axon and the muscle cell is known as the synaptic cleft.

When the nerve impulses reach the end of the axon, the chemical neurotransmitter **acetylcholine** is released. Acetylcholine diffuses across the synaptic cleft and attaches to receptors on the sarcolemma. The sarcolemma then becomes temporarily permeable to sodium ions ($Na+$) which go rushing into the muscle cell. This gives the muscle cell excessive positive ions which upset and change the electrical condition of the sarcolemma. This electrical upset causes an action potential (an electric current).

Skeletal muscle contraction begins with the action potential which travels along the muscle fiber length. The basic source of energy is from glucose and the energy derived is stored in the form of ATP and phosphocreatinine. The latter serves as a trigger mechanism by allowing energy transfer to the protein molecules, actin and myosin, within the muscle fibers. Once begun, the action potential travels over the entire surface of the sarcolemma conducting the electric impulse from one end of the cell to the other. This results in the contraction of the muscle cell. The movement of electrical current along the sarcolemma causes calcium ions ($Ca++$) to be released from storage areas inside the muscle cell. When calcium ions attach to the action myofilaments (contractile elements of skeletal muscle), the sliding of the myofilaments is triggered and the whole cell shortens. The sliding of the myofilaments is energized by ATP.

Effects of Aging on The Muscle System

As an individual ages, the muscle undergoes a great amount of atrophy and there is a gradual decrease in both the number of muscle fibers and their individual bulk. Fibrous tissue replaces the muscle tissue. There is a decrease in muscular strength and endurance associated with a decrease in muscle fibers. A diminished storage of muscular glycogen may cause a loss of energy reserve, which contributes to a rapid onset of fatigue.

Regular exercise improves strength and stamina. Generally, a man of 70 years has 50% the strength of a man of 30 years.

The events that return the cell to a resting phase include the diffusion of potassium and sodium ions back to their initial positions outside the cell. When the action potential ends, calcium ions are reabsorbed into their storage areas and the muscle cell relaxes and returns to its original length. The amazing part is that this entire activity takes place in just a few thousandths of a second.

While the action potential is occurring, acetylcholine (which began the process) is broken down by enzymes on the sarcolemma. For this reason, a single nerve impulse produces only one contraction at a time. The muscle cell relaxes until it is stimulated by the next release of acetylcholine, Figure 7-5.

MUSCLE FATIGUE

Muscle fatigue is caused by an accumulation of lactic acid in the muscles. During periods of vigorous

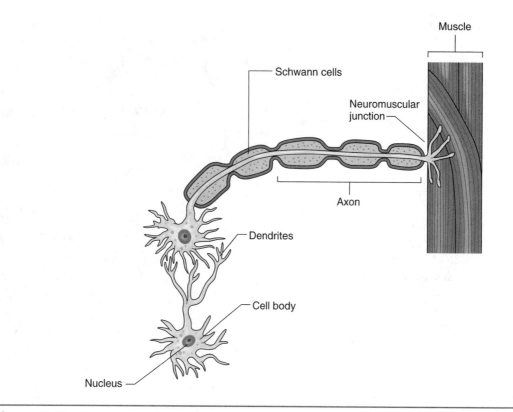

Figure 7-5 *A neuron stimulating muscle*

exercise, the blood is unable to transport enough oxygen for the complete oxidation of glucose in the muscles. This causes the muscles to contract anaerobically (without oxygen).

The lactic acid normally leaves the muscle, passing into the bloodstream; but if vigorous exercise continues, the lactic acid level in the blood rises sharply. In such cases, lactic acid accumulates within the muscle. This impedes muscular contraction, causing muscle fatigue and cramps. After exercise, a person must stop, rest, and take in enough oxygen to change the lactic acid back to glucose and other substances to be used by the muscle cells. The amount of oxygen needed is called the oxygen debt. When the debt is paid back, respirations resume a normal rate.

MUSCLE TONE

To function, muscles should always be slightly contracted and ready to pull. This is **muscle tone.** Muscle tone can be achieved through proper nutri-

tion and regular exercise. Muscle contractions may be **isotonic** or **isometric.** When muscles contract and shorten, it is called an isotonic contraction. This occurs when we walk, talk, and so on. When the tension in a muscle increases but the muscle does not shorten, it is called an isometric contraction. This occurs with exercises such as tensing the abdominal muscles. If we fail to exercise, our muscles become weak and flaccid. Muscles may also shrink from disuse. This is called **atrophy.** If we overexercise, muscles will become enlarged. This is known as **hypertrophy.** In hypertrophy, the size of the muscle fiber (cell) enlarges.

PRINCIPLE SKELETAL MUSCLES

The skeletal or voluntary muscles are the muscles that are attached to, and help to move, the skeleton. These muscles line the walls of the oral, abdominal, and pelvic cavities. Skeletal muscles also control the movement of the eyeballs, eyelids, lips, tongue, and skin.

Naming of Skeletal Muscles

Muscles are named by location, size, direction, number of origins, location of origin and insertion, and action; however, not *all* muscles are named in this manner.

- Location . . . . frontalis—forehead
- Size . . . . gluteus maximus—largest muscle in buttock
- Direction of fibers . . external abdominal oblique—edge of the lower rib cage
- Number of origins . . biceps—two-headed muscle in humerus
- Location of origin and insertion . . . . . sternocleidomastoid —origin in sternum
- Action flexor . . . . . . flexor carpi ulnaris—flexes the wrist
- Extensor . . . . extensor carpi ulnaris —extends the wrist
- Levator and depressor . . . . depressor anguli oris —depresses the corner of the mouth; raises or lowers body parts

Look at Figures 7-6 and 7-7 and find other muscles named by location, size, direction, number of origins, and action.

There are 656 muscles in the human body. This breaks down to 327 antagonistic muscle pairs and two unpaired muscles. These two unpaired muscles are the orbicularis oris and the diaphragm. The 656 muscles can be divided and subdivided into the following muscle regions.

A. *Head muscles*
1. Muscles of expression
2. Muscles of mastication (chewing)
3. Muscles of the tongue
4. Muscles of the pharynx
5. Muscles of the soft palate

B. *Neck muscles*
1. Muscles moving the head
2. Muscles moving the hyoid bone and the larynx
3. Muscles moving the upper ribs

C. *Trunk and extremity muscles*
1. Muscles that move the vertebral column
2. Muscles that move the scapula
3. Muscles of breathing
4. Muscles that move the humerus
5. Muscles that move the forearm
6. Muscles that move the wrist, hand, and finger digits
7. Muscles that act on the pelvis
8. Muscles that move the femur
9. Muscles that move the leg
10. Muscles that move the ankles, feet, and toe digits

Tables 7-2 through 7-7 list some representative skeletal muscles that are involved in various types of bodily movements.

MUSCLES OF THE HEAD AND NECK

Muscles of the head and neck control human facial expressions such as anger, fear, grief, joy, pleasure, and pain. Refer to Table 7-2 and Figure 7-8.

Muscles of mastication control the mandible (lower jaw), raising it to close the jaw and lowering it to open the jaw. Refer to Table 7-3 and Figure 7-8.

Muscles that move the head cause extension, flexion, and rotation. Refer to Table 7-4 and Figure 7-8.

MUSCLES OF THE UPPER EXTREMITIES

Muscles of the upper extremity help to move the shoulder (scapula) and arm (humerus) and the forearm, wrist, hand, and fingers. Refer to Table 7-5 and Figure 7-9.

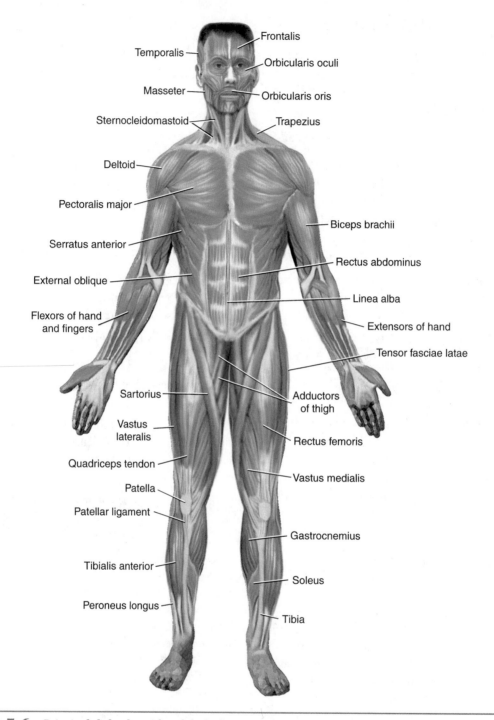

Figure 7-6 *Principal skeletal muscles of the body—anterior view*

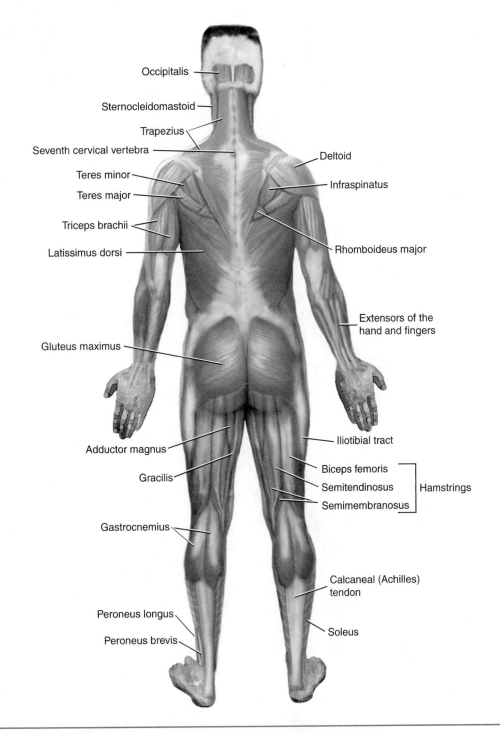

Figure 7-7 *Principal skeletal muscles of the body—posterior view*

Table 7-2 Muscles of Facial Expression

MUSCLE	EXPRESSION	LOCATION	FUNCTION
Frontalis	Surprise	On either side of the forehead	Raises eyebrow and wrinkles forehead
Depressor anguli oris	Doubt, disdain, contempt	Found along the side of the chin	Depresses corner of mouth
Orbicularis oris	Doubt, disdain, contempt	Ring-shaped muscle found around the mouth	Compresses and closes the lips
Platysma (broad sheet muscle)	Horror	Broad, thin muscular sheet covering the side of the neck and lower jaw	Draws corners of mouth downward and backward
Zygomaticus major	Laughing or smiling	Extends diagonally upward from corner of mouth	Raises corner of mouth
Nasalis	Muscles of the nose	Found over the nasal bones	Closes and opens the nasal openings
Orbicularis oculi	Sadness	Surrounds the eye orbit underlying the eyebrows	Closes the eyelid and tightens the skin on the forehead

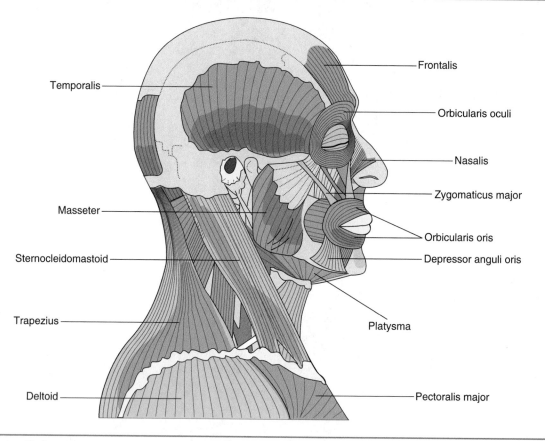

Figure 7-8 *Head and neck muscle arrangement*

Table 7-3 Muscles of Mastication

MUSCLE	LOCATION	FUNCTION
Masseter	Covers the lateral surface of the ramus (angle) of the mandible	Closes the jaw
Temporalis	Located on the temporal fossa of the skull	Raises the jaw, closes the mouth, and draws the jaw backward

Table 7-4 *Muscles of the Neck*

MUSCLE	LOCATION	FUNCTION
Sternocleidomastoid (two heads)	Large muscles extending diagonally down sides of neck	Flexes head; rotates the head toward opposite side from muscle

Table 7-5 *Muscles of the Upper Extremities*

MUSCLE	LOCATION	FUNCTION
*Trapezius	A large triangular muscle located on the upper surface of the back	Moves the shoulder; extends the head
*Deltoid	A thick triangular muscle that covers the shoulder joint	Abducts the upper arm
*Pectoralis major	Anterior part of the chest	Flexes the upper arm and helps to abduct the upper arm
Serratus	Anterior chest	Moves scapula forward and helps to raise the arm
*Biceps brachii	Upper arm to radius	Flexes the lower arm
*Triceps brachii	Posterior arm to ulna	Extends the lower arm
Extensor and flexor carpi muscle groups	Extends from the anterior and posterior forearm to the hand	Moves the hand
Extensor and flexor digitorum muscle groups	Extends from the anterior and posterior forearm to the fingers	Moves the fingers

*Major prime movers

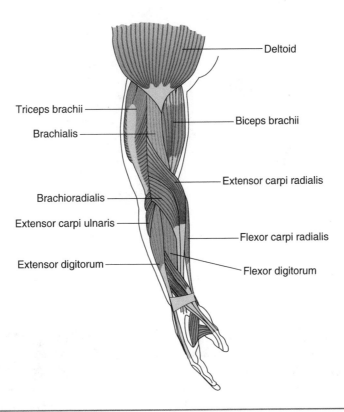

Figure 7-9 *Muscles of the upper extremity*

Table 7-6 *Muscles of the Trunk*

MUSCLE	LOCATION	FUNCTION
External intercostals	Found between the ribs	Raises the ribs to help in breathing
Diaphragm	A dome-shaped muscle separating the thoracic and abdominal cavities	Helps to control breathing
Rectus abdominis	Extends from the ribs to the pelvis	Compresses the abdomen
External oblique	Anterior inferior edge of the last eight ribs	Depresses ribs, flexes the spinal column, and compresses the abdominal cavity
Internal oblique	Found directly beneath the external oblique, its fibers running in the opposite direction	Same as above

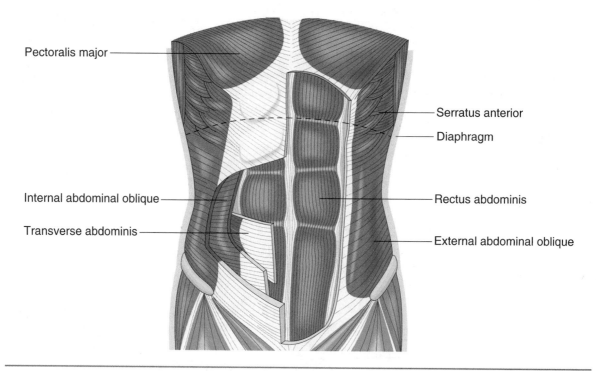

Pectoralis major

Serratus anterior

Diaphragm

Internal abdominal oblique

Rectus abdominis

Transverse abdominis

External abdominal oblique

Figure 7-10 *Muscles of the trunk*

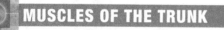

MUSCLES OF THE TRUNK

The trunk muscles control breathing and the movements of the abdomen and the pelvis. Refer to Table 7-6 and Figure 7-10.

MUSCLES OF THE LOWER EXTREMITIES

Muscles of the lower extremities, Figure 7-11, assist in the movement of the thigh (femur), leg, an-

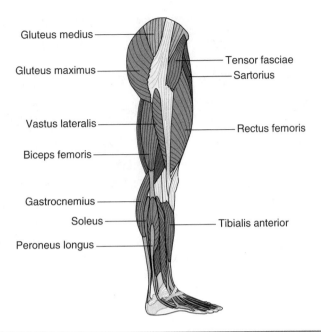

Figure 7-11 *Muscles of the lower extremity*

Table 7-7 *Muscles of the Lower Extremities*

MUSCLE	LOCATION	FUNCTION
*Gluteus maximus	Muscle forms the buttocks	Extends femur and rotates it outward
Gluteus medius	Extends from the deep femur to the buttocks	Abducts and rotates the thigh
Tensor fasciae	A flat muscle found along the upper lateral surface of the thigh	Flexes, abducts, and medially rotates the thigh
*Rectus femoris	Anterior thigh	Flexes thigh and extends the lower leg
*Sartorius (Tailor's muscle)	A long, straplike muscle that runs diagonally across the anterior and medial surface of the thigh	Flexes and rotates the thigh and leg
*Tibialis anterior	In front of the tibia bone	Dorsiflexes the foot; permits walking on the heels
*Gastrocnemius	Calf muscle	Points toes and flexes the lower leg
*Soleus	A broad flat muscle found beneath the gastrocnemius	Extends foot
Peroneus longus	A superficial muscle found on the lateral side of the leg	Extends and everts the foot and supports arches

*Major prime movers

kle, foot, and toes, Table 7-7. Athletes often pull what are known as the hamstrings. The group of muscles that comprise the hamstrings are the semitendinosus, biceps femoris, and semimembranosus muscles. The tendons of these muscles attach posteriorly to the tibia and fibula. They can be felt behind the knee. The hamstring muscle group is responsible for flexing the knee.

Medical Highlight

Benefits of Massage

Massage: Does it have therapeutic value or does it just make you feel good? Some researchers indicate that the feel-good effects of massage can translate into striking improvements in medical conditions ranging from asthma to rheumatoid arthritis to burns.

Researchers are also shedding light on what massage can do for healthy people who want to ward off colds and viruses, cope more effectively with stress and pain, and sleep more soundly. Stress causes a flight-or-fight response from the body. Massage intervenes by convincing the body that the emergency is over. "Massage mechanically forces muscle tension to decrease," says Robert Sapolsky, a Stanford University neurobiologist. As the pressure of the therapist's hands loosens tight muscles, the body produces few stress hormones, such as cortisol and norepinephrine. Once the muscles start to relax, tension seems to ease.

Massage therapists believe that a regular laying on of hands can tune up the immune system, making people less susceptible to colds and viruses. The theory is that deep massage strokes push lymph fluid more quickly through the network of vessels that deliver it throughout the body. Because lymph fluid carries immune cells, massage is thought to give those cells more opportunities to seek out and neutralize disease invaders.

Massage can help produce sound sleep by turning off the sympathetic nervous system, which makes us alert and vigilant, and switching on the parasympathetic, which calms things down. Massage seems to help relieve serious back pain as well as pain associated with rheumatoid arthritis, fibromyalgia, and burns. The theory seems to be that massage may raise the levels of enkephalins, one of the body's natural painkillers. As more research is done, massage may be an alternative way to treat some common diseases.

HOW EXERCISE AND TRAINING CHANGE MUSCLES

Exercise and training will alter the size, structure, and strength of a muscle.

Size and Muscle Structure

Skeletal muscles that are not used will atrophy and those that are used excessively will hypertrophy. The hypertrophy is caused by change in the sarcoplasm (cytoplasm found in the individual skeletal muscle fibers) and *not* to an increase in the number of muscle fibers (cells). Muscles that have been injured can regenerate only to a limited degree. If the muscle damage is extensive, then the muscle tissue is replaced by connective (scar) tissue. Muscles that are overexercised or worked will have a tremendous increase of connective tissue between the muscle fibers. This causes the skeletal muscle to become tougher.

Effect of Training on Muscle Efficiency

The following will occur due to the effects of training.

- Improved coordination of all muscles involved in a particular activity
- Improvement of the respiratory and circulatory system to supply the needs of an active muscular system
- Elimination or reduction of excess fat
- Improved joint movement involved with that particular muscle activity.

Effect of Training on Muscle Strength

Strength (capacity to do work) is increased by proper training. Training can have the following effects on skeletal muscles.

- Increase in muscle size
- Improved antagonistic muscle coordination, where antagonistic muscles are relaxed at the right moment and do not interfere with the functioning of the working muscle.
- Improved functioning in the cortical brain region, where the nerve impulses that start muscular contraction

MASSAGE MUSCLES

Occasionally a health care professional must give a patient either a total body massage or a massage to a specific body area. The correct type of massage is essential in either providing the proper **physiotherapy** or a general sense of comfort and well-being to a patient.

The health care professional must be aware of the specific skeletal muscles involved in therapeutic massage. The importance of these skeletal muscles comes from their proximity to the body's surface and their relatively large size. Table 7-8 gives the names of these superficial skeletal muscles and their general locations. It is essential for the health care professional to be able to locate these skeletal muscles not only on the muscle diagrams but also on the living bodies of patients with different physiques: scrawny, muscular, thin, fat, male, and female.

ELECTRICAL STIMULATION

Passing electrical currents through skin into the body for therapeutic uses have been used for a number of years. As with any electrical modality, physical therapists and physicians are the primary users.

Electrical modalities achieve their effect by stimulating nerve tissue, and do not produce heat or cold. A larger number of different electrical stimulators have been developed over the years. Most of the stimulation units have a pulsed direct current or an altering current.

Electrical stimulation is a commonly used modality in physical therapy, and has proven to be effective for many purposes including increasing

Table 7-8 *Skeletal Muscles Involved in Massage*

NAME OF SKELETAL MUSCLE	LOCATION
Sternocleidomastoid	Side of neck
Trapezius	Back of the neck and upper back
Latissimus dorsi	Lower back
Pectoralis major	Chest
Serratus anterior	Lateral ribs
External oblique	Anterior and lateral abdomen
Deltoid	Shoulder
Biceps brachii	Anterior aspect of arm
Triceps brachii	Posterior aspect of arm
Brachioradialis	Anterior and proximal forearm
Gluteus maximus	Buttock
Tensor fascia latae	Lateral and proximal thigh
Sartorius	Anterior thigh
Quadriceps femoris group (rectus femoris, vastus lateralis, vastus medialis, vastus intermedius)	Anterior thigh
Hamstring group (biceps, femoris, semitendinosus, semimembranosus)	Posterior thigh
Gracilis	Medial thigh
Tibialis anterior	Anterior leg
Gastrocnemius	Posterior leg
Soleus	Posterior (deep) leg
Peroneus longus	Lateral leg

range of motion (ROM), increasing muscle strength, muscle re-education, improving muscle tone, enhancing function, pain control, accelerating wound healing, and muscle spasm reduction.

INTRAMUSCULAR INJECTIONS

A health care professional occasionally has to administer an **intramuscular** (into the muscle) injection into the patient. Therefore, a working knowledge of the major skeletal muscles and the underlying anatomy of the area to be injected is needed. The most common sites for an intramuscular injection are the **deltoid** muscle of the upper arm, vastus lateralis (anterior thigh), dorsal gluteal area or ventral gluteal area of the buttocks.

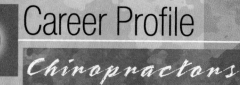

Career Profile
Chiropractors

Chiropractors, also known as chiropractic doctors, diagnose and treat patients whose health problems are associated with the body's muscular, nervous, or skeletal systems. The chiropractic approach to health care is holistic, stressing the patient's overall well-being. Chiropractors use natural, nonsurgical health treatments such as water, heat, light, and massage. With difficulties involving the muscular system, the chiropractor manually manipulates or adjusts the spinal column.

Education required is a bachelor's degree or at least 2 years of college in addition to completion of a 4-year course of study at a chiropractic college. All states require licensure. To qualify, a candidate must meet educational requirements and pass the state boards. Job prospects are excellent and employment is expected to grow faster than the average for all other occupations.

MUSCULOSKELETAL DISORDERS

Muscle and skeletal systems work as a team to move the body. Muscular coordination is vital if a person is to perform daily functions efficiently. Injuries and diseases, which may affect the musculoskeletal system, sometimes interfere with these functions. The retraining of injured or unused muscles is a type of **rehabilitation** called therapeutic exercise.

Muscle atrophy can occur to muscles used infrequently. They shrink in size and lose muscle strength; an example is in a stroke (cerebrovascular accident). The muscles are understimulated and thus gradually waste away. Muscle atrophy due to nerve paralysis may reduce a muscle up to 25% of its normal size. Muscle atrophy can also be caused by prolonged bed rest or the immobilization of a limb in a cast. Muscle atrophy can be minimized by massage or special exercise.

A muscle **strain** is a tear in the muscle resulting from excessive use. Limited bleeding inside the muscle can result in pain and swelling. Ice packs will help to stop bleeding and reduce swelling.

Muscle spasm, or cramp, is a sustained contraction of the muscle. These contractions may occur because of overuse of the muscle.

Myalgia is a term used to describe muscle pain. **Fibromyalgia** disease is a collection of symptoms (syndrome). In fibromyalgia, the most definite symptom is chronic muscle pain lasting 3 or more months in specific muscle points. Other symptoms may include fatigue, headache, feelings of numbness and tingling, and feelings of joint pain. Treatment is directed at pain relief and instructions to get enough sleep, exercise regularly, and utilize massage therapy, chiropractic procedures, relaxation techniques, stretching exercises, and medication prescribed by a physician.

Hernia occurs when an organ protrudes through a weak muscle. **Abdominal hernia** occurs when organs protrude through the abdominal wall. **Inguinal hernia** occurs in the inguinal area (see Figure 1-4, Chapter 1) and **hiatal hernia** occurs when the stomach pushes through the diaphragm.

Flatfeet (**talipes**) result from a weakening of the leg muscles that support the arch. The downward pressure on the foot eventually flattens out the arches. The condition can be helped by exercise, massage, and corrective shoes.

Tetanus (lockjaw) is an infectious disease characterized by continuous spasms of the voluntary muscles. It is caused by a toxin from the bacillus, *Clostridium tetani,* a bacterium that can enter the body through a puncture wound. This disease can be prevented by a tetanus antitoxoid vaccine.

Torticollis, or wry neck, may be due to an inflammation of the trapezius and/or sternocleidomastoid muscle.

Muscular dystrophy is a group of diseases in which the muscle cells deteriorate. The most common type is Duchenne's muscular dystrophy, which is caused by a genetic defect. At birth, the child appears normal; as growth occurs and muscle cells die, the child becomes weak. The child loses the ability to walk between the ages of 9 and 11. Progressive deterioration of muscle, and death, will occur in the late teens or early 20s unless mechanical breathing is instituted.

Myasthenia gravis leads to progressive muscular weakness and paralysis. The cause is still unknown, but many researchers believe it may be due to a defect in the immune system, affecting myoneural function. In extreme cases, it can be fatal due to the paralysis of the respiratory muscles.

Recreation Injuries

The need to exercise can sometimes lead to excessive stress on the tendons. The tendons are cords of connective tissue that attach the muscles to bone. They are not able to contract and return to their original place; therefore, they are more susceptible to straining and tearing. For example, a sudden severe muscle contraction needed for playing tennis can cause the tendons to tear.

Tennis elbow, or lateral epicondylitis, occurs at the bony prominence (lateral epicondyle) on the sides of the elbow. The tendon that connects the arm muscle to elbow becomes inflammed because the repetitive use of the arm and under conditioning, Figure 7-12. This can occur from carrying luggage, playing tennis, swinging a golf club, or pounding a hammer. Treatment consists of relief of pain and ice packs to reduce the inflammation. Sleeping on the affected arm should be avoided. Surgery is used as a last resort.

Shin splints occur when there is injury to the muscle tendon in the front of the shin. This occurs when jogging. To prevent shin splints, choose a running shoe that is comfortable and has proper arch support.

Rotator cuff disease is an inflammation of a group of tendons that fuse together and surround the shoulder joint. This injury can occur because of repetitive overhead swinging, such as swinging a tennis racquet or pitching a ball. The most common complaint is aching in the top and front of the shoulder. Pain increases when the arm is lifted overhead. Treatment includes rest and physical therapy.

Torsion strain occurs when one end of some tissue is twisted while the other end remains

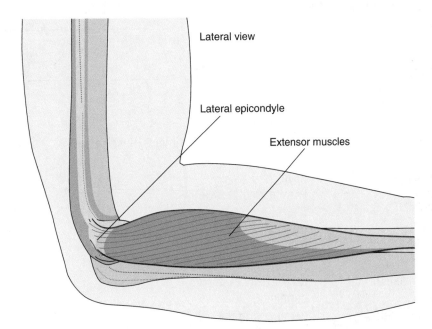

Figure 7-12 Tennis elbow

motionless or is twisted in the opposite direction. For example, the boxer who receives a blow to one side or the mandible will receive torsion forces to the spine as his or her head pivots rapidly in the op- posite direction. The result may be torsion injuries to the spinal cord or vertebrae. Approximately 40–50% of all rotation injuries to the cervical spine occur at the C1–C2 level and are often fatal.

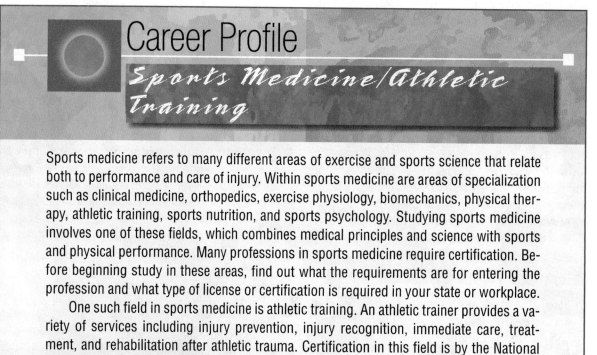

Career Profile

Sports Medicine/Athletic Training

Sports medicine refers to many different areas of exercise and sports science that relate both to performance and care of injury. Within sports medicine are areas of specialization such as clinical medicine, orthopedics, exercise physiology, biomechanics, physical therapy, athletic training, sports nutrition, and sports psychology. Studying sports medicine involves one of these fields, which combines medical principles and science with sports and physical performance. Many professions in sports medicine require certification. Before beginning study in these areas, find out what the requirements are for entering the profession and what type of license or certification is required in your state or workplace.

One such field in sports medicine is athletic training. An athletic trainer provides a variety of services including injury prevention, injury recognition, immediate care, treatment, and rehabilitation after athletic trauma. Certification in this field is by the National Athletic Trainers Association (NATA) Board of Certification. This certification identifies for the public all quality healthcare professionals through a system of certification, adjucation, standards of practice, and continuing competency programs. Most states and places of employment require athletic trainers to be certified.

Medical Terminology

a	without
troph	nourishment
-y	process of
a/troph/y	muscle without nourishment, muscles shrink
bi	two
-ceps	head
bi/ceps	two-headed muscle
fibro	fiber
myl	muscle
-agia	pain
fibro/myl/agia	pain in the muscle fiber
gastrocnemi	calf or belly of the leg
-us	pertaining
gastrocnemi/us	pertaining to the calf of the leg
hyper	excessive

hyper/troph/y	pertaining to excessive nourishment; causes enlargement
intra	into
muscul	muscle
-ar	pertaining to
intra/muscul/ar	pertaining to inside the muscle
myl/agia	muscle pain
my	muscle
asthenia	weakness
gravis	heavy, grave
myasthenia gravis	grave muscle weakness
neuro	nerve
neuro/muscul/ar	pertaining to the nerve and muscle
physio	nature
physiotherapy	treatment with natural means
sarc	flesh
lemma	husk or covering
sarc/o/lemma	covering around muscle flesh
plasm	tumor
sarco/plasm	tumor of the flesh

REVIEW QUESTIONS

Select the letter of the choice that best completes the statement.

1. The muscle system is responsible for:
   a. producing red blood cells
   b. providing a framework
   c. moving the body
   d. conducting impulses

2. Skeletal muscle is also known as:
   a. involuntary
   b. voluntary
   c. cardiac
   d. smooth

3. The muscle responsible for action in a single direction is called:
   a. prime mover
   b. antagonist
   c. synergistic
   d. adduction

4. The constant state of partial contraction of muscles is called:
   a. muscle atrophy
   b. muscle tone
   c. tetanus
   d. muscle hypertrophy

5. The muscle you use to turn your head is the:
   a. trapezius
   b. sternocleidomastoid
   c. orbicularis
   d. temporalis

6. The muscle in the upper arm that is used as an injection site is the:
   a. triceps
   b. biceps
   c. trapezius
   d. deltoid

7. The muscle used in breathing is the:
   a. oblique
   b. diaphragm
   c. rectus abdominus
   d. serratus

8. A muscle located on the chest wall is the:
   a. trapezius
   b. frontalis
   c. pectoralis major
   d. rectus abdominus

9. Muscle fatigue is caused by a buildup of:
   a. glycogen
   b. oxygen
   c. lactic acid
   d. ATP

10. The muscle on the calf portion of the leg is the:
   a. gastrocnemius
   b. sartorius
   c. rectus femoris
   d. tibialis anterior

APPLYING THEORY TO PRACTICE

1. Your body feels very warm after exercising. What has happened?

2. After running up a hill, you are out of breath and have a cramp in your leg. What caused the cramp? How can you relieve it? When will your breathing return to normal?

3. While looking at yourself in the mirror, look surprised. Name and locate the muscle you used. Place your fingers on the muscle and feel it contract. Do the same exercise making a frown and a smile.

4. Name the leg muscles that you would use to kick a soccer ball.

5. A friend who was involved in an accident is wearing a leg cast. Describe the condition that will occur without exercise. How can you prevent this condition?

6. A patient comes to the office and explains that she is on the school all-star tennis team, but her entire right shoulder and arm are hurting. The doctor states that her condition is known as rotator cuff disease. Explain recreation injuries to the patient and the details of this disease.

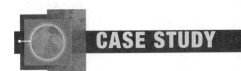

CASE STUDY

Carolyn is a 36-year-old mother of three young children. She had an accident while skiing. After 4 months, she is still experiencing pain in her right knee and is walking with a limp. Carolyn visits the orthopedic physician and is told she needs an arthroscopy examination. While doing the arthroscopy, the physician also removes scar tissue in her knee joint. The follow-up care requires intensive physical therapy.

1. What leg muscles were affected by Carolyn's injury?

2. Explain what an arthroscopy examination is.

3. What condition may result from limited mobility?

4. Name the health care professionals who will be involved with the physical therapy.

5. What are the benefits of a regular exercise program?

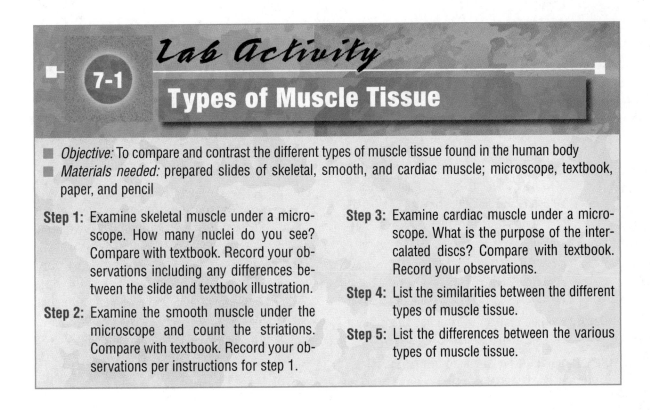

Lab Activity

7-1 Types of Muscle Tissue

- *Objective:* To compare and contrast the different types of muscle tissue found in the human body
- *Materials needed:* prepared slides of skeletal, smooth, and cardiac muscle; microscope, textbook, paper, and pencil

Step 1: Examine skeletal muscle under a microscope. How many nuclei do you see? Compare with textbook. Record your observations including any differences between the slide and textbook illustration.

Step 2: Examine the smooth muscle under the microscope and count the striations. Compare with textbook. Record your observations per instructions for step 1.

Step 3: Examine cardiac muscle under a microscope. What is the purpose of the intercalated discs? Compare with textbook. Record your observations.

Step 4: List the similarities between the different types of muscle tissue.

Step 5: List the differences between the various types of muscle tissue.

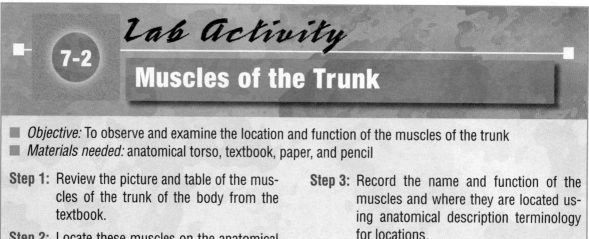

Lab Activity 7-2

Muscles of the Trunk

■ *Objective:* To observe and examine the location and function of the muscles of the trunk
■ *Materials needed:* anatomical torso, textbook, paper, and pencil

Step 1: Review the picture and table of the muscles of the trunk of the body from the textbook.

Step 2: Locate these muscles on the anatomical torso.

Step 3: Record the name and function of the muscles and where they are located using anatomical description terminology for locations.

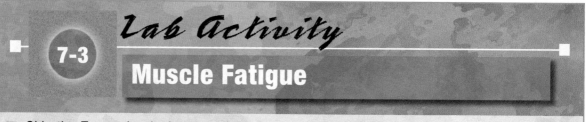

Lab Activity 7-3

Muscle Fatigue

■ *Objective:* To examine the function of the muscle and the effects work has on the muscle
■ *Materials needed:* textbook, stopwatch, blood pressure cuff, paper, and pencil

Step 1: Perform this activity with a lab partner. Rest your elbow on the lab table or desk, with your hand facing you. Open and close your hand making a fist as many times as you can in 30 seconds. Have your lab partner count and record the number of times you open and close your hand.

Step 2: Repeat this activity three more times. Have your lab partner record the number of times you can make the fist in each cycle.

Step 3: Has the number of fists you made in the 30-second period changed?

Step 4: Do you have any sign of muscle aches? Record your answer.

Switch places with your lab partner and repeat steps 1 through 4. Are there any differences in the numbers? Record your answer.

Step 5: Stand up; hold the textbook in your left arm with the arm hanging straight down. Keep your arm straight and raise your arm with the book to shoulder level, lower it, and then count the number of times you can raise and lower the book in 30 seconds. Have your lab partner record the number of times you lifted the textbook.

Step 6: Repeat this activity three more times.

continues

continued

Step 7: Has the number of times you raised and lowered the textbook changed? Record your results.

Step 8: Do you have any sign of muscle aches? Record your answer.

Switch places with your lab partner and repeat steps 5 through 8. Are there any differences in the numbers between you and your lab partner?

Step 9: Apply a blood pressure cuff to your left arm. Inflate the blood pressure cuff to place tension on the muscle. Repeat steps 5 through 8.

Step 10: What differences occur when tension is applied to the muscle?

Step 11: What has occurred in your muscles during these activities that may have caused muscle fatigue? Write a brief paragraph to describe the events including how the muscle returns to its normal state after muscle activity.

This lab activity can be done at home with different family members or friends. Are there differences that might be related to age, gender, or physical fitness of the individual?

Chapter 8

CENTRAL NERVOUS SYSTEM

Key Words

Alzheimer's disease
anticonvulsant
arachnoid (mater)
associative neuron
autonomic nervous
  system
axons
blood-brain barrier
brain stem
brain tumor
central nervous
  system
cerebellum
cerebral aqueduct
cerebral cortex
cerebral palsy
cerebral ventricles
cerebrospinal fluid
cerebrum
choroid plexus
corpus callosum
dementia
dendrites
diencephalon
dura mater

encephalitis
epilepsy
fibers
fissures
fourth ventricle
frontal lobe
gyri (convolutions)
hematoma
hydrocephalus
hypothalamus
interneuron
interventricular
  foramen
lateral ventricle
lumbar puncture
medulla oblongata
membrane
  excitability
memory
meninges
meningitis
motor neuron
  (efferent)
multiple sclerosis
  (MS)

myelin sheath
  (neurilemma)
neuroglia
neuron
nystagmus
occipital lobe
parietal lobe
Parkinson's disease
peripheral nervous
  system
pia mater
poliomyelitis
pons
sensory neuron
  (afferent)
spastic
  quadriplegia
spinal cord
sulci
synapse
synaptic cleft
temporal lobe
thalamus
third ventricle

INTRODUCTION TO THE CENTRAL NERVOUS SYSTEM

The study of body functions reveals that the body consists of millions of small structures that perform a multitude of different activities; these are coordinated and integrated into one harmonious whole. The two main communications systems are the endocrine system and the nervous system. They send chemical messengers and nerve impulses to all of the structures. The endocrine system and hormonal regulation are discussed in other chapters. Hormonal regulations are slow, whereas neural regulation is comparatively rapid.

Functions of the central nervous system are as follows:

1. It is the communication and coordination system in the body.

   - It receives messages from stimuli all over the body.

   - The brain interprets the message.

   - The brain responds to the message and carries out an activity.

2. The brain is also the seat of intellect and reasoning.

The central nervous system is the most highly organized system of the body, consisting of the brain and spinal cord. The nerve cell, or **neuron,** is specially constructed to carry out its function: transmitting a message from one cell to the next. In addition to the nucleus, cytoplasm, and cell membrane, the neuron has extensions of cytoplasm from the cell body. These extensions, or processes, are called **dendrites** and **axons.** There may be several dendrites, but only one axon in each cell. These processes, or **fibers,** are paths along which nerve impulses travel, Figure 8-1. The axon has a specialized covering called **neurilemma** or **myelin sheath,** Figure 8-1. This covering speeds up the nerve impulse as it travels along the axon. The myelin sheath produces a fatty substance called myelin, which protects the axon; this substance is also called white matter. The nodes of Ranvier is the area where no myelin is present. This is important in the conduction of a nerve impulse. Axons carry messages away from the cell body. Dendrites carry messages to the cell body.

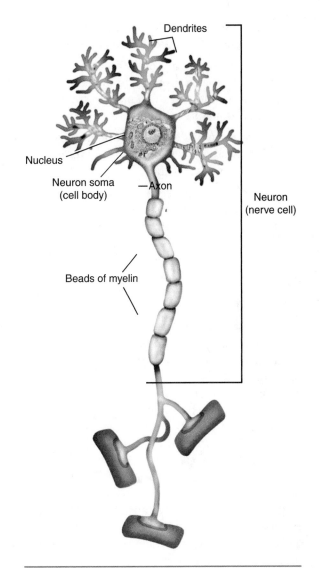

Figure 8-1 *A neuron*

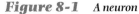

Nervous Tissue

Nerve tissue consists of two major types of nerve cells: **neuroglia** and neurons. Neuroglia is the type of cells that insulate, support, and protect the neurons. They are sometimes referred to as "nerve glue."

All neurons possess the characteristics of being able to react when stimulated and of being able to pass the nerve impulse generated on to other neurons. These characteristics are irritability (the ability to react when stimulated) and conductivity (the ability to transmit a disturbance to distant points). The dendrites receive the impulse and transmit it to the cell body, and then to the axon where it is passed on to another neuron or to a muscle or gland. There are three types of neurons:

1. **Sensory neurons** or **afferent** neurons, which emerge from the skin or sense organs and carry messages or impulses toward the spinal cord and brain

2. **Motor neurons** or **efferent** neurons, which carry messages from the brain and spinal cord to the muscles and glands

3. **Associative neurons** or **interneurons**, which carry impulses from the sensory neuron to the motor neuron

Function of the Nerve Cell/ Membrane Excitability

Nerves carry impulses by creating electric charges in a process known as **membrane excitability.** Neurons have a membrane that separates the cytoplasm inside from the extracellular fluids outside the cell, thereby creating two chemically different areas. Each area has differing amounts of potassium and sodium ions and some other charged substances, with the inside part of the cell being more negatively charged than the outside. When a neuron is stimulated, ions move across the membrane creating a current which, if large enough, will briefly cause the inside of the neuron to be more positive than the outside area. This state is known as action potential. Neurons and other cells that produce action potentials are said to have membrane excitability.

To understand how impulses are carried along nerves or throughout a muscle when it contracts, we need to learn a little more about membrane excitability. Ions cross a membrane through channels, some of which are open and allow ions to "leak" (diffuse) continuously. Other channels are called "gated" and open only during action potential. Another membrane opening is called a sodium-potassium pump which, by active transport, maintains the flow of ions from higher to lower concentration levels across the membrane and restores the cytoplasm and extracellular fluid to their original electrical state, after an action potential occurs. This action is in response to the imbalance between the cytoplasm and the extracellular fluid. When diffusion takes place,

ions move from an area of greater concentration to an area of lesser concentration.

The following simplified description explains how this process works.

1. A neuron membrane is "at rest." There are large amounts of potassium (K+) ions inside the cells but not many sodium (Na+) ions. The reverse is true outside the cell in the extracellular fluid. Most of the open channels are for potassium to pass through, so it leaks out of the cell.

2. As the K+ ions leave, the inside becomes relatively more negative until some K+ ions are attracted back in and the electrical force balances the diffusion force and movement stops. The inside is still more negative and the amount of energy between the two differently charged areas is ready to work (carry an impulse). This state is called resting membrane potential, Figure 8-2A. The membrane is now polarized. The sodium ions are not able to move "in," because their channels are closed during the resting state; however, if a few leak in, the membrane pump sends out an equal number.

3. Now suppose a sensory neuron receptor is stimulated by something (e.g., a sound). This will cause a change in the membrane potential. The stimulus energy is converted to an electrical signal and if it is strong enough, it will depolarize a portion of the membrane and allow the gated Na+ ion channels to open, initiating an action potential, Figure 8-2B.

4. The Na+ ions move through the gated channels into the cytoplasm and the inside becomes more positive until the membrane potential is reversed and the gates close to Na+ ions.

5. Next the K+ gates open and large amounts of potassium leave the cytoplasm resulting in the repolarization of the membrane, Figure 8-2C. After repolarization, the sodium-potassium pump restores the initial concentrations of Na+ and K+ ions inside and outside the neuron.

This entire process occurs in a few milliseconds. When this action occurs in one part of the cell membrane, it spreads to adjacent membrane regions, continuing away from the original site

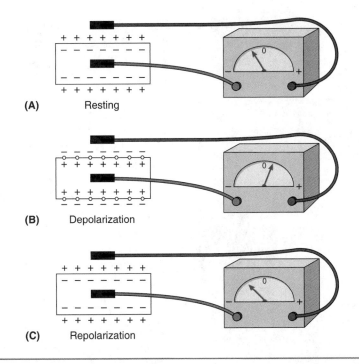

Figure 8-2 *Sequence of events in membrane potential and relative positive and negative states: (A) normal resting potential (negative inside/positive outside); (B) depolarization (positive inside/negative outside); and (C) repolarization (negative inside/positive outside)*

of stimulation, sending "messages" over the nerve. This cycle is completed millions of times a minute throughout the body, day after day, year after year.

Synapse

A **synapse** is where the messages go from one cell to the next cell. The nerve cell has both an axon and a dendrite. Messages go from the axon of one cell to the dendrite of another; they never actually touch. The space between them is known as the **synaptic cleft.** The conduction is accomplished through neurotransmitters at the end of each axon, which are special chemicals, namely epinephrine, norepinephrine, and acetylcholine.

An impulse travels along the axon to the end where the neurotransmitter is released. This helps the impulse to "jump" the space between and the impulse is sent to the dendrite of the next nerve cell: The neurotransmitter between muscle cells and the nervous system cells is acetylcholine.

DIVISIONS OF THE NERVOUS SYSTEM

The nervous system can be divided into three divisions: the central, peripheral, and autonomic nervous system.

1. The **central nervous system** consists of the brain and spinal cord.

2. The **peripheral nervous system** consists of nerves of the body: 12 pairs of cranial nerves extending out from the brain and 31 pairs of spinal nerves extending out from the spinal cord.

3. The **autonomic nervous system** includes peripheral nerves and ganglia (a group of cell bodies outside the central nervous system that carry impulses to involuntary muscles and glands).

Where decision is called for and action must be considered, the central and peripheral nervous systems are involved. They carry information to the brain where it is interpreted, organized, and

Effects of Aging on The Nervous System

As an individual ages, there is a general slowing of nerve conduction due to a decrease in the number of functioning neurons and a degeneration of the existing nerves.

Changes in the nervous system are primarily due to diminished blood supply to the brain and loss of neurons. Slow, progressive loss in brain size in the cerebral cortex leads to impairment in thinking, reasoning, and remembering. There is a decrease in motor and sensory nerve conduction and a slowing of reaction time. Nervous system changes basically affect all voluntary and automatic nervous system functions.

Alterations also occur in the sleep patterns of the aging. They are more easily wakened, take longer to fall asleep, awaken more frequently through the night, spend more time in bed lying awake, and are more susceptible to stress-related sleep disturbances; yet, they do not have a decreased need for sleep. Napping, which increases with aging, is a normal pattern.

stored. An appropriate command is sent to organs or muscles. The autonomic nervous system supplies heart muscle, smooth muscle, and secretory glands with nervous impulses as needed. It is usually involuntary in action.

THE BRAIN

The adult human brain is a highly developed, complex, and intricate mass of soft nervous tissue. It weighs about 1400 g (3 lb) and consists of 100 billion neurons. The brain is protected by the bony cranial cavity. Further protection is afforded by three membranous coverings called **meninges,** and the cerebrospinal fluid. The brain is white and gray matter. The outer cortex, known as the **cerebral cortex,** is gray. This is the highest center of reasoning and intellect. You may have heard people say when trying to resolve a problem, "I need to use my gray matter." The deeper part of the cerebral cortex consists of myelinated nerve tracts and it is called the white matter. An adequate blood supply to the brain is critical. Without oxygen, brain damage will occur within 4 to 8 minutes. The brain is divided into four major parts: the cerebrum, diencephalon, cerebellum, and brain stem, see Figure 8-3.

Memory

The brain is our warehouse that stores "old" information we have learned and packages and stores new information. We call this process **memory.** To create a memory, nerve cells are thought to form new interconnections. No one area of the brain stores all memories, because the storage site depends on the type of memory. For example, how to swim would be held in the motor area of the brain, whereas visual memories would be stored in the visual area of the brain. Scientists believe that the hippocampus of the limbic system acts like a receptionist, deciding the significance of the event and determining where in the brain the information should be stored.

Memory may be short term or long term—depending on how much attention we pay to an event, how many times we repeat an activity, and the kinds of memory associations. People frequently recall what took place during a traumatic event, such as their first day at school. Compare that with how many times you see a commercial before you can remember it.

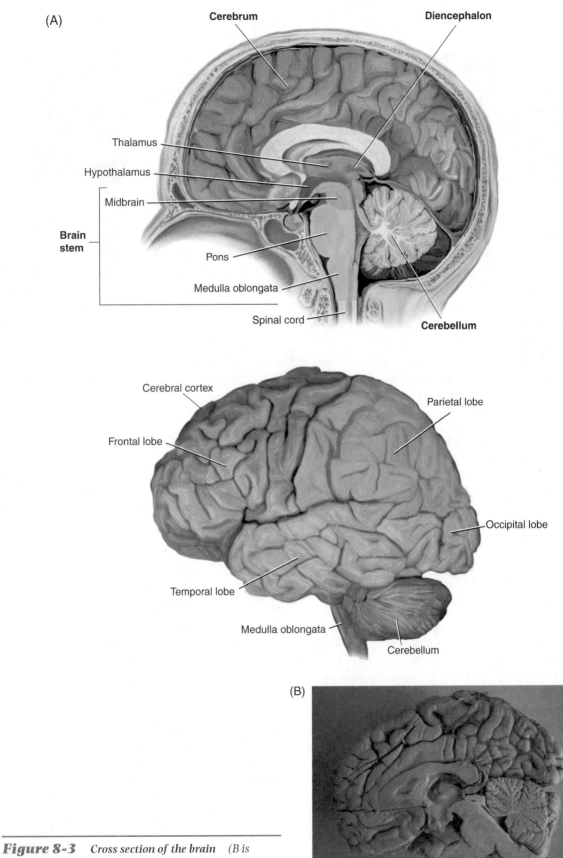

(A)

Cerebrum

Diencephalon

Thalamus

Hypothalamus

Brain stem

Midbrain

Pons

Medulla oblongata

Spinal cord

Cerebellum

Cerebral cortex

Parietal lobe

Frontal lobe

Occipital lobe

Temporal lobe

Medulla oblongata

Cerebellum

(B)

Figure 8-3 *Cross section of the brain* *(B is courtesy of Theodore King, University of Wisconsin, Milwaukee, WI)*

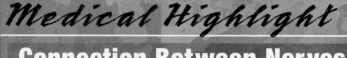

Medical Highlight

Connection Between Nerves and Muscles

Scientists have unraveled the secret of how a nerve communicates with a muscle. Dr. George Yancopoulos and another team working independently have produced the most detailed picture of this incredibly complex system. Their reports were published in the journal *CELL*.

Nerve cells communicate with each other and give orders to muscles by sending messages across gaps called *synapses.* Nerves and muscles create chemically intricate synapses in just the right places. The secret is two proteins: one is called agrin and another is known as muscle-specific receptor kinase, or MuSK. In working with mice, the researchers found that both proteins were necessary during embryonic development to make working connections between nerves and muscles. If either protein was missing, the mice were unable to breathe and died soon after birth.

During development it appears that nerve cells grow toward muscles and release agrin. On the muscle side of the gap, the agrin is received by MuSK, which works in combination with another protein called muscle-associated-specificity component. This connection starts a complicated chain reaction that eventually results in changes in both the nerve and the muscle, which add up to a working synapse. The nerve cells talk to the muscle cells by releasing the neurotransmitter acetylcholine. Agrin is the first step; it signals the muscle to pull together the chemicals it needs to construct acetylcholine receptors so that it can receive these messages.

This discovery may offer insight into how cell-to-cell communication goes on inside the brain and it could also lead to new treatments for nerve injuries and a variety of diseases.

Coverings of the Brain

The three meninges are the dura mater, arachnoid, and pia mater, see Figure 8-4. The **dura mater** is the outer brain covering, which lines the inside of the skull. This is a tough, dense membrane of fibrous connective tissue containing an abundance of blood vessels. The **arachnoid (mater)** is the middle layer. It resembles a fine cobweb with fluid-filled spaces. Covering the brain surface itself is the **pia mater,** consisting of blood vessels held together by fine areolar connective tissue. The space between the arachnoid and pia mater is filled with cerebrospinal fluid, produced within the ventricles of the brain. This fluid acts both as a shock absorber and a source of nutrients for the brain.

Ventricles of the Brain

The brain contains four lined cavities filled with cerebrospinal fluid. These cavities are called **cerebral ventricles,** Figure 8-5. The ventricles lie deep within the brain. The two largest, located within the cerebral hemispheres, are known as the right and left **lateral ventricles.**

The **third ventricle** is placed behind and below the lateral ventricles. It is connected to the two lateral ventricles via the **interventricular foramen.** The **fourth ventricle** is situated below the third, in front of the cerebellum, and behind the pons and the medulla oblongata (brain stem). The third and fourth ventricles are interconnected via a narrow canal called the **cerebral aqueduct.**

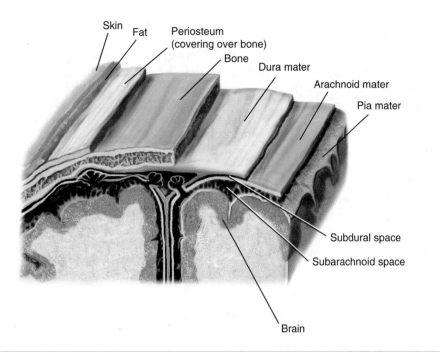

Figure 8-4 *The meninges*

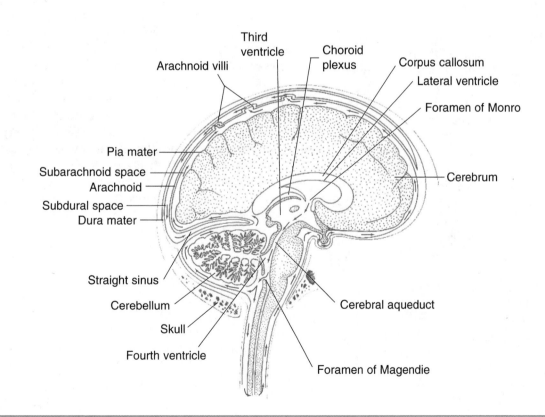

Figure 8-5 *Circulation of the cerebrospinal fluid*

Each of the four ventricles contains a rich network of blood vessels of the pia mater, referred to as the **choroid plexus.** The choroid plexus is in contact with the cells lining the ventricles, which helps in the formation of cerebrospinal fluid.

Cerebrospinal Fluid and Its Circulation.
Cerebrospinal fluid is a substance that forms inside the four brain ventricles from the blood vessels of the choroid plexuses. This fluid serves as a liquid shock absorber protecting the delicate brain and spinal cord. It is formed by filtration from the intricate capillary network of the choroid plexuses. The fluid transports nutrients to, and removes metabolic waste products from, the brain cells.

Choroid plexus capillaries differ significantly in their selective permeability from capillaries in other areas of the body. As a result, drugs carried in the bloodstream may not effectively penetrate brain tissue, rendering infections (such as meningitis) difficult to cure. This phenomenon is commonly referred to as the **blood-brain barrier.**

After filling the two lateral ventricles of the cerebral hemispheres, the cerebrospinal fluid seeps into the third ventricular through the foramen (opening). From here it flows through the cerebral aqueduct into the fourth ventricle. The fluid then passes through the foramen of the fourth ventricle and the two lateral foramina of the fourth ventricle into the small, tubelike central canal of the cord and into the subarachnoid spaces. The subarachnoid spaces are thus filled with cerebrospinal fluid which bathes the brain and the spinal cord. Ultimately the cerebrospinal fluid returns to the bloodstream via the venous structures in the brain, called arachnoid villi.

The formation and circulation of cerebrospinal fluid is used by members of the health team to detect some defects or disease of the brain. For example, inflammation of the cranial meninges quickly spreads to the meninges of the spinal cord. This leads to an increased secretion of cerebrospinal fluid which collects in the confined bony cavity of the brain and spinal column. The accumulation of excess fluid causes headaches, reduced pulse rate, slow breathing, and partial or total unconsciousness.

Removal of cerebrospinal fluid for diagnostic purposes is accomplished with a **lumbar puncture.** The needle used to withdraw the cerebrospinal fluid is inserted between the third and fourth lumbar vertebrae. The fluid or exudate withdrawn contains by-products of the inflammation and organisms causing it. Therefore, a lumbar puncture is helpful in diagnosing such diseases as cerebral hemorrhage, increased pressure, intracranial tumors, meningitis, and syphilis. It also serves to alleviate the pressure caused by meningitis, and especially hydrocephalus.

CEREBRUM

The **cerebrum** is the largest part of the brain. It occupies the whole upper part of the skull and weighs about 2 pounds. Covering the upper and lower surfaces of the cerebrum is a layer of gray matter called the cerebral cortex.

The cerebrum is divided into two hemispheres—right and left—by a deep groove known as the longitudinal fissure. The cerebral surface is completely covered with furrows and ridges. The deeper furrows, or grooves, are referred to as **fissures;** the shallower ones are called **sulci.**

The elevated ridges between the sulci are the **gyri,** or **convolutions,** Figure 8-6. These convolutions serve to increase the surface area of the brain, resulting in a proportionately larger amount of gray matter. The arrangement of the gyri and sulci on the brain's surface varies from one brain to another. Certain fissures, however, are constant and represent important demarcations. They help to localize specific functional areas of the cerebrum, and to divide each hemisphere into four lobes.

Each cerebral hemisphere is divided into a frontal, parietal, occipital, and temporal lobe. These lobes correspond to the cranial bones by which they are overlaid, see Figure 8-6.

The five major fissures dividing the cerebral hemispheres include:

1. *Longitudinal fissure*—a deep groove divides the cerebrum into two hemispheres. The middle region of the two hemispheres is held together by a wide band of axonal fibers called the **corpus callosum.**

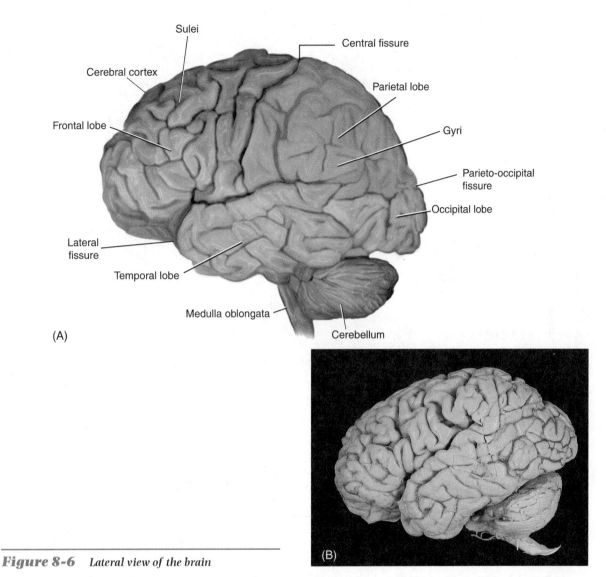

Sulei

Cerebral cortex

Frontal lobe

Central fissure

Parietal lobe

Gyri

Parieto-occipital fissure

Occipital lobe

Lateral fissure

Temporal lobe

Medulla oblongata

Cerebellum

(A)

(B)

Figure 8-6 *Lateral view of the brain*

2. *Transverse fissure*—divides the cerebrum from the cerebellum.

3. *Central fissure,* or *fissure of Rolando*—located beneath the coronal suture of the skull, dividing the frontal from the parietal lobes.

4. *Lateral fissure* or *fissure of Sylvius*—situated on the side of the cerebral hemispheres, dividing the frontal and temporal lobes.

5. *Parieto-occipital fissure*—the least obvious of all the fissures, serves to separate the occipital lobe from the parietal and temporal lobes, although no definite demarcation between these two lobes exists.

Cerebral Functions

Each lobe of the cerebral hemispheres controls different types of functions, Figure 8-7.

1. **Frontal lobe**—The cerebral cortex of the frontal lobe controls the motor functions of humans. The motor area occupies a long band of cortex, just in front of the central fissure in the posterior part of the frontal lobe. This motor area controls the voluntary muscles. Cells in the right hemisphere activate voluntary movements which occur in the left side of the body; the left hemisphere controls voluntary movements of the right side. The

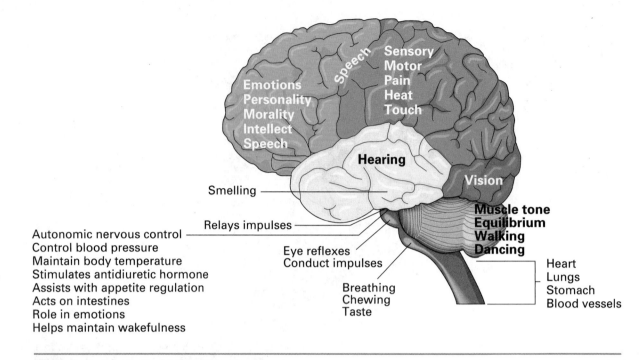

Emotions
Personality
Morality
Intellect
Speech

Speech

Sensory
Motor
Pain
Heat
Touch

Hearing

Smelling

Vision

Relays impulses

Muscle tone
Equilibrium
Walking
Dancing

Autonomic nervous control
Control blood pressure
Maintain body temperature
Stimulates antidiuretic hormone
Assists with appetite regulation
Acts on intestines
Role in emotions
Helps maintain wakefulness

Eye reflexes
Conduct impulses

Breathing
Chewing
Taste

Heart
Lungs
Stomach
Blood vessels

Figure 8-7   *Cerebral functions*

frontal lobe also includes two areas which control speech. The speech area, located anterior to the central fissure usually in the left hemisphere, is also called Broca's area. This area is associated with our ability to speak. Damage to this area means that you may know what to say, but you cannot vocalize the words. The speech area which allows us to recognize words and to interpret the meaning, spoken or read, is located at the junction of the temporal, parietal, and occipital lobes.

2. **Parietal lobe**—The parietal lobe comprises the sensory (somesthetic) area. It is found behind the fissure of Rolando, in front of the parietal lobe. This area receives and interprets nerve impulses from the sensory receptors for pain, touch, heat, and cold. It further helps in the determination of distances, sizes, and shapes.

3. **Occipital lobe**—The occipial lobe, located over the cerebellum, houses the visual area, controlling eyesight.

4. **Temporal lobe**—The upper part of the temporal lobe contains the auditory area (including specific tones); the anterior part of the lobe is occupied by the olfactory (smell) area.

The cerebral cortex also controls conscious thought, judgment, memory, reasoning, and willpower. This high degree of development makes the human the most intelligent of all animals.

DIENCEPHALON

The **diencephalon** is located between the cerebrum and the midbrain. It contains two major structures, the **thalamus** and the **hypothalamus.** The thalamus is a spherical mass of gray matter. It is found deep inside each of the cerebral hemispheres, lateral to the third ventricle. The thalamus acts as a relay station for incoming and outgoing nerve impulses. It receives direct or indirect nerve impulses from the various sense organs of the body (with the exception of olfactory sensations). These nerve impulses are then relayed to the cerebral cortex. The thalamus also receives nerve impulses from the cerebral cortex, cerebellum, and other areas of the brain. Damage to the thalamus may result in increased sensitivity to pain, or total loss of consciousness.

The hypothalamus lies below the thalamus. It forms part of the lateral walls and floor of the third ventricle. A bundle of nerve fibers connects

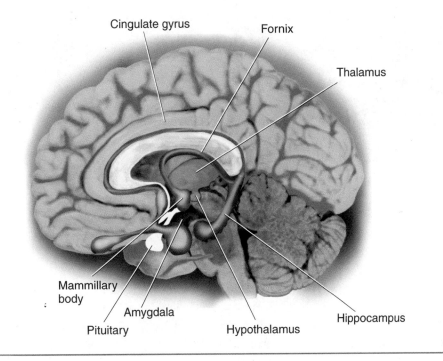

Figure 8-8   *The limbic system*

the hypothalamus to the posterior pituitary gland, the thalamus, and the midbrain. The limbic system is that part of the brain associated with emotional control, Figure 8-8. The hippocampal gyri of the limbic system helps to store and retain short-term memory. The hypothalamus is part of the limbic system and is considered to be the "brain" of the brain. Through the use of feedback, the hypothalamus stimulates the pituitary to release its hormones. Nine vital functions are performed by the hypothalamus.

1. *Autonomic nervous control*—Regulates the parasympathetic and sympathetic systems of the autonomic nervous system.

2. *Cardiovascular control*—Controls blood pressure, regulating the constriction and dilation of blood vessels and the beating of the heart.

3. *Temperature control*—Helps in the maintenance of normal body temperature (37°C or 98.6°F).

4. *Appetite control*—Assists in regulating the amount of food we ingest. The "feeding center," found in the lateral hypothalamus, is stimulated by hunger "pangs," which prompt us to eat. In turn, the "satiety center" in the medial hypothalamus becomes stimulated when we have eaten enough.

5. *Water balance*—Within the hypothalamus, certain cells respond to the osmotic pressure of the blood. When osmotic pressure is high, due to water deficiency, the antidiuretic hormone (ADH) is secreted. A "thirst area" is found near the satiety area, becoming stimulated when the blood's osmolality is high. This causes us to consume more liquids.

6. *Manufacture of oxytocin*—Contracts the uterus during labor.

7. *Gastrointestinal control*—Increases intestinal peristalsis and secretion from the intestinal glands.

8. *Emotional state*—Plays a role in the display of emotions such as fear and pleasure.

9. *Sleep control*—Helps keep us awake when necessary.

CEREBELLUM

The **cerebellum** is located behind the pons and below the cerebrum (see Figure 8-6). It consists of two hemispheres or wings: the right cerebellar hemisphere and the left cerebellar hemisphere. These two hemispheres are connected to a central portion

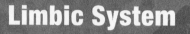

Limbic System

The limbic system influences unconscious, instinctive behaviors that relate to survival. This behavior is modified by the action of the cerebral cortex. Our primitive brain says, "I want it now"; our higher functioning brain says, "You can't have it now. You have to wait until later."

The limbic system encircles the top of the brain stem almost like a covering (the word *limbic* means "border"), linking the cerebral cortex and the midbrain areas with the lower centers that control the automatic functions of the body.

The limbic system plays a role in the expression of instincts, drives, and emotions; mediates the effects of the moods on external behavior; and influences internal changes in bodily functions. The association of feelings with sensations such as sight and smell and the formation of memories are influenced by the limbic system.

Parts of the limbic system include the following:

- *Septum pellucidum*—Connects the fornix to the corpus callosum.
- *Mammillary body*—This nucleus transmits messages between the fornix and thalamus.
- *Olfactory bulbs*—This connection may explain why the sense of smell evokes forgotten memories (think of good smells from your childhood).
- *Amygdala*—This structure influences behavior appropriate to meet the body's needs, which include feeding, sexual interest, and emotional reactions such as anger.
- *Parahippocampal gyrus*—Helps to modify strong emotions such as rage and fright.
- *Hippocampus*—Involves learning and memory, recognizes new information, and recalls spatial relationships.
- *Fornix*—Pathway of nerve fibers transmits information from the hippocampus to the mammillary body.
- *Cingulate gyrus*—This area, with others, comprises the limbic cortex which modifies behavior and emotion.

called the vermis. The cerebellum consists of gray matter on the outside and white matter on the inside. The white matter is marked with a treelike pattern called *arbor vitae* (meaning "tree of life").

The cerebellum communicates with the rest of the central nervous system by three pairs of tracts called peduncles. These three peduncles are composed of "incoming" axons that carry nerve messages into the cerebellum, and "outgoing" axons that transmit messages out of the cerebellum. The incoming axons carry messages to the cerebellum regarding movement within joints, muscle tone, position of the body, and tightness of ligaments and tendons. Any and all information relating to skeletal muscle activity is carried to the cerebellum. This information reaches the cerebel-

lum directly from sensory receptors including the inner ear, the eye, and the proprioceptors in skeletal muscle. The "outgoing" axons carry nerve messages to the different parts of the brain that control skeletal muscles.

Cerebellar Function

The cerebellum controls all body functions that have to do with skeletal muscles.

- *Maintenance of balance.* If the body is imbalanced, sensory receptors in the inner ear send nerve messages to the cerebellum. There the cerebellum carries impulses to the motor-controlling areas of the brain. These brain areas, in turn, stimulate muscle contraction that restores balance.

▨ *Maintenance of muscle tone.* The cerebellum transmits nerve impulses to the red nucleus that, in turn, relays them to the spinal cord and then to the skeletal muscles.

▨ *Coordination of muscle movements.* Any voluntary movement is initiated in the cerebral cortex. However, once the movement is started, its smooth execution is the role of the cerebellum. The cerebellum allows each muscle to contract at the right time, with the right strength, and for the right amount of time so that the overall movement is smooth and flowing. This is important when doing complex or skilled movements such as speaking, walking, writing; even simple movements need the coordinating abilities of the cerebellum. A simple action such as raising the hand to the face to avoid a blow requires the synchronized action of 50 or more muscles. These muscles then act on 30 separate bones of the arm and hand.

The removal of or injury to the cerebellum results in motor impairment.

BRAIN STEM

The **brain stem** is made up of three parts: the midbrain, pons, and the medulla, Figure 8-9. The brain

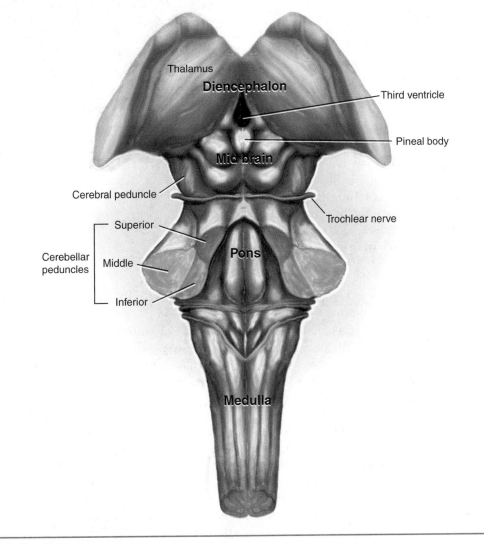

Figure 8-9   The brainstem

stem provides a pathway for the ascending and descending tracts (messages going to the cerebrum and messages coming back from the cerebrum). Extending the length of the brain stem is the gray matter of the reticular formation system. These are the neurons that are involved in the sleep-wake cycle. If there is damage to this area, coma results. The **pons** is located in front of the cerebellum, between the midbrain and the medulla oblongata. It contains interlaced transverse and longitudinal myelinated, white nerve fibers mixed with gray matter. The pons serves as a two-way conductive pathway for nerve impulses between the cerebrum, cerebellum, and other areas of the nervous system. The pons is also the site for the emergence of four pairs of cranial nerves, and it contains a center that controls respiration.

The midbrain extends from mammillary bodies to the pons. The cerebral aqueduct travels through the midbrain. It contains the nuclei for reflex centers involved with vision and hearing.

The **medulla oblongata** is a bulb-shaped structure found between the pons and the spinal cord. It lies inside the cranium and above the foramen magnum of the occipital bone. The medulla is white on the outside, like the pons, because of the myelinated nerve fibers that serve as a passageway for nerve impulses between the brain and spinal cord. It contains the nuclei for vital functions such as the heart rate, the rate and the depth of respiration, the vasoconstrictor center which affects blood pressure, and the center for swallowing and vomiting.

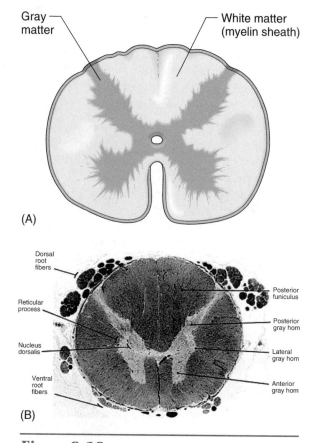

(A)

(B)

Figure 8-10 *Cross sections of the spinal cord. (B is from Atlas of Microscopic Anatomy: A Functional Approach: Companion to Histology and Neuroanatomy, by R. Bergman, A. Afifi, and P. Heidger, 1999, www.vh.org/ Providers/Textbooks/MicroscopicAnatomy.html. Reprinted with permission.)*

SPINAL CORD

The **spinal cord** continues down from the brain. It begins at the foramen magnum of the occipital bone and continues to the second lumbar vertebrae. It is white and soft and lies within the vertebrae of the spinal column. Like the brain, the spinal cord is submerged in cerebrospinal fluid and is surrounded by the three meninges. The gray matter in the spinal cord is located in the internal section; the white matter composes the outer part, Figure 8-10. In the gray matter of the cord, connections can be made between incoming and outgoing nerve fibers which provide the basis for reflex action. The spinal cord functions as both a reflex center and a conduction pathway to and from the brain.

DISORDERS OF THE CENTRAL NERVOUS SYSTEM

Meningitis is the inflammation of the linings of the brain and spinal cord. The cause may be bacterial or viral. The disease has outbreaks at times, appearing in high school or college age students. Symptoms include headache, fever, and stiff neck. In severe form, it may lead to paralysis, coma, and death. If the cause is bacterial, it may be treated with antibiotics.

Encephalitis is an inflammation of the brain. The disease may be caused by a virus; in certain conditions, the cause may be chemical. The symptoms of this disorder usually are fever, lethargy, extreme weakness, and visual disturbances.

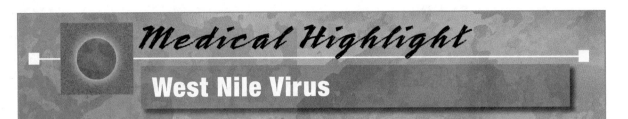

Medical Highlight

West Nile Virus

West Nile is a mosquito-borne virus that can cause encephalitis or meningitis. It is spread to humans by the bite of an infected mosquito. The mosquito becomes infected by biting a bird that carries the virus. Most people infected either have no symptoms or experience mild flulike symptoms. Some people may develop a mild rash or swollen lymph glands.

In some individuals, particularly the elderly, the virus may cause encephalitis or meningitis. There is no specific therapy; supportive therapy is given in most cases to prevent the risk of becoming infected.

To prevent the virus, take the following precautions. If outside from dusk to dawn when mosquitoes are most active or during the day in an area where there are weeds, tall grass, or bushes, wear protective clothing such as long pants, loose-fitting long-sleeve shirts, and socks. Consider use of an insect repellant containing DEET. To protect the home and reduce exposure to mosquitoes, drain water from pool covers, change the water in birdbaths every 3 to 4 days, eliminate any standing water, and make sure all windows and doors have tight-fitting screens.

Replace all screens that have tears or holes. If a mosquito has bitten you, see a doctor if you develop symptoms such as high fever, confusion, muscle weakness, severe headaches, stiff neck, or if your eyes become sensitive to light.

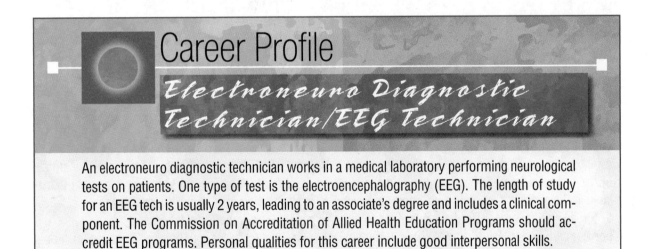

Career Profile

Electroneuro Diagnostic Technician/EEG Technician

An electroneuro diagnostic technician works in a medical laboratory performing neurological tests on patients. One type of test is the electroencephalography (EEG). The length of study for an EEG tech is usually 2 years, leading to an associate's degree and includes a clinical component. The Commission on Accreditation of Allied Health Education Programs should accredit EEG programs. Personal qualities for this career include good interpersonal skills.

Epilepsy is a seizure disorder of the brain, characterized by a recurring and excessive discharge from neurons. Approximately 1 in 200 persons in the United States suffers from some form of epilepsy. Epileptic seizures are believed to be a result of spontaneous, uncontrolled cycles of electrical activity in the neurons of the brain. The cause is uncertain. One portion of the brain stimulates another, setting off a cycle of activity that accelerates and runs its course until the neurons become fatigued. The subject may suffer hallucinations, a seizure (convulsion), and loss of consciousness. Grand mal, or severe, seizure is less frequent than the petit mal (milder) seizure. In petit mal, some victims seem to be staring or daydreaming. Medications used to control seizures are referred to as **anticonvulsants.** Examples are phenobarbital, dilantin, and tegretol.

Cerebral palsy is a disturbance in voluntary muscular action due to brain damage. Definite causes are unknown; it may be due to birth injury or abnormal brain development. The most pronounced characteristic is **spastic quadriplegia,** which involves spastic paralysis of all four limbs. The person with cerebral palsy frequently exhibits head rolling, grimacing, and difficulty in speech and swallowing. In cerebral palsy, there is usually no impairment of the intellect; the person frequently has normal or above normal intelligence.

Poliomyelitis is a disease of the nerve pathways of the spinal cord which causes paralysis. Since the Sabin and Salk vaccines are now used, this dis-

ease has been almost eliminated in the United States. However, the disease still occurs in other countries.

Hydrocephalus is a condition that involves an increased volume of cerebrospinal fluid within the ventricles of the brain. The usual cause is a blockage somewhere in the third or fourth ventricles. Enlargement of the head occurs. This condition is usually noted at birth. A bypass or shunt operation is performed to divert the cerebrospinal fluid around the blocked area. This operation prevents a buildup of pressure on brain tissue.

Parkinson's disease is characterized by tremors, a shuffling gait, pill-rolling (movement of the thumb and index finger), and muscular rigidity. The patient with Parkinson's has difficulty initiating movement. The cause may be a decrease of the neurotransmitter dopamine. Persons with Parkinson's disease are treated with the drug L-dopa and

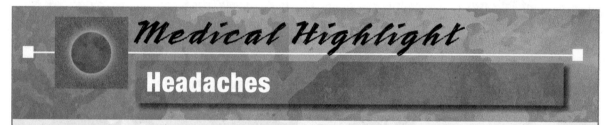

Medical Highlight

Headaches

Most Americans have headaches. The three most common types of headaches are tension, migraine, and cluster headaches. All cause different types of pain. In most cases, headache pain is not related to a separate underlying disease.

A tension headache is usually a dull, squeezing pain that builds slowly and may involve the forehead, scalp, back of the neck, and both sides of the head. Researchers believe the cause is related to levels of the chemical serotinin and endorphins in the brain. Triggers may be stress, poor posture, depression, and anxiety. Treatment involves pain relievers, rest, ice packs, warm compresses, and relaxation techniques.

Migraine headaches affect 28 million Americans; women are three times more likely than men to be affected. They often run in families. Pain may last from a few hours to days. The throbbing pain occurs on one side of the head

and gradually spreads. Migraines may be accompanied by nausea and vomiting. Lights, sounds, and odors may aggravate the migraine. In some people, a migraine is preceded by a visual distortion or aura. The cause is not fully understood. Trigger mechanisms for women may include a change in hormonal levels, dietary factors, lifestyle factors, and certain medications. Treatment includes prescription pain medications to prevent or stop the pain, exercise, and rest in a darkened, quiet room.

Cluster headache pain is worse than migraine pain. This type of headache occurs more frequently in men, usually 50% to 70%. Cluster headaches can occur one or more times daily for weeks—often at the same time each day—and then will disappear for months. Treatment includes 100% oxygen and prescription medications for pain.

Source: Mayo Health Clinic Letter, September 2001

other drugs which help to control the symptoms of the disease.

Multiple sclerosis (MS) is a chronic inflammatory disease of the central nervous system in which immune cells attack the myelin sheath of nerve cell axons. The myelin sheaths are destroyed, leaving scar tissue on the nerve cells. This destruction delays or completely blocks the transmission of nerve impulses in the affected areas. The cause is unknown. There is no definitive test for MS. The diagnosis is symptoms and signs of impairment to more than one area of the central nervous system, occurring at more than one time.

Symptoms include weakness of extremities, numbness, double vision, **nystagmus** (tremorous movement of the eye), speech problems, loss of coordination, and possible paralysis. It typically strikes young adults between the ages of 20 and 40; about two-thirds are women. With MS there are outbreaks of the symptoms and then the disease may go into remission for a long period of time. This disease is classified in the autoimmune category and drugs such as interferon and Avonex are used, which can slow progression of the disease and decrease the number of flare-ups. Adequate rest, exercise, and minimal stress may also lessen the effects of MS.

Dementia is a general term that includes specific disorders such as Alzheimer's disease, vascular dementia, and others. Dementia is defined as a loss in at least two areas of complex behavior, such as language, memory, visual and spatial abilities, or judgment that significantly interferes with a person's daily life. *Note:* Everyone has weak areas and people are frequently forgetful. This does not necessarily mean that the person is experiencing dementia.

Alzheimer's disease is a progressive disease in which the initial symptom is usually a problem with remembering recently learned information. With Alzheimer's disease, the nerve endings in the cortex of the brain degenerate and block the signals that pass between nerve cells. These areas of degeneration have a unique appearance and are called plaques. The nerve cells undergo further change and abnormal fibers build up, creating neurofibrillary tangles, like a group of telephone lines getting tangled.

The cause of Alzheimer's is unknown. The cells that produce the neurotransmitter acetylcholine are sometimes destroyed in this disease. The cause of the disease may be virus related, involve environmental factors, or be associated with a gene defect on chromosome 21.

Alzheimer's disease usually has three stages. The first may last from 2 to 4 years and involves confusion, short-term memory loss, anxiety, and poor judgment. In the second stage, which may last from 2 to 10 years, there is an increase in memory loss, difficulty in recognizing people, motor problems, logic problems, and loss of social skills. The third stage includes the inability to recognize oneself, weight loss, seizures, mood swings, and aphasia (loss of speech). This stage may last from 1 to 3 years.

Factors that may help prevent Alzheimer's disease are continued education, cardiovascular exercise, estrogen replacement therapy, antioxidants such as vitamins C, E, and betacarotene, and the use of anti-inflammatory agents.

Brain tumors may develop in any area of the brain. The symptoms depend on which area of the brain is involved. Early detection, surgery, and chemotherapy may cure some cases of brain tumors.

Hematoma is a localized mass of blood collection and may occur in the spaces between the meninges. The cause may be a traumatic blow to the head; the person may have a subdural hematoma (located between the dura mater and arachnoid layer).

Medical Terminology

arach	spider's web
-oid	resembling
arach/noid	structure resembling a spider's web
cerebell	little brain
-um	presence of

cerebell/um	presence of little brain
cerebr	brain
-al	pertaining to
aqua	water
duct	channel
cerebr/al aqueduct	channel pertaining to brain fluid
cerebr	brain
cerebr/um	presence of brain
en	within
cephal	head
-itis	inflammation
en/ceph/al/itis	presence of inflammation within the head
hema	blood
-toma	tumor
hema/toma	blood tumor
hydro	water
-us	presence of
hydro/cephal/us	presence of water in the head
mening	membrane
mening/itis	inflammation of the membranes
neuro	nerve
-glia	glue
neuro/glia	nerve glue

REVIEW QUESTIONS

Select the letter of the choice that best completes the statement.

1. Each nerve cell has only one:
   a. axon
   b. neurilemma
   c. dendrite
   d. myelin

2. The fatty substance that helps to protect the axon is called:
   a. neurotransmitter
   b. myelin
   c. dendrite
   d. nodes of Ranvier

3. The junction between the axon of one cell and the dendrite of another is called:
   a. neurilemma
   b. myelin
   c. synaptic cleft
   d. nodes of Ranvier

4. The neurons that carry messages to the brain are called:
   a. motor
   b. associate
   c. connective
   d. sensory

5. The nervous system that consists of 12 pairs of cranial nerves and 31 pairs of spinal nerves is called:
   a. central
   b. peripheral
   c. sympathetic
   d. parasympathetic

6. The outermost covering of the meninges is:
   a. arachnoid
   b. arachnoid villa
   c. dura mater
   d. pia mater

7. The lumbar puncture must be done below the:
   a. first lumbar vertebrae
   b. second lumbar vertebrae
   c. third lumbar vertebrae
   d. sacrum

8. The frontal, parietal, temporal, and occipital lobes make up the:
   a. cerebrum
   b. cerebellum
   c. midbrain
   d. brain stem

9. The part of the brain associated with muscle movement is:
   a. midbrain
   b. thalamus
   c. cerebrum
   d. medulla

10. The thalamus and hypothalamus are parts of the:
   a. cerebrum
   b. cerebellum
   c. diencephalon
   d. brain stem

MATCHING

Match each term in Column I with its correct description in Column II.

Column I	Column II
_____ **1.** frontal lobe—cerebrum	a. auditory
_____ **2.** occiptal lobe—cerebrum	b. receptor for pain, touch, and so on
_____ **3.** hypothalamus	c. reflex center
_____ **4.** temporal lobe	d. speech area
_____ **5.** parietal lobe	e. maintain balance
_____ **6.** cerebellum	f. eyesight
_____ **7.** thalamus	g. respiratory center
_____ **8.** spinal cord	h. appetite control
_____ **9.** medulla	i. site for four pairs of cranial nerves
_____**10.** pons	j. relay station for nerve impulses

APPLYING THEORY TO PRACTICE

1. The central nervous system serves as the communication center of our bodies. Explain how your hand touches something cold and you know it; refer to a sensory neuron and the correct lobe of the cerebrum.

2. A blow to the head can cause a loss of consciousness. What centers in the brain are associated with alertness?

3. You frequently hear the expression, "I have early Alzheimer's"; explain what this means. Do you think this illness will have an impact on the cost of health care? Explain your answer.

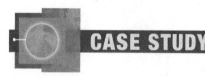

CASE STUDY

Mr. Anwari, age 73, is brought to the doctor's office by his daughter, Lucy, who is an LPN. She states her concerns about her father: During the past 2 months he has been found wandering in the neighborhood because he forgets where he lives. Neighbors would see him, note that he appears confused, and bring him home. Lucy is worried that her father is showing signs of early Alzheimer's disease.

1. Describe the physical changes that occur in the cortex of the brain.

2. How long may each stage of Alzheimer's disease last?

3. Describe the physiological and psychological changes that occur during these stages of Alzheimer's disease.

4. What are the functions of the frontal lobe of the cerebral cortex?

5. What parts of the limbic system may be affected in Alzheimer's disease?

6. What would be the concerns of the family when a person is diagnosed with this disease?

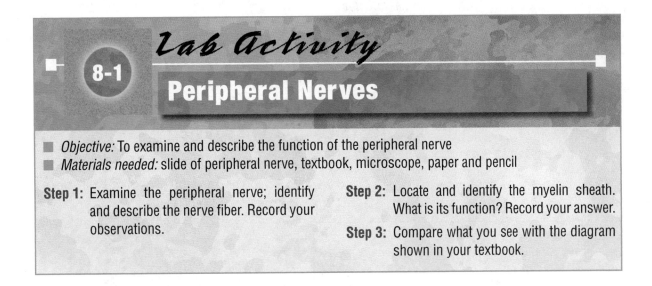

■ *Objective:* To examine and describe the function of the peripheral nerve
■ *Materials needed:* slide of peripheral nerve, textbook, microscope, paper and pencil

Step 1: Examine the peripheral nerve; identify and describe the nerve fiber. Record your observations.

Step 2: Locate and identify the myelin sheath. What is its function? Record your answer.

Step 3: Compare what you see with the diagram shown in your textbook.

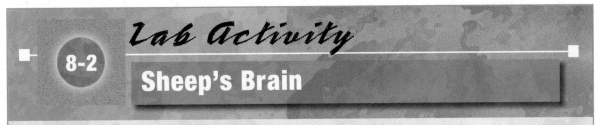

■ *Objective:* To compare and contrast the sheep's brain with the human brain and to identify the structures of the brain
■ *Materials needed:* anatomical human brain model, preserved sheep's brain, dissecting tray and instruments, disposable gloves, paper and pencil

Step 1: Put on disposable gloves.

Step 2: Examine the structures of the sheep's brain. Locate and describe the cerebral cortex, cerebellum, and brain stem. Record your observations of the location and appearance of these structures.

Step 3: Is there a difference in the structure and size of the cerebral cortex, cerebellum, and brain stem between the human brain and the sheep brain? Record your answer.

Step 4: Locate the dura mater on the sheep brain. Describe how it looks and feels. Record your observations.

Step 5: Place the sheep brain ventral side down on the dissecting pan.

Step 6: Using your dissecting knife, carefully cut along the longitudinal fissure of the sheep brain (it separates the two cerebral hemispheres); separate the sheep brain into right and left hemispheres.

continues

continued

Step 7: Examine the right portion of the sheep brain.

Step 8: Locate the arachnoid mater and pia mater in the right hemisphere. Describe the differences between these two meninges layers. Record your observations.

Step 9: Locate and describe the sizes and structures of the following: lateral ventricle, corpus callosum, midbrain, medulla, pons, and pituitary gland. Record your observations and describe the functions of these structures.

Step 10: Observe the anatomical model of the human brain. Compare the size and structure of the lateral ventricle, corpus callosum, midbrain, medulla, pons, and pituitary gland. Record your observations of the similarities and differences.

Step 11: Dispose of the sheep brain in the appropriate disposal containers.

Step 12: Clean all equipment.

Step 13: Remove your gloves and wash your hands.

Step 14: Compare your observations with those of your lab partner.

Chapter

9

THE PERIPHERAL AND AUTONOMIC NERVOUS SYSTEM

Objectives

- Describe a mixed nerve
- Describe the functions of the cranial and spinal nerves
- Relate the functions of the sympathetic and parasympathetic nervous system
- Explain the simple reflex arc pattern
- Describe common disorders of the peripheral nervous system
- Define the key words that relate to this chapter

Key Words

analgesic
Bell's palsy
carpal tunnel
    syndrome
cranial nerves
effector
electromyograph
    (EMG)
ergonomics
femoral nerve
mixed nerve
motor (efferent)
    nerve

neuralgia
neuritis
parasympathetic
    system
paresthesia
phrenic nerve
plexus
radial nerve
receptor
reflex
sciatica

sciatic nerve
sensory (afferent)
    nerve
shingles (herpes
    zoster)
spinal nerves
stimulus
sympathetic
    system
trigeminal
    neuralgia

PERIPHERAL NERVOUS SYSTEM

The peripheral nervous system includes all the nerves of the body and ganglia (groups of cell bodies), see Figure 9-1. It connects the central nervous system to the various body structures. The autonomic nervous system is a specialized part of the peripheral system; it controls the involuntary, or automatic, activities of the vital internal organs.

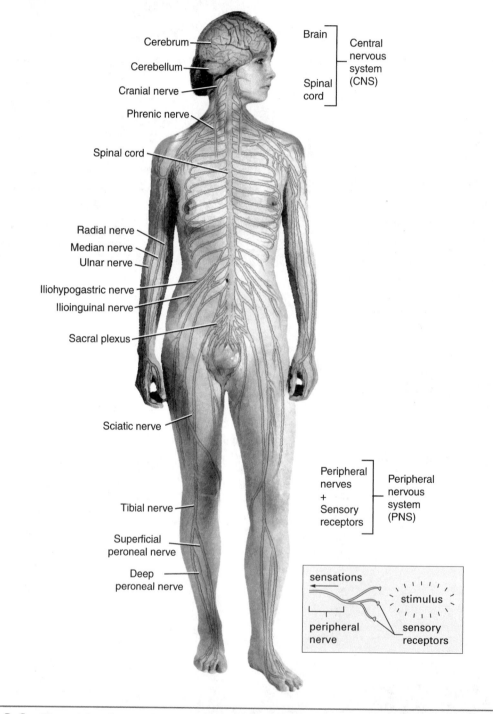

Cerebrum

Cerebellum

Cranial nerve

Phrenic nerve

Spinal cord

Radial nerve

Median nerve

Ulnar nerve

Iliohypogastric nerve

Ilioinguinal nerve

Sacral plexus

Sciatic nerve

Tibial nerve

Superficial peroneal nerve

Deep peroneal nerve

Brain

Spinal cord

Central nervous system (CNS)

Peripheral nerves + Sensory receptors

Peripheral nervous system (PNS)

sensations

stimulus

peripheral nerve

sensory receptors

Figure 9-1   *The peripheral nervous system connects the central nervous system to structures of the body*

Functions of the peripheral nervous system are as follows:

1. To control the automatic or involuntary activities of the body
2. To act as the reflex center of the body

NERVES

A nerve is bundles of nerve fibers enclosed by connective tissue. If the nerve's fibers carry impulses from the sense organs to the brain or spinal cord, it is called a **sensory, or afferent, nerve;** if its fibers carry impulses from the brain or spinal cord to muscles or glands, it is known as a **motor, or efferent, nerve;** and if it contains both sensory and motor fibers, it is called a **mixed nerve.**

CRANIAL AND SPINAL NERVES

Cranial and spinal nerves are part of the peripheral nervous system.

The **cranial nerves** are 12 pairs which begin in areas of the brain. The cranial nerves are designated by number and name; the name may give a clue to its function, Table 9-1. For example, the olfactory nerve, cranial nerve I, is responsible for the sense of smell. The optic nerve, cranial nerve II, is responsible for vision. The functions of the cranial nerves are concerned mainly with the activities of the head and neck, with the exception of the vagus nerve. The vagus nerve, cranial nerve X, is responsible for activities involving the throat as well as regulating the heart rate; it also affects the smooth muscle of the digestive tract. Most of the cranial nerves are mixed nerves: They carry both sensory and motor fibers. The olfactory, optic, and vestibulocochlear nerves, however, carry only the sensory fibers, meaning they pick up only the stimuli.

The **spinal nerves** originate at the spinal cord and go through openings in the vertebrae. There are 31 pairs of spinal nerves, and all are mixed nerves. The spinal nerves are named in relation to their location on the spinal cord. They carry messages to and from the spinal cord and brain and to all parts of the body. In a spinal cord injury, there is no sensation or movement. Each of these spinal nerves divides and branches. They go either directly to a particular body segment or they form a network with adjacent spinal nerves and veins called a **plexus,** Figure 9-2 and Table 9-2.

AUTONOMIC NERVOUS SYSTEM

The autonomic nervous system includes nerves, ganglia, and plexuses which carry impulses to all smooth muscle, secretory glands, and heart muscle, Figure 9-3. It regulates the activities of the visceral organs (heart and blood vessels, respiratory

Table 9-1 *Cranial Nerves*

NUMBER	NAME	FUNCTION
I	Olfactory	Smell
II	Optic	Vision, eyesight
III	Oculomotor	Movement of eye muscle
IV	Trochlear	Movement of eye muscle
V	Trigeminal	Face and teeth muscles, chewing
VI	Abducens	Movement of eye muscle
VII	Facial	Facial expressions, taste
VIII	Vestibulocochlear	Hearing and balance
IX	Glossopharyngeal	Movement of throat muscle, taste
X	Vagus	Movement of throat, affects heart, digestive system
XI	Accessory	Movement of neck muscles
XII	Hypoglossal	Movement of tongue muscles

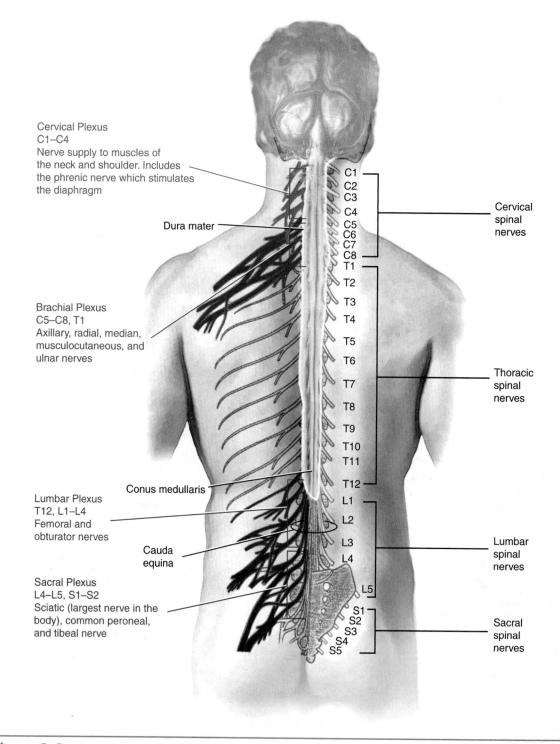

Cervical Plexus
C1–C4
Nerve supply to muscles of
the neck and shoulder. Includes
the phrenic nerve which stimulates
the diaphragm

Dura mater

Cervical
spinal
nerves

C1
C2
C3
C4
C5
C6
C7
C8
T1
T2
T3
T4
T5
T6
T7
T8
T9
T10
T11
T12
L1
L2
L3
L4
L5
S1
S2
S3
S4
S5

Brachial Plexus
C5–C8, T1
Axillary, radial, median,
musculocutaneous, and
ulnar nerves

Thoracic
spinal
nerves

Conus medullaris

Lumbar Plexus
T12, L1–L4
Femoral and
obturator nerves

Cauda
equina

Lumbar
spinal
nerves

Sacral Plexus
L4–L5, S1–S2
Sciatic (largest nerve in the
body), common peroneal,
and tibeal nerve

Sacral
spinal
nerves

Figure 9-2 *Spinal nerve plexus and important nerves*

Table 9-2 *Spinal Nerve Plexus*

NAME	LOCATION	FUNCTION
Cervical plexus	C1–C4	Supplies motor movement to muscles of neck and shoulders and receives messages from these areas. **Phrenic nerve** is part of this group and stimulates the diaphragm.
Brachial plexus	C5–C8, T1	Supplies motor movement to shoulder, wrist, and hand and receives messages from these areas. **Radial nerve** is part of this group and stimulates the wrist and hand.
Lumbar plexus	T12, L1–L4	Supplies motor movement to buttocks, anterior leg, and thighs and receives messages from these areas. **Femoral nerve** is part of this group and stimulates the hip and leg.
Sacral plexus	L4–L5, S1–S2	Supplies motor movement to posterior of leg and thighs and receives messages from these areas. **Sciatic nerve** is the largest nerve in the body and is part of this group. It passes through the gluteus maximus and down the back of the thigh and leg. It extends the hip and flexes the knee. (You must avoid this nerve when you are giving an IM injection.)

organs, alimentary canal, kidneys, urinary bladder, and reproductive organs). The activities of these organs are usually automatic—not subject to conscious control

The autonomic system has two divisions: the sympathetic and the parasympathetic. These two divisions may be antagonistic in their action. The sympathetic system may accelerate the heartbeat in response to fear, whereas the parasympathetic slows it down. Normally the two divisions are in balance; the activity of one or the other becomes dominant as dictated by the needs of the organism.

The **sympathetic system** consists primarily of two cords, beginning at the base of the brain and proceeding down both sides of the spinal column. These consist of nerve fibers and ganglia of nerve cell bodies. The cord between the ganglia is a cable of nerve fibers, closely associated with the spinal cord. Sympathetic nerves extend to all the vital internal organs, including the liver and pancreas, heart, stomach, intestines, blood vessels, the iris of the eye, sweat glands, and the bladder, Figure 9-3A. The sympathetic nervous system is often referred to as the "fight or flight system." When the body perceives it is in danger or under stress, it prepares to run away or stand and fight. The sympathetic nervous system sends the message to the adrenal medulla which secretes its hormones to prepare the body for this action. Think

about how you feel when you are facing a major test, or when you are waiting in the doctor's office for test results. You can feel your heart beating faster and your mouth going dry—all results of the automatic response to danger. When the danger passes, the parasympathetic nervous system will help restore the balance to the body system. If the system gets too much of the "stress hormones," health problems may result. Learning to live with stress is the key to a healthier body.

The **parasympathetic system** has two important active nerves: the vagus and the pelvic nerves. The vagus nerve, which extends from the medulla and proceeds down the neck, sends branches to the chest and neck. The pelvic nerve, emerging from the spinal cord around the hip region, sends branches to the organs in the lower part of the body, Figure 9-3B.

Both the sympathetic and parasympathetic nerves are strongly influenced by emotion. During periods of fear, anger, or stress, the sympathetic division acts to prepare the body for action. The effects of the parasympathetic are generally to counteract the effects of the sympathetic. For example, the sympathetic nervous system increases the rate of heart muscle contraction, and the parasympathetic decreases the rate. The two systems operate as a pair, striking a nearly perfect balance when the body is functioning properly.

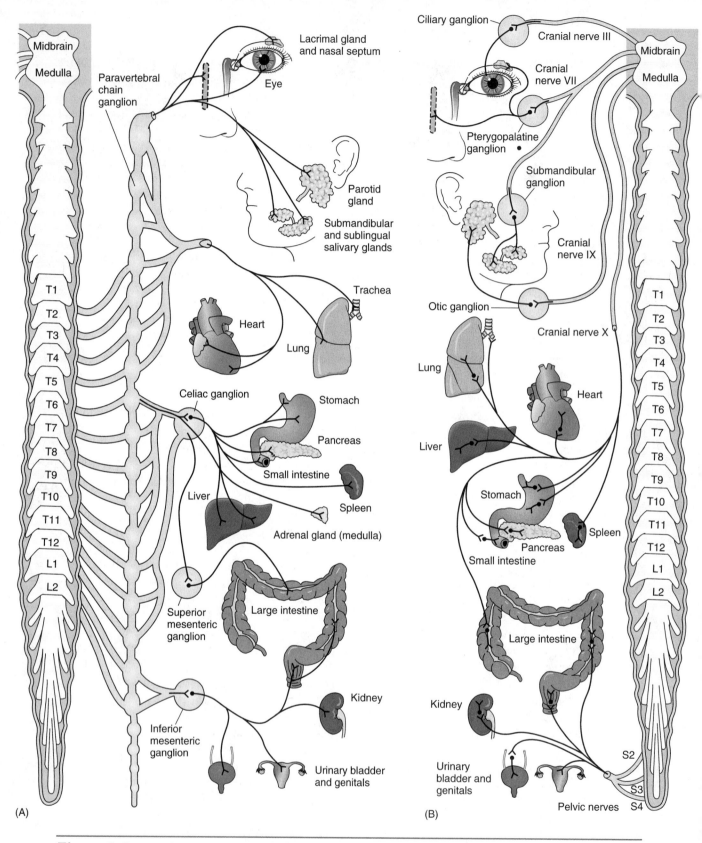

Figure 9-3 *A. The sympathetic division of the autonomic nervous system. B. The parasympathetic division of the autonomic nervous system.*

Reflex Act

The simplest type of nervous response is the **reflex** act, which is unconscious and involuntary. The blinking of the eye when a particle of dust touches it, the removing of the finger from a hot object, the secretion of saliva at the sight or smell of food, the movements of the heart, stomach, and intestines, are all examples of reflex actions.

Every reflex act is preceded by a change in the environment, called a **stimulus.** Examples of stimuli are sound waves, light waves, heat energy, and odors. Special structures called **receptors** pick up these stimuli. For example, the retina of the eye is the receptor for light; special cells in the inner ear are receptors for sound waves; and special structures in the skin are the receptors for heat and cold.

A simple reflex is one in which there is only a sensory nerve and a motor nerve involved. The classic example is the knee-jerk reflex. The knee is tapped and the leg extends, Figure 9-4. This test is used by physicians to test both the muscle and nervous systems.

Reaction to a stimulus is called the response. The response may be in the form of movement; in which case, the muscles are the **effectors,** or responding organs. If the response is in the form of a secretion, the glands are the effectors. Reflex actions, or autonomic reflexes, involving the skeletal muscles are controlled by the spinal cord. They also may be called somatic reflexes.

Biofeedback

Biofeedback is a measurement of physiological responses that yields information about the relationships between the mind and the body and helps people learn how to manipulate those responses through mental activity. While attached to sensitive devices that measure such bodily responses as skin temperature, blood pressure, galvanic skin resistance, and electrical activity in the muscles, the individual imagines stressful experiences. The person's physiological responses are then measured and recorded. The individual receives an interpretation of these responses and is taught methods for practicing relaxation to aid the maintenance of homeostasis.

Biofeedback is used as a restorative method in rehabilitation to help people who have lost sensation and function as the result of illness or injury. Biofeedback also enhances relaxation in tense muscles, relieves tension headaches, reduces bruxism (grinding of the teeth), reduces the pain of temporomandibular joint syndrome, and relieves backache.

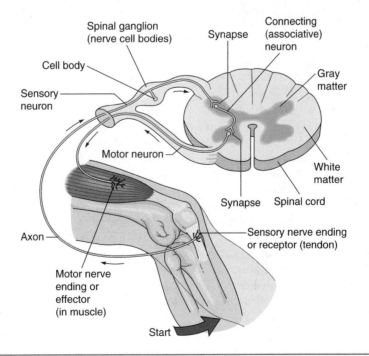

Figure 9-4 *In this example, tapping the knee (patellar tendon) results in extension of the leg, producing the knee-jerk reflex*

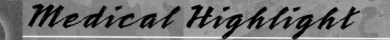

Medical Highlight
Cumulative Trauma Disorders

Computerization of the workplace has created not only a new way of life for many workers, but it has also contributed to one of the fastest growing occupational disorders. Cumulative trauma disorder (CTD) or repetitive motion disorder results from the repeated type of muscle use required for an activity such as using a computer keyboard.

A U.S. Bureau of Labor statistics report shows that CTD accounted for more than half of all occupational illnesses in the United States. This tissue inflammation and pain occurs in workers who spend many hours of the day repeating the same motion. This disorder has given rise to a new area of expertise called **ergonomics**,

which is the study of the application of biology and engineering to the relationship between workers and their environment.

Workers must be educated in the causes and symptoms of CTD. Additionally, workers must be educated in the proper use of tools and lifting techniques to prevent this disorder. For example, wrist disorders may be prevented by making changes in the computer work station such as adjusting the height of the keyboard and screens, and making sure that chairs are well suited to both the job and the individual worker.

Carpal tunnel syndrome is an example of CTD.

DISORDERS OF THE PERIPHERAL NERVOUS SYSTEM

Neuritis is an inflammation of a nerve or a nerve trunk. Symptoms may be severe pain, hypersensitivity, loss of sensation, muscular atrophy, weakness, and **paresthesia** (tingling, burning, and crawling of the skin). The causes of neuritis may be infectious, chemical, or due to other conditions such as chronic alcoholism. In the patient who is diagnosed with alcoholism, neuritis usually occurs because of a lack of vitamin B or improper diet.

In the treatment of neuritis it is necessary to determine the cause to eliminate the symptoms. The pain of neuritis may be relieved with **analgesics** (painkillers).

Sciatica is a form of neuritis that affects the sciatic nerve. The cause may be a rupture of a lumbar disc or arthritic changes. The most common symptom is pain which radiates through the buttock and behind the knee down to the foot. The person may have difficulty walking. Treatment includes traction, physiotherapy, exercises, and possible surgery to alleviate the symptoms.

Neuralgia is a sudden severe, sharp, stabbing pain along the pathway of a nerve. The pain

is often brief; it may be a symptom of a disease. The various forms of neuralgia are named according to the nerve they affect.

Trigeminal neuralgia is a condition that involves the fifth cranial nerve (trigeminal). The cause is unknown and the onset is rapid. The pain is severe. The spasm of pain can be brought on by so slight a stimulus as a breeze, a piece of food in the mouth, or even a change in temperature. The term "tic douloureux" is sometimes applied to this condition, because the pain lasts only 2 to 5 seconds. The treatment may be analgesics or partial removal of the fifth cranial nerve.

Bell's palsy is a condition that involves the seventh cranial nerve (facial). The patient seems to have had a stroke on one side of the face. Bell's palsy affects only one side of the face. The eye does not close properly, the mouth droops, and there is numbness on the affected side. The cause is unknown. Treatment consists of massage and heat application. The patient must do exercises such as whistling to prevent atrophy of the cheek muscles. The symptoms usually disappear within a few weeks, with no residual effects.

Shingles or **herpes zoster** is an acute viral nerve infection. It is characterized by a unilateral (one-sided) inflammation of a cutaneous nerve. The intercostal nerves are the ones most commonly affected. The course of nerve inflammation can spread to any nerve. For more discussion on shingles or herpes zoster, see Chapter 5.

Carpal tunnel syndrome is a condition that affects the median nerve and the flexor tendons that attach to the bones of the wrist (carpal). At the base of the palm is a tight canal or "tunnel" through which tendons and nerves pass on their way from the forearm to the hand and fingers. The median nerve and flexor tendon passes through this tunnel. The syndrome develops because of repetitive movement of the wrist, in which the hands are held in an unusual position. Swelling (edema) develops around the carpal tunnel, the edema causes pressure on the nerve, which results in pain, muscle weakness, and tingling sensations of the hand. The diagnostic test for carpal tunnel syndrome is an **electromyograph (EMG).** Electromyograph is the instrument used to determine the electrical activity of the muscle. Measurements can be made as to muscle strength. Treatment consists of immobilizing the wrist joint. If this treatment is not effective, surgery may be done.

Medical Terminology

anal	without
-gesic	sensitivity to pain
anal/gesic	without sensitivity to pain
crani	skull
-al	pertaining to
crani/al nerve	pertaining to a nerve in the skull
electro	electrical activity
myo	muscle
-graphy	process of recording
electro/myo/graphy	process of recording electrical activity in the muscle
neuro	nerve
-algia	pain
neur/algia	nerve pain
-itis	inflammation
neur/itis	inflammation of a nerve
par	near, beyond, beside
esthesia	abnormal condition of feeling sensation
par/esthesia	an abnormal condition of feeling sensation

REVIEW QUESTIONS

Select the letter of choice that best completes the statement.

1. A nerve that contains fibers that both send and receive messages is called:
   a. sensory nerve
   b. afferent nerve
   c. efferent nerve
   d. mixed nerve

2. The cranial nerve responsible for chewing is:
   a. trochlear
   b. facial
   c. glossopharyngeal
   d. trigeminal

3. The cranial nerves responsible for eye muscle movement are the oculomotor, trochlear, and:
   a. abducens
   b. vestibulocochlear
   c. accessory
   d. hypoglossal

4. A network of spinal nerves is called:
   a. mixed
   b. efferent
   c. plexus
   d. afferent

5. The autonomic nervous system is also called:
   a. voluntary
   b. involuntary
   c. neuralgic
   d. carpal

6. The autonomic nervous system is part of the:
   a. central nervous system
   b. peripheral nervous system
   c. sympathetic nervous system
   d. parasympathetic nervous system

7. The sympathetic nervous system that acts in the same manner as adrenalin, does the following:
   a. increases the heart rate and dilates the pupils
   b. increases the heart rate and constricts the pupils
   c. slows the heart rate and dilates the pupils
   d. slows the heart rate and constricts the pupils

8. The nerve that activates the diaphragm is called:
   a. sciatic
   b. phrenic
   c. radial
   d. femoral

9. The simplest type of nervous system response is called:
   a. stimulus
   b. effector action
   c. reflex
   d. affector action

10. The acute viral infection that usually affects the intercostal nerves is called:
   a. Bell's palsy
   b. neuralgia
   c. sciatica
   d. shingles

COMPLETION

Complete the following statements.

1. A nerve consists of small blood vessels and bundles of fibers enclosed by _____.

2. A nerve composed of fibers carrying impulses from sense organs to the brain or spinal cord is called a _____ or _____ nerve.

3. A nerve composed of fibers carrying impulses from the brain or spinal cord to muscles or glands is called a _____ or _____ nerve.

4. A mixed nerve contains both _____ and _____ fibers.

5. The autonomic nervous system is a specialized part of the peripheral system and controls _____.

6. The autonomic nervous system has two parts which counterbalance each other; these are the _____ and _____ systems.

LABELING

Study the following diagram and name the numbered structures.

1. _____

2. _____

3. _____

4. _____

5. _____

6. _____

7. _____

8. _____

9. _____

10. _____

11. _____

12. _____

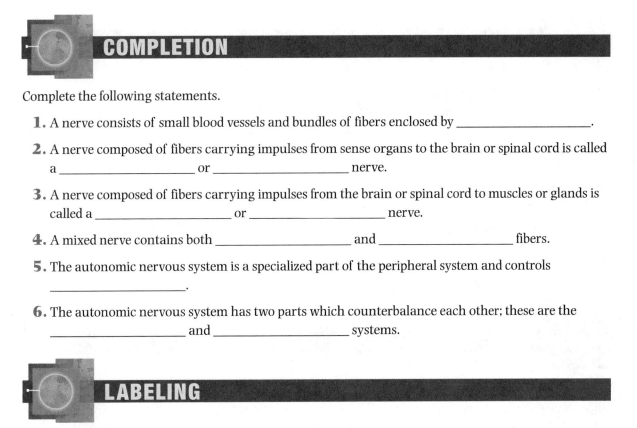

APPLYING THEORY TO PRACTICE

1. You are passing by a pizzeria and smell the pizza cooking. Describe what happens to your salivary glands. What other feelings do you notice? Relate these reactions to your peripheral nervous system.

2. The knee jerk is the most common reflex we know about in health care. You are born with certain reflexes and you learn some reflexes. Name at least five reflexes that you were born with and five reflexes you have learned.

3. A doctor has a patient who is experiencing facial and cheek pain, sometimes called trigeminal neuralgia. Describe this condition and the appropriate treatment.

4. After a lengthy car ride, your elderly uncle gets out of the car and complains, "I can hardly walk. It must be sciatica." Explain what this means.

5. Carpal tunnel syndrome is affecting many Americans in the workplace. What types of jobs increase the risk of this disease?

CASE STUDY

Paula is a 38-year-old administrative assistant. She visits the medical assistant at ABC Company's health office. During the interview, Paula explains she has been waking up at night with pains in both wrists. Paula also states the wrist pain becomes worse after she has been working on the computer. Paula says she has been using wrist supports but they do not seem to help. The medical assistant refers Paula to the physician.

1. The diagnosis is carpal tunnel syndrome. Name the nerves and bones involved in this disorder.

2. Explain the test that will be done to confirm the diagnosis.

3. Describe the symptoms that occur in carpal tunnel syndrome.

4. What is the treatment for this disorder?

5. What is the fastest growing occupational disease?

6. Describe the aspects of CTD.

7. Describe a training program that the medical assistant can present to help prevent CTD.

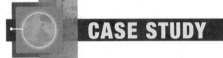

Lab Activity
9-1 Simple Reflex

- *Objective:* To observe the response of the simple knee-jerk reflex
- *Materials needed:* reflex hammer, stopwatch, textbook, paper and pencil

continues

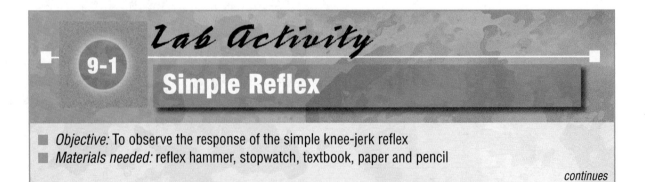

continued

Step 1: Work in groups of three; the third person is needed to do the timing. Have your lab partner sit on the lab bench or chair and cross the right knee over the left knee.

Step 2: Tap the right knee with the reflex hammer (see Figure 9-4 in textbook).

Time the response. Observe the action that occurred. What leg muscle and nerves were involved? Record the timing, your observations, and answers.

Step 3: Reverse the process, and have your lab partner cross the left knee over the right knee.

Step 4: Tap the left knee with the reflex hammer. Distract your partner by reciting the multiplication table for 5 while you are doing the experiment. Time the response. What action occurred? Was there a difference between the response times in the left and right knees? Record your answer.

Step 5: Switch places with your lab partner and have your lab partner conduct steps 1 through 4 on you.

Step 6: Was there any difference in the timing of the responses between you and your partner? Explain the differences, if any. Record your answer.

Lab Activity

9-2

Salivary Reflex Response

■ *Objective:* To observe the response of the salivary reflexes
■ *Materials needed:* lemon juice, measuring cup, paper cup, pH paper, stopwatch, paper and pencil

Step 1: Have your lab partner not swallow for 2 minutes.

Step 2: After 2 minutes, have the partner spit saliva into a paper cup.

Step 3: Measure the amount of saliva and use the pH paper to determine the pH of the saliva.

Step 4: Place two drops of lemon juice on your lab partner's tongue.

Step 5: Allow the lemon juice to mix with the saliva for 5 to 10 seconds.

Step 6: After 5 to 10 seconds, touch a piece of the pH paper to your lab partner's tongue. Record the results.

Step 7: Have your lab partner not swallow for 2 minutes.

Step 8: After 2 minutes, have the partner spit saliva into a paper cup. Measure the amount of saliva. Use pH paper to determine the pH of the saliva. Record your findings.

Step 9: Does the amount and pH of the saliva secretions differ between the ordinary saliva and the saliva that was mixed with lemon juice? Record the differences, if any.

SPECIAL SENSES

Objectives

- Describe the function of the sensory receptors all over the body

- Identify the parts of the eye and describe their functions

- Trace the pathway of light from outside to the occipital lobe

- Identify the parts of the ear and describe their functions

- Trace the pathway of sound from pinna to temporal lobe

- Describe the process involved with the sense of smell

- Describe common disorders of the eye, ear, and nose

- Define the key words that relate to this chapter

Key Words

amblyopia
anterior chamber
anvil (incus)
aqueous humor
astigmatism
cataracts
choroid coat
ciliary body
cochlea
cochlear duct
cones
conjunctivitis
cornea
detached retina
deviated nasal
    septum
diplopia
eustachian tube
extrinsic muscle
fovea centralis
glaucoma

hammer (malleus)
hyperopia
    (farsightedness)
intrinsic muscle
iris
lens
macular
    degeneration
Meniere's disease
miotic
myopia (near-
    sightedness)
myringotomy
nasal polyp
optic disc (blind
    spot)
organ of Corti
otitis media
otosclerosis
pinna

posterior chamber
presbycusis
presbyopia
pupil
retina
rhinitis
rods
sclera
semicircular canals
stirrup (stapes)
strabismus (cross
    eyes)
sty
suspensory
    ligament
tinnitus
tympanic
    membrane
vertigo
vitreous humor

The special senses are those organs and receptors that are associated with touch (sensory receptors), vision, hearing, smell, and taste. Sight, hearing, and smell are distance senses; they bring information from far away. Touch can only reveal information about things you actually come in direct contact with. Functions of the special senses are to receive stimuli from the sensory receptors, the eye, the ear, the nose, and the tongue and to transmit these impulses to the brain for interpretation.

 SENSORY RECEPTORS

Sensory receptors are structures which are stimulated by changes in the environment. Sensory receptors for touch, pain, temperature, and pressure (proprioceptors) are found all over the body in the skin, connective tissue, and muscle. In addition are special sensory receptors which include the taste buds of the tongue, special cells in the nose, the retina of the eye, and the special cells in the inner ear which make up the organ of Corti. When a sense organ is stimulated, the impulse travels along nerve pathways to the brain, where it is registered in a certain area. Sensation actually takes place in the brain, but it is mentally referred back to the sense organ. This is called projection of the sensation.

THE EYE

The human eye is a tender sphere about 1 inch (2.5 cm) in diameter. It is protected by the orbital socket of the skull, the eyebrows, eyelids, and eyelashes, Figure 10-1. The eyes are continuously bathed in fluid by tears secreted from lacrimal glands, which are located above the lateral area of each eye. The tears flow across the eye into the lacrimal duct. The lacrimal duct is located in the corner of the eye and empties into the nasal cavity. This explains why, when we cry, we may also need to blow the nose. Lacrimal secretions have some antibiotic properties: Tears cleanse and moisten the eyes on a continuous basis.

Along the border of each eyelid are glands that secrete an oily substance which lubricates the eye. An infection of this gland is called a **sty.**

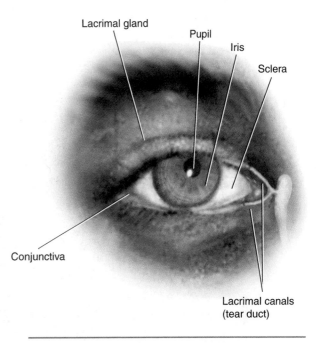

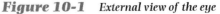

Figure 10-1 *External view of the eye*

The conjunctiva is the thin membrane that lines the eyelids and covers part of the eye. The conjunctiva secretes mucus which helps to lubricate the eye.

The location of the eyes in front of the head allows for superimposition of images from each eye. This enables us to see stereoscopically in three dimensions (length, width, and depth).

The wall of the eye is made up of three concentric layers, or coats, each with its specific function. These three layers are the sclera, choroid, and retina, Figure 10-2.

Sclera

The outer layer is called the **sclera,** or white of the eye. It is a tough, unyielding fibrous capsule which maintains the shape of the eye and protects the delicate structures within. Muscles responsible for moving the eye within the orbital socket are attached to the outside of the sclera. These muscles are referred to as the **extrinsic muscles,** Figure 10-3. They include the superior, inferior, lateral, medial rectus, and the superior and inferior oblique. See Table 10-1 for a listing of the extrinsic eye muscles and their functions.

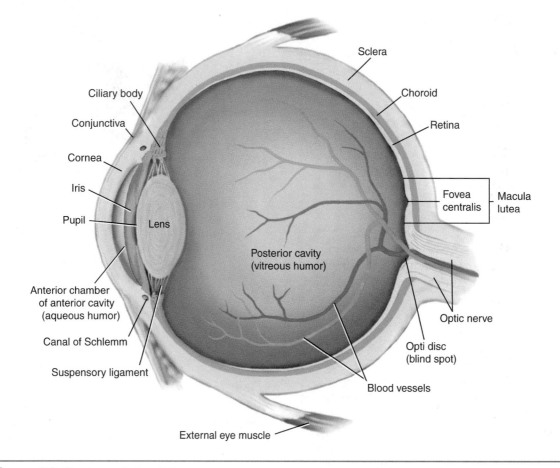

Figure 10-2 *Internal view of the eye*

Cornea

In the very front center of the sclerotic coat lies a circular clear area called the **cornea.** The cornea is sometimes referred to as the "window" of the eye. It is transparent to permit the passage of light rays. This transparency is due to the lack of blood vessels. Thus, corneal cells are fed by the movement of lymph through interstitial or lymph spaces. The cornea consists of five layers of flat cells arranged much like sheets of plate glass. Possessing pain and touch receptors, it is sensitive to any foreign particles that come in contact with its surface. An injury to the cornea may cause scarring and impaired vision.

Choroid Coat and the Iris

The middle layer of the eye is the **choroid coat.** It contains blood vessels to nourish the eye, and a nonreflective pigment rendering it dark and opaque. The pigment provides the choroid coat with a deep, red-purple color; this darkens the eye chamber, preventing light reflection within the eye. In front, the choroid coat has a circular opening called the **pupil.** A colored, muscular layer surrounds the pupil; this is the **iris,** or colored part of the eye. The iris may be blue, green, gray, brown, or black. Eye color is related to the number and size of melanin pigment cells in the iris. If there is little melanin present, the eye is blue, because light is scattered to a greater extent. With increasing quantities of melanin, eye color ranges from green to black. The total absence of melanin results in a pink eye color, characteristic of albinism. Such irises are pink because the blood inside the choroid blood vessels shows through the iris.

Within the iris are two sets of antagonistic smooth muscles, the sphincter and the dilator pupillae. These **intrinsic muscles** help the iris to

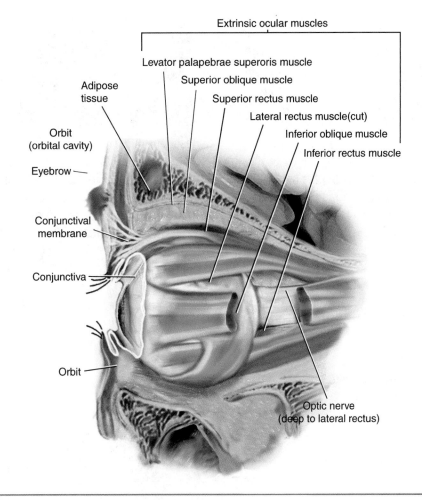

Figure 10-3 *Extrinsic eye muscles*

Table 10-1 Extrinsic and Intrinsic Eye Muscles	
EYE MUSCLE	**FUNCTION**
A. Extrinsic	
1. Superior rectus	Rolls eyeball upward
2. Inferior rectus	Rolls eyeball downward
3. Lateral rectus	Rolls eyeball laterally
4. Medial rectus	Rolls eyeball medially
5. Superior oblique	Rolls eyeball on its axis, moves cornea downward and laterally
6. Inferior oblique	Rolls eyeball on its axis, moves cornea upward and laterally
B. Intrinsic	
1. Sphincter pupillae	Constricts pupil
2. Dilator pupillae	Dilates pupil

control amounts of light entering the pupil. When the eye is focused on a close object or stimulated by bright light, the sphincter pupillae muscle contracts, rendering the pupil smaller. Conversely, when the eye is focused on a distant object or stimulated by dim light, the dilator pupillae muscle contracts. This causes the pupil to grow larger, permitting as much light as possible to enter the eye.

Lens and Related Structures

The **lens** is a crystalline structure located behind the iris and pupil. It has concentric layers of fibers and crystal-clear proteins in solution. It is an elastic, disc-shaped structure with anterior and posterior convex surfaces, thus forming a biconvex lens. However, the posterior surface is more curved than that of the anterior. The curvature of each surface alters with age. During infancy, the lens is spherical; in adulthood, it is medium convexed; in the elderly it is almost flattened. The capsule surrounding the lens also loses its elasticity over time. The lens is held in place behind the pupil by **suspensory ligaments** from the **ciliary body** of the choroid body.

The lens is situated between the **anterior** and **posterior chambers.** The anterior chamber is filled with a watery fluid called **aqueous humor,** and it is constantly replenished by blood vessels behind the iris, Figure 10-4. **Vitreous humor,** a transparent jellylike substance, fills the posterior chamber. Both of these substances help to maintain the eyeball's spherical shape, refracting (bending) light rays as they pass through the eye.

Retina

The **retina** of the eye is the innermost, or third coat of the eye. It is located between the posterior chamber and the choroid coat. The retina does not extend around the front portion of the eye. It is upon this light-sensitive layer that light rays from an object form an image. After the image is focused on the retina, it travels via the optic nerve to the visual part of the cerebral cortex (occipital

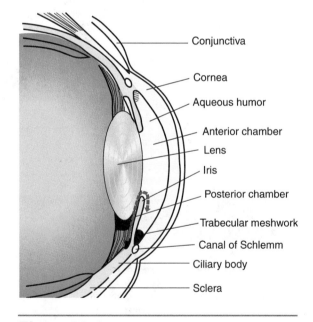

Conjunctiva
Cornea
Aqueous humor
Anterior chamber
Lens
Iris
Posterior chamber
Trabecular meshwork
Canal of Schlemm
Ciliary body
Sclera

Figure 10-4   *Flow of aqueous humor*

lobe). If light rays do not focus correctly on the retina, the condition may be corrected with properly fitted contact lenses, or eyeglasses, which bend the light rays as required.

The retina contains pigment and specialized cells known as **rods** and **cones,** Figure 10-5, which are sensitive to light. The rod cells are sen-

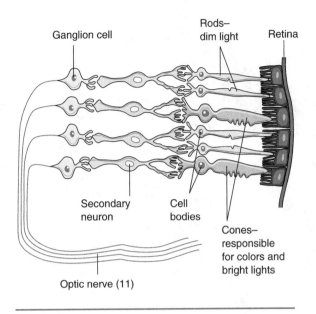

Figure 10-5 *Diagram of visual neurons showing rods and cones*

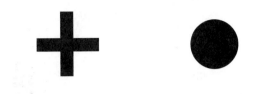

1. Close your left eye and focus your right eye on the <u>cross</u>.
2. Move the page slowly away from your eye and then slowly toward your eye.
3. At a distance of about 6–8 inches the black <u>circle</u> "disappears."

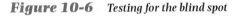

Figure 10-6 *Testing for the blind spot*

sitive to dim light and the cones are sensitive to bright light. The cones are also responsible for color vision. There are three varieties of cone cells. Each type is sensitive to a special color. The part of the retina where the nerve fibers enter the optic nerve to go to the brain does not have these specialized cells.

The Optic Disc and the Fovea. Viewing the retina through an ophthalmoscope, one can observe a yellow disc called the macula lutea. Within this disc is the **fovea centralis,** which contains the cones for color vision, see Figure 10-2. The area around the fovea centralis is the extrafoveal or peripheral region. This is where the rods for dim and peripheral vision can be found.

Slightly to the side of the fovea lies a pale disc called the **optic disc** or **blind spot.** Nerve fibers from the retina gather here to form the nerve. The optic disc contains no rods or cones; therefore, it is devoid of visual reception.

See Figure 10-6 to help you locate your blind spot.

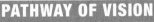

PATHWAY OF VISION

Images in the light → cornea → pupil → lens → where the light rays are bent or refracted → retina → rods and cones (nerve cells) pick up the stimulus → optic nerve → optic chiasma (where the two optic nerves cross) → optic tracts → occipital lobe of the brain for interpretation, Figure 10-7.

EYE DISORDERS

Conjunctivitis is an inflammation of the conjunctival membranes in front of the eye. Redness, pain, swelling, and discharge of mucus occur. Conjunctivitis, or "pink eye," usually begins in one eye and spreads rapidly to the other by a washcloth or hands. Because it is highly contagious, other family members should not share the same washcloths or towels with the infected person. Good handwashing is important to prevent the spread to others. Treatment includes eye washes or eye irrigations which will cleanse the conjunctiva and relieve the inflammation and pain. Bacterial conjunctivitis responds to antibiotic drug therapy.

Glaucoma is a condition of excessive intraocular pressure resulting in the destruction of retina and atrophy of the optic nerve. The condition results from overproduction of aqueous humor, or the obstruction of its outflow through the canal of Schlemm for absorption into the venous circulation. Symptoms are gradual. They include mild aching, a loss of peripheral vision, and a halo around the light.

Glaucoma may occur with aging and has no initial symptoms. It is important for people to be tested for glaucoma annually after age 40. Tonometry, opthalmoscopy with visualization of the optic

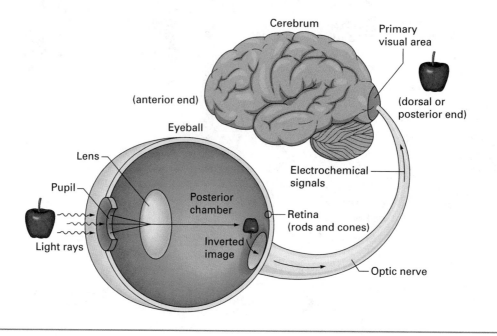

Figure 10-7 *Pathway of vision*

nerve, and central field testing are three prime tests for the diagnosis and continued evaluation of glaucoma.

Treatment involves **miotic** drugs which constrict the pupil and thus increase the outflow of aqueous humor, or drugs which reduce the amount of aqueous fluid produced by the eye. Today, laser surgery or incisional surgery helps to increase the flow of aqueous humor. All treatments are focused on lowering the intraocular pressure.

Cataracts is a condition where the lens of the eye gradually becomes cloudy Figure 10-8. This frequently occurs in people over 70 years of age. The condition causes a painless, gradual blurring and loss of vision. The pupil appears to change color from black to milky white. People with cataracts may complain of seeing halos around lights or being blinded at night by oncoming headlights.

Cataracts are treated by laser surgery or the surgical removal of the lens and postoperative substitution of contact lenses or eyeglasses. There may also be an intraocular lens implanted directly behind the cornea.

Macular degeneration is another eye disorder that occurs as a person ages. In the central part of the retina is the macula which is responsible for sharp central vision. Symptoms include a

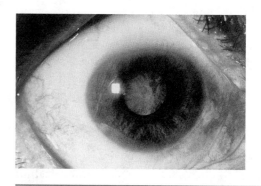

Figure 10-8 *Cataract* *(Courtesy of the National Eye Institute, NIH)*

dimming or distortion of vision that is most obvious when reading. In one form of the disease, straight lines look wavy and blind spots may develop in the visual field. The two types of macular degeneration are dry and wet. In the dry type, the main defect is a gradual thinning of the retina. This is slowly progressive and there is no known treatment. Central vision will be greatly reduced but usually there is not total blindness.

In the wet type, leakage develops under the retina causing blister formation which may involve blood vessels. Laser treatment may be used with this type of macular degeneration. The good news about macular degeneration is that the majority of

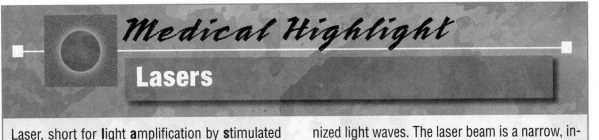

Medical Highlight

Lasers

Laser, short for **l**ight **a**mplification by **s**timulated **e**mission of **r**adiations, is based on the principle that certain atoms, molecules, or ions can be excited by absorption of thermal, electrical, or light energy. After such energy absorptions, the atoms, molecules, or ions give off a beam of synchronized light waves. The laser beam is a narrow, intense, and monochromatic (single color) light beam that can be used for a variety of purposes. For example, it can stop bleeding, make incisions, or remove tissue.

people who develop it will be able to maintain their independence of movement with low-vision aids.

Detached retina is another problem which may occur with aging. It may also occur as the result of a traumatic accident at a younger age. The vitreous fluid contracts as it ages and pulls on the retina, causing a tear Figure 10-9. Symptoms include loss of peripheral vision and then loss of central vision. Early detection is important as it can be repaired with laser or a freezing technique. **NOTE:** It is important to have annual eye examinations. Early detection of eye problems can save your vision.

Sty (hordeolum) is a tiny abscess at the base of an eyelash. The eye is red, painful, and swollen, Figure 10-10. It is due to the inflammation of a tiny sebaceous gland of the eyelid. Treatment consists of warm, wet compresses to relieve pain and promote drainage.

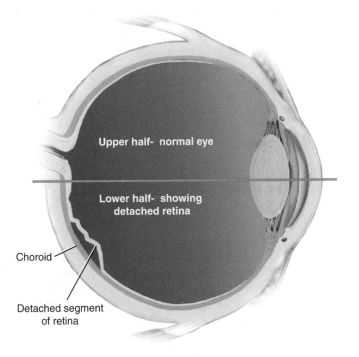

Upper half- normal eye

Lower half- showing detached retina

Choroid

Detached segment of retina

Figure 10-9   *Retinal detachment*

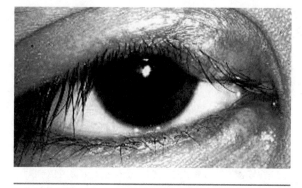

Figure 10-10   *Sty*   *(Courtesy of Eye MAC Development, LLC, Green Bay, WI, www.eyemac.com)*

Eye Injuries

In most cases of simple eye irritation, the natural flow of tears will help to cleanse the eye. In cases when pieces of glass or other fragments get into the eye, do not attempt to remove the object. Patch both eyes and get medical treatment.

Corneal abrasions and scarring may occur as a result of an accident or irritation. The cornea is avascular; that is, there are no blood vessels present. Therefore, corneal transplants can be done readily without fears of tissue rejection.

Eye irritations can be caused by chemicals or fragments that get into the eye. Rinse eyes with water for at least 15 minutes and seek medical treatment.

Vision Defects

Night blindness is a condition that makes it difficult to see at night. The rod cells in the retina are affected in this condition.

Color blindness is the inability to distinguish colors. There are three specific types of cone cells in the retina related to the primary colors: blue, red, and green. The cone cells are affected in color blindness. Color blindness is identified as a hereditary characteristic.

Presbyopia is a condition in which the lenses lose their elasticity resulting in a decrease in ability to focus on close objects. It usually occurs after age 40. There is difficulty in focusing with this condition.

Hyperopia (farsightedness) is a condition in which the focal point is beyond the retina

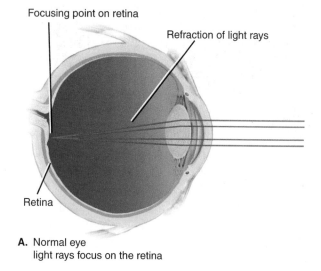

A. Normal eye
light rays focus on the retina

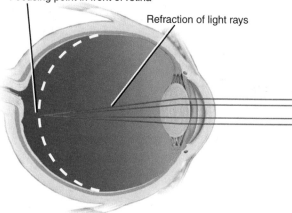

B. Myopia (nearsightedness)
light rays focus in front of the retina

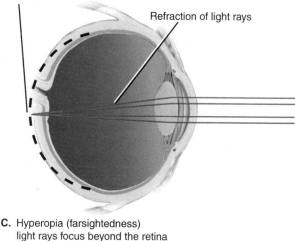

C. Hyperopia (farsightedness)
light rays focus beyond the retina

Figure 10-11   *Vision defects*

because the eyeball is shorter than normal, Figure 10-11B. Objects must be moved farther away from the eye to be seen clearly. Convex lenses help correct this situation.

Myopia (nearsightedness) is a condition in which the focal point is in front of the retina, because the eyeball is elongated, see Figure 10-11C. Objects must be brought close to the eye to be seen clearly. Concave lenses help correct this condition. Various surgical techniques can be used to correct refraction errors, particularly myopia (nearsightedness). One such procedure is photo refractive keratectomy, a laser therapy used to reshape the anterior cornea of the eye and correct the condition.

Amblyopia is a reduction, or dimness, of vision.

Astigmatism is a condition in which there is an irregular curvature of the cornea or lens, which causes blurred vision and possible eyestrain. A special prescription eyeglass helps this condition.

Diplopia is blurred vision.

Strabismus (cross-eyes) is a condition in which the muscles of the eyeball do not coordinate their action. This condition is usually seen early in children and can be corrected by eye exercises or surgery.

THE EAR

The ear is a special sense organ that is especially adapted to pick up sound waves and send these impulses to the auditory center of the brain. The auditory center is located in the temporal area just above the ears. The receptor for hearing is the delicate **organ of Corti,** which is located within the cochlea of the inner ear.

The ear is also involved with equilibrium. The receptors in the inner ear send a message to the cerebellum in the brain about head position, to help maintain balance. Other receptors include proprioceptors in our eyes and receptors located around our joints. The information picked up by these receptors is processed by the cerebellum and cerebral cortex to enable the body to cope with changes in equilibrium.

The ear has three parts: the outer or external ear, the middle ear, and the inner ear, see Figure 10-12.

Effects of Aging on The Eye

The loss of elasticity, opacity of the lens, and atrophy of the ciliary muscle decreases the ability to focus on fine details (presbyopia). This change compromises the accommodation of the lenses. Older adults need more time for the eyes to adjust from light to dark; thus, they have a loss of night vision.

Peripheral vision and depth perception decline with age. An adequate visual field is necessary for driving and walking in crowded places. The depth perception loss leads to falls and mobility problems because of miscalculations about the distance and height of objects.

Loss of visual acuity occurs from changes in the lenses. Cataract formation, glaucoma, and macular degeneration occur more often as one ages.

The Outer Ear

The **pinna,** or outer ear, collects sound waves and directs them into the auditory canal. The auditory canal is lined with sebaceous or ceruminous glands which secrete a waxlike or oily substance called cerumen. This substance protects the ear. The auditory canal leads to the eardrum or **tympanic membrane,** which separates the outer and middle ear.

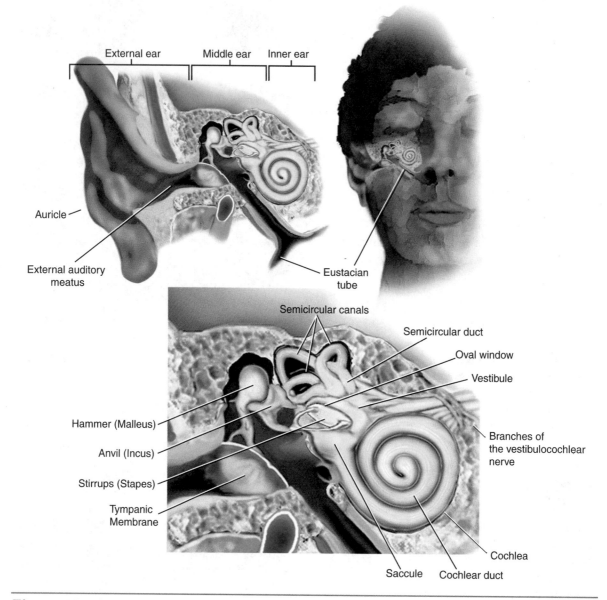

Figure 10-12 *The ear and its structures*

The Middle Ear

The middle ear is really the cavity in the temporal bone. It connects with the pharynx (throat) by means of a tube called the **eustachian tube.** This tube serves to equalize the air pressure in the middle ear with that of the outside atmosphere. A chain of three tiny bones is found in the middle ear: the **hammer** (**malleus**), the **anvil** (**incus**), and the **stirrup** (**stapes**); they transmit sound waves from the ear drum to the inner ear.

The Inner Ear

The inner ear consists of several membrane-lined channels which lie deep within the temporal bone. The special organ of hearing is a spiral-shaped passage known as the **cochlea,** which contains a membranous tube called the **cochlear duct.** The duct is filled with fluid that vibrates when the sound waves from the stirrup bone strike against it. Located in the cochlear duct are delicate cells which make up the organ of Corti.

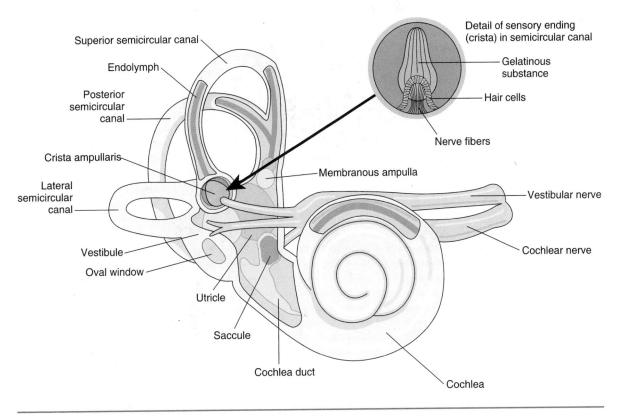

Detail of sensory ending
(crista) in semicircular canal

— Gelatinous substance

— Hair cells

Nerve fibers

Superior semicircular canal

Endolymph

Posterior semicircular canal

Crista ampullaris

Lateral semicircular canal

— Membranous ampulla

— Vestibular nerve

— Cochlear nerve

Vestibule

Oval window

Utricle

Saccule

Cochlea duct

Cochlea

Figure 10-13   *Enlargement of the inner ear showing the three semicircular canals*

These hairlike cells pick up the vibrations caused by sound waves against the fluid, then they transmit them through the auditory nerve to the hearing center of the brain.

Three **semicircular canals** also lie within the inner ear, Figure 10-13. They contain a liquid, and delicate hairlike cells which bend when the liquid is set in motion by head and body movements. These impulses are sent to the cerebellum, helping to maintain body balance, or equilibrium. They have nothing to do with the sense of hearing.

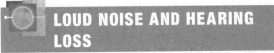

PATHWAY OF HEARING

Sound waves → *pinna*, or outer ear → *auditory canal* → *tympanic membrane* → *ear ossicles* (hammer, anvil, and stirrup) → stimulate the receptors in the *cochlea* → *cochlear nerve* (part of the vestibulocochlear nerve) → *temporal lobe* of the brain for interpretation, Figure 10-14.

When the same sound keeps reaching the ears, the auditory receptors adapt to the sound and we do not hear it.

PATHWAY OF EQUILIBRIUM

Movement of head → stimulates equilibrium receptors in the semicircular and vestibule areas of the inner ear → vestibular nerve (part of the vestibulocochlea nerve) → cerebellum of the brain for interpretation.

LOUD NOISE AND HEARING LOSS

Hearing is both sensitive and fragile. Loud noise heard for too long will damage your hearing. If the delicate hair cells in the organ of Corti in the inner ear become overstimulated, they will become damaged. Repeated exposure to the loud noise causes the loss to become permanent as more cells and their nerve receptors are destroyed.

The alarming increase of hearing loss in young people is most likely caused by loud music usually heard through headphones. The symptoms of hearing loss may be tinnitus (ringing in

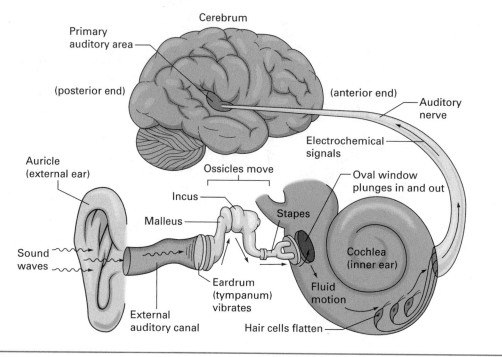

Figure 10-14   *Pathway of hearing*

the ears) or difficulty in understanding what people are saying (they seem to be mumbling). Words with high-frequency sounds such as *pill, hill* and *fill* may sound alike.

Sound is measured in decibels. The scale runs from the faintest sound the human ear can hear, labeled 0dB, to the scream of a jet engine or a shotgun blast at over 165 dB. Exposure to more than 90 decibels for 8 hours (busy city traffic noise) may be dangerous to your hearing. At 100 dB, the noise level of a chain saw, it would take 2 hours to do the same damage to your hearing. ***NOTE:*** Noise heard long enough and loud enough over time will cause damage.

To protect your hearing, turn down the volume on the stereo, find a quiet place, and wear earplugs or ear muffs.

EAR DISORDERS

Otitis media is an infection of the middle ear. It usually causes earache. This disorder is often a complication of the common cold in children. Treatment with antibiotics will cure the infection. In some cases, there may be a buildup of fluid or pus which can be relieved by a **myringotomy** (an opening made in the tympanic membrane). Tubes may be placed in the ear to allow fluids to drain off, especially in cases of chronic otitis media.

Otosclerosis is an inherited disorder in which the bone stapes of the middle ear first become sponge and then harden. This causes the stirrup or stapes to become fixed or immovable. Otosclerosis is a common cause of deafness in young adults. Stapedectomy, a total replacement of the stapes, is the treatment of choice.

Tinnitus is a sensation of ringing or buzzing that is perceived in the ear in the absence of an actual sound stimulus. It may be caused by impacted wax, otitis media, otosclerosis, loud noise, blockage of normal blood supply to the cochlea, or the effects of various drugs such as the salicylates (painkillers).

Presbycusis is a condition that causes deafness due to the aging process. This can be helped with the use of hearing aids.

Meniere's disease is a condition that affects the semicircular canals of the inner ear, causing marked **vertigo** (dizziness). Vertigo can occur at any time and without warning, causing the patient to be very frightened. In addition, vertigo is

Effects of Aging on Hearing

The physiologic changes of aging result in three major types of hearing deficit: conductive, sensorineural, and mixed. Conductive hearing loss occurs when there is an interference with conduction of sound waves. In the outer ear, cerumen (earwax) becomes imbedded and drier because of a decrease in the number and activity of ceruminal glands. The tympanic membrane becomes fibrotic, reducing the transmission of sound. There is a degeneration of ear bones, vestibular structure, cochlea, and organ of Corti affecting sensitivity to sound, understanding of speech, and maintenance of equilibrium.

Sensorineural hearing loss (presbycusis) involves changes in neural, sensory, and mechanical structure of the inner ear. It is characterized by loss of hearing of high-pitched frequencies and diminished ability to hear consonants. These changes result in the inability to hear as result of impaired recognition of words as opposed to a loss of volume. The speech of others sounds garbled and a normal conversation is difficult to follow.

Mixed hearing loss is a combination of both types.

accompanied by nausea, vomiting, and a ringing sensation in the ears. Bed rest is sometimes necessary during an acute attack. Medication may be given to relieve vertigo and nausea. The patient should avoid any sudden movement, because it may precipitate an attack. The cause is unknown and the symptoms subside; however, an attack occurs without warning.

Types of Hearing Loss

- *Conductive hearing loss* occurs when sounds to the inner ear are blocked by ear wax or there is fluid in the middle ear or abnormal bone growth.

- *Sensorineural damage* to parts of the inner ear of auditory nerve results in a partial or complete deafness. In cases of profound deafness, cochlear implants improve communication ability which leads to positive psychological and social changes. At the present time, children after the age of 2 and adults with profound deafness are candidates for cochlear implants.

THE NOSE

The human nose can detect about 10,000 different smells. Smell accounts for about 90% of what we think of as taste. Hold your nose and see if you can tell the difference between eating a piece of orange and a piece of pear. Odor molecules inhaled through the nose get warmed and moistened as they pass through the nasal cavity.

In the nasal cavity, Figure 10-15, is a patch of tissue about the size of a postage stamp called the olfactory epithelium, which has a plentiful supply of nerve cells with specialized receptors. The receptors send signals to the adjoining olfactory bulbs, an extension of the brain. The stimulus is transmitted by the olfactory nerve to the limbic system, thalamus, and frontal cortex. The limbic system generates our basic emotions such as affection, aggression, and fear. This relationship may explain why odors are tied to feelings. For example, we may associate the smell of something cooking usually with a good experience.

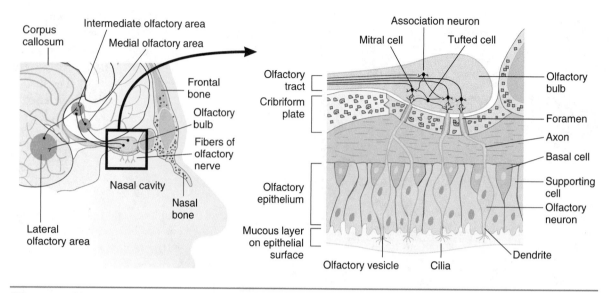

Figure 10-15   *The nasal cavity*

Scientists are starting to do research on how smells may affect learning, weight loss, aggression levels, and behavior.

DISORDERS OF THE NOSE

Rhinitis is an inflammation of the lining of the nose which may cause nasal congestion, nasal drainage, sneezing, or itching. The cause may be allergies, infection, or other factors such as fumes, odors, emotional changes, or drugs. Treatment includes eliminating the allergens, if possible, or reducing exposure to them. Some antihistamines are effective for short periods of time.

Nasal polyps are growths in the nasal cavity associated with rhinitis, Figure 10-16. In severe cases, surgery may be necessary to remove the polyps.

Deviated nasal septum is a condition in which there is a bend in the cartilage structure of the septum. Symptoms that result are a blockage in the airflow through one nostril, difficulty sleeping, headaches, loud breathing or snoring, dry nose, and nose bleeds. Treatment has been surgical correction. An external adhesive strip placed across the nose can provide temporary relief of breathing problems associated with a deviated

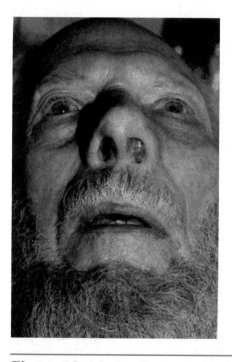

Figure 10-16   *Nasal polyp*

nasal septum. This product improves breathing by reducing nasal airflow resistance. It can be effective in reducing snoring and in the temporary relief of nasal congestion.

Effects of Aging on Smelling

A decrease in the number of olfactory neurons during aging reduces the awareness of odors. This decrease in the sense of smell can affect appetite, social relationships, and detection of warning smells such as gas. Senile rhinitis is a clear, continuous watery discharge from the nose that is not associated with underlying disease.

Effects of Aging on Tasting

Older persons experience a diminished number of taste buds. Increased amounts of salt, sweet, sour, and bitter are needed for the person to identify the food. Wearing full upper dentures diminishes taste sensation because they cover the taste buds in the upper palate.

THE TONGUE

The tongue is a mass of muscle tissue which has structures called papillae. Located on the papilla are the taste buds for sweet, sour, salty, and bitter, which are stimulated by the flavors of foods, see Figure 18-3. The receptors in the taste buds send stimuli through three cranial nerves to the cerebral cortex for interpretation.

Career Profile
Audiologists

Audiologists assess and treat patients with hearing and hearing-related disorders. They use audiometers and other testing devices to measure the loudness at which a person begins to hear sounds, the ability to distinguish between sounds, and the extent of the hearing loss. Audiologists coordinate the results with medical and educational information to make a diagnosis and determine a course of treatment. Treatment may consist of cleaning the ear canal, fitting a hearing aid, auditory training, and instruction in speech or lip reading.

A master's degree is the standard credential in this field. Patience and compassion are critical traits because the client's progress may be very slow. Job outlook is higher than average because hearing loss is associated with the aging process.

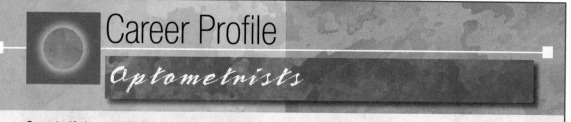

Career Profile

Optometrists

Over half the people in the United States wear glasses. Optometrists (doctors of optometry) provide most of the primary vision care people need.

Optometrists examine eyes to diagnose vision problems and eye disease. Optometrists use instruments and observations to examine eye health and to test patients' visual acuity, depth and color perception, and their ability to focus and coordinate the eyes. They analyze test results and develop a treatment plan. Optometrists prescribe eyeglasses, contact lenses, and vision therapy. They prescribe drugs for other eye problems such as conjunctivitis, glaucoma, and corneal infection.

Optometrists differ from opthamologists. Opthamologists diagnose and treat eye diseases, perform surgery, and prescribe drugs. All states require optometrists to be licensed. Applicants must have a doctor of optometry degree from an accredited school and pass a licensing examination.

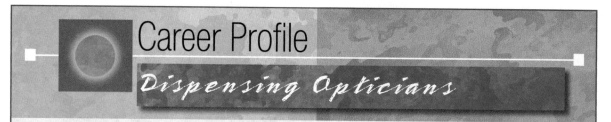

Career Profile

Dispensing Opticians

Dispensing opticians fit eyeglasses and contact lenses. Dispensing opticians help customers select appropriate frames, order the necessary opthalmic laboratory work, and adjust the finished eyeglasses. They examine written prescriptions to determine lens specification and measure the client's eyes. They prepare work orders which give the laboratory technicians information needed to grind and insert lenses.

Dispensing opticians keep records, work orders, and payments as well as track inventory and perform other administrative duties.

Employers generally hire individuals with no background in opticianry and then provide the required training. Mechanical drawing is particularly useful because training in this field usually includes instruction in optical mathematics, optical physics, and the use of precision measuring instruments and other machinery and tools. Formal training may be offered in community colleges. Job outlook is greater than average in response to rising demand for corrective lenses. Fashion also influences demand, encouraging people to buy more than one pair of eyeglasses.

Medical Terminology

ambly	dull or dim
op	eyes
-ia	condition of
ambly/op/ia	condition of dim eyes
cochle	snail shell
-a	relating to, pertaining to
cochle/a	relating to snail shell
conjunctiv	eyelid lining
-itis	inflammation of
conjunctiv/itis	inflammation of eyelid lining
corne	tough, hornlike
corne/a	relating to a tough structure
tympan	eardrum
-ic	relating to
tympan/ic	relating to eardrum
dipl	double
dipl/op/ia	condition of seeing double
hyper	over, excessive
hyper/op/ia	condition of excessive eye vision, farsightedness
lacrim	tears
-al	pertaining to
lacrim/al gland	tear gland
my	squinting
my/op/ia	condition of squinting, nearsightedness
myring	eardrum
-otomy	opening into
myring/otomy	opening into eardrum
ot	ear
media	middle
ot/itis media	inflammation of middle ear
oto	ear
sclerosis	hardening
oto/sclerosis	hardening of the ear
strabism	distorted squinting, cross-eyed
-us	presence of
strabism/us	presence of cross-eyes

REVIEW QUESTIONS

Select the letter of the choice that best completes the statement.

1. The outer tough coat of the eye is the:
   a. retina
   b. sclera
   c. choroid
   d. lens

2. The clear anterior portion of the sclera is called:
   a. cornea
   b. lens
   c. pupil
   d. iris

3. The muscle that regulates how much light enters the eye is called:
   a. conjunction
   b. iris
   c. cornea
   d. lens

4. The posterior chamber of the eye is filled with fluid called:
   a. tears
   b. ciliary body
   c. vitreous humor
   d. aqueous humor

5. The area of the eye that contains the rods and cones is called:
   a. retina
   b. choroid
   c. sclera
   d. cornea

6. The tube that connects the throat to the ear is called:
   a. pinna
   b. eustachian
   c. cochlear
   d. auditory

7. Hardening of the bones of the middle ear is called:
   a. otitis media
   b. presbycusis
   c. otosclerosis
   d. presbyopia

8. Nearsightedness is also known as:
   a. myopia
   b. hyperopia
   c. presbyopia
   d. strabismus

9. A clouding of the lens is called:
   a. myopia
   b. glaucoma
   c. hyperopia
   d. cataract

10. An infectious disease known as pink-eye is also called:
   a. kernicterus
   b. otitis
   c. conjunctivitis
   d. strabismus

LABELING

Study the following diagram of the eye and name the numbered structures.

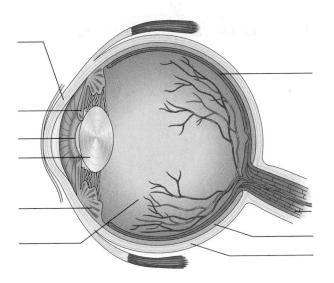

1. _____   6. _____

2. _____   7. _____

3. _____   8. _____

4. _____   9. _____

5. _____   10. _____

APPLYING THEORY TO PRACTICE

1. Explain how you see and track the pathway of light from the cornea to the occipital lobe of the brain.

2. Explain to a friend how your outer ear catches a sound and where in the brain it is interpreted.

3. A patient comes to the doctor's office for treatment of glaucoma. She states, "I am so tired of taking these eyedrops. I don't want to use them anymore." How would you respond and what instructions would you give her?

4. The phrase "stop and smell the roses" means slow down and enjoy life. What conditions may interfere with your ability to smell the roses?

5. Map your tongue. Try locating where the taste buds are on your tongue: Try a little sugar to locate the sweet taste buds; try a little salt for the salt taste buds; use a piece of lemon to locate the sour taste buds; and apply a few coffee grinds for bitter taste buds.

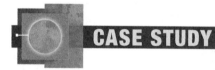

CASE STUDY

Wayne is a 75-year-old retired teacher who comes to the physician's office feeling quite upset. He tells Rebecca, the LPN, that he does not know what is happening to him. When people speak to him, their speech seems garbled and lately he is having difficulty reading. After an examination, the doctor tells him he has a conductive hearing loss because of accumulated cerumen.

1. What is a conductive hearing loss?

2. What is cerumen?

3. Describe other causes of conductive hearing loss.

4. What is the role of an audiologist?

5. Explain the pathway of sound.

The doctor tells Rebecca to make an appointment for Wayne to be seen by the optometrist for his vision problem. The optometrist tells Wayne he has the beginning of macular degeneration.

6. Describe the duties of the optometrist.

7. Explain and describe the symptoms of macular degeneration.

8. What is the treatment for macular degeneration?

9. What reassurance can the optometrist give Wayne regarding macular degeneration?

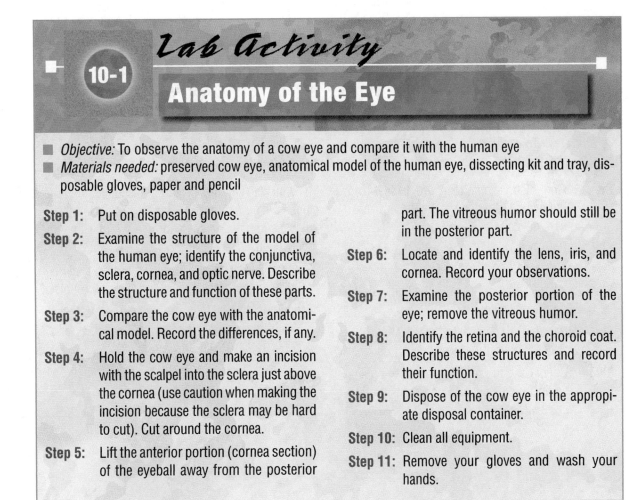

Lab Activity

10-1 Anatomy of the Eye

- *Objective:* To observe the anatomy of a cow eye and compare it with the human eye
- *Materials needed:* preserved cow eye, anatomical model of the human eye, dissecting kit and tray, disposable gloves, paper and pencil

Step 1: Put on disposable gloves.

Step 2: Examine the structure of the model of the human eye; identify the conjunctiva, sclera, cornea, and optic nerve. Describe the structure and function of these parts.

Step 3: Compare the cow eye with the anatomical model. Record the differences, if any.

Step 4: Hold the cow eye and make an incision with the scalpel into the sclera just above the cornea (use caution when making the incision because the sclera may be hard to cut). Cut around the cornea.

Step 5: Lift the anterior portion (cornea section) of the eyeball away from the posterior part. The vitreous humor should still be in the posterior part.

Step 6: Locate and identify the lens, iris, and cornea. Record your observations.

Step 7: Examine the posterior portion of the eye; remove the vitreous humor.

Step 8: Identify the retina and the choroid coat. Describe these structures and record their function.

Step 9: Dispose of the cow eye in the appropiate disposal container.

Step 10: Clean all equipment.

Step 11: Remove your gloves and wash your hands.

Lab Activity
10-2

Test for Visual Acuity

■ *Objective:* To observe the function of the eye
■ *Materials needed:* Snellen eye chart, measuring device card, paper and pencil

Step 1: Find a lab partner. Measure 20 feet from the eye chart, which is where your partner will stand.

Step 2: Have your partner cover the left eye with one hand or a card.

Step 3: Have your partner read each line with the right eye; check for accuracy.

Step 4: Record the line with the smallest number read for the right eye.

Step 5: Repeat the process to record the visual acuity for the left eye. Record the number.

If your lab partner wears glasses or contact lenses, have the person do the test first with the glasses/contact lenses and then without the corrective lenses.

Step 6: Switch places and have your lab partner repeat steps 1 to 5 with you as the subject.

Step 7: Is there a difference between your test results and your lab partner's results? Record your answers.

Lab Activity
10-3

Anatomy of the Ear

■ *Objective:* To observe the anatomical structure of the ear
■ *Materials needed:* anatomical model of the ear, paper and pencil

Step 1: Using the anatomical model, locate and identify the structures of the outer ear. List them, describe them, and state their function.

Step 2: Locate and identify the structures of the middle ear. Record their description and function the same as in step 1.

Step 3: Locate and identify the structures of the inner ear. Again, record their description and function the same as in step 1. What fluid fills the inner ear and what is the function of this fluid?

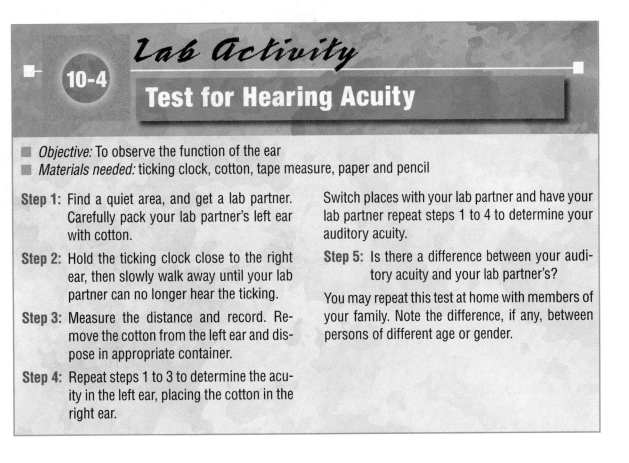

Lab Activity 10-4
Test for Hearing Acuity

- *Objective:* To observe the function of the ear
- *Materials needed:* ticking clock, cotton, tape measure, paper and pencil

Step 1: Find a quiet area, and get a lab partner. Carefully pack your lab partner's left ear with cotton.

Step 2: Hold the ticking clock close to the right ear, then slowly walk away until your lab partner can no longer hear the ticking.

Step 3: Measure the distance and record. Remove the cotton from the left ear and dispose in appropriate container.

Step 4: Repeat steps 1 to 3 to determine the acuity in the left ear, placing the cotton in the right ear.

Switch places with your lab partner and have your lab partner repeat steps 1 to 4 to determine your auditory acuity.

Step 5: Is there a difference between your auditory acuity and your lab partner's?

You may repeat this test at home with members of your family. Note the difference, if any, between persons of different age or gender.

Lab Activity 10-5
Sense of Taste and Smell

- *Objective:* To observe the function of the nose and mouth
- *Materials needed:* cubes of apple, pear, orange, cheese; blindfold; spoon; paper towels; paper and pencil.

Step 1: Blindfold your lab partner.

Step 2: Have your partner pinch the nostrils together.

Step 3: Using the spoon, place one of the four foods in your partner's mouth.

Step 4: Have your partner chew the food and then spit it out into the paper towel.

Step 5: Identify the food and record the information.

Step 6: Repeat steps 3 to 5 for the remaining three foods.

Step 7: Leave the blindfold in place but do not pinch the nostrils this time and repeat steps 3 to 5.

Step 8: Is there a difference in the identification of food? Can food be identified by taste alone?

Chapter 11

ENDOCRINE SYSTEM

Key Words

A gland is any organ that produces a secretion. **Endocrine glands,** Figure 11-1, are organized groups of tissues which use materials from the blood or lymph to make new compounds called hormones. Endocrine glands are also called ductless glands and glands of internal secretion; the hormones are secreted directly into the bloodstream as the blood circulates through the gland. The secretions are transported to all areas of the body where they have a special influence on cells, tissues, and organs. There is another type of gland called an **exocrine gland,** in which the secretions from the gland must go through a duct. This duct then carries the secretion to a body surface or organ. Exocrine glands include sweat, salivary, lacrimal, and pancreas. Their functions are included in chapters on the relevant body systems. See Figure 11-2.

One of the endocrine glands, the pancreas, performs both as an exocrine gland and an endocrine gland. The pancreas produces pancreatic juices which go through a duct into the small intestines. The pancreas also has a special group of cells known as **islets of Langerhans** which secrete the hormone insulin directly into the bloodstream.

FUNCTION OF THE ENDOCRINE SYSTEM

The function of the endocrine system is to secrete hormones or chemical messengers which coordinate and direct the activities of target cells and target organs, Table 11-1.

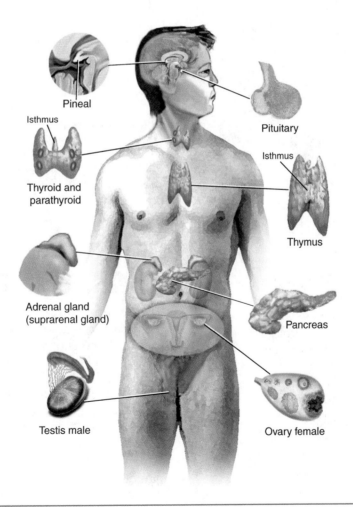

Pineal

Isthmus

Thyroid and parathyroid

Adrenal gland (suprarenal gland)

Testis male

Pituitary

Isthmus

Thymus

Pancreas

Ovary female

Figure 11-1 *Locations of the endocrine glands*

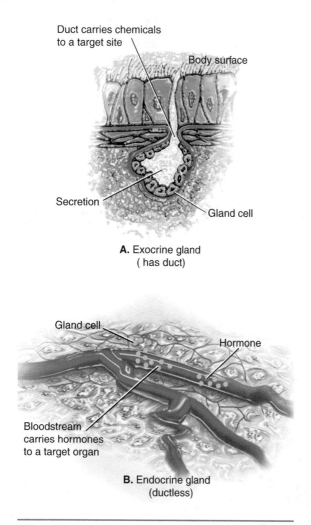

Duct carries chemicals to a target site

Body surface

Secretion

Gland cell

A. Exocrine gland (has duct)

Gland cell

Hormone

Bloodstream carries hormones to a target organ

B. Endocrine gland (ductless)

Figure 11-2 (A) Exocrine gland; (B) endocrine gland

The major glands of the endocrine system include pituitary, pineal, thyroid, parathyroid, thymus, adrenals, pancreas, and the gonads (ovaries in the female and testes in the male).

Figure 11-1 shows the locations of the endocrine glands in the body. Each has specific functions to perform. Any disturbance in the functioning of these glands may cause changes in the appearance or functioning of the body.

HORMONAL CONTROL

The secretion of the hormones operates on a negative feedback system or under the control of the nervous system.

Negative Feedback

Negative feedback occurs when there is a drop in the level of a hormone. This drop triggers a chain reaction of responses to increase the amount of hormone in the blood. A description follows of how the negative feedback system functions as it relates to the thyroid gland.

1. The blood level of thyroxine (thyroid hormone) falls.→
2. The hypothalamus in the brain gets the message.→
3. The hypothalamus responds by sending a releasing hormone for TSH.→
4. This goes to the anterior pituitary gland which responds by releasing TSH.→
5. TSH stimulates the thyroid gland to produce thyroxine.→
6. Thyroxine blood level rises which in turn causes the hypothalmus to shut off the releasing hormone for TSH.

Nervous Control

The nervous system controls the glands which are stimulated by nervous stimuli, as in the adrenal medulla where the gland is stimulated by the sympathetic nervous system. For example, when we are frightened, the adrenal medulla secretes adrenalin.

PITUITARY GLAND

The **pituitary gland** is a tiny structure having a diameter of about 10 mm and a weight of approximately 0.5 g, about the size of a grape. It is located at the base of the brain within the sella turcica, a small bony depression in the sphenoid bone of the skull, Figure 11-3. The pituitary gland is connected to the hypothalamus by a stalk called the infundibulum. The pituitary gland is divided into an anterior lobe and a posterior lobe, Figure 11-4.

Figure 11-5 highlights the hormones of the pituitary gland and the structures they act upon. The pituitary gland is known as the *master gland* because of its major influence on the body's activities. See Table 11-2. It is even more amazing

Table 11-1 Endocrine Glands

GLAND	LOCATION	HORMONE	PRINCIPAL EFFECTS
PITUITARY Anterior lobe	Undersurface of the brain in the sella turcica of the skull	Growth hormone (GH)	Normal growth of body tissues
		Thyroid-stimulating hormone (TSH) (Thyrotropin)	Stimulates growth and activity of thyroid cells to produce thyroid hormone
		Adrenocorticotropic hormone (ACTH)	Stimulates the cortex of the adrenal gland
		Melanocyte-stimulating hormone (MSH)	Increases skin pigmentation
		Follicle-stimulating hormone (FSH)	Stimulates the maturity of the graafian follicle to rupture and to produce estrogen in the female. In the male it stimulates the development of the testes and the production of sperm.
		Luteinizing hormone (LH) Interstitial cell–stimulating hormone (ICSH)	Causes the development of the corpus luteum, which then secretes progesterone in the female. ICSH in the male stimulates the interstitial cells of the testes to produce testosterone.
		Prolactin	Develops breast tissue and stimulates production of milk after childbirth.
Posterior lobe		Oxytocin	Stimulates contraction of uterus, especially during child-birth; causes ejection of milk from mammary glands
		Vasopressin or Antidiuretic hormone (ADH)	Acts on cells of kidney tubules to concentrate urine and conserve fluid in the body. Also acts to constrict blood vessels.
THYROID	Lower portion of anterior neck	Thyroxine (T_4) and Triiodothyronine (T_3)	Increases metabolism; influences both physical and mental activity; promotes normal growth and development
		Thyrocalcitonin	Causes calcium to be stored in bones; reduces blood level of calcium
PARATHYROID	Posterior surface of thyroid gland	Parathormone	Regulates exchange of calcium between the bones and blood
ADRENAL Medulla	Superior surface of each kidney	Adrenaline (Epinephrine)	Increases heart rate, blood pressure, and flow of blood; decreases intestinal activity
Cortex		Glucocorticoids	Affect the metabolism of protein, fat, and glucose, thereby increasing blood sugar
		Aldosterone (Mineral corticoid)	Controls electrolyte balances by regulating the reab-sorption of sodium and the excretion of potassium
		Sex hormones (Androgens)	Govern sex characteristics, especially those that are masculine
PANCREAS	Behind the stomach	Insulin	Essential to the metabolism of carbohydrates; reduces the blood sugar level
		Glucagon	Stimulates the liver to release glycogen and converts it to glucose to increase blood sugar levels
THYMUS	Under the sternum	Thymosin	Reacts upon lymphoid tissue to produce T lymphocyte cells to develop immunity to certain disease
PINEAL BODY	Base of brain	Melatonin	Relates to the sleep cycle
OVARIES	Female pelvis	Estrogen	Promotes growth of primary and secondary sexual characteristics
		Progesterone	Develops excretory portion of mammary glands; aids in maintaining pregnancy
TESTES	Male scrotum	Testosterone	Develops primary and secondary sexual characteristics; stimulates maturation of sperm

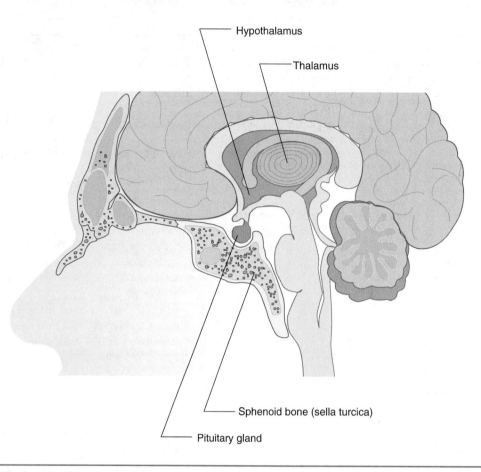

Hypothalamus

Thalamus

Sphenoid bone (sella turcica)

Pituitary gland

Figure 11-3 *The pituitary gland in relation to the brain*

when you consider the size of this incredible gland.

Pituitary-Hypothalamus Interaction

The hormones of the anterior pituitary are controlled by the releasing chemicals or factors produced by the hypothalamus in the brain. As the pituitary hormones are needed by the body, the hypothalamus releases a specific releasing factor for each hormone. See Figure 11-4. For example, the thyroid-stimulating hormone (TSH) has a TSH releasing factor. In addition, when a sufficient amount of the hormone is released, a different releasing factor will inhibit the anterior pituitary from secreting TSH.

The hypothalamus is considered part of the nervous system. However, it produces two hormones: vasopressin, which converts to antidiuretic hormone (ADH), and oxytocin. These hormones are stored in the posterior lobe of the pituitary and are released into the bloodstream in response to nerve impulses from the hypothalamus.

HORMONES OF THE PITUITARY GLAND

The pituitary gland is divided into two lobes. The larger anterior pituitary lobe produces seven hormones. The smaller posterior pituitary lobe consists primarily of nerve fibers and neuroglial cells

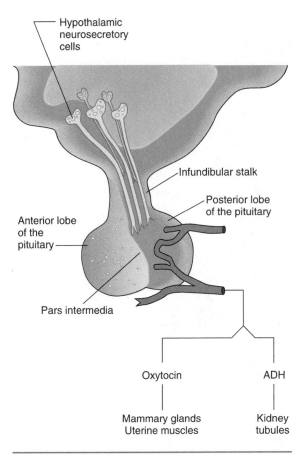

Hypothalamic neurosecretory cells

Infundibular stalk

Posterior lobe of the pituitary

Anterior lobe of the pituitary

Pars intermedia

Oxytocin

ADH

Mammary glands Uterine muscles

Kidney tubules

Figure 11-4 Pituitary gland

that support the nerve fibers. Neurons in the hypothalamus produce hormones secreted by the posterior pituitary lobe.

Anterior Pituitary Lobe

The **anterior pituitary lobe** secretes the following hormones.

1. **Growth hormone (GH)** (or **somatotropin**) is responsible for growth and development. This hormone also helps fat to be used for energy, saving glucose and helping to maintain blood sugar levels.

2. **Prolactin hormone (PRL)** develops breast tissue and stimulates the production of milk after childbirth. The function in males is unknown.

3. **Thyroid-stimulating hormone (TSH)** stimulates the growth and secretion of the thyroid gland.

4. **Adrenocorticotropic hormone (ACTH)** stimulates the growth and secretion of the adrenal cortex.

5. **Follicle-stimulating hormone (FSH)** stimulates the growth of the graafian follicle and the production of estrogen in females, and stimulates the production of sperm in the male.

6. **Luteinizing hormone (LH)** stimulates ovulation and the formation of the corpus luteum, which produces progesterone in females.

7. **Interstitial cell–stimulating hormone (ICSH)** is necessary for the production of testosterone by the interstitial cells of the testes in men.

8. **melanocyte-stimulating hormone (MSH)** is responsible for increasing skin pigmentation.

Posterior Pituitary Lobe

The hormones produced by the hypothalamus are stored in the **posterior pituitary lobe.**

1. **Vasopressin** converts to antidiuretic hormone or ADH in the bloodstream. The name vasopressin may cause confusion because it causes little or no vasoconstriction. ADH maintains the water balance by increasing the absorption of water in the kidney tubules. Sometimes drugs called diuretics are used to inhibit the action of ADH. The result is an increase in urinary output and a decrease in blood volume, thus decreasing blood pressure.

2. **Oxytocin** is released during childbirth, causing strong contractions of the uterus. It also causes strong contractions when a mother is breastfeeding. A synthetic form of oxytocin is called pitocin and is given to help start labor or make uterine contractions stronger.

THYROID AND PARATHYROID GLANDS

The thyroid and parathyroid glands are located in the neck, close to the cricoid cartilage (or the "Adam's apple"). The thyroid regulates body metabolism. The parathyroid maintains the calcium-phosphorus balance.

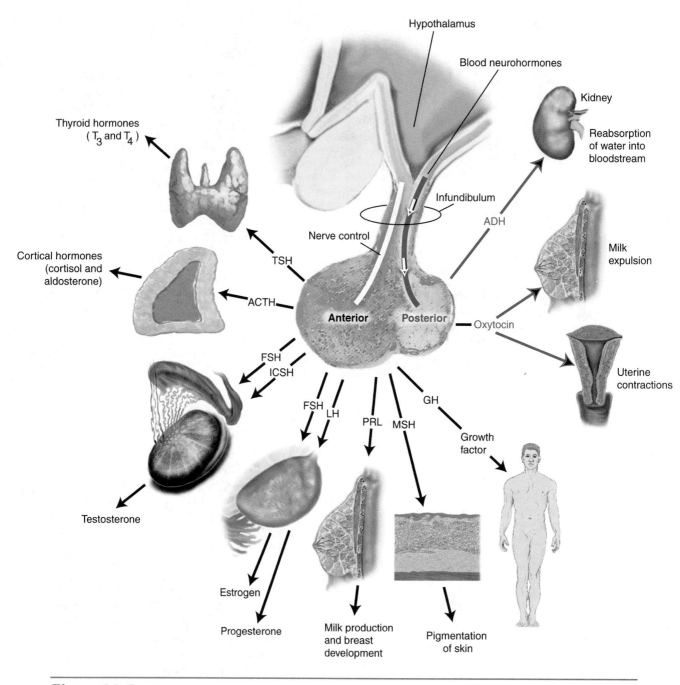

Figure 11-5 *The pituitary gland and its hormonal secretions*

Thyroid Gland

The **thyroid gland** is a butterfly-shaped mass of tissue located in the anterior part of the neck, Figure 11-6. It lies on either side of the larynx, over the trachea. Its general shape is that of the letter *H.* It is about 2 inches long, with two lobes joined by strands of thyroid tissue called the isthmus. Coming from the isthmus is a fingerlike lobe of tissue known as the intermediate lobe. This intermediate lobe projects upward toward the floor of the mouth, as far up as the hyoid bone. The thyroid gland has a rich blood supply. In fact, it has been

Table 11-2 *Pituitary Hormones and Their Known Functions*

PITUITARY HORMONE	KNOWN FUNCTION
Anterior Lobe	
TSH—thyroid-stimulating hormone (thyrotropin)	Stimulates the growth and the secretion of the thyroid gland.
ACTH—adrenocorticotropic hormone	Stimulates the growth and the secretion of the adrenal cortex.
FSH—follicle-stimulating hormone	Stimulates growth of new graafian (ovarian) follicle and secretion of estrogen by follicle cells in the female and the production of sperm in the male.
LH—luteinizing hormone (female)	Stimulates ovulation and formation of the corpus luteum. Corpus luteum secretes progesterone.
ICSH—interstitial cell–stimulating hormone (male)	Stimulates testosterone secretion by the interstitial cells of the testes.
PRL—prolactin	Stimulates secretion of milk in females. Function in males is unknown.
GH—growth hormone (somatotropin, STH)	Accelerates body growth and causes fat to be used for energy; this helps to maintain blood sugar.
MSH—melanocyte-stimulating hormone	Increases skin pigmentation
Posterior Lobe—Hormones Produced by the Hypothalamus	
Vasopressin—antidiuretic hormone (ADH)	Maintains water balance by reducing urinary output. It acts on kidney tubules to reabsorb water into the blood more quickly. In large amounts, it causes constriction of arteries.
Oxytocin	Promotes milk ejection and causes contraction of the smooth muscles of the uterus.

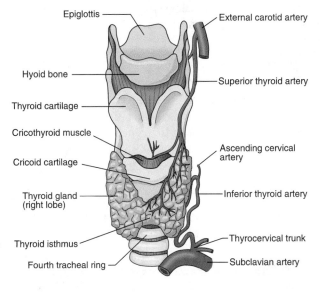

Epiglottis
External carotid artery
Hyoid bone
Superior thyroid artery
Thyroid cartilage
Cricothyroid muscle
Ascending cervical artery
Cricoid cartilage
Thyroid gland (right lobe)
Inferior thyroid artery
Thyroid isthmus
Thyrocervical trunk
Fourth tracheal ring
Subclavian artery

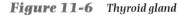

Figure 11-6   *Thyroid gland*

estimated that about 4 to 5 liters (some 8.5 to 10.5 pints) of blood pass through the gland every hour.

The thyroid gland secretes three hormones: thyroxine, triiodothyronine, and calcitonin. The first two are iodine-bearing derivatives of the amino acid, tyrosine. Triiodothyronine is 5 to 10 times more active than thyroxine, but its activity is less prolonged. However, the two have the same effect. Both hormones are produced in the follicle cells of the thyroid gland. These cells are stimulated to secretory activity by a hormone from the anterior lobe of the pituitary gland. This thyroid-stimulating hormone (TSH) controls the production and secretion of the thyroid hormones from the thyroid gland. The thyroid hormones contain iodine. Most of the iodine needed for their synthesis comes from the diet. Iodides are circulated to the thyroid gland, where they are "trapped." Here the iodides combine with the amino acid tyrosine to form the hormones **triiodothyronine (T_3)** and **thyroxine (T_4).** The concentration of these two hormones in the bloodstream is controlled by the negative feedback system previously discussed. The consequences of hyposecretion and hypersecretion of the thyroid hormones is discussed later in this chapter.

Thyroxine controls the rate of metabolism, heat production, and oxidation of all cells, with the possible exception of the brain and spleen cells. It can speed up or slow down the activities of the body as needed. In the liver, the two thyroid hormones affect the conversion of glycogen from sources other than sugar. It also helps to change glycogen into glucose, raising the glucose level of the blood.

The functions of thyroxin (T_4) and triiodothyronine (T_3) are as follows:

1. Controls the rate of metabolism in the body; how cells use glucose and oxygen to produce heat and energy.

2. Stimulates protein synthesis and thus helps in tissue growth.

3. Stimulates the breakdown of liver glycogen.

Calcitonin. Another hormone produced and secreted by the thyroid gland is **calcitonin.** It controls the calcium ion concentration in the body by maintaining a proper calcium level in the bloodstream.

Calcium is an essential body mineral. Approximately 99% of the calcium in the body is stored in the bones. The rest is located in the blood and tissue fluids. Calcium is necessary for blood clotting, holding cells together, and neuromuscular functions. The constant level of calcium in the blood and tissues is maintained by the action of calcitonin and parathormone (produced by the parathyroid gland).

When blood calcium levels are higher than normal, calcitonin secretion is increased. Calcitonin lowers the calcium concentration in the blood and body fluids by decreasing the rate of the bone resorption or osteoclastic activity and by increasing the calcium absorption by bones or osteoblastic activity. Proper secretion of calcitonin into the bloodstream prevents hypercalcemia, a harmful rise in the blood calcium level.

Parathyroid Glands

The **parathyroid glands,** usually four in number, are tiny glands the size of grains of rice. These are attached to the posterior surface of the thyroid gland, and secrete the hormone **parathormone.** Parathormone, like calcitonin, also controls the concentration of calcium in the bloodstream. When the blood calcium level is lower than normal, parathormone secretion is increased.

Parathormone stimulates an increase in the number and size of specialized bone cells referred to as osteoclasts. Osteoclasts quickly invade hard bone tissue, digesting large amounts of the bony material containing calcium. As this process continues, calcium leaves the bone and is released into the bloodstream, increasing the calcium blood level.

Bone calcium is bonded to phosphorus in a compound called calcium phosphate ($CaPO_4$). When calcium is released into the bloodstream, phosphorus is released along with it. Parathormone stimulates the kidneys to excrete any excess phosphorus from the blood; at the same time, it inhibits calcium excretion from the kidneys. Consequently, the concentration of blood calcium rises.

Thus, parathormone and calcitonin of the thyroid have opposite, or antagonistic, effects to one another (see Figure 11-7 for a summary of their actions). Parathormone, however, acts much more slowly than calcitonin. It may be hours before the effects of parathormone become apparent. In this manner, the secretion of parathormone and calcitonin serve as complementary processes controlling the level of calcium in the bloodstream.

THYMUS GLAND

The **thymus** gland is both an endocrine gland and lymphatic organ. It is located under the sternum, anterior and superior to the heart. Fairly large during childhood, it begins to disappear at puberty. Research has discovered that the thymus gland secretes a large number of hormones. The major hormone is thymosin, which helps to stimulate the lymphoid cells that are responsible for the production of T cells, which fight certain diseases.

ADRENAL GLANDS

The two **adrenal glands** are located on top of each kidney, one gland on each kidney, Figure 11-8. Each gland has two parts: the cortex and the medulla. Adrenocorticotrophic hormone (ACTH) from the pituitary glands stimulates the activity of the cortex of the adrenal gland. The hormones secreted by the adrenal cortex are known as cor-

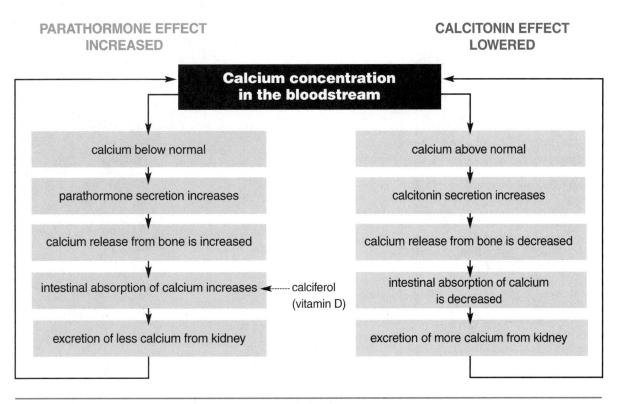

PARATHORMONE EFFECT INCREASED

CALCITONIN EFFECT LOWERED

Calcium concentration in the bloodstream

calcium below normal	calcium above normal
parathormone secretion increases	calcitonin secretion increases
calcium release from bone is increased	calcium release from bone is decreased
intestinal absorption of calcium increases ◀----- calciferol (vitamin D)	intestinal absorption of calcium is decreased
excretion of less calcium from kidney	excretion of more calcium from kidney

Figure 11-7 *Effects of parathormone and calcitonin on the level of calcium in the blood*

ticoids. The corticoids are very effective as anti-inflammatory drugs.

The cortex secretes three groups of corticoids, each of which is of great importance.

1. **Mineralocorticoids**—mainly aldosterone, affects the kidney tubules by speeding up the reabsorption of sodium into the blood circulation and increasing the excretion of potassium from the blood. They also speed up the reabsorption of water by the kidneys. Aldosterone (M-C) is used in the treatment of Addison's disease to replace deficient secretion of mineralocorticoids.

2. **Glucocorticoids**—namely cortisone and cortisol, increase the amount of glucose in the blood. This is done by (1) the conversion of proteins and fats to glycogen in the liver, followed by (2) breakdown of the glycogen into glucose. These glucocorticoids also help the body resist the aggravations caused by various everyday stresses. In addition, these hormones seem to de-

crease edema in inflammation and reduce pain by inhibiting pain-causing **prostaglandin.**

3. Sex hormones for both males and females—**androgens** are male sex hormones which, together with similar hormones from the gonads, bring about masculine characteristics. Some estrogens are also present.

Medulla of the Adrenal Gland

The medulla of the adrenal gland secretes **epinephrine** and **norepinephrine,** Table 11-3. Epinephrine or (**adrenalin**), is a powerful cardiac stimulant. It functions by bringing about a release of more glucose from stored glycogen for muscle activity and increasing the force and rate of the heartbeat. This chemical activity increases cardiac output and venous return, and raises the systolic blood pressure. The adrenal medulla responds to the sympathetic nervous system. The hormones produced are referred to

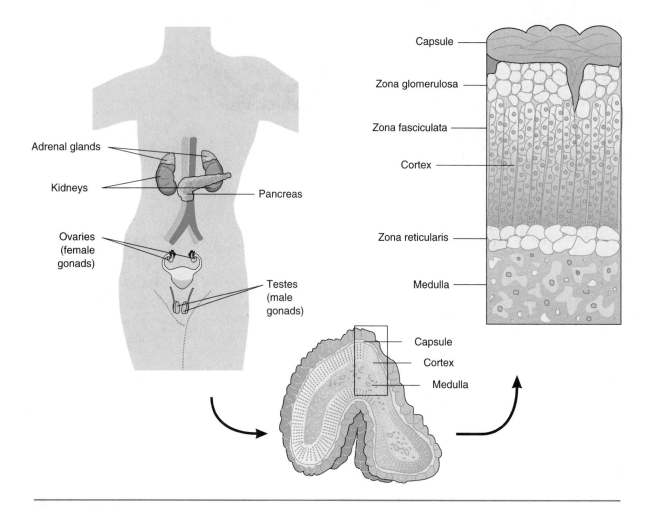

Figure 11-8 *Locations of adrenal glands and gonads*

Table 11-3 *Comparison of the Effects Between Epinephrine and Norepinephrine*

EPINEPHRINE	NOREPINEPHRINE
1. Bronchial relaxation	No effect
2. Dilation of iris	No effect
3. Excitation of central nervous system	No effect
4. Increased conversion of stored glycogen to glucose	Much less effect
5. Increased heart rate	Little effect
6. Increased cardiac output and venous return	Slight effect
7. Increased blood flow to muscles	Vasoconstriction in muscle
8. Increased myocardial strength	About the same
9. Increased basal metabolic rate (BMR)	Much less effect
10. Increased systolic blood pressure	Raises both systolic and diastolic blood pressure
11. Increased lipolytic effects; frees fatty acids from fat deposits	Slightly greater effects
12. Relaxation of uterine myometrial muscles	Pilomotor contraction

as the fight-or-flight hormones, because they prepare the body for an emergency situation.

GONADS

The **gonads,** or sex glands, include the ovaries in the female and the testes in the male. The ovary is responsible for producing the ova or egg and the hormones **estrogen** and **progesterone.** The testes are responsible for producing sperm and the hormone **testosterone.**

Female Hormones— Estrogen and Progesterone

Estrogen is produced by the graafian follicle cells of the ovary. It stimulates the development of the reproductive organs, including the breast, and secondary sex characteristics such as pubic and axillary hair.

Progesterone is produced by the cells of the corpus luteum of the ovary. Progesterone works with estrogen to build up the lining of the uterus for the fertilized egg. If no fertilization occurs, menstruation takes place. This cycle depends on the secretion of the anterior pituitary gland (see Chapter 21).

Male Hormone—Testosterone

Testosterone is produced by the interstitial cells of the testes and is responsible for the development of the male reproductive organs and secondary sex characteristics. Testosterone influences the growth of a beard and other body hair, deepening of the voice, increase in musculature, and the production of sperm. The secretion of the hormone depends on the pituitary gland (see Chapter 21).

PANCREAS

The **pancreas** is located behind the stomach and functions as both an exocrine and an endocrine gland. The exocrine portion secretes pancreatic juices which are excreted through a duct into the small intestines. There they become part of the digestive juices. The endocrine portion is involved in the production of insulin by the B cells of the islets of Langerhans on the pancreas.

The islet cells are distributed throughout the pancreas. These cells were named the islets of Langerhans after the doctor who discovered them, Figure 11-9. B cells produce **insulin,** which (1) promotes the utilization of glucose in the cells, necessary for maintenance of normal levels of blood glucose, (2) promotes fatty acid transport and fat deposition into cells, (3) promotes amino acid transport into cells, and (4) facilitates protein synthesis. Lack of insulin secretion by the island (islet) cells causes diabetes mellitus.

The A cells contained in the islets of Langerhans secrete the hormone **glucagon.** The action of glucagon may be antagonistic or opposite to that of insulin. Glucagon's function is to increase the level of glucose in the bloodstream. This is done by stimulating the conversion of liver glycogen to glucose. The control of glucagon secretion

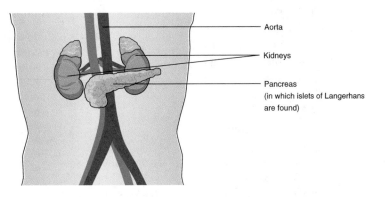

Aorta

Kidneys

Pancreas
(in which islets of Langerhans
are found)

Figure 11-9   *Location of islets of Langerhans*

is achieved by negative feedback (refer to "Negative Feedback" earlier in the chapter). Low glucose levels in the bloodstream stimulate the A cells to secrete glucagon, which quickly increases the glucose level in the bloodstream.

PINEAL GLAND

The **pineal gland** or body is a small pinecone-shaped organ attached by a slim stalk to the roof of the third ventricle in the brain. The hormone produced by the pineal gland is called **melatonin.** The pineal gland is stimulated by a group of nerve cells called the suprachiasmatic nucleus (SCN), which are located in the brain over the pathway of fibers of the optic nerve. The amount of light entering the eye stimulates the SCN which then stimulates the pineal gland to release its hormone. The amount of light affects the amount of melatonin secreted. The darker it is, the more melatonin is produced; the lighter it is, the less melatonin is produced. There are no clear answers to the function of melatonin; however, melatonin causes body temperature to drop. For example, falling asleep is associated with lowered body temperature, whereas waking up is associated with rising body temperature.

OTHER HORMONES PRODUCED IN THE BODY

Prostaglandins

In various tissues throughout the body, hormones are secreted which are called prostaglandins. Their activity depends on which tissue secretes them. Some prostaglandins can cause constriction of the blood vessels; others may cause dilation. Prostaglandins can be used to induce labor and cause severe muscular contractions of the uterus. The exact nature and function of the prostaglandins are being extensively studied by scientists.

A host of hormones are produced throughout the body. They can originate from many different glands or other organs. A complete description of all the hormones in the body is beyond the intent of this anatomy textbook.

Effects of Aging on The Endocrine System

As the body ages, the glands of the endocrine system undergo changes. An example is the reduction of aldosterone and cortisol from the adrenal glands. In addition, in women after menopause there is a sharp decline in estrogen and progesterone. In the male the prostate gland enlarges, and there is a reduction in testosterone from the testes. The physician may prescribe hormones if these endocrine changes create a disorder.

DISORDERS OF THE ENDOCRINE SYSTEM

Endocrine gland disturbances may be caused by several factors such as disease of the gland itself, infections in other parts of the body, autoimmune causes, and dietary deficiencies. Most disturbances result from (1) hyperactivity of the glands, causing oversecretion of hormones, or (2) hypoactivity of the gland, resulting in undersecretion of hormones. Health care workers most often see these patients in a doctor's office.

PITUITARY DISORDERS

Disturbances of the pituitary gland may produce a number of body changes. This gland is chiefly involved in the growth function. However, as the master gland, the pituitary indirectly influences other activities.

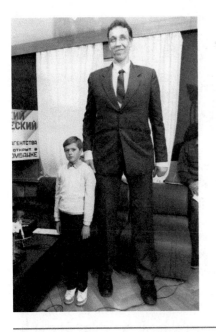

Figure 11-10   *Gigantism caused by excessive secretion of growth hormone from the anterior pituitary gland*

Hyperfunction of Pituitary

Hyperfunctioning of the pituitary gland (often due to a pituitary tumor) causes hypersecretion of the pituitary growth hormone. This can lead to two conditions: gigantism and acromegaly.

Hyperfunctioning during preadolescence causes **gigantism,** an overgrowth of the long bones leading to excessive tallness, Figure 11-10.

If hypersecretion of the growth hormone occurs during adulthood, **acromegaly** results. This is an overdevelopment of the bones of the face, hands, and feet, Figure 11-11. In adults whose long bones have already matured, the growth hormone attacks the cartilaginous regions and the bony joints. Thus, the chin protrudes, and the lips, nose, and extremities enlarge disproportionately. Lethargy and severe headaches frequently set in as well.

Treatment of acromegaly and gigantism is drug therapy (which inhibits GH), and radiation therapy.

Hypofunction of Pituitary

Hypofunctioning of the pituitary gland during childhood leads to pituitary **dwarfism.** Growth of the long bones is abnormally decreased by an

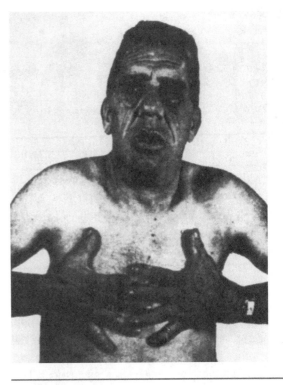

Figure 11-11   *Acromegaly*   (*Photo courtesy of Dr. Matthew Leinung, Acting Head, Division of Endocrinology, Albany Medical College, Albany, NY*)

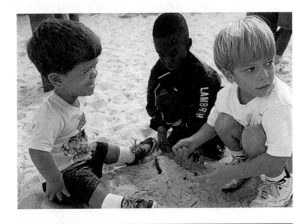

Figure 11-12   *Dwarfism*

inadequate production of growth hormone. Despite the small size, however, the body of a dwarf is normally proportioned and intelligence is normal. Unfortunately, the physique remains juvenile and sexually immature, Figure 11-12. Treatment involves early diagnosis and injections of human growth hormone. The treatment period is 5 years or more.

Medical Highlight

Sunshine Disorder

It is called "cabin fever" or "winter blues." It is the depression or anxiety many people feel during the dark days of winter. To feel better many people look for a winter vacation in the sunshine. Scientists have identified this phenomena and call it seasonal affective disorder or SAD. Scientists at the National Institute of Mental Health described SAD and documented preliminary findings regarding a form of treatment with light.

They conducted a study to observe how a group of people reacted to amounts of daylight. As daylight began decreasing during the fall, people started to develop symptoms of lethargy, anxiety, mood changes, appetite increases (especially a craving for carbohydrates), and a decrease in physical activity. As winter progressed and the days shortened, the symptoms increased. When spring arrived, the symptoms diminished; by the end of May almost everyone in the study group exhibited no symptoms.

During this study, scientists found that they could reverse the symptoms by supplying light. They used two different kinds of light: The dimmer yellow light had no effect, but the brighter light (with a frequency spectrum more or less simulating the frequencies in sunlight) produced a marked change in mood in most of the patients who received this treatment.

Our bodies have evolved to respond to a biological clock, being alert by daylight and sleepy as the sun fades into the night. A small cluster of brain cells called the suprachiasmatic nucleus (SCN) has been identified as the probable site for the biological clock in our bodies. One type of information concerns the amount of light coming in through the eyes. **Note:** *Supra* means "over"; *chiasmatic* refers to "optic chiasma," which is the site where the fibers (nerve endings) from the retinas of the right and left eye cross. The SCN nerve cluster is located directly above a part of our vision system.

The SCN sends its message about the amount of light through the sympathetic nervous system to the pineal gland. The pineal gland secretes melatonin.

For people affected by SAD, the suggested treatment is bright light exposure for 0.5 to 3 hours, usually in the morning. In addition, prepare for the change in daylight hours by planning special activities for shorter days of winter. Expose yourself to as much bright light as possible. On sunny days go outside; on dark days use bright lights. Proper diagnosis is essential for proper treatment. If these symptoms develop, seek professional advice.

Diabetes Insipidus

Another disorder caused by posterior lobe dysfunction is **diabetes insipidus.** In this condition, there is a drop in the amount of ADH, which causes an excessive loss of water and electrolytes. The affected person complains of excessive thirst (**polydypsia**).

THYROID DISORDERS

Because the thyroid gland controls metabolic activity, any disorder will affect other structures besides the gland itself. Persons at risk include those with other immune system problems, such as arthritis sufferers. Signs and symptoms of the disorders most frequently seen are discussed in this section.

Diagnostic Tests for Thyroid

To diagnose thyroid function, a blood test is done; blood levels of TSH, T_3, and T_4 are checked to see if they are within normal limits.

A thyroid scan is another diagnostic tool used to determine the activity of the thyroid gland. The patient takes radioactive iodine; after the dye is taken, a scan measures how the radioactive iodine is taken up by the thyroid gland. A large uptake indicates hyperthyroidism.

A similiar test is the radioactive iodine uptake test measures the activity of the thyroid gland. Dilute radioactive iodine is given orally. The amount which accumulates in the thyroid gland is calculated by use of a scan.

Hyperthyroidism

Hyperthyroidism is due to the overactivity of the thyroid gland. Too much thyroxin is secreted (hypersecretion), leading to enlargement of the gland. People with hyperthyroidism consume large quantities of food, but nevertheless suffer a loss of body fat and weight. Symptoms include feeling too hot, fast growing and rougher fingernails, and weakened muscles. They may suffer from increased blood pressure and heartbeat, hand tremors, perspiration, and irritability. In addition, the liver releases excess glucose into the bloodstream, increasing the blood sugar level and causing a mild case of glycosuria. The most pronounced symptoms of hyperthyroidism include enlargement of the thyroid gland (**goiter**), bulging of the eyeballs (**exophthalmos**), dilation of the pupils, and wide-opened eyelids, Figure 11-13. In the United States, 70% to 80% of people who have hyperthyroidism have the type also known as Graves' disease.

The immediate cause of exophthalmos is not completely known. It is not directly caused by the hyperthyroidism, because removal of the thyroid does not always cause the eyeballs to return to their normal state. Treatment of hyperthyroidism includes total or partial removal of the thyroid

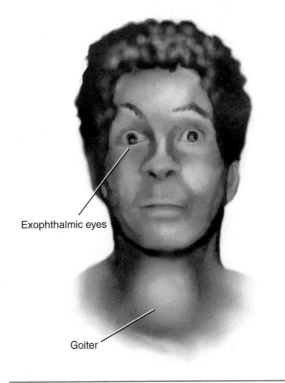

Exophthalmic eyes

Goiter

Figure 11-13   *Hyperthyroidism*

and administration of drugs such as propylthiouracil and methylthiouracil to reduce the thyroxin secretion. The use of radioactive iodine to suppress the activity of the thyroid gland is another treatment for hyperthyroidism.

Hypothyroidism

Hypothyroidism is a condition in which the thyroid gland does not secrete sufficient thyroxin (hyposecretion). This is manifested by low T_3 or T_4 levels or increased TSH blood levels.

Adult hypothyroidism may occur because of iodine deficiency. A simple goiter may indicate this condition. Because iodized salt is commonly used in the United States, that is not the usual cause of a hypothyroid condition. The major cause is an inflammation of the thyroid which destroys the ability of the gland to make thyroxine. This inflammation is an autoimmune disease that attacks the body's own thyroid gland. Symptoms include dry and itchy skin, dry and brittle hair, constipation, and muscle cramps at night. If this condition goes untreated, a condition known as myxedema occurs.

Depending on the time hypothyroidism strikes its victims, two different sets of disorders may occur: myxedema or cretinism.

Myxedema. The face becomes swollen, weight increases, and initiative and memory fail for a person experiencing **myxedema.** Treatment is daily medication of thyroid hormone. It is important for the health care worker to be sure the patient understands the necessity of taking the medication. Follow-up tests to measure TSH blood levels are also important.

Cretinism. Developing early in infancy or childhood, **cretinism** is characterized by a lack of mental and physical growth, resulting in mental retardation and malformation (dwarfism or cretinism). The sexual development and physical growth of cretins do not proceed beyond that of 7- or 8-year-old children.

In treating cretinism, thyroid hormones or thyroid extract may restore a degree of normal development if administered in time. In most cases, however, normal development cannot be completely restored once the affliction has set in.

○─ PARATHYROID DISORDERS

The parathyroid glands regulate the use of calcium and phosphorus. Both of these minerals are involved in many of the body systems.

Hyperfunctioning of the parathyroid glands may cause an increase in the amount of blood calcium, increasing the tendency for the calcium to crystallize in the kidneys as kidney stones. Excess amounts of calcium and phosphorus are withdrawn from the bones; this may lead to eventual deformity. So much calcium can be removed from the bones that they become honeycombed with cavities. Afflicted bones become so fragile that even walking can cause fractures.

Hypofunctioning of the parathyroid glands leads to a condition known as **tetany.** In this case, severely diminished calcium levels affect the normal function of nerves. Convulsive twitchings develop, and the afflicted person dies of spasms in the respiratory muscles. Treatment consists of ad-

ministering vitamin D, calcium, and parathormone to restore a normal calcium balance.

○─ ADRENAL DISORDERS

The adrenal glands produce glucocorticoid hormones. Therefore, disorders of the adrenal glands result in either an abundance or a deficiency of these hormones. Changes in glucocorticoid hormone levels always affect blood glucose levels.

Hyperfunction of Adrenal

Cushing's syndrome results from the hypersecretion of the glucocorticoid hormones from the adrenal cortex, Figure 11-14. This hypersecretion may be caused by an adrenal cortical tumor or the prolonged use of prednisone. (Oddly enough, more women than men tend to develop this endocrine disorder.) Symptoms include high blood pressure, muscular weakness, obesity, poor healing of skin lesions, a tendency to bruise easily, hirsutism (excessive hair growth), menstrual disorders in women, and hyperglycemia. The most noticeable characteristics are a rounded "moon" face and a "buffalo hump" that develops from the redistribution of body fat. Therapy consists of surgical removal of the adrenal cortical tumor.

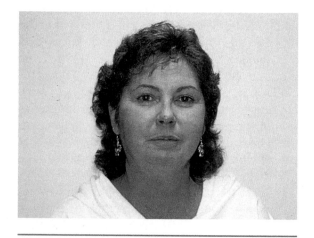

Figure 11-14 *Cushing's syndrome (Photo courtesy of Dr. Matthew Leinung, Acting Head, Division of Endocrinology, Albany Medical College, Albany, NY)*

Hypofunction of Adrenal Cortex

Hypofunctioning of the adrenal cortex also leads to **Addison's disease.** Persons with the disease exhibit the following symptoms: excessive pigmentation prompting the characteristic "bronzing" of the skin, decreased levels of blood glucose, hypoglycemia, low blood pressure which falls further when standing, pronounced muscular weakness and fatigue, diarrhea, weight loss, vomiting, and a severe drop of sodium in the blood and tissue fluids, causing a serious imbalance of electrolytes.

The medical treatment of Addison's disease is focused on the replacement of the deficient hormones.

STEROID ABUSE IN SPORTS

Athletes of today have turned to the use of androgenic anabolic steroids to build bigger, stronger muscles and thus hope to achieve status in the world of sports.

The risks of taking steroids far outweigh any temporary improvement that an athlete may hope to gain. Effects on males who abuse steroids include liver changes, decrease in spleen production, atrophy of the testicles, breast enlargement, and increased risk of cardiovascular disease. Effects on females include amenorrhea (loss of menstrual cycle), abnormal placement of body hair, baldness, and voice changes. In addition, both sexes complain of headaches, dizziness, hypertension, mood swings, and aggressiveness.

GONAD DISORDERS

Disturbances in the ovaries may consist of cysts and tumors, abnormal menstruation, and menopausal changes. Turner's syndrome may occur in either the male or female; this is a chromosomal disorder (see Chapter 21).

PANCREATIC DISORDERS

Diabetes mellitus is a condition caused by decreased secretion of insulin from the islets of Langerhans cells of the pancreas or by the ineffective use of insulin. Insulin is necessary for the cells to use glucose. Carbohydrate metabolism in diabetes mellitus is disturbed and thus has an adverse effect on protein and fat metabolism.

Diabetes is divided into two main types: Type I and Type II. Type I, also known as juvenile diabetes, is usually exhibited in children or young adults. The cause of Type I is thought to be an autoimmune reaction, which involves genetic and virus factors that destroy the islets of Langerhans cells. Patients who have Type I diabetes must take insulin and monitor daily blood glucose levels.

Symptoms of Type I diabetes include the following:

- Polyuria—excessive urination
- Polydipsia—excessive thirst
- Polyphagia—excessive hunger
- Weight loss
- Blurred vision
- Possible diabetic coma

Insulin deficiency causes glucose to accumulate in the bloodstream, rather than be transported to the cells and converted into energy. Eventually the excess becomes too much for the kidneys to reabsorb, and the excess glucose is excreted in the urine. Excretion of excess glucose requires an accompanying excretion of large amounts of water. This occurs to ensure that the sugar concentration does not rise too high. Diabetics are constantly thirsty because the lost water must be replaced.

Because sufficient glucose is not available for cellular oxidation in diabetes mellitus, the body starts to burn up protein and fats. The diabetic is constantly hungry and usually eats voraciously, but loses weight nonetheless.

When fats are utilized as a fuel source, they are rapidly but incompletely oxidized. One product of this abnormal rate of fat oxidation is ketone bodies. Ketone bodies are highly toxic; the type most commonly formed is acetoacetic acid. These ketone acids accumulate in the blood, promoting the development of acidosis, giving the breath and urine an odor of "sweet" acetone. If acidosis is severe, diabetic coma and death may result. Prolonged diabetes leads to atherosclerosis, heart disease, blindness, and kidney damage. Therapy consists of daily insulin injections and a controlled diet.

Patient education is critical in the treatment of diabetes. Insulin-dependent diabetes requires education in the signs of **hypoglycemia** (low blood sugar; insulin shock) and **hyperglycemia** (high blood sugar; diabetic coma), as illustrated in Table 11-4.

Characteristics and symptoms of Type II diabetes include the following:

- Gradual onset
- Most common in adults over age 45
- Feelings of tiredness or illness
- Frequent urination, especially at night
- Unusual thirst
- Frequent infections and slow healing of sores

Type II diabetes makes up 90% to 95% of diabetics. Diabetes is most common in adults over age 45, people who are overweight, individuals who have an immediate family member with diabetes, and people of certain ethnic or cultural groups. The incidence of Type II diabetes in younger people is growing; scientists believe the major cause is obesity. In this condition, insulin is secreted but in lowered amounts.

Treatment of Diabetes Mellitus

Diabetes is recognized as a leading cause of death and disability in the United States. Diabetes can damage the coronary arteries and blood vessels. Persons with diabetes also have higher cholesterol and triglyceride blood levels. This combination acts to cause the damaged vessels to trap cholesterol from the blood; in time, the blood vessels fill with fatty buildup, leading to heart disease, high blood pressure, and poor circulation. Heart and blood vessel damage occurs three times more often and at an earlier age in persons with diabetes. Diabetes is also associated with blindness, kidney failure, amputations, and nerve damage.

The treatment focus is on diet, weight reduction, glucose monitoring, and medication. Individuals who have diabetes need instruction on how to use their glucose monitoring system, how to inject insulin, how to exercise, how to use their calculated diet, and how to take prescribed medications as instructed. Oral hypoglycemic agents

Table 11-4 *Signs of Hypoglycemia and Hyperglycemia*

	HYPOGLYCEMIA (↓ BLOOD SUGAR)	HYPERGLYCEMIA (↑ BLOOD SUGAR)
Onset	Sudden	Slow
Reason	Too much insulin Too much exercise Not enough food	Not enough insulin Not enough exercise Too much food
Skin	Pale, moist to wet Sweating	Flushed, dry, hot No sweating
Symptoms	Nervous, trembling, confusion, irritable	Drowsy, lethargic, weak, lapses into unconsciousness
Breath	Normal odor	Fruity odor
Respiration	Normal to rapid	Kussmaul breathing (air hunger)
Glycosuria	Little to none	High amount
Ketonuria	None	Present
Blood sugar	Low—below 80	High—above 150
Treatment	Rapid response; give sugar in form of soft drink or orange juice Glucagon (IM); glucose 50% IV	Slow response IV fluids Regular insulin

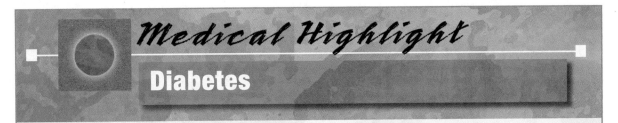

Medical Highlight

Diabetes

There are about 16 million Americans who have diabetes mellitus, a serious lifelong disorder that is yet incurable. About one-half of these people do not know they have the disease and are not under medical care. Researchers have made advances in managing diabetes and treating its complications. Major advances include:

- Development of better ways for patients to monitor blood glucose levels at home
- Development of external and implantable insulin pumps which deliver appropriate amounts of insulin and replace daily injections
- Use of laser treatment for diabetic eye disease, reducing the risk of blindness
- Successful transplantation of kidneys in diabetics with kidney failure
- Better ways of managing diabetic pregnancies and improving chances of a successful outcome
- Proof that intensive management of blood glucose levels reduces and may prevent development of microvascular complications of diabetes, such as peripheral vascular disease
- Use of glargine (insulin drug) that needs to be injected only once daily
- Benefits of taking aspirin for patients with diabetes and coronary artery disease

- Development of noninvasive blood glucose monitoring systems (e.g., use of laser beam and infrared technology)
- New oral medications for better control in Type II diabetes.

In the future, insulin may be administered through nasal sprays or taken in the form of a pill.

Researchers continue to look for the exact cause of diabetes and methods to prevent and cure the disease. Researchers have identified 20 genes involved in Type I diabetes, which makes its inheritance patterns complicated. Other scientists are studying environmental factors that may trigger Type I diabetes. If they can determine what causes the immune system to attack the cells that produce insulin, they may discover how to prevent the condition from developing. At the National Institute of Health, researchers believe stem cell research has the potential to help people with Type I diabetes. Researchers attribute most cases of Type II diabetes to obesity. Researchers are investigating the exact role that extra weight plays in preventing the proper utilization of insulin and why some overweight people develop the disease but others do not.

used by Type II diabetics can stimulate the pancreas to produce more insulin, increase the effectiveness of the insulin that is produced, slow the digestion of carbohydrates, and control liver production of glucose. In addition, some Type II diabetics may need insulin.

Patients with diabetes can lead normal, productive lives if they follow their treatment. They

should wear a medic-alert bracelet, stating that they are diabetic.

Tests for Diabetes Mellitus

The diagnostic tests to determine the presence of glucose are done on urine and blood samples. The most common test done is a finger prick to

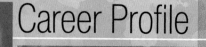

Career Profile
Medical Assistant

The medical assistant is an important allied health professional in the ambulatory care setting. The medical assistant performs both administrative and clinical tasks under the direction of licensed medical professionals. Medical assistants are great communicators acting as liaisons between the physician, patient, hospital staff, and other health professionals.

The medical assistant serves in many capacities—receptionist, secretary, transcriptionist, bookkeeper, insurance coder and biller, patient educator, and clinical assistant.

Education for this career may be in a vocational school or college program leading to a degree. The Certified Medical Assistant (CMA) or Registered Medical Assistant (RMA) organizations provide certification for this area. To be eligible for certification, the candidate must pass certain criteria. With the exception of a few states, both credentials are voluntary in that neither the federal government nor the state requires a medical assistant to be certified, although certification can be expected to enhance employment opportunities.

obtain a blood sample that is then measured in a glucometer (glucose monitor). This test may be done by the patient at home. The normal blood sugar is 110 mg (or below) of glucose per 100 ml of blood.

Another blood test for diabetics is glycosylated hemoglobin (HbA1c). The glucose exposed to hemoglobin attaches itself to the protein in a way that reflects the average blood glucose concentration for the preceding 2 to 3 months. The test is done every 3 months.

Urine may also be tested by using a specifically coded dipstick. A urine sample is obtained, then the tape is dipped into the urine and compared with the special coding bar that is found on the outside of the dipstick container.

Medical Terminology

acr/o	body extremity
megaly	enlargement of
acr/o/megaly	enlargement of body extremity
adren	toward the kidney
-al	pertaining to
adren/al	pertaining toward the kidney, above the kidney
dwarf	small by comparison
-ism	abnormal condition of
dwarf/ism	abnormal condition of smallness
exo	outside of

opthalm	eye
-os	one who
exo/phthalm/os	one who has abnormal protrusion of eyeball
gigant	largeness by comparison
gigant/ism	abnormal condition of largeness by comparison
hyper	over, excessive
glycemia	blood sugar
hyper/glycemia	excessive blood sugar
hypo	deficient
hypo/glycemia	deficient blood sugar
poly	many, much
dyspia	thirst
poly/dyspia	much or excessive thirst
phagia	eating
poly/phagia	much or excessive eating
urea	urination
poly/urea	much or excessive urination
ster	solid oil
-oid	resembles
ster/oid	resembles a solid oil
thyr	shield
thyr/oid	resembles a shield

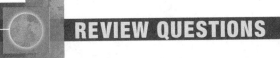

REVIEW QUESTIONS

Select the letter of the choice that best completes the statement.

1. The master gland is known as:
   a. pituitary
   b. thyroid
   c. adrenal
   d. ovary

2. The pituitary hormone which is necessary to govern metabolism is:
   a. FSH
   b. MSH
   c. TSH
   d. ACTH

3. The hormones that affect neuromuscular functioning, blood clotting, and holding the cells together are:
   a. thyroxine and calcitonin
   b. thyroxine and parathormone
   c. calcitonin and thymosin
   d. calcitonin and parathormone

4. The gland that governs the production of antibodies is the:
   a. thymus
   b. thyroid
   c. parathyroid
   d. pituitary

5. The hormone that is responsible for stimulating ovulation is:
   a. TSH
   b. ICSH
   c. FSH
   d. LTH

6. The hormone that prepares us to fight or flee is:
   a. aldosterone
   b. epinephrine
   c. cortisol
   d. corticoid

7. The secretions of the ovaries are:
   a. estrogen and LTH
   b. estrogen and LH
   c. progesterone and LTH
   d. progesterone and estrogen

8. A decrease in the production of insulin causes:
   a. diabetes mellitus
   b. diabetes insipidus
   c. cretinism
   d. exophthalmos

9. A hypofunction of the thyroid gland causes:
   a. exophthalmos
   b. glycosuria
   c. cretinism
   d. Graves' disease

10. An oversecretion of the adrenal cortex is known as:
   a. myxedema
   b. Cushing's syndrome
   c. Addison's disease
   d. dwarfism

COMPLETION

Complete the following chart.

GLAND	HORMONE	NORMAL FUNCTION	DISORDERS
Pituitary			
Pineal			
Thyroid			
Parathyroid			
Thymus			
Adrenals			
Gonads			
Pancreas			

MATCHING

Match each term in Column I with its correct description in Column II.

Column I	Column II
_____ **1.** ACTH	a. master gland of the endocrine system
_____ **2.** adrenals	b. any gland of internal secretion
_____ **3.** cortisone	c. a hormone secreted by adrenals
_____ **4.** gonad	d. regulates use of calcium
_____ **5.** endocrine	e. the secretion of any endocrine gland
_____ **6.** hormone	f. helps body meet emergencies
_____ **7.** insulin	g. sex gland
_____ **8.** parathyroid	h. regulates body metabolism
_____ **9.** pituitary	i. one of the hormones secreted by pituitary gland
_____**10.** thyroid	j. neccessary to maintain levels of blood glucose
	k. hypofunction of endocrine glands

APPLYING THEORY TO PRACTICE

1. You have a thermostat in your house which regulates the furnace or the air conditioner. When a certain temperature is reached, it automatically shuts off. This principle applies also to negative feedback in hormonal control. Explain how this functions in relation to the thyroid gland.

2. A patient comes to the doctor's office and tells the doctor she is experiencing leg cramping, which she has heard is related to calcium. Explain to the patient how calcium is affected by the action of the thyroid gland and parathyroid.

3. When you arrive at your office in the health maintenance organization, a patient calls out to you. He is near hysteria; he tells you he is experiencing heart palpitations and feels he is "jumping out of his skin." You check the records and note this patient has been on thyroid medication. Explain to the patient what you think may be the cause of his symptoms and what action should be taken.

4. Your brother wants to be a football player. He is 5'7"; he heard "steroids" could help him. Explain the action of steroids and why they should not be used.

5. Remember a time when you were frightened; think about it. How did your body react?

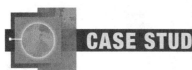

CASE STUDY

Jack, age 52, has been feeling tired lately. He also gets up frequently during the night to urinate and is always thirsty. He makes an appointment with Jodi, the medical assistant, to see his doctor. When Jack arrives at the office, Jodi takes his medical history and weighs and measures him. He is 5'9" and weighs 270 pounds. The doctor suspects Jack is exhibiting signs of diabetes. The doctor orders tests to be done and Jack is to return in 3 days for a follow-up visit. Jodi makes the arrangements for the tests and follow-up visit.

1. Explain the tests that are done to diagnose diabetes mellitus.

When Jack returns to the office, the doctor says his blood sugar is 240 mg and he makes the diagnosis of Type II diabetes. The doctor orders oral medication, prescribes an exercise program, gives Jack a calculated diet, and tells him he must monitor his blood glucose.

2. Describe diabetes mellitus and the cause of Jack's symptoms.

Jodi reviews with Jack the medication, his glucose monitoring system, the exercise program, and his diet requirements.

3. What is the benefit of exercise to patients with diabetes?

4. How do the oral agents help lower the blood glucose level?

5. What are the major complications of diabetes?

6. Explain the relationship between diabetes and heart disease.

7. What do researchers say is the biggest cause of Type II diabetes?

8. Researchers are making many advances in diabetic research. List the advances that may be most helpful to Jack.

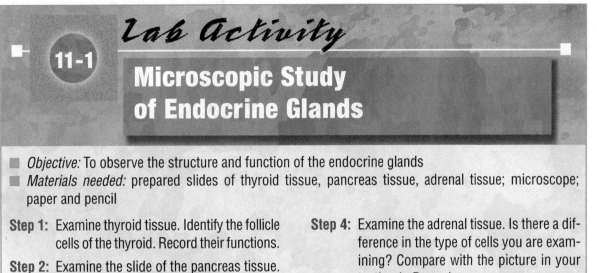

Lab Activity
11-1
Microscopic Study of Endocrine Glands

■ *Objective:* To observe the structure and function of the endocrine glands
■ *Materials needed:* prepared slides of thyroid tissue, pancreas tissue, adrenal tissue; microscope; paper and pencil

Step 1: Examine thyroid tissue. Identify the follicle cells of the thyroid. Record their functions.

Step 2: Examine the slide of the pancreas tissue. Identify the islets of Langerhans. Record their functions.

Step 3: Before placing the adrenal tissue under the microscope, hold the slide up to a light to distinguish between the cortex and medulla areas.

Step 4: Examine the adrenal tissue. Is there a difference in the type of cells you are examining? Compare with the picture in your textbook. Record your answer.

Step 5: Compare the three types of endocrine tissue. Record if you note any differences.

Lab Activity
11-2
Structure and Function of Endocrine Glands

■ *Objective:* To observe and identify placement and function of the endocrine glands
■ *Materials needed:* anatomical chart of the endocrine system, paper and pencil

Step 1: Locate the organs of the endocrine system.

Step 2: What is special about the location of the pituitary gland? What is the function of the pituitary gland? Record your answers.

Step 3: Make sketches of the thyroid, parathyroid, pancreas, and adrenal glands.

Step 4: Describe and record the function of each of these glands.

Step 5: What are the gonads? What is their function? Record your answer.

Chapter 12

BLOOD

Key Words

abscess	erythrocyte	oxyhemoglobin
agranulocyte	erythropoiesis	pathogenic
albumin	fibrin	pernicious anemia
anemia	fibrinogen	plasma
antibody	gamma globulin	polycythemia
anticoagulant	globin	prothrombin
antigen	globulin	pus
antiprothrombin	granulocyte	pyrexia
(heparin)	hematoma	Rh factor
antithromboplastin	hemoglobin	RHO Gam
aplastic anemia	hemolysis	sedimentation rate
B-lymphocyte	hemophilia	septicemia
basophil	inflammation	sickle cell anemia
Carbon monoxide	iron-deficiency	thrombin
(CO) poisoning	anemia	thrombocyte
clotting time	leukemia	thrombocytopenia
coagulation	leukocyte	thromboplastin
Cooley's anemia	leukocytosis	thrombosis
diapedesis	leukopenia	thrombus
embolism	lymphocyte	T-lymphocyte
eosinophil	monocyte	universal donor
erythroblastosis	myeloblast	universal recipient
fetalis	neutrophil	

The average adult's body has 8 to 10 pints of blood. Loss of more than 2 pints at any one time leads to a serious condition.

FUNCTION OF BLOOD

Blood is the transporting fluid of the body. It carries nutrients from the digestive tract to the cells, oxygen from the lungs to the cells, waste products from the cells to the various organs of excretion, and hormones from secreting cells to other parts of the body. It aids in the distribution of heat formed in the more active tissues (such as the skeletal muscles) to all parts of the body. Blood also helps to regulate the acid-base balance and to protect against infection. Consequently, blood is a vital fluid to our life and health, Table 12-1.

Table 12-1 *Summary of the Various Functions of Blood*

FUNCTION	EFFECT ON BODY
Nutritive	Transporting nutrient molecules (glucose, amino acids, fatty acids, and glycerol) from the small intestine or storage sites to the tissues.
Respiratory	Transporting oxygen from the lungs to the tissues and carbon dioxide from the tissue to the lungs.
Excretory	Transporting waste products (lactic acid, urea, and creatinine) from the cells to the excretory organs.
Regulatory	Transporting hormones and other chemical substances that control the proper functioning of many organs.
	Circulating excess heat to the body surfaces and to the lungs, through which it is lost (controls body temperature).
	Maintains water balance and a constant environment for tissue cells.
Protective	Circulating antibodies and defensive cells throughout the body to combat infection and disease.

BLOOD COMPOSITION

Blood is made up of **plasma,** the liquid portion of blood without its cellular elements. Serum is the name given to plasma after a blood clot is formed: serum = plasma − (fibrinogen + prothrombin). Blood also contains cellular elements, including **erythrocytes** or red blood cells (RBCs), **leukocytes** or white blood cells (WBCs), and **thrombocytes** (platelets), Figure 12-1.

BLOOD PLASMA

Plasma is a straw-colored, complex liquid, comprising about 55% of the blood volume and containing the following six substances in solution.

1. *Water*—Water makes up about 92% of the total volume of plasma. This percentage is maintained by the kidneys and by water intake and output.

2. *Plasma proteins*—These three proteins are the most abundant of those found in plasma: fibrinogen, serum albumin, and serum globulin.

   a. **Fibrinogen** is necessary for blood clotting. Without fibrinogen, the slightest cut or wound would bleed profusely. It is synthesized in the liver.

   b. **Albumin** is the most abundant of all the plasma proteins. A product of the liver, albumin helps to maintain the blood's osmotic pressure and volume. It provides the "pulse pressure" needed to hold and pull water from the tissue fluid back into the blood vessels. Normally, plasma proteins do not pass through the capillary walls, as their molecules are relatively large. They are colloidal substances; they can give up, or take up, water-soluble substances, thus regulating the osmotic pressure within the blood vessels.

   c. **Globulin** is formed not only in the liver, but also in the lymphatic system (discussed in Chapter 15). **Gamma globulin** has been fractionated (separated) from globulin. This portion helps in the synthesis of antibodies, which destroy or render harmless various

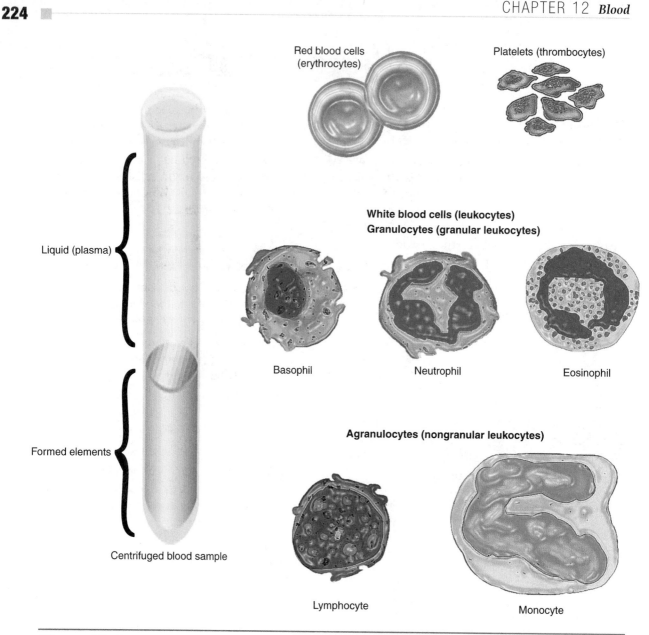

Red blood cells
(erythrocytes)

Platelets (thrombocytes)

Liquid (plasma)

White blood cells (leukocytes)
Granulocytes (granular leukocytes)

Basophil   Neutrophil   Eosinophil

Agranulocytes (nongranular leukocytes)

Formed elements

Centrifuged blood sample

Lymphocyte   Monocyte

Figure 12-1   *Cellular elements of the blood*

disease-causing organisms. **Prothrombin** is yet another globulin, formed continually in the liver, which helps blood to coagulate. Vitamin K is necessary in aiding the process of prothrombin synthesis.

3. *Nutrients*—Nutrient molecules are absorbed from the digestive tract. Glucose, fatty acids, cholesterol, and amino acids are dissolved in the blood plasma.

4. *Electrolytes*—The most abundant electrolytes are sodium chloride and potassium chloride.

These come from foods and chemical processes occurring in the body.

5. *Hormones, vitamins, and enzymes*—These three substances are found in very small amounts in the blood plasma. They generally help the body to control its chemical reactions.

6. *Metabolic waste products*—All of the body's cells are actively engaged in chemical reactions to maintain homeostasis. As a result of this, waste products are formed and subsequently carried by the plasma to the various excretory organs.

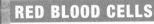 RED BLOOD CELLS

Red blood cells (RBCs), or erythrocytes, are biconcave, disc-shaped cells. They are caved in on both sides, with a thin center and thicker margins. When viewed from above, they appear to have a doughnut shape, see Figure 12-1.

Hemoglobin

Erythrocytes contain a red pigment (coloring agent) called **hemoglobin,** which provides its characteristic color. Hemoglobin is made of a protein molecule called **globin** and an iron compound called heme. A single blood cell contains several million molecules of hemoglobin. Hemoglobin is vital to the function of the red blood cell, helping it to transport oxygen to the tissues and some carbon dioxide away from the tissues. Normal hemoglobin count for men is 14 to 18 g and for women is 12 to 16 g per 100 cc.

Function

In the capillaries of the lung, erythrocytes pick up oxygen from the inspired air. The oxygen chemically combines with the hemoglobin, forming the compound **oxyhemoglobin.** The oxyhemoglobin-laden erythrocytes circulate to the capillaries of tissues. Here oxygen is released to the tissues. The carbon dioxide that is formed in the cells is picked up by the plasma as a bicarbonate. The red blood cells circulate back to the lungs to give up the carbon dioxide and absorb more oxygen. Arteries carry blood away from the heart and veins carry blood toward the heart, but there are exceptions. Blood cells that travel in the arteries (except for pulmonary arteries) carry oxyhemoglobin, which gives blood its bright red color. Blood cells in the veins (except for pulmonary veins) contain carbaminohemoglobin, which is responsible for the dark, reddish-blue color characteristic of venous blood.

Carbon monoxide (CO) poisoning is a serious and sometimes fatal condition. Carbon monoxide is an odorless gas present in the exhaust of gasoline engines. Carbon monoxide rapidly combines with hemoglobin; and binds at the same site on the hemoglobin molecule as oxygen and crowds oxygen out. The cells are deprived of their oxygen supply. Symptoms may include headache, dizziness, drowsiness, and unconsciousness. Death may occur in severe cases of carbon monoxide poisoning. It is important to remember that carbon monoxide gas is odorless. Carbon monoxide is also present in the flue gases of furnaces and gas or oil-fired space heaters. Damaged or improperly installed furnaces and heaters, as well as plugged or defective chimneys and vents, can bring carbon monoxide into the home. Always be certain to allow for proper ventilation of home and work areas. Never allow a car to run in an unventilated garage. Commercial carbon monoxide detectors are available for home use.

Erythropoiesis

Erythropoiesis, or the manufacture of red blood cells, occurs in the red bone marrow of essentially all bones, until adolescence. (In the fetus, red blood cells are also produced by the spleen and liver.) As one grows older, the red marrow of the long bones is replaced by fat marrow; erythrocytes are thereafter formed only in the short and flat bones.

Erythrocytes come from stem cells in the red bone marrow called hemocytosblasts (see Figure 12-1). As the hemocytoblast matures into an erythrocyte, it loses its nucleus and cytoplasmic organelles. The hemocytoblast also becomes smaller, gains hemoglobin, develops a biconcave shape, and enters into the bloodstream. To aid in erythropoiesis, vitamin B_{12}, folic acid, copper, cobalt, iron, and proteins are needed.

Since erythrocytes are enucleated (contain no nucleus), they only live about 120 days. Destruction occurs as the cells age, rendering them more vulnerable to rupturing. They are broken down by the spleen and liver. Hemoglobin breaks down into globin and heme; the iron content of heme is used to make new red blood cells. The normal count of red blood cells ranges from 4.5 to 6.2 million/μl venous blood for men and 4.2 to 5.4 million/μl venous blood for women.

Hemolysis

A rupture or bursting of the red blood cell (erythrocyte) is called **hemolysis.** This sometimes occurs as a result of a blood transfusion reaction or other disease processes.

WHITE BLOOD CELLS

White blood cells (WBCs) are called leukocytes. They are larger than the erythrocytes and granular (with grain appearance) or agranular (no grain appearance). Leukocytes are manufactured in both red bone marrow and lymphatic tissue. Leukocytes are the body's natural defense against injury and disease.

Types of Leukocytes

Leukocytes are classified into two major groups of cells: the **granulocytes** (granular leukocytes) and the **agranulocytes** (agranular leukocytes). This classification is due to the presence of cytoplasmic granules, nuclear structure, and reactions to stains such as Wright's stain. In the laboratory, stains are applied to blood smears so that formed elements may be easily identified. Granulocytes are made in red bone marrow from cells called **myeloblasts.** Granulocytes are destroyed as they age and as a result of participating in bacterial destruction. The lifespan of white blood cells is variable, but most granulocytes live only a few days.

There are three types of granulocytes: neutrophils, eosinophils, and basophils.

Neutrophils, also called polymorphonuclear leukocytes, phagocytize bacteria with lysosomal enzymes. Phagocytosis is a process that surrounds, engulfs, and digests harmful bacteria. **Eosinophils** phagocytize the remains of antibody-antigen reactions. They also increase in great numbers in allergic conditions, malaria, and in worm infestations. **Basophils** perform phagocytosis, and their count increases during chronic inflammation and during the healing from an infection. Basophils produce histamine, a vasodilator, and heparin, an anticoagulant.

Agranulocytes are divided into lymphocytes and monocytes. **Lymphocytes** are further subdivided into **B-lymphocytes,** which are synthesized in the bone marrow, and **T-lymphocytes** from the thymus gland. Still others are formed by the lymph nodes and spleen. Their lifespan ranges

from a few days to several years. They basically help the body by synthesizing and releasing antibody molecules and by protecting against the formation of cancer cells.

Monocytes are formed in bone marrow and the spleen. They assist in phagocytosis, and are able to leave the bloodstream to attach themselves to tissues; here they become tissue macrophages, or histiocytes. During an inflammation, histiocytes help to wall off and isolate the infected area.

The aforementioned types of leukocytes (basophils, neutrophils, eosinophils, and monocytes) that can perform phagocytosis are called phagocytes. Unlike erythrocytes, they can move through the intercellular spaces of the capillary wall into neighboring tissue. This process is known as **diapedesis.**

A normal leukocyte count averages from 3,200 to 9,800/µl.

To summarize, leukocytes help protect the body against infection and injury. This is achieved through (1) phagocytosis and destruction of bacteria, (2) synthesis of antibody molecules, (3) "cleaning up" of cellular remnants at the site of inflammation, and (4) the walling off of the infected area. See Tables 12-2 and 12-3.

INFLAMMATION

If living tissue is damaged in any way, the body usually responds to the damage by either neutralizing or eliminating the cause of the damage. When this happens, the damaged body part goes through an inflammation process. **Inflamma-**

Table 12-2 Types of Leukocytes and Their Number or Percent

MAJOR TYPES OF LEUKOCYTES	SPECIFIC KINDS OF LEUKOCYTES
Granulocytes 60%–70%	Neutrophils Eosinophils Basophils
Agranulocytes Lymphocytes 20%–30% Monocyte 5%–8%	Small Large Mononuclear Transitional

Table 12-3 *Characteristics and Functions of the Leukocytes*

LEUKOCYTE	WHERE FORMED	TYPE OF NUCLEUS	CYTOPLASM	FUNCTION
Agranular leukocytes 1. Lymphocyte	Lymph glands and nodes, bone marrow, spleen	One large, spherical nucleus; may be indented Sharply defined and stains dark blue	Cytoplasm stains a pale blue and contains scattered violet granules	Helps to form antibodies at a site of inflammation; protects against cancer
2. Monocyte (macrophage)	Lymph glands and nodes, bone marrow, spleen	One lobulated or horseshoe-shaped nucleus that stains blue	Abundant cytoplasm that stains a gray-blue	Phagocytosis of cellular debris and foreign particles
Granular leukocytes 1. Neutrophil	Formed in bone marrow from neutrophilic myelocytes	Lobulated: contains 1 to 5 or more lobes, stains deep blue	Cytoplasm has a pink tinge with very fine granules	Displays marked phagocytosis toward bacteria during infections and inflammations. Contributes to pus formation
2. Eosinophil	Formed in bone marrow from eosinophilic myelocytes	Irregularly shaped with 2 lobes, stains blue, but less deeply than neutrophils	Cytoplasm has a sky-blue tinge with many coarse, uniform, round or oval bright-red granules	Marked increase during parasitic, worm infections and allergic attacks
3. Basophil (mast cell)	Formed in bone marrow from basophilic myelocytes	Centrally located, slightly lobulated nucleus, stains a light purple and hidden by granules	Cytoplasm has a mauve color with many large deep-purple granules	Phagocytosis; releases heparin and histamine and promotes the inflammatory response

tion occurs when tissues are subjected to chemical or physical trauma (cut or heat). Invasion by **pathogenic** (disease-causing) microorganisms such as bacteria, fungi, protozoa, and viruses also can cause inflammation.

The characteristic symptoms of inflammation are redness, local heat, swelling, and pain. This is due to irritation by bacterial toxins, to increased blood flow, to congestion of blood vessels, and to the collection of blood plasma in the surrounding tissues (edema) Figure 12-2. Histamine released from the basophil and other chemical substances increase blood flow to the injured area as well as increasing capillary permeability. Thus, large amounts of blood plasma and fibrinogen enter the damaged area. The damaged area is walled off as a result of the clotting action of fibrinogen on the damaged tissue and macrophage action.

Neutrophils move very quickly to the damaged area. The neutrophils move through the capillary walls by diapedesis and begin phagocytosis

of the pathogenic microorganisms. Macrophages also participate in phagocytosis.

In most inflammations, a cream-colored liquid called **pus** forms. Pus is a combination of dead tissue, dead and living bacteria, dead leukocytes, and blood plasma. If the damaged area is below the epidermis, an **abscess** (pus-filled cavity) forms. If it is on the skin or a mucosal surface, it is called an ulcer. In many inflammations, chemical substances called pyrogens are formed, which are circulated to the hypothalamus. In the hypothalamus, the pyrogens affect the temperature control center, which raises the body's temperature causing fever or **pyrexia.**

In inflammation, there is an increased production of neutrophils by bone marrow. If the white blood cell count exceeds 10,000 cells/μl, a condition called **leukocytosis** exists. Following healing, the leukocyte count returns to normal. Sometimes a decrease in the number of white blood cells occurs. This is called **leukopenia.** It

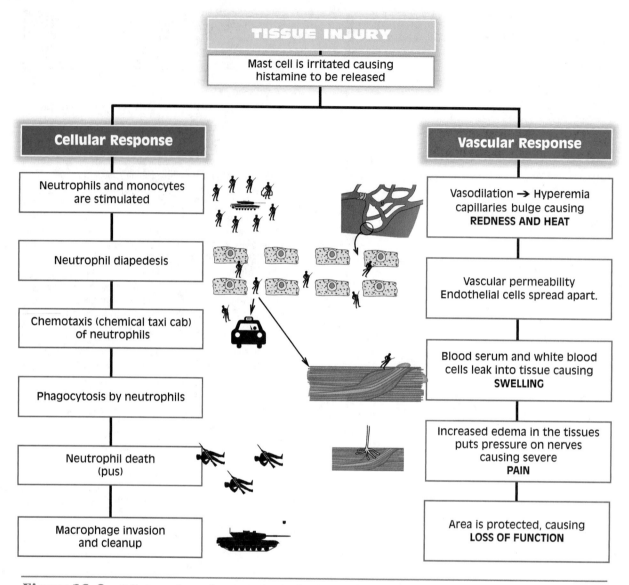

Figure 12-2   *Cellular and vascular response to inflammation*

can be caused by taking marrow-depressant drugs, by pathologic conditions, or by radiation.

THROMBOCYTES (BLOOD PLATELETS)

Thrombocytes are the smallest of the solid components of blood. They are ovoid-shaped structures, synthesized from the larger megakaryocytes in red bone marrow. Thrombocytes are not cells but fragments of the megakaryocytes cytoplasm (see Figure 12-1).

The normal blood platelet count ranges from 250,000 to 450,000 per cubic millimeter of blood. Platelets function in the initiation of the blood-clotting process. When a blood vessel is damaged, as in a cut or wound, the vessel's collagen fibers come into contact with the platelets. The platelets are then stimulated to produce sticky projecting structures, allowing them to stick to the collagen fibers. This reaction occurs countless times, creating a "platelet plug" to stop the bleeding. The platelets secrete a chemical called serotin which causes the blood vessel to spasm and narrow and a decrease in blood loss until the clot forms. Subsequently, the blood clotting process follows to "harden" the platelet plug. Old platelets eventually disintegrate in the bone marrow.

Coagulation

Blood clotting or **coagulation** is a complicated and essential process which depends in large part on thrombocytes. When a cut or other injury ruptures a blood vessel, clotting must occur to stop the bleeding.

Although the exact details of this process are not clear, there is a general agreement that the following reaction occurs. When a blood vessel or tissue is injured, platelets and injured tissue release **thromboplastin.** An injury to a blood vessel makes the lining rough; as blood platelets flow over the roughened area, they disintegrate, releasing thromboplastin.

Thromboplastin is a complex substance that can only cause coagulation if calcium ions and prothrombin are present. Prothrombin is a plasma protein synthesized in the liver.

The thromboplastin and calcium ions act as enzymes in a reaction that converts prothrombin into **thrombin.** This reaction occurs only in the presence of bleeding, because normally there is no thrombin in the blood plasma.

In the next stage of coagulation, the thrombin just formed acts as an enzyme, changing fibrinogen (a plasma protein) into **fibrin.** These gel-like fibrin threads layer themselves over the cut, creating a fine, meshlike network. This fibrin network entraps the red blood cells, platelets, and plasma, creating a blood clot. At first, serum (a pale yellow fluid) oozes out of the cut. As the serum slowly dries, a crust (scab) forms over the fibrin threads, completing the common clotting process.

For coagulation to occur successfully, two **anticoagulants** (substances preventing coagulation) must be neutralized. These are called **antithromboplastin** and **antiprothrombin (heparin);** they are neutralized by thromboplastin.

Prothrombin is dependent on vitamin K. Vitamin K is manufactured in the body by a type of bacteria found in the intestines. See Figure 12-3 for a summary of the coagulation process. It is

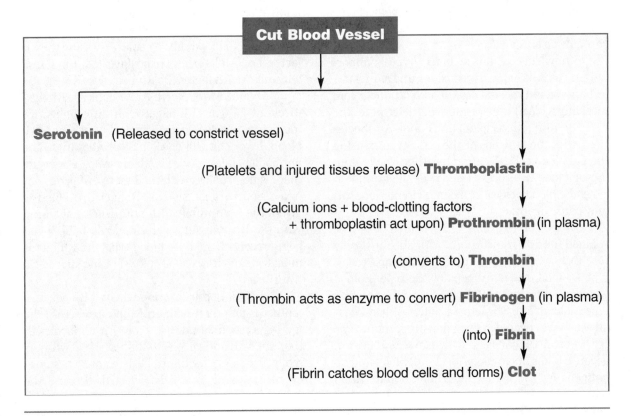

Figure 12-3   *Blood-clotting process*

important to note that prothrombin and fibrinogen are plasma proteins manufactured in the liver; therefore, serious liver disease may interfere with the blood clotting process.

Clotting Time. The time it takes for blood to clot is known as its **clotting time.** The clotting time for humans is from 5 to 15 minutes. This information is quite useful prior to surgery.

BLOOD TYPES

There are four major groups or types of blood: A, B, AB, and O. Blood type is inherited from one's parents. It is determined by the presence—or absence—of the blood protein called agglutinogen or **antigen,** on the surface of the red blood cell. People with type A blood have the A antigen on their red blood cells; type B blood has the type B antigen; type AB has both A and B antigen; and type O has neither of the antigens.

There is a protein present in the plasma known as agglutinin or **antibody.** An individual with type A blood has B antibodies in the blood plasma. Type B blood possesses A antibodies; type O contains *both* A and B antibodies; and type AB contains *no* antibodies.

Knowledge of one's correct type is important in cases of blood transfusions and surgery. A test known as type and crossmatch is done before receiving a blood transfusion. This determines the blood type of both recipient and donor. Antibodies react with the antigens of the same type, causing the red blood cells to clump together. The clumping of blood, a process known as agglutination clogs the blood vessels, impeding circulation; this may cause death.

By way of an example, if a person with type A blood needs a transfusion, he or she must only receive type A blood. Should the person receive type B blood, the B antigens of the type B blood would clump with the B antibodies of the person's type A blood. The Rh factors positive (+) and negative (−) are covered in the following section. Type O Rh-negative is considered the **universal donor,** because it has no antigens for A or B blood and no antigens for the Rh factor. It may donate to all types of blood. Type AB+ is considered the **universal recipient,** because it has both A and B

Table 12-4 *Blood Type Crossmatches*

IF THE PATIENT'S BLOOD TYPE IS:	THE DONOR'S BLOOD TYPE MUST BE:
O+	O+, O−
O− (universal donor)	O−
A+	A+, A−, O+, O−
A−	A−, O−
B+	B+, B−, O+, O−
B−	B−, O−
AB+ (universal recipient)	AB+, AB−, A+, A−, B+, B−, O+, O−
AB−	AB−, A−, B−, O−

antigens and the Rh antigen. See Table 12-4 for blood type crossmatches.

RH FACTOR

Human red blood cells, in addition to containing antigens A and B, also contain the Rh antigen. We know it as the **Rh factor** because it was found in the Rhesus monkey. The Rh factor is found on the surface of red blood cells. People possessing the Rh factor are said to be Rh positive (Rh+). Those without the Rh factor are Rh negative (Rh−).

About 85% of North Americans are Rh positive and 15% are Rh negative. If an Rh negative individual receives a transfusion of Rh positive blood, he or she will develop antibodies to it. The antibodies take 2 weeks to develop. Generally there is no problem with the first transfusion; but if a second transfusion of Rh positive blood is given, the accumulated Rh antibodies will clump with the Rh antigen (agglutinogen) of the blood being received. So, both blood type and Rh factor must be taken into account for safe and successful transfusions.

The same problem arises when an Rh negative mother is pregnant with an Rh positive fetus. The mother's blood can develop anti-Rh antibodies to the fetus's Rh antigens. The first-born child will normally suffer no harmful effects; however, subsequent pregnancies will be affected, because the mother's accumulated anti-Rh antibodies will clump the baby's red blood cells. If the condition is left untreated, the baby will usually be born with the condition known as **erythroblastosis fetalis** (hemolytic disease of newborn). This condition is rare today because of the use of the drug **RHO Gam,** which is a special preparation of immune globulin. RHO Gam is given to the Rh negative (Rh−) mother within 72 hours after delivery of each baby. (Some doctors also give this drug during the last trimester of pregnancy.) The antibodies in the RHO Gam will destroy any Rh positive (Rh+) cells of the baby's which may have entered the mother's bloodstream; therefore, the mother's immune system will not be stimulated to produce antibodies.

BLOOD NORMS

Tests have been devised to use physiological blood norms in diagnosing and following the course of certain diseases. Some of these norms are listed in Table 12-5.

Patients who are taking anticoagulant medications to prolong the clotting time of their blood must have prothrombin time (PT) and a partial thromboplastin test (PTT) done frequently. The dosage of their medication is based on their clotting times.

Sedimentation rate is the time required for erythrocytes to settle to the bottom of an upright tube at room temperature. An elevated sedimentation rate indicates whether disease is present and is valuable in observing the progression of inflammatory conditions.

DISORDERS OF THE BLOOD

Anemia is a deficiency in the number and/or percentage of red blood cells and the amount of hemoglobin in the blood. Anemia results from a large or chronic loss of blood (hemorrhage) which decreases the number of erythrocytes. Extreme erythrocyte destruction and malformation of the hemoglobin of red blood cells also causes this condition. Because these conditions always cause some hemoglobin deficiency, there is never enough oxygen transported to the cells for cellular oxidation. Consequently, not enough energy is being released. Anemia is characterized by varying degrees of dyspnea, pallor, palpitation, and fatigue.

Iron-deficiency anemia is a condition that often exists in women, children, and adolescents. It is caused by a deficiency of adequate amounts of iron in the diet. This leads to insufficient hemoglobin synthesis in the red blood cells. The condition is easily alleviated by ingestion of iron supplements and green, leafy vegetables that contain the mineral iron.

Pernicious anemia is a form of anemia caused by a deficiency of vitamin B_{12} and/or lack of the intrinsic factor. Pernicious anemia is seen in association with some autoimmune endocrine diseases. The intrinsic factor produced by the stomach mucosa is necessary for the absorption and utilization of vitamin B_{12}. Vitamin B_{12} and folic acid are necessary for the development of mature red blood cells. Symptoms such as dyspnea, pallor, and fatigue are present as well as specific neurologic changes. Treatment for pernicious anemia involves injections of vitamin B_{12}.

Aplastic anemia is a disease caused by the suppression of the bone marrow. Suppression can be caused by chemical agents, certain drugs, or radiation therapy. In this condition, bone marrow does not produce enough red blood cells and white blood cells. Treatment consists of removal of the toxic substances or discontinuing the drugs and radiation. In severe conditions, a bone marrow transplant may be performed.

Sickle cell anemia is a chronic blood disease inherited from both parents. The disease

Table 12-5 *Blood Tests*	
TEST	**NORMAL RANGE**
Bleeding time	1 to 3 minutes
Coagulation time	5 to 15 minutes
Hemoglobin count	Men: 14 to 18 gm/dl Women: 12 to 16 gm/dl
Platelet count	150,000 to 350,000/mm^3
Prothrombin time (quick)	9.5 to 11 seconds
Sedimentation rate (Westergren) in first hour	Men: 0 to 10 mm/hour Women: 0 to 20 mm/hour
Red blood cell count	Men: 4.5 to 6.2 million/μl Women: 4.2 to 5.4 million/μl
White blood cell count	3,200 to 9,800/μl
Cholesterol level	below 200 mg/dl

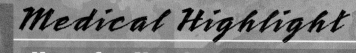

Medical Highlight

Uses for Newborn's Umbilical or Cord Blood

The blood found in the umbilical cord contains the same immunity-producing stem cells found in the bone marrow and is far easier to transplant. While bone marrow transplants require an almost exact match, cord blood stem cells are too young and the brand new donor has not yet developed anti-bodies that turn against the recipient. At this time, these transplants are highly experimental and have been used mainly in children. Proponents of this treatment say it will give a new chance for life to people with some forms of leukemia, anemia, Hodgkin's disease, and other conditions.

Medical Highlight

Treatment for Sickle Cell Anemia

Scientists continue to work to treat and prolong the life expectancy for someone diagnosed with sickle cell anemia. Following are some of the latest developments.

1. *Partial chimerism*—This procedure uses a mixture of the patient's bone marrow and a donor's bone marrow to combine and form healthy new blood cells. It allows for a patient's bone marrow not to be destroyed. This type of mixture will allow more people to be eligible for the transplant. Controlled studies will begin in a few months.

2. Cord blood stem cell transplant—Doctors from Emory University's Department of Pediatrics, Hematology-Oncology Bone Marrow Transplant successfully performed the first cord blood stem cell transplant from an unrelated donor. This type of stem cell transplant is an alternative for a patient who does not have family to provide an immunologic match.

3. Gene cell therapy—Scientists have been able to correct sickle cell disease in mice using gene cell therapy. Researchers inject a gene into the mice and that gene stops the red blood cells from sickling.

Sources: (1) Gentler treatment for sickle cell hailed by Guthree, Patricia, Atlanta Journal Constitution 10/26/2001
(2) Bone Marrow and Cord Blood Stem Cell Transplant-December 13, 1999
(3) Sickle Cell Therapy shows Promise by Kristen Philip Koski-WiredNews-12/19/01 http://www.wired.com/news/medtech/ 0, 1286, 49084, 00.html

causes red blood cells to form in the abnormal crescent shape. These cells carry less oxygen and break easily, causing anemia. The sickling trait, a less serious disease, occurs with inheritance from only one parent. The disease is most prevalent in African-Americans, affecting about 1 in 400. The rigid sickling of the red blood cells causes vaso-occlusion and results in painful crises. A painful crisis is a sudden attack of pain often occurring in bones and joints in adults. Hydroxyurea taken daily prevents painful episodes about 50% of the time. Treatment for sickle cell anemia is bone marrow transplants to eligible candidates and blood transfusions when necessary. Scientists are work-

Career Profile

Clinical Laboratory Technician/Medical Laboratory Technician Clinical Laboratory Technologist/Medical Technologist

The Clinical laboratory testing plays a key role in the detection, diagnosis, and treatmetn of disease. Clinical laboratory personnel obtain, and analyze body fluids, tissue, and cells.

- Clinical laboratory technicians perform routine tests in a medical laboratory and are able to discriminate and recognize factors that directly affect procedures and results. Clinical lab technicians have either an associate's degree or certification from a hospital or vocational-technical school. They work under the supervision of a medical technologist or physician.
- Clinical laboratory technologists physically and chemically analyze and culture all body fluids. Knowledge of specimen collection, anatomy and physiology, biochemistry, and laboratory equipment is essential. Education requirement is at least a bachelor's degree.

The American Society of Clinical Pathology is a professional organization that oversees credentialing and education in the medical laboratory profession.

ing on stem cell research, gene therapy, and new drugs to prevent or lessen the disease condition.

Cooley's anemia, also known as thalassemia major, is a blood disease caused by a defect in hemoglobin formation. It affects people of Mediterranean descent.

Polycythemia is a condition in which too many red blood cells are formed. This may be a temporary condition which occurs at high altitudes because there is less oxygen present. The disease polycythemia vera, cause unknown, is a condition of too many red blood cells. The increase in the number of red blood cells causes a thickening of the blood with possible blood clot formation. Treatment for this condition is phlebotomy—removal of approximately 1 pint of blood or drug therapy.

Embolism is a condition where an embolus is carried by the bloodstream until it reaches an artery too small for passage. An embolus is a substance foreign to the bloodstream. It may be air, a blood clot, cancer cells, fat, bacterial clumps, a needle, or even a bullet that was lodged in tissue and breaks free.

Thrombosis is the formation of a blood clot in a blood vessel. The blood clot formed is called a **thrombus.** It is caused by unusually slow blood circulation, changes in the blood or blood vessel walls, immobility, or a decrease in mobility.

Hematoma is a localized clotted mass of blood found in an organ, tissue, or space. It is caused by a traumatic injury, such as a blow, that can cause a blood vessel to rupture.

Hemophilia is a hereditary disease in which the blood clots slowly or abnormally. This causes prolonged bleeding with even minor cuts and bumps. Although sex-linked hemophilia occurs mostly in males, it is transmitted genetically by females to their sons. The person with hemophilia may be treated with the missing clotting factor. The hemophiliac is taught to avoid trauma, if possible, and report promptly any bleeding, no matter how slight.

Thrombocytopenia is a blood disease in which there is a decrease in the number of platelets (thrombocytes). In this condition, blood will not clot properly.

Leukemia is a cancerous or malignant condition in which there is a great increase in the number of white blood cells. The overabundant immature leukocytes replace the erythrocytes, thus interfering with the transport of oxygen to the tissues. They can also hinder the synthesis of new red blood cells from bone marrow. The acute form of the disease, which develops quickly and runs its course rapidly, occurs most often in children and young adults. Treatment today consists of drug therapy, bone marrow transplants, and radiation therapy which has given people with leukemia remissions lasting for several years.

Septicemia describes the presence of pathogenic (disease-producing) organisms or toxins in the blood.

Medical Terminology

an	without
emia	blood
an/emia	without blood
coagul	clotting
-tion	process of
coagul/a/tion	process of blood clotting
edem	swelling
-a	presence of
edem/a	presence of swelling
embol	plug
-ism	condition of
embol/ism	condition of a plug or blockage
erythro	red
cyte	cell
erythro/cyte	red blood cell
poiesis	formation of
erythro/poiesis	formation of red blood cell
hema	blood
-oma	tumor or swelling
hema/toma	swelling that contains blood
leuko	white blood
leuko/cyte	white blood cell
lympho	clear spring, water
lympho/cyte	clear blood cell

mono	one
mono/cyte	type of white blood cell with one large nucleus
patho	disease
gen	producing
-ic	refers to
patho/gen/ic	refers to disease producing
poly	many
cyth	cells
poly/cyth/emia	many blood cells
thrombo	clot
-sis	condition of
thrombo/sis	condition of a blood clot

REVIEW QUESTIONS

Select the letter of the choice that best completes the statement.

1. Blood of the universal donor is:
   a. type B–
   b. type A–
   c. type AB–
   d. type O–

2. Blood of the universal recipient is:
   a. type B+
   b. type A+
   c. type AB+
   d. type O+

3. Negative Rh blood is found in:
   a. 5% of the population
   b. 10% of the population
   c. 15% of the population
   d. 20% of the population

4. The leukocytes that phagocytize bacteria with lysosomal enzymes are the:
   a. eosinophils
   b. basophils
   c. neutrophils
   d. monocytes

5. The prothrombin in the blood-clotting process is dependent upon:
   a. vitamin A
   b. vitamin K
   c. vitamin P
   d. vitamin D

6. Which of the following is not a blood cell?
   a. erythrocyte
   b. leukocyte
   c. osteocyte
   d. monocyte

7. Erythrocytes contain all but one of the following elements:
   a. Rh factor
   b. leukocytes
   c. hemoglobin
   d. globin and heme

8. What characteristic is not true of normal thrombocytes?
   a. They average 4,500 for each cubic millimeter of blood
   b. They are also called platelets
   c. They are plate-shaped cells
   d. They initiate the blood-clotting process

9. The normal leukocyte cell:
   a. can only be produced in the lymphatic tissue
   b. goes to the infection site to engulf and destroy microorganisms
   c. is too large to move through the intracellular spaces of the capillary wall
   d. exists in numbers which amount to an average of 12,000 cells per cubic millimeter of blood

10. The blood-clotting process:
    a. requires a normal platelet count which is 5,000 to 9,000 for each cubic millimeter of blood
    b. is delayed by the rupture of platelets which produces thromboplastin
    c. occurs in less time with persons having type O blood
    d. requires vitamin K for the synthesis of prothrombin

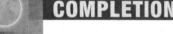

COMPLETION

Briefly answer the following questions.

1. Name the three major types of blood cells.

2. What name is given to the straw-colored liquid portion of the blood?

3. What five proteins are contained in the blood and what are their functions?

4. Describe the process of blood clot formation.

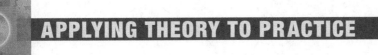

APPLYING THEORY TO PRACTICE

1. You hear that your friend has been in a car accident and needs a blood transfusion; you want to donate blood. You friend has type O+ blood and you have A+ blood. Can your blood be given to your friend? Explain the reason for your answer.

2. Why is blood considered the "gift of life"?

3. A patient comes to the doctor's office. She is pregnant and states she is Rh negative and her husband is Rh positive. She has heard that there may be a problem with the baby. Explain to her about the Rh factor and how this situation is treated today.

4. In the hospital you are caring for a 6-year-old girl with leukemia. The mother asks what she did that caused the disease. What will be your response?

5. You are employed as a medical technologist. A patient comes to the lab and requires a complete blood count and sedimentation rate. The patient asks you to explain these tests and their purpose.

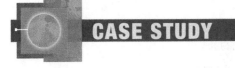

CASE STUDY

John, age 24, is involved in an automobile accident. Ken, a paramedic, arrives on the scene and does emergency first aid. John has multiple lacerations on his hand and arms; the laceration on his right arm is bleeding profusely. Ken applies a pressure bandage and notes that John's blood pressure is 90/60. Ken starts an intravenous line and transports John to the hospital. The ER doctor examines John and notes he also has contusions near his liver. The doctor has the med tech draw blood for a CBC and to type and crossmatch for blood.

1. A severe loss of blood may lead to what condition?

2. Name the blood components and their function.

3. What is a normal blood count for John?

4. Why is the ER doctor concerned about possible liver damage? How does liver damage relate to the blood?

5. Describe the role of a med tech.

6. Explain typing and crossmatching.

7. It is determined that John has type A positive blood. Can John receive blood from Ken who is O negative?

Lab Activity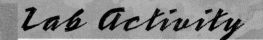

12-1

Red Blood Cells (RBCs) and White Blood Cells (WBCs)

- *Objective:* To observe the structure of red and white blood cells
- *Materials needed:* prepared stained slides of blood cells, microscope, medicine dropper, disposable gloves, safety goggles, disposable autoclave bag, household bleach, textbook, paper and pencil

Note: Remember to use all safety measures when in contact with blood or blood products and dispose of items according to standard precautions.

Step 1: Put on gloves and safety goggles.

Step 2: Examine the stained slide of blood under a microscope. Draw and describe the structure of the RBC. Which is more numerous, RBCs or WBCs? Record your answer.

Step 3: Identify the five types of WBCs. Compare their appearance with the diagram in the textbook. What is the difference between each type of WBC? What is the function of each type of WBC?

Step 4: What is the difference between the RBC and the WBC? Record your answer.

Step 5: Place the blood slides in an autoclave bag, to be autoclaved before disposal.

Step 6: Clean all other equipment with household bleach.

Step 7: Remove goggles and gloves.

Step 8: Wash hands.

Lab Activity

12-2

Blood Simulated Transfusion Compatibility

- *Objective:* To observe the transfusion reactions of blood
- *Materials needed:* at least five paper cups, food coloring, water, medicine dropper, marking pen, paper and pencil.

Note: Prepare chart for recording.

Blood Type of Patient	Potential Blood Types for Transfusion			
	Group A	**Group B**	**Group AB**	**Group O**
Group A				
Group B				
Group AB				
Group O				

continues

continued

Step 1: Fill four cups about 2/3 full with water. Leave the fifth cup empty.

Step 2: Label paper cups with water Group A, Group B, Group AB, Group O. Label the empty cup Patient.

Step 3: Add red color to cup A, blue to cup B, and equal amounts of red and blue to cup AB; do not add food coloring to cup O.

Step 4: Pour a small amount of liquid from cup B into Patient cup. Patient now has that type of blood.

Step 5: Using a medicine dropper, transfer "blood" from Group A to Patient cup. Did the color change in Patient cup? Record your findings as either safe or unsafe.

Step 6: Rinse the Patient cup. Add liquid from Group B to the Patient cup.

Step 7: Repeat step 5 using "blood" from the Group B cup.

Step 8: Repeat step 6.

Step 9: Repeat step 5 using "blood" from the Group AB cup.

Step 10: Repeat step 6.

Step 11: Repeat step 5 using liquid from the Group O cup.

Step 12: Which "blood" groups can safely give blood to the patient who had Group B blood?

As long as the liquid in the Patient cup does not change color, the "transfusion" is safe.

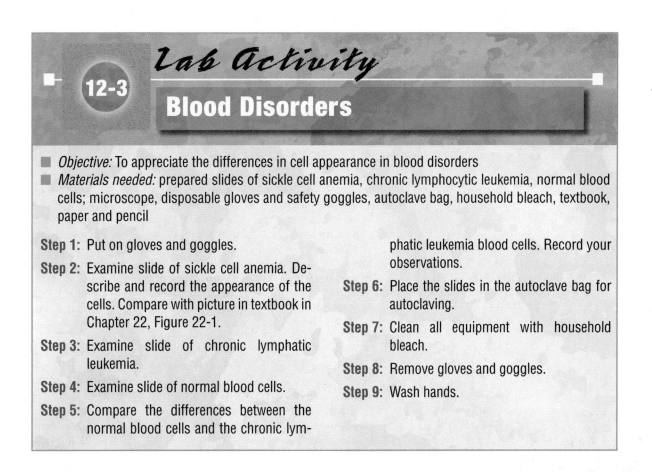

Lab Activity

12-3   Blood Disorders

■ *Objective:* To appreciate the differences in cell appearance in blood disorders

■ *Materials needed:* prepared slides of sickle cell anemia, chronic lymphocytic leukemia, normal blood cells; microscope, disposable gloves and safety goggles, autoclave bag, household bleach, textbook, paper and pencil

Step 1: Put on gloves and goggles.

Step 2: Examine slide of sickle cell anemia. Describe and record the appearance of the cells. Compare with picture in textbook in Chapter 22, Figure 22-1.

Step 3: Examine slide of chronic lymphatic leukemia.

Step 4: Examine slide of normal blood cells.

Step 5: Compare the differences between the normal blood cells and the chronic lymphatic leukemia blood cells. Record your observations.

Step 6: Place the slides in the autoclave bag for autoclaving.

Step 7: Clean all equipment with household bleach.

Step 8: Remove gloves and goggles.

Step 9: Wash hands.

Chapter 13

HEART

Objectives

- Describe the functions of the circulatory system

- List the components of the circulatory system

- Describe the structure of the heart

- Describe the function of the various structures of the heart

- Describe the control of heart contractions

- Discuss the diseases of the heart

- Define the key words that relate to this chapter

Key Words

angina pectoris
angioplasty (balloon surgery)
aorta
aortic semilunar valve
apex
arrhythmia
ascites
atrioventricular bundle (bundle of His)
atrioventricular (AV) node
atrium
bicuspid (mitral) valve
bradycardia
cardiac arrest
cardiac output
cardiac catheterization
cardiac stents
coronary artery disease (CAD)
cardiopulmonary circulation

cardiopulmonary resuscitation (CPR)
cardiotonics
chordae tendinae
conduction defect
congestive heart failure
coronary bypass
coronary sinus
defibrillator
deoxygenated
diuretics
dyspnea
edema
electrocardiogram (ECG or EKG)
endocarditis
endocardium
fibrillation
heart block
heart failure
left ventricle
lubb dupp sound
mitral valve prolapse
murmur

myocardial infarction
myocarditis
myocardium
oxygenated
palpitations
pericarditis
pericardium
pulmonary artery
pulmonary semilunar valve
pulmonary veins
Purkinje fibers
rheumatic heart disease
right ventricle
septum
sinoatrial (SA) node (pacemaker)
stress test
stethoscope
stroke volume
tachycardia
tricuspid valve
vena cava
transmyocardial laser revascularization (TMR)

240

The circulatory system is the longest system of the body. If one were to lay all of the blood vessels in a single human body end to end, they would stretch one fourth the way from earth to the moon, a distance of some 60,000 miles.[1]

FUNCTIONS OF THE CIRCULATORY SYSTEM

1. The heart is the pump that circulates blood to all parts of the body.

2. Arteries, veins, and capillaries are the structures that take blood from the heart to the cells and return blood from the cells back to the heart.

3. Blood carries oxygen and nutrients to the cells and carries the waste products away.

4. The lymph system (see Chapter 15) returns excess fluid from the tissues to the general circulation and manufactures lymphocytes.

ORGANS OF THE CIRCULATORY SYSTEM

The organs of the circulatory system include the heart, arteries, veins, and capillaries. The blood and lymphatic system are part of the circulatory system.

The heart is the muscular pump which is responsible for circulating the blood throughout the body.

MAJOR BLOOD CIRCUITS

Blood leaves the heart through arteries and returns by veins. The blood uses two circulation routes:

1. The general (or systemic) circulation carries blood throughout the body, Figure 13-1.

2. The **cardiopulmonary circulation** carries blood from the heart to the lungs and back, Figure 13-2.

[1] I. Sherman and V. Sherman, *Biology: A Human Approach* (New York: Oxford University Press, 1979).

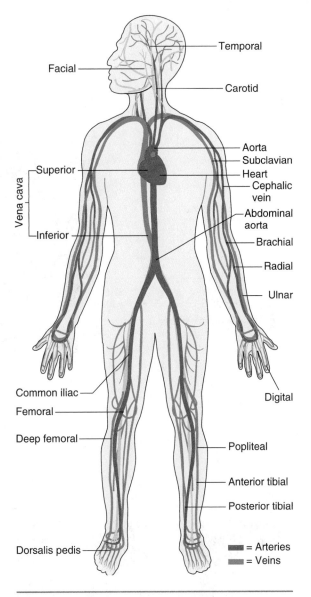

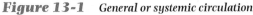

Figure 13-1 *General or systemic circulation*

CHANGES IN THE COMPOSITION OF CIRCULATING BLOOD

The major substances added to and removed from the blood as it circulates through organs along the various sites of the circulatory system are outlined in Table 13-1. This table includes only the major changes in the blood as it passes through certain specialized organs or structures.

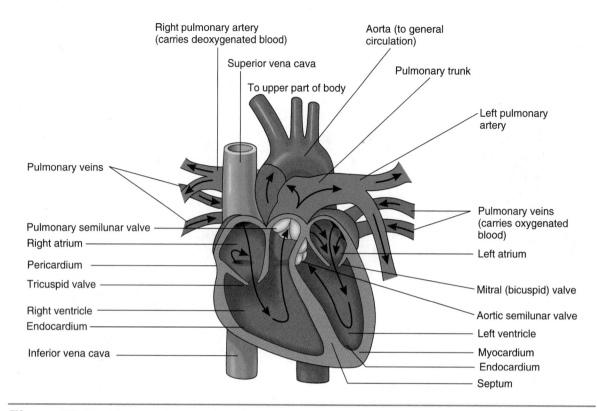

Figure 13-2   *Schematic of heart pulmonary circulation*

Table 13-1 *Changes in the Composition of the Blood*		
ORGANS	**BLOOD LOSES**	**BLOOD GAINS**
Digestive glands	Raw materials needed to make digestive juices and enzymes	Carbon dioxide
Kidneys	Water, urea, and mineral salts	Carbon dioxide
Liver	Excess glucose, amino acids, and worn-out red blood cells	Released glucose, urea, and plasma proteins
Lungs	Carbon dioxide and water	Oxygen
Muscles	Glucose and oxygen	Lactic acid and carbon dioxide
Small intestinal villi	Oxygen	End products of digestion (glucose and amino acids)

THE HEART

The blood's circulatory system is extremely efficient. The main organ responsible for this efficiency is the heart, a tough, simply constructed muscle about the size of a closed fist.

The adult human heart is about 5 inches long and 3.5 inches wide, weighing less than 1 pound (12 to 13 oz), Figure 13-3. The importance of a healthy, well-functioning heart is obvious: to circulate life-sustaining blood throughout the body. When the heart stops beating, life stops as well! To explain further, if the blood flow to the brain ceases for 5 seconds or more, the subject loses consciousness. After 15 to 20 seconds, the muscles twitch convulsively; after 4 to 5 minutes without blood flow, the brain cells are irreversibly damaged.

The heart is located in the thoracic cavity. This places the heart between the lungs, behind

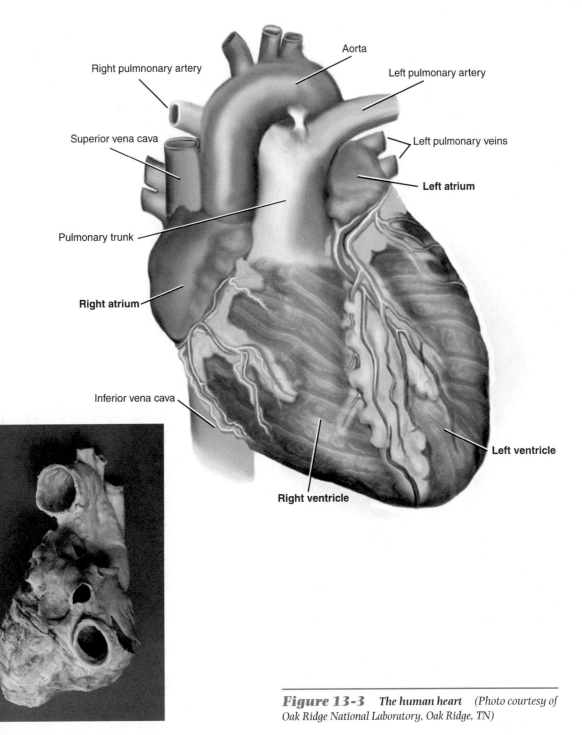

Aorta

Right pulmnonary artery

Left pulmonary artery

Superior vena cava

Left pulmonary veins

Left atrium

Pulmonary trunk

Right atrium

Inferior vena cava

Right ventricle

Left ventricle

Figure 13-3   ***The human heart***   *(Photo courtesy of Oak Ridge National Laboratory, Oak Ridge, TN)*

the sternum, in front of the thoracic vertebrae, and above the diaphragm. Although the heart is centrally located, its axis of symmetry is not along the midline. The heart's **apex** (conical tip) lies on the diaphragm and points to the left of the body. It

is at the apex where the heartbeat is most easily felt and heard through the **stethoscope.**

Try this simple demonstration: Place the disk or bowl of a stethoscope over the heart's apex. This is the area between the fifth and sixth ribs, along an imaginary line extending from the middle of the left clavicle. Since the heartbeat is felt and heard so easily at the apex, this gives rise to the popular but incorrect notion that the heart is located on the left side of the body.

Knowledge of the correct position of the heart can make all the difference in the treatment of **cardiac arrest.** During such a medical emergency, the combination of manual heart compression and artificial respiration can save a life. This lifesaving technique is known as **cardiopulmonary resuscitation (CPR)** and should be performed only by those specifically trained in CPR. All health care workers should have current CPR certification.

STRUCTURE OF THE HEART

The heart is a hollow, muscular, double pump that circulates the blood through the blood vessel to all parts of the body. Surrounding the heart is a double layer of fibrous tissue called the **pericardium,** Figure 13-2. Between these two pericardial layers is a space filled with a lubricating fluid called pericardial fluid. This fluid prevents the two layers from rubbing against each other and creating friction. The thin inner layer covering the heart is the visceral or serous pericardium. The tough outer membrane is the parietal or fibrous pericardium.

Cardiac muscle tissue, or **myocardium,** makes up the major portion of the heart. On the inner lining lies a smooth tissue called the **endocardium.** The endocardium covers the heart valves and lines the blood vessels providing smooth transit for the flowing blood.

A frontal view of the human heart reveals a thick, muscular wall separating it into a right half and a left half. This partition, known as the **septum,** completely separates the blood in the right half from that in the left half. See Figure 13-4a.

Structures leading to and from the heart are:

- Superior **vena cava** and inferior vena cava—the large veinous blood vessels which bring **deoxygenated** blood (which has lesser amounts of oxygen) to the right atrium from all parts of the body

- **Coronary sinus**—from the heart muscle to the right atrium

- **Pulmonary artery**—takes blood away from the right ventricle to the lungs for oxygen

- **Pulmonary veins**—bring **oxygenated** blood from the lungs to the left atrium

- **Aorta**—takes blood away from the left ventricle to the rest of the body

Chambers and Valves

The human heart is separated into right and left halves by the septum. In turn, each half is divided into two parts, thus creating four chambers. The two upper chambers are called the right atrium and the left atrium (pl. atria). The **atrium** may be referred to as the auricle. The lower chambers are the **right ventricle** and the **left ventricle,** Figure 13-4.

The heart has four valves which permit the blood to flow in one direction only. These valves open and close during the contraction of the heart, preventing the blood from flowing backwards, Figure 13-4c.

Atrioventricular valves are located between the atria and the ventricles.

- The **tricuspid valve** is positioned between the right atrium and the right ventricle. Its name comes from the fact that there are three points, or cusps, of attachment. The **chordae tendinae** are small fibrous strands connecting the edges of the tricuspid valve to the papillary muscle that are projections of the myocardium. When the right ventricle contracts the papillary muscle contracts pulling on the chordae tendinae to prevent inversion of the tricuspid valve. See Figure 13-4b. It allows blood to flow from the right atrium into the right ventricle, but not in the opposite direction.

- The **bicuspid** or **mitral valve** (resembles a bishop's hat, called a miter) is located between the left atrium and the left ventricle. Blood flows from the left atrium into the left ventricle, preventing backflow from the left ventricle to the left atrium.

Semilunar valves are located where blood will leave the heart:

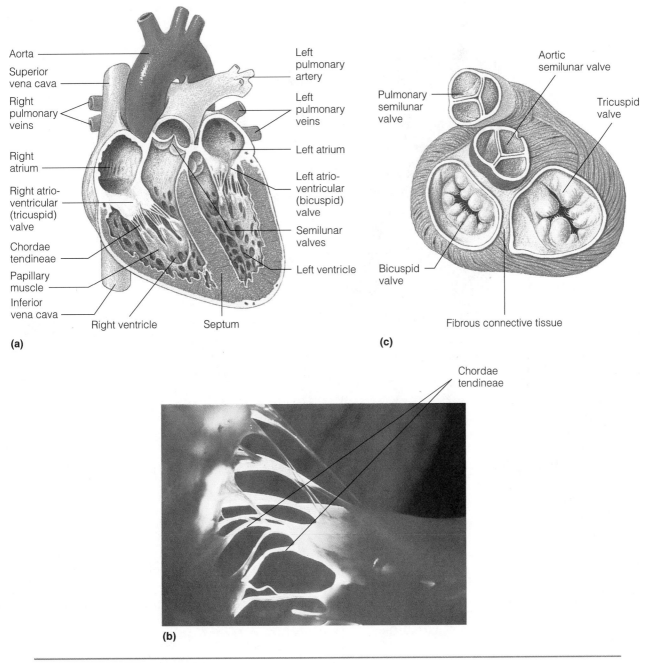

Figure 13-4 *The heart and its valves*

The **pulmonary semilunar valve** is found at the orifice (opening) of the pulmonary artery. It allows blood to travel from the right ventricle into the pulmonary artery, and then into the lungs.

The **aortic semilunar valve** is at the orifice of the aorta. This valve permits the blood to pass from the left ventricle into the aorta, but not backwards into the left ventricle. See Figure 13-4.

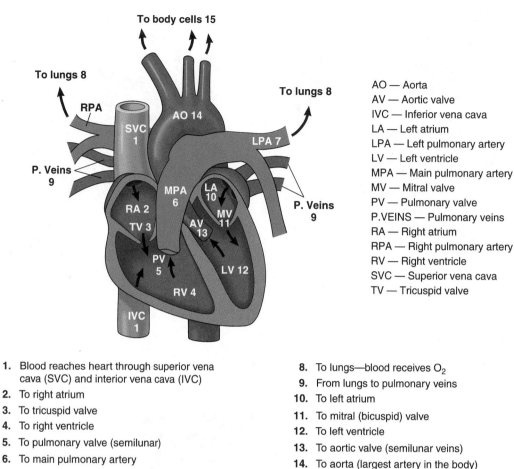

To body cells 15

To lungs 8

RPA

To lungs 8

SVC 1

AO 14

LPA 7

P. Veins 9

MPA 6

LA 10

RA 2

MV 11

TV 3

AV 13

P. Veins 9

PV 5

LV 12

RV 4

IVC 1

AO — Aorta
AV — Aortic valve
IVC — Inferior vena cava
LA — Left atrium
LPA — Left pulmonary artery
LV — Left ventricle
MPA — Main pulmonary artery
MV — Mitral valve
PV — Pulmonary valve
P.VEINS — Pulmonary veins
RA — Right atrium
RPA — Right pulmonary artery
RV — Right ventricle
SVC — Superior vena cava
TV — Tricuspid valve

1. Blood reaches heart through superior vena cava (SVC) and interior vena cava (IVC)
2. To right atrium
3. To tricuspid valve
4. To right ventricle
5. To pulmonary valve (semilunar)
6. To main pulmonary artery
7. To left pulmonary artery and right pulmonary artery

8. To lungs—blood receives O_2
9. From lungs to pulmonary veins
10. To left atrium
11. To mitral (bicuspid) valve
12. To left ventricle
13. To aortic valve (semilunar veins)
14. To aorta (largest artery in the body)
15. Blood with oxygen then goes to all cells of the body

Figure 13-5   *Physiology of the heart*

Physiology of the Heart

The structure of the heart allows it to function as a double pump. (Think of the heart as having a right side and a left side.) Two major functions occur each time the heart beats, Figure 13-5:

▪ *Right heart*—Blood (deoxygenated) flows into the heart from the superior and inferior vena cava to the right atrium to the tricuspid valve to the right ventricle through the pulmonary semilunar valves to the pulmonary artery, which takes blood to the lungs for oxygen.

▪ *Left heart*—Blood (oxygenated) flows into the heart from the lungs by the pulmonary veins to the left atrium through the bicuspid valve (mitral) to the left ventricle to the aorta to general circulation.

It is sometimes hard to imagine this idea of two pumping actions occurring at the same time. Each time the ventricles contract, blood leaves the right ventricle to go to the lungs, and blood leaves the left ventricle to go to the aorta.

Heart Rate and Cardiac Output

The heart, with the individual at rest, beats between 72 and 80 times per minute. With each beat, between 60 and 80 ml of blood are ejected from the ventricles. This is known as the **stroke volume.** The **cardiac output** is the total volume of blood ejected from the heart per minute:

Stroke volume × Heart rate = Cardiac output

$$60 \text{ ml} \times 80 \qquad = 4{,}800 \text{ ml/per minute}$$

The average adult body contains about 5,000 ml of blood. This means all the blood is pumped through the heart about once every minute. Exercise increases cardiac output, because the heart rate is increased. During exercise, muscles receive about 60% of the cardiac output. At rest, the muscles receive only 27% of the cardiac output.

Blood Supply to the Heart

The heart receives its blood supply from the coronary artery, which branches into right and left coronary arteries. (Further discussion on this subject can be found in Chapter 14.)

Heart Sounds

The physician listens at specific locations on the chest wall to hear how the heart is functioning. During the cardiac cycle, the valves make a sound when they close. These are referred to as the **lubb dupp sounds.** The lubb sound is heard first and is made by the valves (tricuspid and bicuspid) closing between the atria and ventricles. The physician refers to it as the S_1 sound. It is heard loudest at the apex of the heart.

The dupp sound is heard second and is shorter and higher pitched. It is caused by the semilunar valves in the aorta and the pulmonary artery closing. The physician refers to it as the S_2 sound. Certain conditions can cause changes in the action of the heart valves.

CONTROL OF HEART CONTRACTIONS

A heart removed from the body will continue to beat rhythmically, which shows that heartbeat generates in the heart muscle itself. The heart rate is also affected by the endocrine and nervous systems. The myocardium contracts rhythmically to perform its duty as a forceful pump.

Control of heart muscle contractions is found within a group of conducting cells located at the opening of the superior vena cava into the right atrium. These cells are known as the **sinoatrial (SA) node,** or **pacemaker.** The SA node sends out an electrical impulse that begins and regulates the heart. The impulse spreads out over the atria, making them contract or depolarize. This causes blood to flow downward from the upper atrial chamber to the atrioventricular openings. The electrical impulse eventually reaches the **atrioventricular (AV) node,** which is another conducting cell group located between the atria and ventricle.

From the AV node, the electrical impulse is carried to conducting fibers in the septum. These conducting fibers are known as the **atrioventricular bundle** or the **bundle of His.** It divides into a right and left branch: Each branch then subdivides into a fine network of branches spreading throughout the ventricles called the Purkinje network. The electrical impulse shoots along the **Purkinje fibers** to the ventricles causing them to contract. The heart then rests briefly (repolarizes). See Figure 13-6.

The combined action of the SA and AV nodes is instrumental in the cardiac cycle. The cardiac cycle comprises one complete heartbeat, with both atrial and ventricular contractions.

1. The SA node stimulates the contraction of both atria. Blood flows from the atria into the ventricles through the open tricuspid and mitral valves. At the same time, the ventricles are relaxed, allowing them to fill with the blood. At this point, since the semilunar valves are closed, the blood cannot enter the pulmonary artery or aorta.

2. The AV node stimulates the contraction of both ventricles so that the blood in the ventricles is pumped into the pulmonary artery and the aorta through the semilunar valves which are now open. At this point the atria are relaxed and the tricuspid and mitral valves closed.

3. The ventricles relax; the semilunar valves are closed to prevent the blood flowing back into the ventricles. The heart rests briefly (repolarization). The cycle begins again with the signal from the SA node.

This action of the heart is known as the cardiac cycle and represents one heart beat. Each cardiac cycle takes 0.8 second. The average person's heart rate is between 72 and 80 beats per minute.

Electrocardiogram (ECG or EKG)

The **electrocardiogram ECG** or **EKG** is a device used to record the electrical activity of the heart that causes the contraction (systole) and the

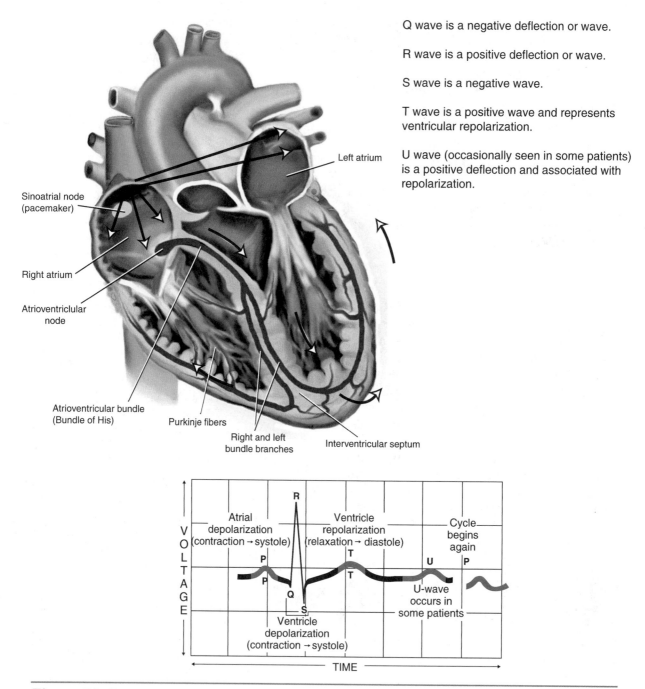

Q wave is a negative deflection or wave.

R wave is a positive deflection or wave.

S wave is a negative wave.

T wave is a positive wave and represents ventricular repolarization.

U wave (occasionally seen in some patients) is a positive deflection and associated with repolarization.

Left atrium

Sinoatrial node
(pacemaker)

Right atrium

Atrioventriclular
node

Atrioventricular bundle
(Bundle of His)

Purkinje fibers

Right and left
bundle branches

Interventricular septum

V
O
L
T
A
G
E

R

Atrial
depolarization
(contraction → systole)

Ventricle
repolarization
(relaxation → diastole)

Cycle
begins
again

P

P

Q

S

Ventricle
depolarization
(contraction → systole)

T

T

U

P

U-wave
occurs in
some patients

TIME

Figure 13-6   *Cardiac cycle and ECG reading*

relaxation (diastole) of the atria and ventricles during the cardiac cycle, Figure 13-6.

The baseline, or isoelectric line, of the ECG is the flat line that separates the various waves. It is present when there is no current flowing in the

heart. The waves are either deflecting upward, known as *positive deflection,* or deflecting downward, known as *negative deflection.* The P, QRS, and T waves recorded during the ECG represent the depolarization (contraction) and repolarization (re-

Effects of Aging
The Heart Muscle

The impact of aging on the heart influences the total cardiovascular system. The heart, as a muscular organ, changes as muscle fibers are replaced by fibrous tissue. This change leads to a diminished contractibility and filling capacity. Heart valves increase in thickness that may modify the normal closing of the valves, causing murmurs. Cardiac output decreases as one ages. The diminished output becomes significant when an elderly person is physically or mentally stressed by illness, strenuous physical activity, or other disabilities.

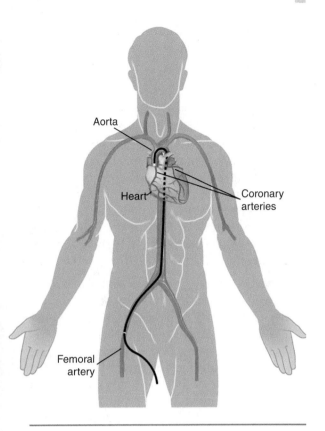

Figure 13-7 *Cardiac catheterization*

laxation) of the myocardial cells. The P wave represents atrial depolarization; QRS represents ventricular depolarization; and the T wave represents ventricular repolarization.

By observing the size, shape, and location of each wave, the physician can analyze and interpret the conduction of electricity through the cardiac cells, the heart's rate, the heart's rhythm, and the general health of the heart.

DIAGNOSTIC TESTS FOR HEART AND CIRCULATORY FUNCTION

Cardiac catherization is the insertion of a catheter usually into the femoral artery or vein. The catheter tip is fed up into the chambers of the heart, Figure 13-7. Dye is inserted and pictures are taken as the fluid moves through the chambers of the heart. The patient may experience a warm or flushing sensation as the dye moves through the circulatory system, but this lasts only a few seconds. This test is useful to determine patency of the coronary blood vessels as well as the efficiency of the structures of the heart. Patients must be asked if they are allergic to shellfish.

Stress tests determine how the physiological stress of vigorous exercise affects the heart. The test is done while a patient is exercising on a bicycle or treadmill under careful supervision. Any abnormalities may be seen on the ECG.

DISEASES OF THE HEART

One of the leading causes of death is cardiovascular disease. Common symptoms of heart disease are as follows:

- **Arrhythmia** or dysrhythmia—the term used to discuss any change or deviation from the normal rate or rhythm of the heart

■ **Bradycardia**—the term used for slow heart rate (less than 60 beats per minute)

■ **Tachycardia**—the term used for rapid heart rate (more than 100 beats per minute)

■ **Murmurs**—indicate some defects in the valves of the heart. When valves fail to close properly, a gurgling or hissing sound will occur. Cardiac murmurs may be classified according to which valve is affected or according to the heart's cardiac cycle: If the murmur occurs when the heart is contracting it is called a systolic murmur; if the heart is at rest it is called a diastolic murmur. A surgical procedure can be done to replace the defective valve.

■ **Mitral valve prolapse**—a condition in which the valve between the left atria and the left ventricle closes imperfectly. Symptoms are thought to occur because of a response to stress. These symptoms include fatigue, **palpitations** (heart feels like it is racing), headache, chest pain, and anxiety. Exercise, restricting sugar and caffeine intake, adequate fluid intake, and relaxation techniques help to alleviate symptoms.

Diseases of the Coronary Artery

Coronary artery disease (CAD) is a narrowing of the arteries that supply oxygen and nutrient-filled blood to the heart muscle. The narrowing usually results from the buildup of plaque on the artery walls (atherosclerosis). If the artery becomes completely blocked, a myocardial infarction may occur. To prevent coronary artery disease, one needs to change lifestyle habits such as no smoking, increased exercise, and reduction of cholesterol levels. Angina is one of the most important symptoms of this disease.

Angina pectoris is the severe chest pain that arises when the heart does not receive enough oxygen. It is not a disease in itself, but a symptom of an underlying problem with the coronary circulation. The chest pain radiates from the precordial area to the left shoulder, down the arm along the ulnar nerve. Victims often experience a feeling of impending death. Angina pectoris occurs quite suddenly; it may be brought on by stress or physical exhaustion. It may be treated with the

drug nitroglycerine which helps to dilate the coronary arteries to permit blood flow to the heart.

Myocardial infarction, commonly known as an "MI" or "heart attack," is caused by a lack of blood supply to the heart muscle, the myocardium. This may be due to blocking of the coronary artery by a blood clot, narrowing of the coronary artery as a result of arteriosclerosis, a loss of elasticity and thickening of the wall, or atherosclerosis (caused by plaque buildup in the arterial walls), Figure 13-8. The heart muscle becomes damaged due to lack of blood supply. The amount of tissue affected depends on how much of the heart area is deprived of blood. Symptoms are crushing, severe chest pain radiating to the left shoulder, arm, neck, and jaw. Patients may also complain of nausea, increased perspiration, fatigue, and dyspnea. Mortality is highest when treatment is delayed; therefore, immediate medical care is critical. Treatment consists of bed rest, oxygen, and medications. Morphine or demerol is given to alleviate the pain, drugs such as tPA are used to dissolve the blood clot, and **cardiotonic** drugs such as digitalis are used to slow and strengthen the heartbeat. Anticoagulant therapy is used to prevent further clots from forming. Angioplasty and bypass surgery may also be necessary.

Infectious Diseases of the Heart

A bacteria or virus is usually the cause of infectious diseases of the heart. These conditions may be treated with antibiotic therapy.

■ **Pericarditis** is an inflammation of the outer membrane covering the heart. The symptoms are pain in the chest area overlying the heart, cough, **dyspnea** (difficulty in breathing), rapid pulse, and fever.

■ **Myocarditis** is an inflammation of the heart muscle. The symptoms may be the same as pericarditis.

■ **Endocarditis** is an inflammation of the membrane that lines the heart and covers the valves. This causes the formation of rough spots in the endocardium, which may lead to the development of a fatal blood clot (thrombus).

■ **Rheumatic heart disease** may be a result of a person having frequent strep throat in-

Cross sections through a coronary artery
undergoing progressive atherosclerosis
and arteriosclerosis

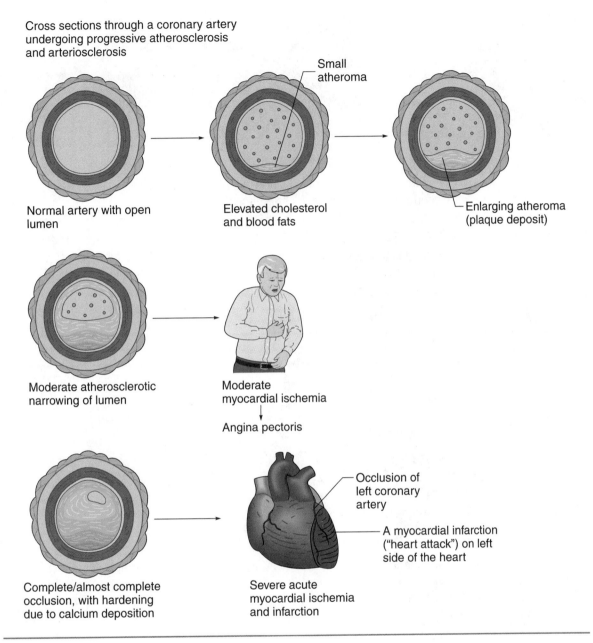

Normal artery with open
lumen

Small
atheroma

Elevated cholesterol
and blood fats

Enlarging atheroma
(plaque deposit)

Moderate atherosclerotic
narrowing of lumen

Moderate
myocardial ischemia

Angina pectoris

Complete/almost complete
occlusion, with hardening
due to calcium deposition

Severe acute
myocardial ischemia
and infarction

Occlusion of
left coronary
artery

A myocardial infarction
("heart attack") on left
side of the heart

Figure 13-8 *Progressive atherosclerosis*

fections during childhood; these infections
may lead to rheumatic fever. The antibodies
which form to protect the child from the
strep throat or rheumatic fever may also attack the lining of the heart, especially the bicuspid or mitral valve. The valve becomes
inflamed and may be scarred, which leads to
narrowing of the valve. The mitral valve is
then unable to close properly, which interferes with the blood flow from the left atrium

to the left ventricle. It is most important that
children who have streptococcal infections
are treated with antibiotic therapy.

Prevention of Heart Disease

The National Institute of Health has stated that
the following lifestyle changes would reduce the
risk of heart attacks. These include not smoking,

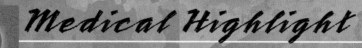

Triglycerides and Cholesterol Levels

The blood contains cholesterol and other fat substances known as triglycerides. High levels of cholesterol are a major contributor to coronary artery disease. The two main types of cholesterol are low density lipoprotein (LDL), or the "bad cholesterol" which causes a buildup of fat in the arteries, and high density lipoprotein (HDL), known as "good cholesterol" because it helps to counter the buildup on artery walls by picking up previously deposited cholesterol and transporting it to the liver for disposal.

Triglycerides are another form of fat. Increasing evidence shows that high triglyceride levels increase the risk for coronary artery disease. Excess dietary fat intake is converted into triglycerides.

CHOLESTEROL AND TRIGLYCERIDE VALUES

	DESIRABLE	BORDERLINE	UNDESIRABLE
Total cholesterol	Below 200	200–239	240 and above
LDL cholesterol	Below 130	130–145	160 and above
HDL cholesterol	Above 45	40–45	Below 40
Triglycerides	Below 150	150–199	Above 200

Levels are given for adults age 20 and older. If you have coronary artery disease, diabetes, or multiple coronary artery disease, the desirable values for total and LDL cholesterol are lower (LDL should be at or below 100).

Source: Mayo Clinic Health Letter, Cholesterol and Triglycerides, July 2001

regular exercise, maintaining ideal weight, estrogen replacement therapy for postmenopausal women, reduction of blood triglyceride and cholesterol levels, and maintaining normal blood pressure. In the blood there are two types of blood cholesterol: high density lipoprotein (HDL) and low density lipoprotein (LDL). The benefits of increasing the HDL ratio to the LDL ratio are significant; medication and diet help to increase HDL.

Heart Failure

Heart failure occurs when the ventricles of the heart are unable to contract effectively and blood pools in the heart. Different symptoms can arise depending on which ventricle fails to beat properly. If the left ventricle fails, dyspnea occurs. If the right ventricle fails, engorgement of organs with venous blood occurs, as well as **edema** (excessive fluid in tissues) and **ascites** (abnormal accumulation of serous fluid in the abdominal cavity). Other symptoms may include lung congestion and coughing.

Congestive Heart Failure

Congestive heart failure is similar to heart failure, but in addition there is edema of the lower extremities. Blood backs up into the lung vessels, and fluid extends into the air passages. Treatment consists of cardiotonics and **diuretics** (drugs that reduce the amount of fluid in the body).

Rhythm/Conduction Defects

A **conduction,** or rhythm, **defect** is said to occur when the conduction system of the heart is affected.

- **Heart block** is the interruption of the AV node message from the SA node. The interruption can occur in varying degrees. The abnormal patterns are seen on an electrocardiograph. *First-degree block* is characterized by a momentary delay at the AV node before the impulse is transmitted to the ventricles. *Second-degree block* can be of two forms. One occurs in cycles of delayed impulses until the SA node fails to conduct to the AV node, then returns to near normal. A second form is characterized by a pattern of only every second, third, or fourth impulse being conducted to the ventricles. This causes a decrease in heart output and usually progresses to the third degree. *Third-degree block* is known as "complete heart block." There is no impulse carried over from the pacemaker. Because the heart is essential to life, there is a built-in safety factor. The atria continue to beat 72 beats per minute while the ventricles contract independently at about half the atrial rate, adequate to sustain life but resulting in a severe decrease in cardiac output. Conduction defects may be treated by medications and/or the use of an artificial pacemaker.

- *Premature contractions* is an arrhythmia disorder which occurs when an area of the heart known as an ectopic (abnormal place) pacemaker (not the SA node) sparks and stimulates a contraction of the myocardium. There are three types identified by the area of their location: atrial, ventricular, or AV junctional. Premature atrial contractions (PACs) cause the atria to contract ahead of the anticipated time. Premature junctional contractions (PJCs) have the ectopic pacemaker focused at the junction of the AV node and the bundle of His. Usually PACs and PJCs are of no clinical significance and are usually caused by stress, nicotine, caffeine, or fatigue. Premature ventricular contractions (PVCs) originate in the ventricles and cause contractions ahead of the next anticipated beat. They can be benign or deadly (ventricular fibrillation). If frequent (five to six per minute) or in pairs, they may require immediate intervention to decrease the irritability of the cardiac muscle and maintain cardiac output.

- In **fibrillation,** the rhythm breaks down and muscle fibers contract at random without coordination. This results in ineffective heart action and is a life-threatening condition. An electrical device called a **defibrillator** is used to discharge a strong electrical current through the patient's heart through electrode paddles held against the bare chest wall. The shock interferes with the uncoordinated action and attempts to shock the SA node to resume its control.

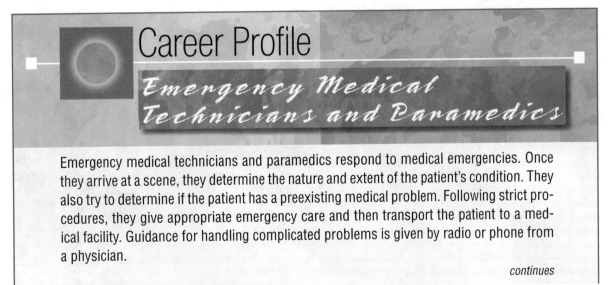

Career Profile
Emergency Medical Technicians and Paramedics

Emergency medical technicians and paramedics respond to medical emergencies. Once they arrive at a scene, they determine the nature and extent of the patient's condition. They also try to determine if the patient has a preexisting medical problem. Following strict procedures, they give appropriate emergency care and then transport the patient to a medical facility. Guidance for handling complicated problems is given by radio or phone from a physician.

continues

continued

EMTs and paramedics may use special equipment such as defibrillators. The specific responsibilities between EMTs and paramedics depend on their level of qualification and training. The National Registry of Emergency Medical Technicians registers emergency medical services at four levels; first responder, EMT-basic, EMT-intermediate and EMT-paramedic.

EMTs and paramedics work both indoors and outdoors in all types of weather. They are required to do considerable kneeling, bending, and heavy lifting. Formal training and certification is needed in all states to become an EMT or paramedic. Job outlook is good, as demand is expected to grow faster than average.

TYPES OF HEART SURGERY

■ **Angioplasty,** or **balloon surgery,** is a procedure to help open clogged vessels. A small deflated balloon is able to be threaded into the coronary artery; when it reaches the blocked area, the balloon is inflated. The balloon is then opened and closed a few times, until the blockage is pushed against the arterial wall and the area is unblocked. The balloon is then deflated and removed, Figure 13-9.

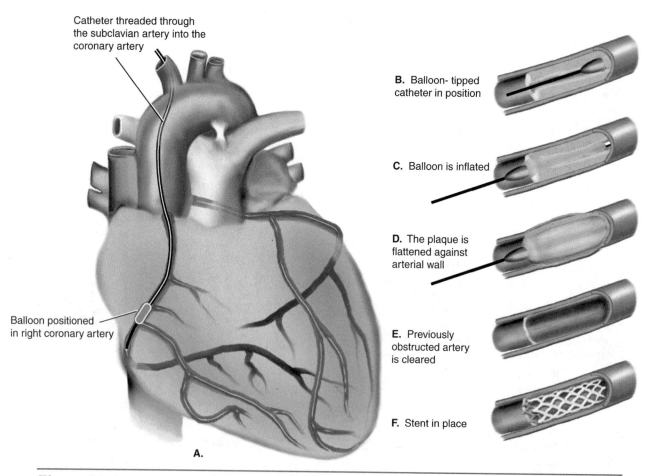

Catheter threaded through the subclavian artery into the coronary artery

Balloon positioned in right coronary artery

A.

B. Balloon- tipped catheter in position

C. Balloon is inflated

D. The plaque is flattened against arterial wall

E. Previously obstructed artery is cleared

F. Stent in place

Figure 13-9   *Balloon angioplasty*

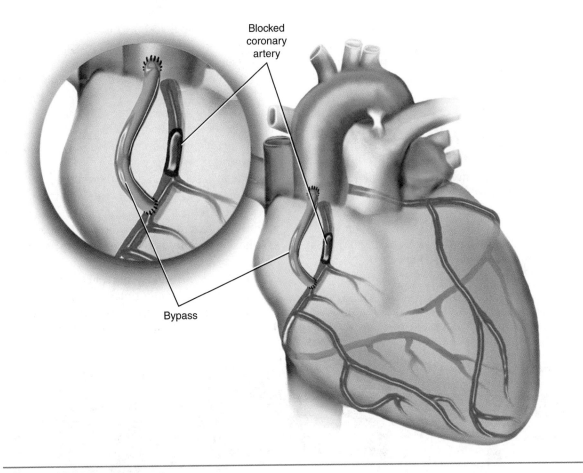

Figure 13-10 *Coronary bypass*

- **Coronary bypass** involves surgically providing a detour or bypass to allow the blood supply to go around the blocked area of the coronary artery, Figure 13-10. A healthy blood vessel, usually a vein from the leg, is used for this purpose. The vein is inserted before the blocked area and provides another route for the blood supply to the myocardium.

- **Cardiac stents** are tiny webbed, stainless steel devices, which hold arteries open after an angioplasty, Figure 13-9. About 25% of the patients who are stented develop restenosis, where scar tissue forms inside the stent and reclogs the arteries. A procedure called brachytherapy, which uses radiation to destroy the scar tissue, may be done. In this procedure, a conventional angioplasty is done and then a radiation source is applied through a tiny balloon inside the stent. While the radioactive material stays in place

just a few minutes, it effectively eliminates the cells that produce the scar tissue. The radiation is used in such a controlled manner that it does not affect other sections of the body. The newest technique uses a specially coated stent that resists the formation of scar tissue.

- **Transmyocardial laser revascularization (TMR)** is the use of lasers to puncture holes in the heart muscle to improve blood flow. This procedure will benefit patients who are not candidates for bypass or angioplasty surgery. The laser instrument is placed on the heart muscle around a blocked artery and the heart muscle is zapped. The laser's energy creates a tiny hole about 1 mm in size through the heart wall to the blood-filled chamber. The outside of the hole heals in a matter of minutes, but the channel created remains. The new channel allows blood from the heart chamber to reach the heart muscle. The trauma caused by the laser beam stimulates the growth of new blood vessels. The full effect of the TMR does not take place until about 2 weeks to 6 months after surgery.

HEART TRANSPLANTS

A heart transplant is needed in cases when the individual's own heart can no longer function properly. This happens when someone has suffered repeated heart attacks and there is irreparable damage to the heart muscle, valves, or blood vessels leading to and from the heart. Occasionally, a baby or young child might need a heart transplant because of a congenital (present at birth) heart defect.

There are always problems that follow even the most "successful" of heart transplants, how-

ever. The problem is one of histocompatibility (matching of tissue type) and organ rejection. Heart transplants that occur between two unrelated people must be monitored carefully. When the heart from the donor is placed into the recipient's body, the recipient's body chemically recognizes the donated heart as a "foreign tissue." Thus, the recipient's immune system starts to reject the transplanted heart.

Medical science has counteracted the rejection by developing chemicals called immunosuppressants. These drugs suppress the recipient's immune system so it will not form antibodies to reject the donated heart. Suppressing the recipient's immune system indefinitely is not medically wise because he or she will be more susceptible to disease and infection. Oftentimes a heart transplant patient dies not from problems arising from the donated heart but from a case of pneumonia.

Medical Highlight

Pacemakers, Defibrillators, and Artificial Hearts

PACEMAKERS

A pacemaker is a surgically implanted electronic device that regulates the patient's heartbeat, Figure 13-11. It may be implanted to regulate irregular contractions of the heart. In addition, a pacemaker is frequently prescribed to speed the heart rate of patients who have a rate under 60 beats per minute (bradycardia).

Patients with cardiac pacemakers should not undergo magnetic resonance imaging (MRI) procedures. Devices that emit electromagnetic fields (including magnets) may alter pacemaker functioning. Researchers have observed interference from cellular phones only when they are held directly over the pacemaker. Patients should avoid carrying a cellular telephone in a shirt pocket over or close to the pacemaker while the telephone is on. Patients with pacemakers should check their

continues

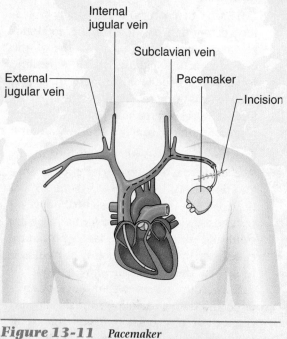

Figure 13-11   *Pacemaker*

continued

pulse rate to determine if the pacemaker is functioning properly.

DEFIBRILLATORS

A defibrillator is a device that shocks the heart to return it to a normal rhythm. The implantable defibrillator protects patients at risk from severe ventricular tachycardia. Medications and pacemakers are the most common treatment for arrhythmias, but for a small proportion of patients the implantable defibrillator can save lives.

The *wearable defibrillator* is a vestlike device worn outside the body for patients with serious heart attack risks. It generates unnecessary shock less frequently than implantable defibrillators do.

The *automated external defibrillator* is a new generation of affordable, easy to use, and extremely portable defibrillators that are being kept where people live and work. Most airlines, sports arenas, community sites, and industries have them available for use.

HEART-ASSIST DEVICES

Ventricular-assist device. A device that helps the heart pump and is used mainly while patients are waiting for a heart transplant.

Artificial hearts. Over the past 50 years, researchers have been searching for an implantable artificial heart. The device must be durable and powerful enough to pump 100,000 times per day. It has to be small enough to be placed inside a person's chest. A battery-powered titanium and plastic model heart was implanted in a patient in 2001. This heart has been approved only for those patients who are too sick to be eligible for a transplant. At present, this device is only expected to prolong the life span by 30 to 60 days. The most that can be expected at present is an artificial heart that would allow a patient to survive until a transplant became available. To date, artificial hearts have had a very small impact. Cardiovascular researchers continue to work toward developing a practical artificial heart that will sustain life over longer periods.

Career Profile

Cardiovascular Technologists and Technicians/ EKG Technicians

Cardiovascular technologists and *technicians* assist physicians in diagnosing and treating cardiac and peripheral vascular disease. Cardiovascular technicians may also be known as *EKG technicians* because they take electrocardiograms. More skilled technicians may also do Holter monitor and stress testing. Cardiovascular technologists who specialize in cardiac catheterization procedures are called *cardiology technologists.*

Education to prepare a technician for EKG, Holter, and stress testing usually requires a one-year certificate program. Training for cardiology technologists involves a two-year program, which is dedicated to core courses and clinical practice. The job prospects for cardiology technologists are excellent. However, cardiovascular technologists' job prospects are not as good because nurses and others may be trained to do procedures such as EKG and stress testing.

Medical Terminology

angin	tightness with pain
-a	presence of
pector	chest
-is	presence
angin/a pector/is	presence of pain in the chest
angio	vessel
plasty	surgical repair
angi/o/plasty	surgical repair of vessels
brady	slow
-card	heart
-ia	condition of
brady/card/ia	condition of slow heart
-ton	strength
-ic	pertaining to
cardi/o/ton/ics	pertaining to heart strengthener
electro	electric current or activity
-gram	recording of
electro/cardio/gram	recording of electric activity of the heart
endo	within, inner
-itis	inflammation of
endo/card/itis	inflammation within the heart
myo	muscle
-al	presence of
myo/cardi/al	presence of heart muscle
infarct	area of tissue death
myo/cardi/al infarct	area of tissue death in the heart muscle
peri	around
peri/card/itis	inflammation around the heart
sept	wall, partition
-um	presence of
sept/um	presence of partition
steth/o	chest
scope	instrument used to examine
steth/o/scope	instrument used to examine the chest
tachy	rapid, fast
tachy/cardia	rapid or fast heart rate

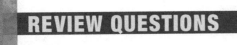

REVIEW QUESTIONS

Select the letter of the choice that best completes the statement.

1. The organs of the circulatory system include the:
   a. heart, blood vessels, and liver
   b. heart, blood vessels, and lungs
   c. heart, blood vessels, and lymph
   d. heart, blood vessels, and kidneys

2. The outer layer of the heart is called the:
   a. myocardium
   b. endocardium
   c. pericardium
   d. pleural lining

3. The muscle layer of the heart is called the:
   a. myocardium
   b. endocardium
   c. pericardium
   d. pleural lining

4. The valve between the right atrium and the right ventricle is called the:
   a. tricuspid valve
   b. aortic semilunar valve
   c. bicuspid valve
   d. pulmonary semilunar valve

5. The blood vessel that brings blood to the right atrium is called the:
   a. pulmonary vein
   b. aorta
   c. pulmonary artery
   d. vena cava

6. The pacemaker of the heart is the:
   a. SA node
   b. AV node
   c. Bundle branches
   d. Purkinje fibers

7. The heart contracts in this fashion:
   a. bundle branches, AV node, SA node
   b. AV node, bundle branches, SA node
   c. SA node, AV node, bundle branches
   d. bundle branches, SA node, AV node

8. The device used to measure the electrical activity of the heart is called an:
   a. EEG
   b. MRI
   c. EKG
   d. EMG

9. A heart rate below 60 is called:
   a. bradycardia
   b. tachycardia
   c. arrhythmia
   d. murmur

10. An inflammation of the inner layer of the heart is called:
   a. pericarditis
   b. myocarditis
   c. endocarditis
   d. phlebitis

11. The term "heart attack" is another name for:
   a. rheumatic heart disease
   b. myocardial infarction
   c. heart block
   d. congestive heart failure

12. The treatment for a heart attack may include all but:
   a. angioplasty
   b. antibiotics
   c. coronary bypass
   d. anticoagulants

13. Another name for stationary blood clot is a:
   a. embolus
   b. stenosis
   c. thrombus
   d. thrombosis

14. The treatment for conduction defect may include:
   a. coronary bypass
   b. cardiotonic
   c. insertion of a pacemaker
   d. angioplasty

15. The circulation that carries blood from the heart to lungs and back to heart is the:
   a. coronary
   b. fetal
   c. cardiopulmonary
   d. portal

LABELING

Locate and label the various structures of the heart. Also include valves, vessels, and nodes. Trace blood from right atrium to aorta.

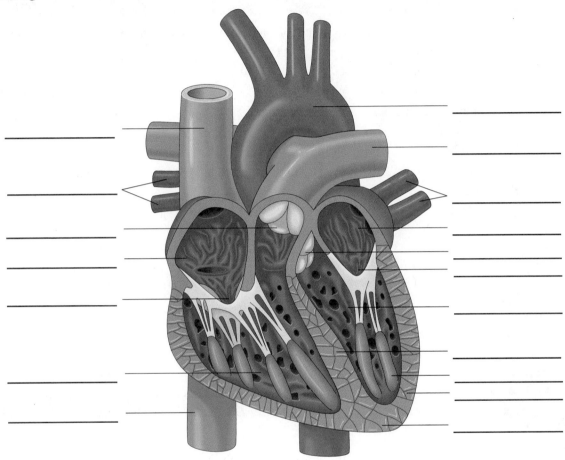

MATCHING

Match each term in Column I with its correct description or function in Column II.

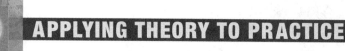

Column I	Column II

_____ **1.** pulmonary artery

_____ **2.** lymphatic system

_____ **3.** pulmonary vein

_____ **4.** septum

_____ **5.** pulmonary circulation

_____ **6.** left ventricle

_____ **7.** general circulation

_____ **8.** right ventricle

_____ **9.** aorta

a. vein that carries freshly oxygenated blood from the lung to the heart

b. circulation route that carries blood to and from the heart and lungs

c. divides the heart into right and left sides

d. artery that carries deoxygenated blood from the heart to the lung

e. system that consists of lymph and tissue fluid derived from the blood

f. blood from the pulmonary vein that re-enters the heart through the left atrium

g. artery that carries blood with nourishment, oxygen, and other materials from the heart to all parts of the body

h. ventricle from which the aorta receives blood

i. circulation that carries blood throughout the body

j. ventricle from which the pulmonary artery leaves the heart

APPLYING THEORY TO PRACTICE

1. Pretend you are a blood cell that has just arrived in the right atrium. Trace the journey you will take to get to the aorta.

2. A child has chronic strep throat. If this condition is not treated, what heart disease can occur? Describe what happens in the heart. How can this be prevented?

3. Your 70-year-old neighbor, Mr. Michael, tells you he has been diagnosed with a second-degree heart block. The doctor told him he would need a pacemaker implanted. He knows you are an RN and he wants you to explain pacemakers to him. He is worried he will not be able to use a cell phone. Describe for Mr. Michael what a pacemaker is and what precautions, if any, he has to take after the pacemaker is implanted.

4. A 50-year-old female patient comes into the doctor's office and states, "People in my family all start to die at 50 from heart disease." What guidelines can you give her to help prevent the disease?

5. Many poems and songs are written about love and the heart. Why do you think there is a connection? Compare your answer with at least two classmates' answers.

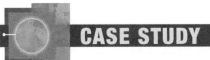

CASE STUDY

Mr. Vincent is a 45-year-old overweight salesman. At work he suddenly develops severe chest pain and is nauseous. A coworker takes him to a nearby hospital. The ER doctor orders an immediate EKG. A diagnosis of acute myocardial infarct is made. Mr. Vincent is scheduled for a balloon angioplasty. The following day the surgery is done and Mr. Vincent recovers with no complications. Margaret, the nurse clinician, is assigned to educate Mr. Vincent regarding his procedure and follow-up care.

1. What is the cause of a myocardial infarct?

2. What is the function of the heart?

3. Describe the cardiac cycle and how it would be affected by a myocardial infarct.

Margaret is explaining to Mr. Vincent the procedure he had done and his follow-up care.

4. Describe a balloon angioplasty.

5. How can Mr. Vincent prevent a future heart attack from occurring?

6. Explain the effect of cholesterol and triglycerides on the arteries. What blood level values for cholesterol and triglycerides should Mr. Vincent maintain?

Mr. Vincent asks Margaret if the blood vessel will close again.

7. Explain restenosis and brachytherapy.

8. What are the effects of cardiotonics and anticoagulant medication?

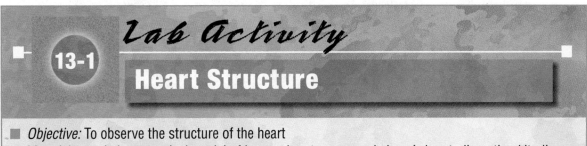

Lab Activity
13-1
Heart Structure

- *Objective:* To observe the structure of the heart
- Materials needed: anatomical model of human heart, preserved sheep's heart, dissecting kit, disposable gloves, paper and pencil

Step 1: Put on disposable gloves.

Step 2: Rinse off sheep's heart in cold water to remove preservatives.

Step 3: Locate the apex and base of the heart. Contrast the size and shape of the sheep's heart with the anatomical model of the heart. Is there a difference? List any differences you see.

Step 4: Describe and record the appearance of the sheep's heart pericardium. Using a scalpel, carefully pull the pericardium away from the myocardium.

Step 5: Using a scalpel, carefully scrape away any accumulation of fat which may surround the heart. This will help you to see the heart chambers and coronary blood vessels.

continues

continued

Step 6: Locate and describe coronary arteries. Record your observations.

Step 7: Identify the right and left atrium. Describe and record their appearance.

Step 8: Locate the ventricles of the heart. Feel both ventricle chambers. Is there a difference between the right and left chamber? Record your answer.

Step 9: Locate and describe the pulmonary artery and aorta. Draw and label a simple sketch to show these features.

Step 10: Using a scalpel or scissors, carefully cut through the aorta and locate the aortic semilunar valve (see Figure 13-2 in textbook). Describe the appearance of the semilunar valve.

Step 11: Examine the heart on its posterior side. Locate and identify the superior and inferior vena cava.

Step 12: Using a scalpel or scissors, carefully cut through the wall of the superior vena cava to view the right atrium. Observe the right tricuspid valve. Sketch the tricuspid valve.

Step 13: Continue to cut carefully through the right atrium into the right ventricle. Observe the walls of the right ventricle and locate pulmonary semilunar valve. Record your observations.

Step 14: Using a scalpel or scissors, carefully cut through the aorta into the left atrium. Observe the bicuspid valve. Record your observations.

Step 15: Continue to cut carefully into the left ventricle. Observe the walls of the left ventricle. Record your observations.

Step 16: Is there a difference between the structure of the right and left ventricle? Record your answer.

Step 17: Dispose of the sheep heart in the appropriate laboratory container.

Step 18: Clean all equipment.

Step 19: Remove gloves and wash hands.

Step 20: Use the anatomical model of a human heart and record any heart features you found in steps 6 through 14.

Chapter 14

CIRCULATION AND BLOOD VESSELS

Key Words

aneurysm	coronary sinus	popliteal artery
aorta	cyanosis	portal circulation
aphasia	diastolic blood	portal vein
arteriole	pressure	pulse
arteriosclerosis	dorsalis pedis	pulse pressure
artery	artery	radial artery
atherosclerosis	ductus arteriosus	stroke
brachial artery	dysphasia	systolic blood
capillary	embolism	pressure
cerebral	femoral artery	temporal artery
hemorrhage	fetal circulation	transient ischemic
cerebral vascular	foramen ovale	attacks (TIA)
accident (CVA)	gangrene	tunica adventitia
claudication	hemiplegia	(externa)
common carotid	hemorrhoids	tunica intima
artery	hepatic vein	tunica media
congenital heart	hypertension	valves
defects	hypotension	varicose veins
coronary artery	peripheral	vein
coronary	vascular disease	venule
circulation	phlebitis	

The blood vessels circulate the blood through two major circulatory systems:

1. *Cardiopulmonary circulation*—blood from the heart to the lungs and back to the heart

2. *Systemic circulation*—blood from the heart to the tissues and cells and back to the heart

Specialized systemic routes are as follows:

1. *Coronary circulation*—brings blood from the heart to the myocardium

2. *Portal circulation*—takes blood from the organs of digestion to the liver through the portal vein

3. *Fetal circulation*—only occurs in the pregnant female. The fetus obtains oxygen and nutrients from the mother's blood.

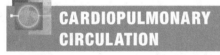

CARDIOPULMONARY CIRCULATION

Cardiopulmonary circulation takes deoxygenated blood from the heart to the lungs where carbon dioxide is exchanged for oxygen. The oxygenated blood returns to the heart. As stated in Chapter 13, blood enters the right atrium, which contracts, forcing the blood through the tricuspid valve into the right ventricle.

The right ventricle contracts to push the blood through the pulmonary valve into the pulmonary trunk. The pulmonary trunk bifurcates (divides in two). It branches into the right pulmonary artery, bringing blood to the right lung, and into the left pulmonary artery, bringing blood to the left lung, Figure 14-1.

Inside the lungs, the pulmonary arteries branch into countless small arteries called **arterioles.** The arterioles connect to dense beds of capillaries lying in the alveoli lung tissue. Here, gaseous exchange takes place: Carbon dioxide leaves the red blood cells and is discharged into the air in the alveoli, to be excreted from the lungs. Oxygen from air in the alveoli combines with hemoglobin in the red blood cells. From these capillaries the blood travels into small veins or **venules,** Figure 14-2.

Venules from the right and left lung form large pulmonary veins. These veins carry oxy-

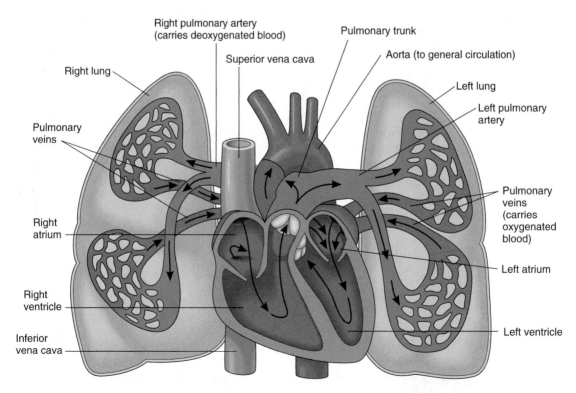

Figure 14-1   *Cardiopulmonary circulation*

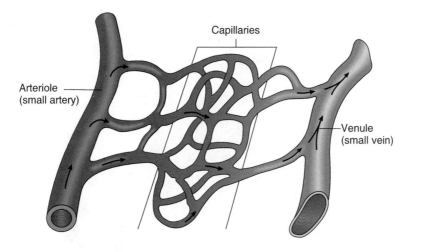

Capillaries

Arteriole
(small artery)

Venule
(small vein)

Figure 14-2 *Arteries deliver oxygenated blood to capillaries, and, once the oxygen has been extracted, the blood is returned to the venous system*

genated blood from the lungs back to the heart and into the left atrium.

The left atrium contracts, sending the blood through the bicuspid, or mitral valve, into the left ventricle. This chamber, then, acts as a pump for newly oxygenated blood. When the left ventricle contracts, it sends oxygenated blood through the aortic semilunar valve, then into the aorta.

SYSTEMIC CIRCULATION

The function of the general (systemic) circulation is fourfold: it circulates nutrients, oxygen, water, and secretions to the tissues and back to the heart; it carries products such as carbon dioxide and other dissolved wastes away from the tissues; it helps equalize body temperature; it aids in protecting the body from harmful bacteria.

The **aorta** is the largest artery in the body. The first branch of the aorta is the **coronary artery** which takes blood to the myocardium (cardiac muscle). As the aorta emerges (ascending aorta) from the anterior (upper) portion of the heart, it forms an arch. This arch is known as the aortic arch. Three branches come from this arch: the brachiocephalic, the left common carotid, and the left subclavian arteries, Figure 14-3. These arteries and their branches carry blood to the arms, neck, and head.

From the aortic arch, the aorta descends along the mid-dorsal wall of the thorax and abdomen. Many arteries branch off from the descending aorta, carrying oxygenated blood throughout the body.

As the descending aorta proceeds posteriorly, it sends off additional branches to the body wall, stomach, intestines, liver, pancreas, spleen, kidneys, reproductive organs, urinary bladder, legs, and so forth. Each of these arteries subdivides into still smaller arteries, then into arterioles, and finally into numerous capillaries embedded in the tissues. This is where hormones, nutrients, oxygen, and other materials are transferred from the blood into the tissue.

In turn, metabolic waste products, such as carbon dioxide and nitrogenous wastes, are picked up by the blood capillaries. Hormones and nutrients from the small intestines and liver, are also absorbed by the blood capillaries. Blood goes from the capillaries first into tiny veins, through increasingly larger veins, and finally into one (or more) of the veins which exit from the organ. Eventually it empties into one of two largest veins in the body. See Figure 14-3.

Deoxygenated venous blood, returning from the lower parts of the body, empties into the inferior vena cava. Venous blood from the upper body parts (arms, neck, and head) passes into the superior vena cava. Both the inferior and superior vena

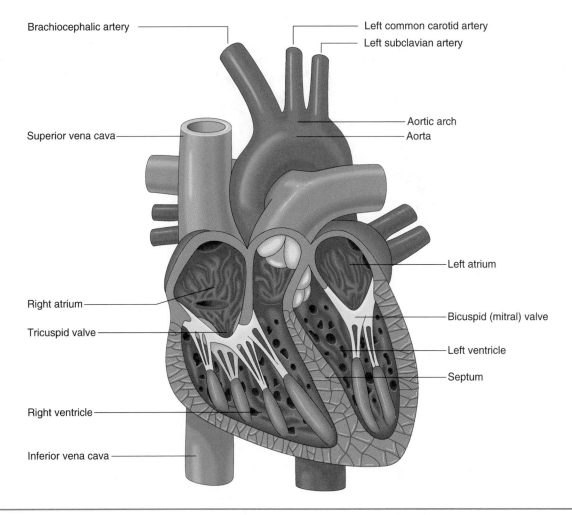

Figure 14-3   *Blood flow into, around, and out of the heart*

cava empty their deoxygenated blood into the right atrium.

Coronary Circulation

The **coronary circulation** brings oxygenated blood to the heart muscle. The coronary artery has a right and left branch. These branches encircle the heart muscle with many tiny branches going to all parts of the heart muscle. The blood circulates to the capillaries where the exchange of gases takes place, and then goes to the veins. Deoxygenated blood returns through the coronary veins to the **coronary sinus.** This is a trough in the posterior wall of the right atrium.

Portal Circulation

The **portal circulation** is a branch of the general circulation. Veins from the pancreas, stomach, small intestine, colon, and spleen empty their blood into the **portal vein** which goes to the liver, see Figure 14-4.

After meals, blood reaching the liver contains a higher than normal concentration of glucose. The liver removes the excess glucose, converting it to glycogen. In the event of vigorous exercise, work or prolonged periods without nourishment, glycogen reserves will be changed back into glucose for energy. The liver ensures that the blood's glucose concentration is kept within a relatively narrow range.

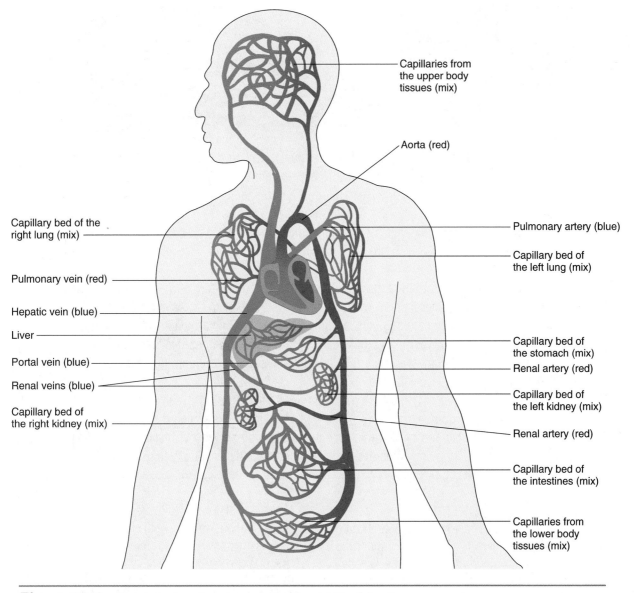

Figure 14-4   *The systemic, pulmonary, renal, and portal blood circuits*

Deoxygenated venous blood leaves the liver through the **hepatic vein,** which carries it to the inferior vena cava. From the inferior vena cava, blood enters the right atrium.

Fetal Circulation

Fetal circulation occurs in the fetus (unborn baby). Instead of using its own lungs and digestive system, the fetus obtains oxygen and nutrients from the mother's blood. The fetal and maternal blood do not mix. The exchange of gases, food, and waste takes place in the structure known as the placenta, located in the pregnant uterus.

In fetal circulation, blood may follow two paths: In the fetal heart there is an opening in the septum called the **foramen ovale,** which permits blood to flow from the right atrium to the left atrium, and/or blood may go from the right ventricle to the pulmonary semilunar valve to the pulmonary artery. Another fetal structure, called the **ductus arteriosus,** allows the blood to flow from the pulmonary artery to the aorta.

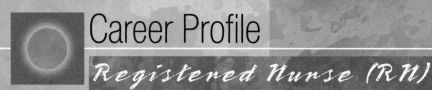

Career Profile

Registered Nurse (RN) and Nurse Practitioner

Registered nurses provide for the physical, mental, and emotional needs of their patients. They observe, assess, and record symptoms, reactions, and progress; they also assist physicians during treatments and examinations, administer medications, and assist in convalescence and rehabilitation. RNs develop nursing care plans, instruct patients and their families in proper care, and help individuals and groups improve and maintain their health.

Registered nurses work in hospitals, the home, offices, nursing homes, public health services, and industries.

In all states, students must graduate from an accredited school of nursing and pass a national licensing examination to become an RN. There are three major educational paths to nursing: associate degree programs (ADN) take 2 years, bachelor of science in nursing (BSN) takes 4 years, and diploma programs given in hospitals last 2 to 3 years.

Employment outlook is expected to be above average in the coming years. Job outlook is best for the nurse with a BSN.

Nurse practitioner or nurse clinician is an RN with a master's degree and clinical experience in a particular branch of nursing. The nurse practitioner has acquired expert knowledge in a specific medical specialty. Nurse practitioners are employed by physicians in private practice or clinics, or they sometimes practice independently, especially in rural areas.

In a fetus the purpose of the blood circulating through the heart is to give the heart and blood vessels oxygen and nutrients to grow. When birth occurs, the foramen ovale closes and the ductus arteriosus collapses and the normal cardiopulmonary circulation begins.

BLOOD VESSELS

The heart pumps the blood to all parts of the body through a remarkable system of three types of blood vessels: arteries, capillaries, and veins.

Arteries

Arteries carry oxygenated blood away from the heart to the capillaries. (There is one exception—the pulmonary arteries—which carry deoxy-genated blood from the heart to the lungs). The arteries transport blood under very high pressure; they are elastic; muscular, and thick walled. The thickness of the arteries makes them the strongest of the three types of blood vessels. Table 14-1 lists the principal arteries and the areas they serve. See also Figure 14-5.

As seen in Figure 14-6, the arterial walls consist of three layers. The outer layer is called the **tunica adventitia** or **externa.** This layer consists of fibrous connective tissue with bundles of smooth muscle cells which lends great elasticity to the arteries. This elasticity allows the arteries to withstand sudden large increases in internal pressure, created by the large volume of blood forced into them at each heart contraction.

The **tunica media** is the middle arterial layer. It consists of muscle cells arranged in a circular pattern. This layer controls the artery's di-

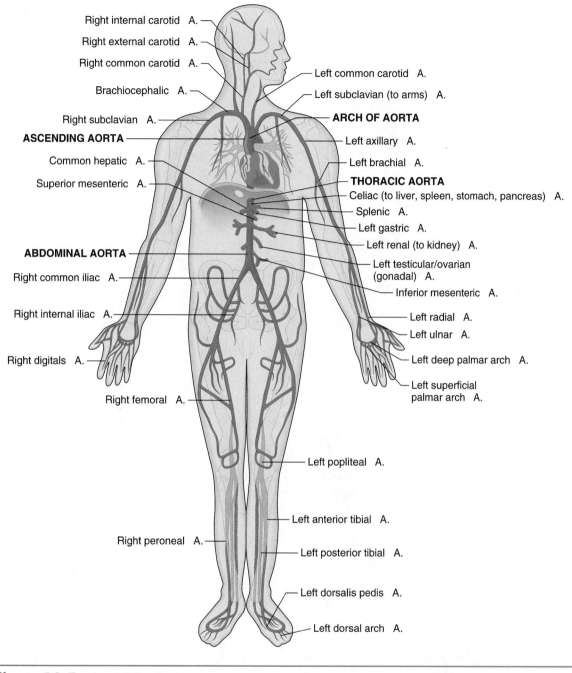

Right internal carotid A.
Right external carotid A.
Right common carotid A.
Brachiocephalic A.
Right subclavian A.
ASCENDING AORTA
Common hepatic A.
Superior mesenteric A.
ABDOMINAL AORTA
Right common iliac A.
Right internal iliac A.
Right digitals A.
Right femoral A.
Right peroneal A.

Left common carotid A.
Left subclavian (to arms) A.
ARCH OF AORTA
Left axillary A.
Left brachial A.
THORACIC AORTA
Celiac (to liver, spleen, stomach, pancreas) A.
Splenic A.
Left gastric A.
Left renal (to kidney) A.
Left testicular/ovarian (gonadal) A.
Inferior mesenteric A.
Left radial A.
Left ulnar A.
Left deep palmar arch A.
Left superficial palmar arch A.
Left popliteal A.
Left anterior tibial A.
Left posterior tibial A.
Left dorsalis pedis A.
Left dorsal arch A.

Figure 14-5   *Arterial distribution*

ameter by dilatation and constriction, which regulates the flow of blood through the artery. This keeps the blood flow steady and even and reduces the heart's work.

An inner layer (**tunica intima**) consists of three smaller layers: endothelium, areolar, and elastic tissue. The endothelium gives the artery a smooth lining which allows for the free flow of blood. See Figure 14-6.

The aorta leads away from the heart and branches into smaller arteries. These smaller arteries, in turn, branch into arterioles, which still

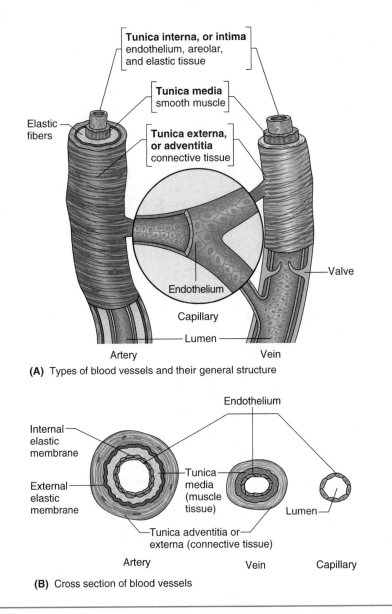

(A) Types of blood vessels and their general structure

(B) Cross section of blood vessels

Figure 14-6   *Different types of blood vessels and their cross-sectional views*

have some smooth muscle in the walls and are also resistant vessels. Arterioles give rise to the capillaries.

Capillaries

Capillaries are the smallest blood vessels and can only be seen through a compound microscope. Capillaries connect the arterioles with venules. Capillaries are branches of the finest arteriole di-

visions, known as metarterioles. The metarterioles have lost most of their connective tissue and muscle layers. Eventually, the last traces of these two tissues disappear and there remains only a simple endothelial cell layer. This endothelial cell layer constitutes the capillaries.

The capillary walls are extremely thin to allow for the selective permeability of various cells and substances. Nutrient molecules and oxygen pass out of the capillaries and into the surround-

Table 14-1 *Principal Arteries*	
PRINCIPAL ARTERIES	**AREA SERVED**
Common carotid	head and face
Internal carotid	brain
External carotid	face (*pulse point*)
Vertebral	spinal column and brain
Brachiocephalic	right arm, head, and shoulder
Subclavian	shoulder
Axillary	axilla area
Brachial	upper arm and elbow area (*pulse point*)
Radial	arm, wrist (*pulse point*)
Thoracic aorta	chest cavity
Celiac	liver, spleen, stomach, and pancreas
splenic	spleen
hepatic	liver
Superior mesenteric	small intestines and colon
Renal	kidney
Common iliac	lower abdominal area
Internal iliac	pelvis and bladder
External iliac	groin and lower leg
Femoral	groin (*pulse point*)
Popliteal	knee area (*pulse point*)
Anterior tibialis	anterior lower leg
Posterior tibialis	posterior lower leg
Dorsalis pedis	ankle (*pulse point*)

Although capillaries are ultimately responsible for transporting blood to all tissues, not all capillaries are open simultaneously. This system allows for regulation of blood flow to so-called active tissues. In the human brain, for instance, most of the capillaries remain open; however, in a resting muscle, only 1/20 to 1/50 of the capillaries transport blood to the muscle cells. Compare this with an actively contracting muscle where as many as 190 capillaries per square millimeter are open. If the same muscle is not active, there may be as few as 5 capillaries open per square millimeter.

Veins

The **veins** carry deoxygenated blood away from the capillaries to the heart. The smallest vein is hardly larger than a capillary, but it contains a muscular layer which is not present within capillaries. Table 14-2 lists the principal veins and the areas they serve. See also Figure 14-7.

The veins are composed of three layers: the tunica externa, tunica media, and tunica intima. Veins are considerably less elastic and muscular than arteries. The walls of the veins are much thinner than those of the arteries, because they do not have to withstand such high internal pressures. The pressure from the heart's contraction is greatly diminished by the time the blood reaches the veins for its return journey. Thus the thinner walled veins can collapse easily when not filled with blood. Finally, veins have **valves** along their length. These valves allow blood to flow only in one direction—toward the heart. This prevents reflux (backflow) of blood toward the capillaries, Figure 14-8. Valves are found in abundance in veins where there is a greater chance of reflux. There are many valves in the lower extremities where blood has to oppose the force of gravity.

Eventually, all the venules converge to make up larger veins, which ultimately form the body's largest veins, the vena cavae. Venous blood from the upper part of the body returns to the right atrium via the superior vena cava; blood from the lower body parts is conducted to the heart via the inferior vena cava.

ing cells and tissues. Metabolic waste products such as carbon dioxide and nitrogenous wastes pass back from the cells and tissues into the bloodstream for excretion at their proper sites (i.e., lungs and kidneys).

Tiny openings in the capillary walls allow white blood cells to leave the bloodstream and enter the tissue spaces to help destroy invading bacteria. In the capillaries, some of the plasma diffuses out of the bloodstream and into the tissue spaces. This fluid is called interstitial fluid and is returned to the bloodstream in the form of lymph via the lymphatic vessels.

Blood flow through the capillaries can be controlled by the action of small muscular bands called precapillary sphincters.

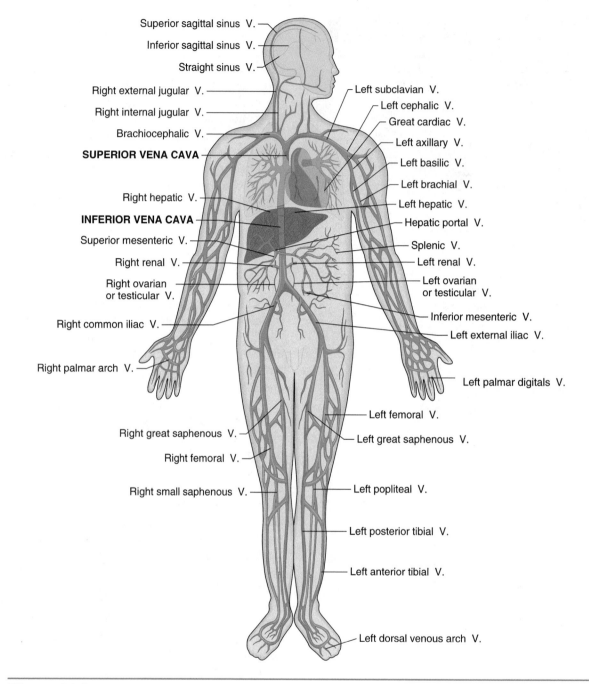

Superior sagittal sinus V.
Inferior sagittal sinus V.
Straight sinus V.
Right external jugular V.
Right internal jugular V.
Brachiocephalic V.
SUPERIOR VENA CAVA
Right hepatic V.
INFERIOR VENA CAVA
Superior mesenteric V.
Right renal V.
Right ovarian or testicular V.
Right common iliac V.
Right palmar arch V.
Right great saphenous V.
Right femoral V.
Right small saphenous V.

Left subclavian V.
Left cephalic V.
Great cardiac V.
Left axillary V.
Left basilic V.
Left brachial V.
Left hepatic V.
Hepatic portal V.
Splenic V.
Left renal V.
Left ovarian or testicular V.
Inferior mesenteric V.
Left external iliac V.
Left palmar digitals V.
Left femoral V.
Left great saphenous V.
Left popliteal V.
Left posterior tibial V.
Left anterior tibial V.
Left dorsal venous arch V.

Figure 14-7   *Venous distribution*

VENOUS RETURN

In addition to valves, the skeletal muscles contract to help push the blood along its path. In the abdominal and thoracic cavity, pressure changes occur when you breathe; this also helps to bring the venous blood back to the heart. Think about sitting for a long period of time, especially on a car ride. Think how sleepy you start to get. The reason may be that blood is not getting back to the heart for oxygen. To reduce the drowsiness, you should pull over, and stop the car, and get out and walk

Table 14-2 *Principal Veins*	
PRINCIPAL VEINS	**AREA(S) SERVED**
External jugular	face
Internal jugular	head and neck
Subclavian	shoulder and upper limbs
Brachiocephalic	right side of head and shoulder
Left cephalic	shoulder and axillary
Axillary	axilla area
Brachial	upper arm
Radial	lower arm and wrist
Superior vena cava	upper part of body
Inferior vena cava	lower part of body and abdominal area
Hepatic	liver
Renal	kidney
Hepatic portal	organs of digestion
Splenic	spleen
Superior mesenteric	small intestine and colon
Common iliac internal iliac external iliac	lower abdominal and pelvis, bladder, and reproductive organs lower limbs
Great saphenous	upper leg
Femoral	upper leg and groin area
Popliteal	knee
Posterior tibialis	posterior leg
Dorsal venous arch	foot

Blood flow toward the heart

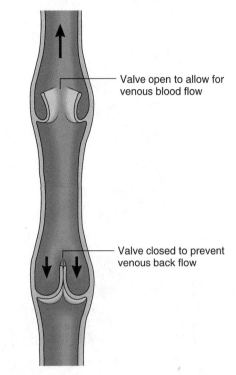

Valve open to allow for venous blood flow

Valve closed to prevent venous back flow

Figure 14-8   *Valves in the veins*

The average systolic pressure measured in the upper arm in an adult is 120 mm/Hg. The average diastolic pressure in an adult is 80 mm/Hg. The blood pressure is recorded as 120/80. **Pulse pressure,** a term associated with blood pressure, is the difference between the systolic and diastolic; if blood pressure is 120/80, the pulse pressure is 40.

around for a while. This will improve circulation and the drowsiness should pass.

BLOOD PRESSURE

When the heart pumps blood into the arteries, the surge of blood filling the vessels creates pressure against their walls. The pressure measured at the moment of contraction is the **systolic blood pressure.** The lessened force of the blood (measured when the ventricles are relaxed) is called **diastolic pressure.** The pressure in arteries that are closest to the heart is greatest and gradually decreases as the blood travels further away from the heart.

PULSE

If you touch certain areas (pulse points) of the body, such as the radial artery at the wrist, you will feel alternating, beating throbs. These throbs represent your body's pulse. A **pulse** is the alternating expansion and contraction of an artery as blood flows through it. The pulse rate usually is the same as the heart rate.

Try this simple demonstration: Place your fingertips (except for the thumb that has its own pulse point) over an artery which is near the surface of the skin and over a bone. The seven paired

Effects of Aging
The Circulation and Blood Vessels

The arteries that are pliable and elastic when young become less elastic, dilated, and elongated with age. These physiological changes mean the heart has to work harder to push blood through the less elastic arteries. Overall, arterial changes appear to be widespread and result in a diminished circulation to all organs and tissues.

A frequent cardiovascular measure is blood/pressure. It is debatable how aging affects this measure of cardiovascular status. Some researchers believe normal B/P for older persons is typically 140 mm/Hg systolic and 90 diastolic (140/90).

Some researchers think that systolic increases are due to aortic elasticity, whereas others believe that peripheral resistance in the vessels causes an increase in both systolic and diastolic.

The baro receptors in the carotid arteries (neural receptors sensitive to blood/pressure) become rigid and less sensitive to pressure changes with aging. This results in a slow response to posture changes. Changes in position may cause dizziness and fainting. This hypotensive response is called orthostatic hypotension.

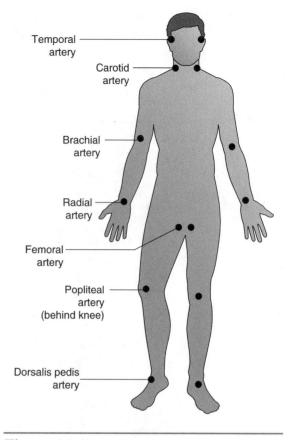

Figure 14-9   *Pulse points/pressure points*

locations where you can conveniently feel your pulse are as follows (see Figure 14-9):

1. **Brachial artery**—located at the crook of the elbow, along the inner border of the biceps muscle

2. **Common carotid artery**—found in the neck, along the front margin of the sternocleidomastoid muscle, near the lower edge of the thyroid cartilage

3. **Femoral artery**—in the inguinal or groin area

4. **Dorsalis pedis artery**—on the anterior surface of the foot, below the ankle joint

5. **Popliteal artery**—behind the knee; may be hard to palpate

6. **Radial artery**—at the wrist, on the same side as the thumb

7. **Temporal artery**—slightly above the outer edge of the eye

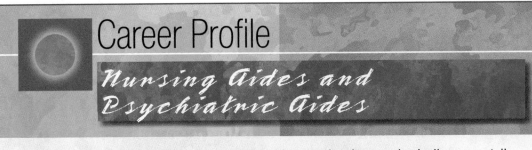

Career Profile
Nursing Aides and Psychiatric Aides

Nursing aides and psychiatric aides help care for people who are physically or mentally ill, injured, disabled, or confined to hospitals, nursing, or residential care facilities.

Nursing aides work under the supervision of nursing and medical staff. They answer call bells, deliver messages, serve meals, make beds, and help patients to eat, dress, and bathe. Aides may also provide skin care, take vital signs, and assist patients in and out of bed. They observe patients' physical, mental, and emotional states and report any changes to the nursing or medical staff. Nursing aides employed in nursing homes are often the principal caregiver, having far more contact with the residents than other staff members.

Psychiatric aides care for the mentally impaired and work under a health care team. In addition to helping patients with the activities of daily living, they socialize with the patients and lead them in educational and recreational activities. Because they have the closest contact with the patients, psychiatric aides have a great deal of influence on patients' outlook and treatment.

Most states require a nursing aide to have training. Nursing aides employed in the nursing homes must complete a minimum of 75 hours of mandatory training and pass a competency examination within 4 months of employment. Aides who complete the course are placed on the state registry of nursing aides.

In response to the aging population, job outlook is good and is expected to grow faster than the average.

A pressure point is where the main artery to the injured part lies near the skin surface over a bone. The seven locations where you can feel your pulse may also serve as pressure points. If direct pressure cannot be applied to a wound to stop bleeding, pressure should be applied to the closest pulse point.

 CONGENITAL HEART DEFECTS

Congenital heart defects occur when there is a malformation of the heart during fetal development. In addition to malformation, other conditions may exist because of the unique structure of the fetal heart. As mentioned in fetal circulation, when the baby is born the lungs begin to function, the foramen ovale closes, and the ductus arteriosus collapses. If this does not occur, proper oxygenation will not occur. The most common symptom of heart disease is **cyanosis,** which is a bluish discoloration to the skin and mucous membrane. Microscopic surgery today can be used to correct many congenital heart defects.

DISORDERS OF BLOOD VESSELS

Aneurysm is the ballooning out of an artery, accompanied by a thinning arterial wall, caused by a weakening of the blood vessel (almost like having a

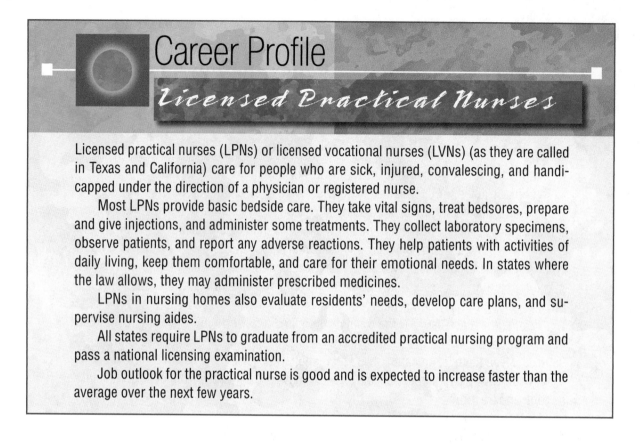

Career Profile
Licensed Practical Nurses

Licensed practical nurses (LPNs) or licensed vocational nurses (LVNs) (as they are called in Texas and California) care for people who are sick, injured, convalescing, and handicapped under the direction of a physician or registered nurse.

Most LPNs provide basic bedside care. They take vital signs, treat bedsores, prepare and give injections, and administer some treatments. They collect laboratory specimens, observe patients, and report any adverse reactions. They help patients with activities of daily living, keep them comfortable, and care for their emotional needs. In states where the law allows, they may administer prescribed medicines.

LPNs in nursing homes also evaluate residents' needs, develop care plans, and supervise nursing aides.

All states require LPNs to graduate from an accredited practical nursing program and pass a national licensing examination.

Job outlook for the practical nurse is good and is expected to increase faster than the average over the next few years.

bubble on a tire). The aneurysm pulsates with each systolic beat. The symptoms are pain and pressure, but sometimes there are no symptoms. The most common aneurysm site is in the aorta.

Arteriosclerosis is the disease that occurs when the arterial walls thicken because of a loss of elasticity as aging occurs. **Atherosclerosis** is the disease that occurs when deposits of fatty substances form along the walls of the arteries. See Chapter 13. Exercise, low-fat diet, and cholesterol-lowering drugs are recommended to prevent this disease. In both arteriosclerosis and atherosclerosis, there is a narrowing of the blood vessel opening. This interferes with the blood supply to the body parts and causes hypertension. Symptoms develop where the circulation is impaired (numbness and tingling of the lower extremities or loss of memory indicates interference with circulation). See Figure 14-10.

Gangrene is death of body tissue due to an insufficient blood supply caused by disease or injury.

Phlebitis is an inflammation of the lining of a vein, accompanied by clotting of blood in the vein. Symptoms include edema (swelling) of the affected area, pain, and redness along the length of the vein.

Embolism is a traveling blood clot. A pulmonary embolism is a blood clot in the lungs.

Varicose veins are the swollen veins that result from a slowing of blood flow back to the heart, Figure 14-11. Blood backs up in the veins if the muscles do not massage them. The weight of the stagnant blood distends the valves; the continued pooling of blood then causes distention and inelasticity of the vein walls. This condition develops due to hereditary weakness in vein structure. In addition the human posture, prolonged periods of standing, and physical exertion can cause valves in the superficial leg veins to enlarge and weaken. Age and pregnancy are other factors responsible for varicose veins.

Hemorrhoids are varicose veins in the walls of the lower rectum and the tissues around the anus.

Cerebral hemorrhage refers to bleeding from blood vessels within the brain. It can be caused by arteriosclerosis, disease, or injury, such as a blow to the head.

Peripheral vascular disease is caused by blockage of the arteries, usually in the legs. Symptoms are pain or cramping in the legs or buttocks while walking. This pain is called **claudication**.

AFFECTED SITE

COMPLICATION

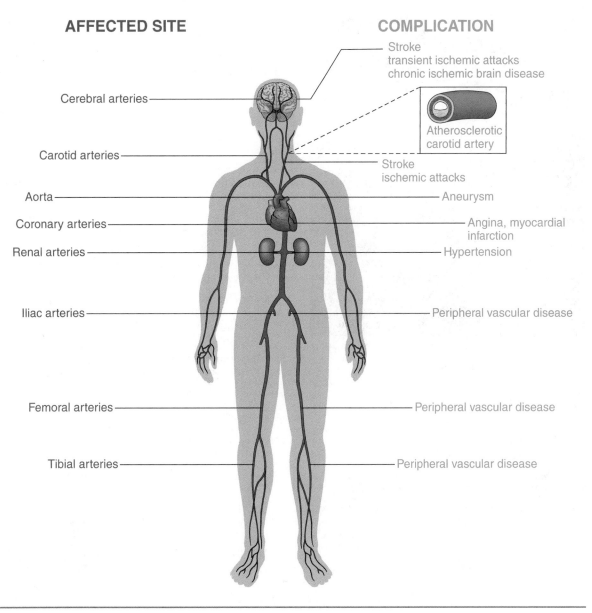

Figure 14-10 *Arteries affected by and resulting complications of atherosclerosis*

As the condition worsens, symptoms may include pain in the toes or feet while at rest, numbness, paleness, and cyanosis in the foot or leg. The condition must be treated or amputation may be necessary. Treatments include medication to reduce cholesterol, improved and/or modified diet, and other treatments to improve circulation.

Hypertension or high blood pressure is frequently called the "silent killer," because there are usually no symptoms of the disease. This condition leads to strokes, heart attacks, and kidney failure. Most people discover that they have the condition during a routine physical. Hypertension means that blood pressure is 140/90 or higher. One in five Americans has hypertension. Incidence of hypertension is higher in black Americans and postmenopausal women. Risk factors for hypertension are stress, smoking, overweight, diets high in fat, and a family history of the disease. Treatment consists of relaxation techniques, reducing fat in the diet, exercise, weight loss, and medication to control blood pressure. In the treatment of hypertension, patients do not understand the disease and its risks. They frequently stop taking their medication because of costs and side effects. Health care workers must realize that better

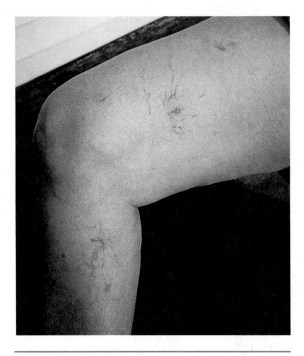

Figure 14-11   *Varicose veins*

education and communication will lead to more effective treatment and a higher level of compliance by patients.

Hypotension is low blood pressure; usually, the systolic reading is under 100 mm/Hg.

Transient ischemic attacks (TIAs) are temporary interruptions of the blood flow (ischemia) to the brain. The cause is usually a narrowing of the carotid artery due to an accumulation of fat. Patients may experience strokelike symptoms such as dizziness, weakness, or temporary paralysis which lasts less than 24 hours. About 50% of people who have TIAs have a major stroke within the following year.

Cerebral vascular accident (CVA) or **stroke** is the sudden interruption of the blood supply to the brain. This results in a loss of oxygen to brain cells causing impairment of the brain tissue and/or death, Figure 14-12. Stroke is the third leading cause of death in the United States. Based on statistics from the American Heart Association, about 730,000 Americans are affected per year with about 160,000 resulting in death.

Risk factors include smoking, hypertension, heart disease, and family history. About 90% of strokes are caused by blood clots. The clots become lodged in the carotid arteries, choking off the blood supply to the brain. The remaining 10% of

strokes called hemorrhagic strokes are caused when blood vessels within the brain rupture.

Symptoms depend on which side of the brain has its blood supply interrupted. Loss of blood supply to the right cerebrum can affect spatial and perceptual abilities and cause weakness or **hemiplegia** (paralysis) on the left side of the body. Loss of blood supply to the left cerebrum will result in **aphasia,** a loss of speech and memory, as well as right-sided hemiplegia. Although no two stroke patients will experience the same injuries or disabilities, symptoms common to many stroke patients include vision problems, communication difficulties, **dysphasia** (inability to say what one wishes to say), emotional lability (uncontrolled, unexplained outward displays of crying, anger, or laughter which have no connection to patient's emotional state), depression, coma, and possible death.

For treatment to be effective it should begin as soon as possible and within 4 hours after the stroke. On arrival at the hospital, a CT scan is done to determine if the cause is a blood clot or a ruptured blood vessel. If the cause is a blood clot, a drug such as tPA is used to dissolve the clot, restoring the blood supply to the brain.

Physicians are exploring ways to prevent strokes. Patients who have had TIAs are being examined to check the patency of the carotid artery to see if they would benefit from a balloon angioplasty. In 39% of patients who have had TIA, one aspirin per day seems to have prevented a stroke. Other drugs are currently being tested to determine if they can prevent or reverse the damage by a stroke. To reduce risk factors, encourage patients to stop smoking, get exercise, and control hypertension. Be aware of the signs and symptoms of stroke and get to a hospital immediately if they occur. A stroke occurs suddenly and a patient who wakes up paralyzed and unable to speak will be very frightened. A health care worker must be very supportive to the patient.

HYPOPERFUSION

Hypoperfusion means inadequate flow of blood carrying oxygen to the organs and body systems. Hypoperfused tissue is no longer being given enough oxygen and will stop working optimally. The most sensitive organ to a decrease in blood supply and oxygenation is the brain. After just 4 minutes of decreased blood flow to the brain, brain cells will be irreversibly damaged. One cause

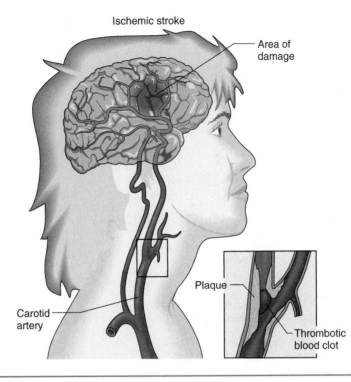

Figure 14-12 *Stroke is caused by a sudden blockage of blood to the brain, thus depriving an area of the brain of oxygen*

of hypoperfusion is inadequate blood supply which can be caused by excessive blood or fluid loss. Another cause of hypoperfusion is due to a change in the size of the arteries and veins. Blood vessels may dilate thus causing decreased amounts of blood flow to the organs in cases of severe allergic reaction, severe infection, and loss of smooth muscle control. The main cause of hypoperfusion is inadequate pumping of the heart. Hypoperfusion can lead to shock. The body will attempt to compensate for hypoperfusion by increasing respiratory rate, increasing the heart rate, or sacrificing organs to protect blood flow to the brain.

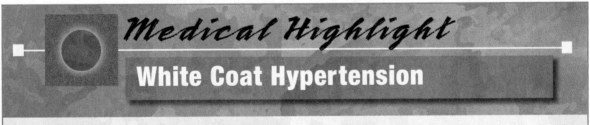

Medical Highlight

White Coat Hypertension

White coat hypertension is so called because it is an increase in a patient's blood pressure that occurs only when a professional in a white coat takes the blood pressure. It is thought that the stress of a medical examination causes the B/P to rise, resulting in an inaccurate diagnosis of hypertension. This phenomenon is also known as resistant hypertension, because blood pressure-lowering medication does not help the problem.

The best way to differentiate between white coat hypertension and true hypertension is to ask the patient to wear a device that measures blood pressure over 24 hours. Of patients who wore this device, more than 25% were found to have normal blood pressure.

Medical Terminology

a	without
-phas	speech
-ia	abormal condition of
a/phas/ia	abnormal condition of being without speech
arterio	arteries
-sclerosis	hardening
arterio/sclerosis	hardening of the arteries
athero	fatty
athero/sclerosis	hardening of the arteries by fat
cerebr	main brain
-al	pertaining to
vascular	blood vessels
cerebr/al vascular accident	accident pertaining to the blood vessels in the main brain
cyan	blue
-osis	process of becoming
cyan/osis	process of becoming blue
diastol	relaxation
-ic	pertaining to
diastol/ic pressure	pertaining to the relaxation phase of the heart cycle
dys	difficult
dys/phas/ia	pertaining to difficulty in speech
embol	plug or clot
-ism	condition of
embol/ism	condition of having a blood clot
hemi	half
-plegia	paralysis
hemi/plegia	condition of paralysis on one side or half
hyper	over or excessive
-tens	condition of tension or pressure
-ion	process of
hyper/tens/ion	condition of excessive blood pressure
hypo	under
hypo/tens/ion	condition of low blood pressure
phleb	vein
-itis	inflammation of
phleb/itis	inflammation of a vein
systol	contraction
systol/ic pressure	pertaining to the contraction phase of the heart cycle

REVIEW QUESTIONS

Select the letter of choice that best completes the statement.

1. The name of the blood vessel that supplies the myocardium is the:
   a. coronary artery
   b. brachial artery
   c. aorta
   d. subclavian artery

2. Special circulation that collects blood from the organs of digestion and takes it to the liver is the:
   a. coronary
   b. fetal
   c. cardiopulmonary
   d. portal

3. In fetal circulation, the opening between the right atrium and the left atrium is the:
   a. umbilical artery
   b. foramen ovale
   c. umbilical vein
   d. ductus asteriosus

4. The blood vessel that carries blood away from the heart to the lungs is called:
   a. pulmonary artery
   b. pulmonary vein
   c. coronary sinus
   d. coronary artery

5. The inner layer of the artery is called:
   a. tunica adventitia
   b. tunica intima
   c. tunica media
   d. externa

6. The blood supply to the brain is carried by the:
   a. external carotid artery
   b. popliteal artery
   c. internal carotid artery
   d. coronary artery

7. The blood supply returns from the legs through the:
   a. saphenous vein
   b. external jugular vein
   c. superior vena cava vein
   d. hepatic vein

8. A buildup of fat in the arterial walls can cause the disease of:
   a. gangrene
   b. atherosclerosis
   c. arteriosclerosis
   d. aneurysm

9. An inflammation of the lining of the vein is called:
   a. hemorrhoid
   b. thrombus
   c. embolism
   d. phlebitis

MATCHING

Match each term in Column I with its correct description in Column II.

Column I	Column II
_____ **1.** arteries	a. small arteries that lead to capillaries
_____ **2.** capillaries	b. permit blood to flow in only one direction
_____ **3.** valves	c. blood vessels that carry blood back to the heart
_____ **4.** veins	d. connect arterioles with venules
_____ **5.** arterioles	e. large, thick, muscle-walled blood vessels that carry blood away
_____ **6.** aorta	from the heart
_____ **7.** atria	f. lower chambers of the heart
_____ **8.** cardiac	g. loss of elasticity in the artery
_____ **9.** coronary	h. referring to the lungs
_____ **10.** hypertension	i. largest artery in body
_____ **11.** atherosclerosis	j. traveling blood clot
_____ **12.** aneurysm	k. upper chambers of heart
_____ **13.** arteriosclerosis	l. enlargement of a blood vessel
_____ **14.** pericardium	m. circulation through kidneys
_____ **15.** portal circulation	n. blood pressure over 140/90
_____ **16.** pulmonary	o. arteries that nourish heart
_____ **17.** embolism	p. largest vein in body; returns to right atrium
_____ **18.** vena cava (superior and inferior)	q. deposit of fatty substance in the arteries
	r. pertaining to the heart
_____ **19.** ventricles	s. goes to liver from small intestine
	t. covering of heart
	u. membrane that lines the chest cavity

APPLYING THEORY TO PRACTICE

1. You are a red blood cell and you are leaving the arch of the aorta. Trace your journey to the right great toe. Name all the blood vessels through which you will travel.
2. You are a red blood cell in the left finger. You need oxygen and you must get to the lungs. Trace your journey from the finger to the lungs. Name the blood vessels and structures through which you will travel.
3. You have just heard about a friend's grandmother who has arteriosclerosis of the brain. Your friend asks you to explain the disease and how her grandmother will act.
4. The fetal heart is unique. Why is it different? Describe the structures of the fetal heart that change at birth.
5. Take the pulse and blood pressure of a 20-year-old, a 40-year-old, and a 70-year-old. Compare the results; if they are different, why are they different?

CASE STUDY

Mrs. Frances arrives in the ER with her son George. She cannot speak and there is weakness and numbness on her right side. She is seen by Victoria, the nurse practitioner, who also notices a drooping on the right side of Mrs. Frances's face. George states that his mother was fine, eating her breakfast when this occurred. Victoria checks the woman's B/P and it is 180/100. The ER doctor and Victoria examine the patient and make the diagnosis of a cerebral vascular accident (CVA).

1. Describe what a CVA is. What is the other name given to a CVA?
2. What is the correlation between Mrs. Frances's B/P and her CVA?
3. What other body systems will be affected because of the CVA?
4. What is the major cause of strokes?
5. Explain the simple tests Victoria will do to determine Mrs. Frances's state of paralysis.
6. Mrs. Frances cannot speak. Which side of her brain was affected?
7. List some of the therapies Mrs. Frances will need.
8. Explain some of the actions people can take to avoid a CVA.

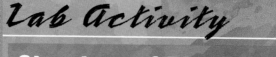

(14-1) *Lab Activity*
Structure of Blood Vessels

■ *Objective:* To observe the structure of the various blood vessels in the human body
■ *Materials needed:* microscopic slides of cross sections of a normal artery, vein, and an atherosclerotic artery; microscope, textbook, disposable gloves, autoclave bag, household bleach, paper and pencil

Step 1: Put on gloves.

Step 2: Observe the slide of the structure of the normal artery. Record a brief description of the features you see.

Step 3: Observe the slide of the structure of a vein. Record a brief description of the features you see.

Step 4: What is the difference between the artery and the vein? Record your observations.

Step 5: Observe the slide of the sclerotic artery. Compare with the diagram in the textbook. Record your observations. Contrast the appearance of the normal artery with the appearance of the arterosclerotic artery.

Step 6: Place slides in the autoclave bag for autoclaving.

Step 7: Clean all equipment with household bleach.

Step 8: Remove your gloves and wash your hands.

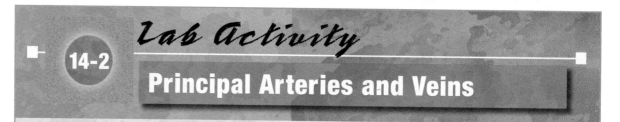

(14-2) *Lab Activity*
Principal Arteries and Veins

■ *Objective:* To locate and identify the major arteries and veins within the body
■ *Materials needed:* Unlabeled anatomical charts of the major arteries and veins, magnetic labels with the names of the arteries and veins, textbook, paper and pencil

Step 1: Locate and name the arteries on the anatomical chart that supply the following organs or body regions with blood: brain, face, pectoral girdle, upper arm, radius, ulna, heart, lungs, liver, stomach, spleen, kidney, intestines, femur, tibia, fibula, and pelvic girdle. Place the names of the arteries in their appropriate places on the chart.

Step 2: Compare your answers to the diagrams in Chapter 14 in the textbook.

Step 3: Locate and name the veins that return the blood to the heart from the following organs or body regions: brain, face, pectoral girdle, upper arm, radius, ulna, heart, lungs, liver, stomach, spleen, kidney, intestines, femur, tibia, fibula, and pelvic girdle. Place the names of the veins in their appropriate places on the chart.

Step 4: Compare your answers to the diagrams in Chapter 14 in the textbook.

Step 5: Do the arteries and veins that supply these locations have the same or similar names? Record your answer.

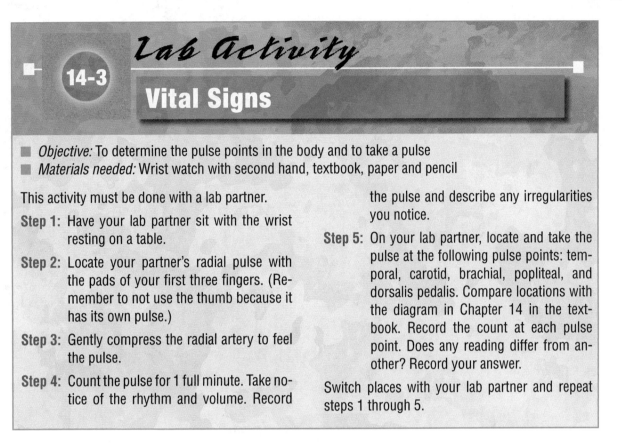

Lab Activity

14-3

Vital Signs

- *Objective:* To determine the pulse points in the body and to take a pulse
- *Materials needed:* Wrist watch with second hand, textbook, paper and pencil

This activity must be done with a lab partner.

Step 1: Have your lab partner sit with the wrist resting on a table.

Step 2: Locate your partner's radial pulse with the pads of your first three fingers. (Remember to not use the thumb because it has its own pulse.)

Step 3: Gently compress the radial artery to feel the pulse.

Step 4: Count the pulse for 1 full minute. Take notice of the rhythm and volume. Record the pulse and describe any irregularities you notice.

Step 5: On your lab partner, locate and take the pulse at the following pulse points: temporal, carotid, brachial, popliteal, and dorsalis pedalis. Compare locations with the diagram in Chapter 14 in the textbook. Record the count at each pulse point. Does any reading differ from another? Record your answer.

Switch places with your lab partner and repeat steps 1 through 5.

THE LYMPHATIC SYSTEM AND IMMUNITY

Objectives

- Describe the lymphatic system

- Define the components of the lymphatic system

- Outline the function of the lymph nodes

- Explain what is meant by immunity

- Identify the causative agents of AIDS

- List the symptoms of AIDS

- Describe the modes of AIDS transmission and measures used to prevent its transmission

- Define the key words that relate to this chapter

Key Words

acquired immunity
acquired immuno-
    deficiency
    syndrome (AIDS)
active acquired
    immunity
adenitis
adenoids
allergen
anaphylactic shock
anaphylaxis
artificial acquired
    immunity
autoimmune
    disorder
autoimmunity
axillary node

human immuno-
    deficiency virus
    (HIV)
Hodgkin's disease
hypersensitivity
immunity
immunization
immunoglobulin
infectious
    mononucleosis
interstitial fluid
lingual
lupus
lymph
lymphadenitis
lymphatic system

lymph nodes
lymph vessels
natural acquired
    immunity
natural immunity
palatine
passive acquired
    immunity
right lymphatic
    duct
scleroderma
spleen
thoracic duct (left
    lymphatic duct)
tonsillitis
tonsils

The **lymphatic system** can be considered a supplement to the circulatory system. It is composed of lymph, lymph nodes, lymph vessels, the spleen, the thymus gland, lymphoid tissue in the intestinal tract, and the tonsils. Unlike the circulatory system, it has no muscular pump or heart.

FUNCTIONS OF THE LYMPHATIC SYSTEM

1. *Lymph fluid* acts as an intermediary between the blood in the capillaries and the tissue.

2. *Lymph vessels* transport the excess tissue fluid back into the circulatory system.

3. *Lymph nodes* produce lymphocytes and filter out harmful bacteria.

4. *Spleen*

   - produces lymphocytes and monocytes.

   - acts as a reservoir for blood in case of emergency.

   - works as a recycling plant, destroying and removing old red blood cells, preserving the hemoglobin.

5. *Thymus gland* produces T-lymphocytes necessary for the immune system.

LYMPH

Lymph is a straw-colored fluid, similar in composition to blood plasma. Lymph is what diffuses from the capillaries into the tissue spaces. Since lymph fills the surrounding spaces between tissue cells it is also referred to as intercellular, **interstitial fluid** or tissue fluid. Lymph is composed of water, lymphocytes, some granulocytes, oxygen, digested nutrients, hormones, salts, carbon dioxide, and urea. It does not contain red blood cells or protein molecules which are too large to diffuse through the capillaries.

Lymph acts as an intermediary between the blood in the capillaries and the tissues. It carries digested food, oxygen, and hormones to the cells. It also carries metabolic waste products (carbon dioxide, urea wastes) away from the cells and back into the capillaries for excretion.

Because the lymphatic system has no pump, other factors operate to push lymph through the lymph vessels. The contractions of the skeletal muscles against the lymph vessels cause the lymph to surge forward into larger vessels. The breathing movements of the body also cause lymph to flow. Valves located along the lymph vessels prevent backward lymph flow.

LYMPH VESSELS

The **lymph vessels** accompany and closely parallel the veins. They form an extensive, branchlike system throughout the body which may be considered as an auxiliary to the circulatory system.

Lymph vessels are located in almost all the tissues and organs that have blood vessels. They are not found in the cuticle, nails, and hair. Lymphatic capillaries are not in the cartilage, central nervous system, epidermis, eyeball, the inner ear, or the spleen.

The lymph surrounding tissue cells enters small lymph vessels, Figure 15-1. These, in turn, join to form larger lymph vessels called lymphatics. They continue to unite, forming larger and larger lymphatics, until the lymph flows into one of two large, main lymphatics. They are the **thoracic duct** and the **right lymphatic duct.**

The thoracic duct, also called the **left lymphatic duct,** receives lymph from the left side of the chest, head, neck, abdominal area, and lower

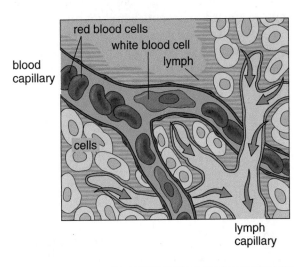

Figure 15-1   Lymph circulation

limbs. Lymph in the thoracic duct is carried to the left subclavian vein, and from there to the superior vena cava and the right atrium. In this manner, lymph carrying digested nutrients and other materials can return to the systemic circulation. Lymph from the right arm, right side of the head, and upper trunk enters the right lymphatic duct. From there, it enters the right subclavian vein at the right shoulder, then flows into the superior vena cava, Figure 15-2.

Unlike the circulatory system, which travels in closed circuits through the blood vessels, lymph travels in only one direction: from the body organs to the heart. It does not flow continually through vessels forming a closed circular route.

LYMPH NODES

Lymph nodes are tiny, oval-shaped structures ranging from the size of a pinhead to that of an almond, Figure 15-3. They are located alone or grouped in various places along the lymph vessels throughout the body. Their function is to provide a site for lymphocyte production and to serve as a filter for screening out harmful substances (such as bacteria or cancer cells) from the lymph. If the harmful substances occur in such large quantities that they cannot be destroyed by the lymphocytes before the lymph node is injured, the node becomes inflamed. This causes a swelling in the lymph glands, a condition known as **adenitis.**

An example of care based on knowledge may be applied to patients with breast cancer. In such cases, lymph nodes under the arms (**axillary nodes**) and near the breasts may contain entrapped cancer cells. These cancer cells are filtered out of the lymph that comes from the breast area.

Early detection of unusual lumps in the breast is possible through monthly self-examination and routine mammography. Early detection and treatment are *vital.* If discovered too late, the cancer cells may have spread (metastasized) to other areas. It is the lymphatic vessels that spread the cancer cells.

TONSILS

Tonsils are masses of lymphatic tissues which are capable of producing lymphocytes and filtering

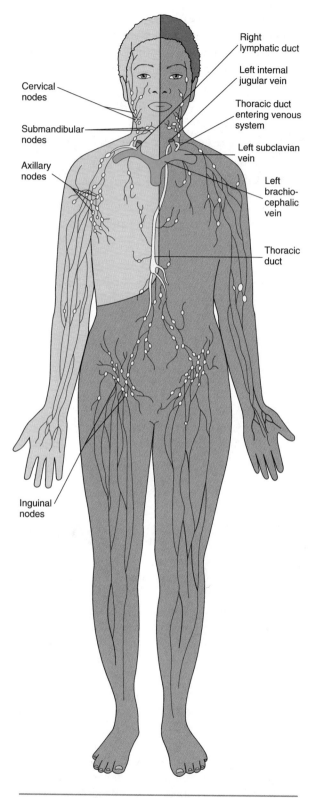

Figure 15-2 *Lymphatic trunks pass their lymph into two main collecting ducts, the thoracic duct and the right lymphatic duct*

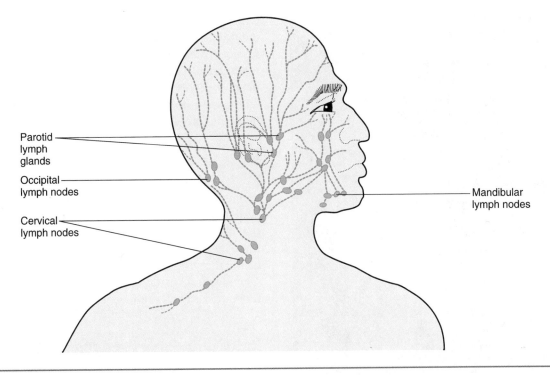

Figure 15-3 *Lymph nodes and lymph vessels found in the head*

bacteria. There are three pairs of tonsils. The most common tonsils are the **palatine,** which are located on the sides of the soft palate. The tonsils located in the upper part of the throat are more commonly known as **adenoids.** The third pair, **lingual,** may be found at the back of the tongue.

During childhood the tonsils frequently become infected, enlarged, cause difficulty in swallowing, severe sore throat, elevated temperature, and chills. This condition is known as **tonsillitis.** Surgery is done in only extreme cases, because the tonsils have an important role in the line of defense against infection. The tonsils get smaller in size as a person gets older.

SPLEEN

The **spleen** is a saclike mass of lymphatic tissue. It is located near the upper left area of the abdominal cavity, just beneath the diaphragm. The spleen forms lymphocytes and monocytes. Blood passing through the spleen is filtered, as in any lymph node.

The spleen stores large amounts of red blood cells. During excessive bleeding or vigorous exercise, the spleen contracts, forcing the stored red

blood cells into circulation. It also destroys and removes old or fragile red blood cells, and forms erythrocytes in the embryo.

THYMUS GLAND

The **thymus gland** is located in the upper anterior part of the thorax, above the heart. Its function is to produce lymphocytes. These lymphocytes are called T-lymphocytes. The thymus is often classified with the lymphatic organs because it consists largely of lymphatic tissue. It is also considered an endocrine gland because it secretes a hormone called thymosin which stimulates production of lymphoid cells.

DISORDERS OF THE LYMPH SYSTEM

Lymphadenitis is an enlargement of the lymph nodes. This frequently occurs when an infection is present and the body is attempting to fight the infection. The term "swollen glands" is used frequently for this condition.

Effects of Aging on The Immune System

Aging causes a decline in immune function, which leaves every organ and every tissue throughout the body more vulnerable to infectious diseases. The ultimate consequence of any age-related decline in the immune function is an increase in the incidence and severity of infectious diseases such as pneumonia, gastrointestinal diseases, urinary tract infections, skin infections, and cancers. The major problem with aging in the immune system appears to be the loss of the ability of the specific immune system cells (T-cells and B-cells) to undergo rapid cell division. As a result, the immune system has trouble keeping up with the rate of cell division performed by bacteria and viruses. The end result is older people tend to be more ill more often. This is why the elderly are encouraged to receive annual flu vaccinations.

Hodgkin's disease is a form of cancer of the lymph nodes. The most common early symptom of this disease is painless swelling of the lymph nodes. Treatment of Hodgkin's disease with chemotherapy and radiation produces good results.

Infectious mononucleosis is a disease caused by the Epstein-Barr virus. It frequently occurs in young adults and children. This disease is spread by oral contact and is frequently called the "kissing disease" or "mono." The symptoms are enlarged lymph nodes, fever, and physical and mental fatigue. There is a marked increase in the number of leukocytes. This illness is treated symptomatically (you treat the symptoms as they appear). Bed rest is essential in the treatment of mono. In some cases the liver may be affected and hepatitis can result.

IMMUNITY

Sometimes pathogens and foreign materials succeed in penetrating a person's first line of defense, the unbroken skin. The body's ability to resist these invaders and the diseases they cause is called **immunity.** Individuals differ in their ability to resist infection. In addition, an individual's resistance varies at different times.

Natural and Acquired Immunities

The two general types of immunity are natural and acquired, Table 15-1. **Natural immunity** is the immunity with which we are born. It is inherited and is permanent. This inborn immunity consists of anatomical barriers, such as the unbroken skin, and cellular secretions, such as mucus and tears. Blood phagocytes and local inflammation are also part of one's natural immunity.

When the body encounters an invader, it tries to kill the invader by creating a specific substance to combat it. The body also tries to make itself permanently resistant to these intruders. **Acquired immunity** is the reaction that occurs as a result of exposure to these invaders. This is the immunity developed during an individual's lifetime. It may be passive or active.

Passive acquired immunity is borrowed immunity. It is acquired artificially by injecting antibodies from the blood of other individuals or animals into a person's body to protect him or her from a specific disease. The immunity produced is immediate in its effect. However, it lasts only from 3 to 5 weeks. After this period, the antibodies will be inactivated by the individual's own macrophages.

Because it is immediate, passive immunity is used when one has been exposed to a virulent disease, such as measles, tetanus, and infectious hepatitis, and has not acquired active immunity to

Table 15-1 *Types of Immunity*

NATURAL IMMUNITY	ACQUIRED IMMUNITY		
Lasts a lifetime Born with it Inherited	Reaction as a result of exposure		
	ACTIVE: Lasts a long time.		**PASSIVE:** Borrowed; lasts a short time.
	Natural—Get the disease and recover or mild form of disease with no symptoms and recovery.		*Natural*—baby gets from mother's placenta or mother's milk.
	Artificial—vaccination; immunization.		*Artificial*—Serum from another; immunoglobulin; antitoxin.

that disease. The borrowed antibodies will confer temporary protection.

A baby has temporary passive immunity from the mother's antibodies. These antibodies pass through the placenta to enter the baby's blood. In addition, the mother's milk also offers the baby some passive immunity. Thus, a newborn infant may be protected against poliomyelitis, measles, and mumps. Measles and mumps immunity may last for nearly a year. Then the child must develop his or her own active immunity.

Active acquired immunity is preferable to passive immunity because it lasts longer. There are two types of active acquired immunity: natural acquired immunity and artificial acquired immunity. Here is how these two types of immunity are acquired.

- **Natural acquired immunity** is the result of having had and recovered from the disease. For example, a child who has had measles and has recovered will not ordinarily get the measles again because the child's body has manufactured antibodies. This form of immunity is also acquired by having a series of unnoticed or mild infections. For example, a person who has had a mild form of a disease one or more times and has fought it off, sometimes unnoticed, is later immune to the disease.

- **Artificial acquired immunity** comes from being inoculated with a suitable vaccine, antigen, or toxoid. For example, a child vaccinated for measles has been given a very mild form of the disease; the child's body will thus be stimulated to manufacture its own antibodies.

Immunization (see Table 15-2 and Table 15-3) is the process of increasing an individual's resistance to a particular infection by artificial means. An antigen may be a substance that is injected to stimulate production of antibodies. For example, toxins produced by bacteria, dead or weakened bacteria, viruses, and foreign proteins are examples of antigens. These weakened toxins stimulate the body to produce antibodies.

An **immunoglobulin** is a protein that functions specifically as an antibody. There are five classes of immunoglobulins; immunoglobulin G (IgG), and the others, IgM, IgA, IgD, and IgE.

Autoimmunity

Autoimmunity is when a person's own immune system mistakenly targets the normal cells, tissues, and organs of a person's own body. This is known as an **autoimmune disorder.**

There are many different autoimmune diseases and they can affect the body in different ways. For example, the autoimmune reaction is directed against the nervous system in multiple sclerosis and the skin in psoriasis. In other autoimmune diseases such as systemic lupus erythematosus (**lupus**), affected tissues and organs may vary among individuals with the same disease. One person with lupus may have affected skin and joints, whereas another may be affected with the blood-clotting problems.

Causes of autoimmune disease may be from genetic familial predisposition, viruses, or even sunlight, which can act as a trigger for lupus.

Table 15-2 *Summary of Adolescent/Adult Immunization Recommendations*

AGENT	INDICATIONS	PRIMARY SCHEDULE	CONTRAINDICATIONS	COMMENTS
Hepatitis B Vaccine	a. Persons with occupational risk of exposure to blood or blood-contaminated body fluids. b. Clients and staff of institutions for the developmentally disabled. c. Hemodialysis patients. d. Recipients of clotting-factor concentrates. e. Household contacts and sex partners of those chronically infected with HBV. f. Family members of adoptees from countries where HBV infection is endemic, if adoptees are HBsAg⁺. g. Certain international travelers. h. Injecting drug users. i. Men who have sex with men. j. Heterosexual men and women with multiple sex partners or recent episode of a sexually transmitted disease. k. Inmates of long-term correctional facilities. l. All unvaccinated adolescents.	Three doses: second dose 1–2 months after the first, third dose 4–6 months after the first. No need to start series over if schedule interrupted. Can start series with one manufacturer's vaccine and finish with another. Dose (*Adult*): intramuscular (IM) Recombivax HB®: 10 μg/1.0 mL (green cap) Engerix-B®: 20 μg/1.0 mL (orange cap) Dose (*Adolescents 11–19 years*): intramuscular (IM) Recombivax HB®: 5 μg/0.5 mL (yellow cap) Engerix-B®: 10 μg/0.5 mL (light blue cap) Two doses (*Only for Adolescents 11–15 years*): intramuscular (IM), 4–6 months apart. Restricted to Recombivax HB®: 10 μg/1.0 mL (green cap) Booster: None presently recommended.	Anaphylactic allergy to yeast.	a. Persons with serologic markers of prior or continuing hepatitis B virus infection do not need immunization. b. For hemodialysis patients and other immunodeficient or immunosuppressed patients, vaccine dosage is doubled or special preparation is used. c. *Pregnant women should be sero-screened for HBsAg and, if positive, their infants should be given post-exposure prophylaxis beginning at birth.* d. Post-exposure prophylaxis: consult ACIP recommendations, or state or local immunization program.
Poliovirus Vaccine: IPV - Inactivated Vaccine: OPV - Oral (live) Vaccine Give IM or Sc	Routine vaccination of those ≥18 years of age residing in the U.S. is not necessary. Vaccination is recommended for the following high-risk adults: a. Travelers to areas or countries where poliomyelitis is epidemic or endemic. b. Members of communities or specific population groups with disease caused by wild polioviruses. c. Laboratory workers who handle specimens that may contain polioviruses. d. Health care workers who have close contact with patients who may be excreting wild polioviruses. e. Unvaccinated adults whose children will be receiving OPV.	Unimmunized adolescents/adults: IPV is recommended—two doses at 4–8 week intervals, third dose 6–12 months after second (can be as soon as 2 months) Dose: 0.5 mL subcutaneous (SC) or intramuscular (IM). Partially immunized adolescents/adults: Complete primary series with IPV (IPV schedule shown above). OPV is no longer recommended for use in the United States.	*IPV:* Anaphylactic reaction following previous dose or to streptomycin, polymyxin B, or neomycin.	In instances of potential exposure to wild poliovirus, adults who have had a primary series of OPV or IPV may be given 1 more dose of IPV. Although no adverse effects have been documented, vaccination of pregnant women should be avoided. However, if immediate protection is required, pregnant women may be given IPV in accordance with the recommended schedule for adults.

(continues)

Table 15-2 *(continued)*

AGENT	INDICATIONS	PRIMARY SCHEDULE	CONTRAINDICATIONS	COMMENTS
Varicella Vaccine	a. Persons of any age without a reliable history of varicella disease or vaccination, or who are seronegative for varicella. b. Susceptible adolescents and adults living in households with children. c. All susceptible health care workers. d. Susceptible family contacts of immunocompromised persons. e. Susceptible persons in the following groups who are at high risk for exposure: - persons who live or work in environments in which transmission of varicella is likely (e.g., teachers of young children, day care employees, residents and staff in institutional settings) or can occur (e.g., college students, inmates and staff of correctional institutions, military personnel) - nonpregnant women of childbearing age - international travelers	For persons <13 years of age, one dose. For persons 13 years of age and older, two doses separated by 4–8 weeks. If >8 weeks elapse following the first dose, the second dose can be administered without restarting the schedule. Dose: 0.5 mL subcutaneous (SC)	a. Anaphylactic allergy to gelatin or neomycin. b. Untreated, active TB. c. Immunosuppressive therapy or immunodeficiency (including HIV infection). d. Family history of congenital or hereditary immunodeficiency in first-degree relatives, unless the immune competence of the recipient has been clinically substantiated or verified by a laboratory. e. Immune globulin preparation or blood/blood product received in preceding 5 months. f. Pregnancy.	Women should be asked if they are pregnant before receiving varicella vaccine, and advised to avoid pregnancy for one month following each dose of vaccine.
Hepatitis A Vaccine	a. Persons traveling to or working in countries with high or intermediate endemicity of infection. b. Men who have sex with men. c. Injecting and non-injecting illegal drug users. d. Persons who work with HAV-infected primates or with HAV in a research laboratory setting. e. Persons with chronic liver disease. f. Persons with clotting factor disorders. g. Consider food handlers, where determined to be cost-effective by health authorities or employers.	HAVRIX®: Two doses, separated by 6–12 months. Adults (18 years of age and older)—Dose: 1.0 mL intramuscular (IM); Persons 2–17 years of age: Dose: 0.5 mL (IM). VAQTA®: Adults (18 years of age and older): Two doses, separated by 6 months. Dose: 1.0 mL intramuscular (IM); Persons 2–17 years of age: Two doses, separated by 6–18 months; Dose: 0.5 mL (IM)	A history of hypersensitivity to alum or the preservative 2-phenoxyethanol	The safety of hepatitis A vaccine during pregnancy has not been determined, though the theoretical risk to the developing fetus is expected to be low. The risk of vaccination should be weighed against the risk of hepatitis A in women who may be at high risk of exposure to HAV.

(continues)

Table 15-2 *(continued)*

AGENT	INDICATIONS	PRIMARY SCHEDULE	CONTRAINDICATIONS	COMMENTS
Tetanus and Diphtheria Toxoids Combined (Td)	All adults. All adolescents should be assessed at 11–12 or 14–16 years of age and immunized if no dose was received during the previous 5 years.	Two doses 4–8 weeks apart, third dose 6–12 months after the second. No need to repeat doses if the schedule is interrupted. Dose: 0.5 mL intramuscular (IM) Booster: At 10 year intervals throughout life.	Neurologic or severe hypersensitivity reaction to prior dose.	WOUND MANAGEMENT: Patients with three or more previous tetanus toxoid doses: (a) give Td for clean, minor wounds only if more than 10 years since last dose; (b) for other wounds, give Td if over 5 years since last dose. Patients with less than 3 or unknown number of prior tetanus toxoid doses; give Td for clean, minor wounds and Td and TIG (Tetanus Immune Globulin) for other wounds.
Influenza Vaccine	a. Adults 50 years of age and older. b. Residents of nursing homes or other facilities for patients with chronic medical conditions. c. Persons ≥6 months of age with chronic cardiovascular or pulmonary disorders, including asthma. d. Persons ≥6 months of age with chronic metabolic diseases (including diabetes), renal dysfunction, hemoglobinopathies, immunosuppressive or immunodeficiency disorders. e. Women in their 2nd or 3rd trimester of pregnancy during influenza season. f. Persons 6 mo.–18 years of age receiving long-term aspirin therapy. g. Groups, including household members and care givers, who can infect high risk persons.	Dose: 0.5 mL intramuscular (IM) Given annually each fall and winter.	Anaphylactic allergy to eggs. Acute febrile illness.	Depending on season and destination, persons traveling to foreign countries should consider vaccination. Any person ≥ 6 months of age who wishes to reduce the likelihood of becoming ill with influenza should be vaccinated. Avoiding subsequent vaccination of persons known to have developed GBS within 6 weeks of a previous vaccination seems prudent; however, for most persons with a GBS history who are at high risk for severe complications, many experts believe the established benefits of vaccination justify yearly vaccination.

(continues)

Table 15-2 *(continued)*

AGENT	INDICATIONS	PRIMARY SCHEDULE	CONTRAINDICATIONS	COMMENTS
Pneumococcal Polysaccharide Vaccine (PPV)	a. Adults 65 years of age and older. b. Persons ≥ 2 years with chronic cardiovascular or pulmonary disorders including congestive heart failure, diabetes mellitus, chronic liver disease, alcoholism, CSF leaks, cardiomyopathy, COPD or emphysema. c. Persons ≥ 2 years with splenic dysfunction or asplenia, hematologic malignancy, multiple myeloma, renal failure, organ transplantation or immunosuppressive conditions, including HIV infection. d. Alaskan Natives and certain American Indian populations.	One dose for most people* Dose: 0.5 mL intramuscular (IM) or subcutaneous (SC) *Persons vaccinated prior to age 65 should be vaccinated at age 65 if 5 or more years have passed since the first dose. For all persons with functional or anatomic asplenia, transplant patients, patients with chronic kidney disease, immunosuppressed or immunodeficient persons, and others at highest risk of fatal infection, a second dose should be given – at least 5 years after first dose.	The safety of PPV during the first trimester of pregnancy has not been evaluated. The manufacturer's package insert should be reviewed for additional information.	If elective splenectomy or immunosuppressive therapy is planned, give vaccine 2 weeks ahead, if possible. When indicated, vaccine should be administered to patients with unknown vaccination status. All residents of nursing homes and other long-term care facilities should have their vaccination status assessed and documented.
Measles and Mumps Vaccines**	a. Adults born after 1956 without written documentation of immunization on or after the first birthday. b. Health care personnel born after 1956 who are at risk of exposure to patients with measles should have documentation of two doses. c. Women born outside the U.S. in 1957 or later	At least one dose. (Two doses of measles - containing vaccine if in college, in health care profession or traveling to a foreign country with second dose at least 1 month after the first). Dose 0.5 ml subcutaneous (SC)	a. Immunosuppressive therapy or immunodeficiency including HIV-infected persons with severe immunosuppression.	Women should be asked if they are pregnant before receiving vaccine, and advised to avoid pregnancy for 28 days after immunization.

*Adapted from the recommendations of the Advisory Committee on Immunization Practices (ACIP).
**Foreign travel and less commonly used vaccines such as typhoid, rabies, and meningococcal are not included.
***These vaccines can be given in the combined form measles-mumps-rubella (MMR). Persons already immune to one or more components can still receive MMR.

Table 15-3 Recommended Childhood Immunization Schedule United States, 2002

Recommended Childhood Immunization Schedule
United States, 2002

	range of recommended ages			catch-up vaccination			preadolescent assessment			

Vaccine ▼ / Age ▶	Birth	1 mo	2 mos	4 mos	6 mos	12 mos	15 mos	18 mos	24 mos	4-6 yrs	11-12 yrs	13-18 yrs
Hepatitis B[1]	Hep B #1	only if mother HBsAg (-)								Hep B series		
		Hep B #2			Hep B #3							
Diphtheria, Tetanus, Pertussis[2]			DTaP	DTaP	DTaP		DTaP			DTaP	Td	
Haemophilus influenzae Type b[3]			Hib	Hib	Hib	Hib						
Inactivated Polio[4]			IPV	IPV		IPV				IPV		
Measles, Mumps, Rubella[5]						MMR #1				MMR #2	MMR #2	
Varicella[6]						Varicella				Varicella		
Pneumococcal[7]			PCV	PCV	PCV	PCV				PCV / PPV		
Hepatitis A[8]										Hepatitis A series		
Influenza[9]						Influenza (yearly)						

Vaccines below this line are for selected populations

This schedule indicates the recommended ages for routine administration of currently licensed childhood vaccines, as of December 1, 2001, for children through age 18 years. Any dose not given at the recommended age should be given at any subsequent visit when indicated and feasible. ▨ Indicates age groups that warrant special effort to administer those vaccines not previously given. Additional vaccines may be licensed and recommended during the year. Licensed combination vaccines may be used whenever any components of the combination are indicated and the vaccine is other components are not contraindicated. Providers should consult the manufacturers' package inserts for detailed recommendations.

Approved by the Advisory Committee on Immunization Practices (www.cdc.gov/nip/acip) the American Academy of Pediatrics (www.aap.org), and the American Academy of Family Physicians (www.aafp.org).

1. Hepatitis B vaccine (Hep B). All infants should receive the first dose of hepatitis B vaccine soon after birth and before hospital discharge; the first dose may also be given by age 2 months if the infant's mother is HBsAg-negative. Only monovalent hepatitis B vaccine can be used for the birth dose. Monovalent or combination vaccine containing Hep B may be used to complete the series; four doses of vaccine may be administered if combination vaccine is used. The second dose should be given at least 4 weeks after the first dose, except for Hib-containing vaccine which cannot be administered before age 6 weeks. The third dose should be given at least 16 weeks after the first dose and at least 8 weeks after the second dose. The last dose in the vaccination series (third or fourth dose) should not be administered before age 6 months.

Infants born to HBsAg-positive mothers should receive hepatitis B vaccine and 0.5 mL hepatitis B immune globulin (HBIG) within 12 hours of birth at separate sites. The second dose is recommended at age 1–2 months and the vaccination series should be completed (third or fourth dose) at age 6 months.

Infants born to mothers whose HBsAg status is unknown should receive the first dose of the hepatitis B vaccine series within 12 hours of birth. Maternal blood should be drawn at the time of delivery to determine the mother's HBsAg status; if the HBsAg test is positive, the infant should receive HBIG as soon as possible (no later than age 1 week).

2. Diphtheria and tetanus toxoids and acellular pertussis vaccine (DTaP). The fourth dose of DTaP may be administered as early as age 12 months, provided 6 months have elapsed since the third dose and the child is unlikely to return at age 15–18 months.

Tetanus and diphtheria toxoids (Td) is recommended at age 11–12 years if at least 5 years have elapsed since the last dose of tetanus and diphtheria toxoid-containing vaccine. Subsequent routine Td boosters are recommended every 10 years.

3. *Haemophilus influenzae* type b (Hib) conjugate vaccine. Three Hib conjugate vaccines are licensed for infant use. If PRP-OMP (PedvaxHIB® or ComVax® [Merck]) is administered at ages 2 and 4 months, a dose at age 6 months is not required. DTaP/Hib combination products should not be used for primary immunization in infants at age 2, 4 or 6 months, but can be used as boosters following any Hib vaccine.

4. Inactivated poliovirus vaccine (IPV). An all-IPV schedule is recommended for routine childhood poliovirus vaccination in the United States. All children should receive four doses of IPV at age 2 months, 4 months, 6–18 months, and 4–6 years.

5. Measles, mumps, and rubella vaccine (MMR). The second dose of MMR is recommended routinely at age 4–6 years but may be administered during any visit, provided at least 4 weeks have elapsed since the first dose and that both doses are administered beginning at or after age 12 months. Those who have not previously received the second dose should complete the schedule by the visit at 11–12 years.

6. Varicella vaccine. Varicella vaccine is recommended at any visit at or after age 12 months for susceptible children (i.e. those who lack a reliable history of chickenpox). Susceptible persons aged ≥13 years should receive two doses, given at least 4 weeks apart.

7. Pneumococcal vaccine. The heptavalent **pneumococcal conjugate vaccine (PCV)** is recommended for all children aged 2–23 months and for certain children aged 24–59 months. **Pneumococcal polysaccharide vaccine (PPV)** is recommended in addition to PCV for certain high-risk groups. See *MMWR* 2000;49(RR-9);1–37.

8. Hepatitis A vaccine. Hepatitis A vaccine is recommended for use in selected states and regions, and for certain high-risk groups; consult your local public health authority. See *MMWR* 1999;48(RR-12); 1–37.

9. Influenza vaccine. Influenza vaccine is recommended annually for children age ≥ 6 months with certain risk factors (including but not limited to asthma, cardiac disease, sickle cell disease, HIV, and diabetes; see *MMWR* 2001;50(RR-4); 1–44), and can be administered to all others wishing to obtain immunity. Children aged ≤12 years should receive vaccine in a dosage appropriate for their age (0.25 mL if age 6–35 months or 0.5 mL if aged ≥ 3 years). Children aged ≤ 8 years who are receiving influenza vaccine for the first time should receive two doses separated by at least 4 weeks.

For additional information about vaccines, vaccine supply, and contraindications for immunization, please visit the National Immunization Program Website at www.cdc.gov/nip or call the National Immunization Hotline at 800-232-2522 (English) or 800-232-0233 (Spanish).

Following are examples of autoimmune diseases and where in the textbook they are discussed in more detail.

- Multiple sclerosis, Chapter 8
- Myasthenia gravis, Chapter 7
- Pernicious anemia, Chapter 12
- Psoriasis, Chapter 5
- Crohn's disease, Chapter 18
- Ulcerative colitis, Chapter 18
- Type I diabetes mellitus, Chapter 11
- Rheumatoid arthritis, Chapter 6
- Lupus, Chapter 15
- Scleroderma, Chapter 15

Lupus is a chronic inflammatory autoimmune disease. Patients with systemic lupus erythematosus (SLE) most commonly experience profound fatigue, rashes, and joint pains. In severe cases, the immune system may attack and damage several organs such as the kidney, brain, blood, or lung. For many individuals, symptoms and damage from the disease can be controlled with anti-inflammatory medication and symptomatic prescribed medication.

Scleroderma is a disease that results in thickening of the skin and blood vessels, Figure 15-4. Almost every patient with scleroderma has Raynaud's, which is a spasm of the blood vessels of the fingers and toes. Symptoms of Raynaud's include increased sensitivity of the fingers and toes to the cold, changes in skin color, pain, and occasionally ulcers of the fingertips or toes. For people with scleroderma, the thickening of skin and blood vessels can result in loss of movement and dyspnea.

Hypersensitivity

Hypersensitivity occurs when the body's immune system fails to protect itself against foreign material. Instead, the antibodies formed irritate certain body cells. A hypersensitive or allergic individual is generally more sensitive to certain allergens than most people.

An **allergen** is an antigen that causes allergic responses. Examples of allergens include grass, ragweed pollen, ingested food, peanuts,

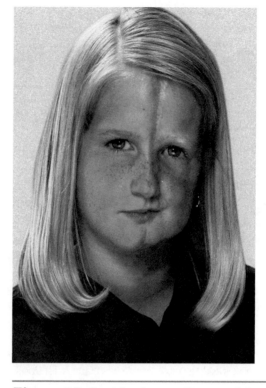

Figure 15-4 *Scleroderma* (*Courtesy of the Scleroderma Foundation, www.scleroderma.org*)

penicillin, and other antibiotics, and bee and wasp stings. Such allergens stimulate antibody formation, some of which are known as the IgE antibodies. Antibodies are found in individuals who are allergic, drug sensitive, or hypersensitive. The antibodies bind to certain cells in the body, causing a characteristic allergic reaction.

In asthma, the IgE antibodies bind to the bronchi and bronchioles; in hay fever they bind to the mucous membranes of the respiratory tract and eyes, causing runny nose and itchy eyes. In hives and rashes, they bind to the skin cells.

An even more severe and sometimes fatal allergic reaction is called **anaphylaxis** or **anaphylactic shock.** It is the result of an antigen-antibody reaction that stimulates a massive secretion of histamine. Anaphylaxis can be caused by insect stings and injected drugs such as penicillin. A person suffering from anaphylaxis experiences breathing problems, headache, facial swelling, falling blood pressure, stomach cramps, and vomiting. The antidote is an injection of either adrenaline or antihistamine. If proper care is not given immediately, death may occur in minutes.

Health care professionals should always ask patients if they are sensitive to any allergens or drugs. This precaution is necessary to prevent negative and sometimes fatal allergic responses to injected drugs. People with such hypersensitivities should wear a medic-alert tag to alert health professionals in the event of an emergency. Such tags have saved the lives of patients rendered unconscious or otherwise unable to communicate.

AIDS/HIV

Acquired immunodeficiency syndrome (AIDS) was first reported in the United States in 1981, and has since become a worldwide epidemic. AIDS is a disease that suppresses the body's natural immune defense system. The term AIDS is derived from the following meanings.

- Acquired—the disease is not inherited.

- Immune—refers to the body's natural defenses against cancers, disease, and infections.

- Deficiency—lacks cellular immunity.

- Syndrome—involves the set of diseases or conditions that are present to signal the diagnosis.

The **human immunodeficiency virus (HIV)** causes AIDS. HIV progressively destroys the body's T4-lymphocyte cells, which are the immune system's key infection fighters, Figure 15-5. The virus initially disables or destroys these cells without causing symptoms. Individuals diagnosed with AIDS are susceptible to life-threatening diseases called *opportunistic* infection, because they are caused by organisms that do not normally produce life threats. There are three possible outcomes that can result from infection with HIV. One is the actual development of AIDS, the second is the development of a condition called AIDS-related complex (ARC), and the third condition is known as asymptomatic infection.

HIV Statistics

Through June 2000, a total of 753,900 U.S. cases were reported to the Centers for Disease Control (CDC—National Center for HIV, STS, and TP prevention). The worldwide figure based on the UN-AID program, indicates approximately 47 million people have been infected with HIV. UNAIDS estimates that there are almost 16,000 new AIDS cases per day.

Transmission of AIDS

The transmission of AIDS occurs in the following ways.

1. Sexual contact with an infected partner—the virus can enter the body through the lining of the vagina, vulva, penis, rectum, or mouth during sex.

2. Sharing hypodermic needles among IV drug users—infected blood is injected into the body. *Transmission from patient to health care worker or health care worker to patient via accidental sticks with contaminated needles or other medical instruments are rare.*

3. In utero or at birth from an infected mother

4. Transmission of HIV through transfusion of blood. This mode of transmission has been almost eliminated because blood banks now test all blood donors to determine if they have been exposed to HIV.

Scientists have found no evidence that HIV is spread through sweat, tears, urine, or feces. The virus is fragile and does not survive outside the body. Even close, nonsexual contact such as coughing, sneezing, embracing, shaking hands, and sharing eating utensils cannot spread the virus.

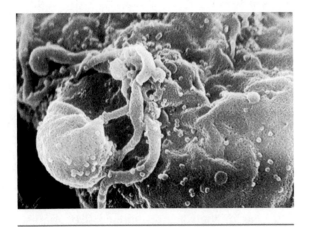

Figure 15-5 *HIV budding from lymphocyte (Courtesy of the CDC Public Health Image Library)*

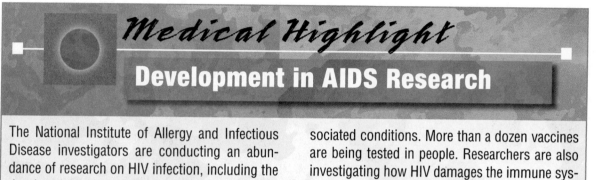

Medical Highlight

Development in AIDS Research

The National Institute of Allergy and Infectious Disease investigators are conducting an abundance of research on HIV infection, including the development and testing of HIV vaccines, and new therapies for the disease and some of the associated conditions. More than a dozen vaccines are being tested in people. Researchers are also investigating how HIV damages the immune system. This research is suggesting new and more effective targets for drugs and vaccines.

Source: HIV Infection and AIDS, January 15, 2002 http://content.health.msn.com/content/dmk/dmk_article_5462568

Screening Tests for HIV/AIDS

Because early HIV infection often causes no symptoms, it is primarily detected by testing a person's blood for the presence of antibodies to HIV. HIV antibodies do not reach detectable levels until 1 to 3 months after the infection. A positive result may indicate that the person has either fought off the infection and is now immune to AIDS, the person is carrying the infection but is not sick, or the person may be developing or already has AIDS.

Two different types of antibody tests are as follows:

- Enzyme-linked immunosorbent assay (ELISA) is an AIDS antibody indicator. It detects the antibodies for AIDS but not the virus itself.

- Western blot is a follow-up to confirm the ELISA results.

Blood sample kits for anonymous HIV testing may now be used at home. Home-based test kits are available by telephone or over the counter at pharmacies. The sample is collected and then sent and analyzed at a laboratory. The confidential results are provided in response to a request, which must have the correct security identification of the sender.

Symptoms of HIV/AIDS

In the early stages of HIV/AIDS, some people experience flulike symptoms, including fever, headache, malaise, and enlarged lymph glands. The symptoms then disappear within a week to a month. More persistent symptoms may not occur

for another 10 years; however, even though there are no symptoms present, the HIV-infected person can still transmit the disease. As the immune system begins to deteriorate, a variety of symptoms appear, which include lymph glands that may be enlarged for more than 3 months. Other symptoms experienced before the onset of AIDS include a lack of energy, weight loss, frequent fevers and sweats, persistent yeast infections (oral or vaginal), persistent skin rashes, flaky skin, pelvic inflammatory disease that does not respond to treatment, and short-term memory loss.

As the disease progresses, the AIDS patient is now susceptible to opportunistic infections. The opportunistic infections common to people with AIDS produce such symptoms as coughing, shortness of breath, seizures, mental symptoms, persistent diarrhea, fever, vision loss, severe headaches, weight loss, extreme fatigue, nausea, vomiting, lack of coordination, coma, abdominal cramps, or difficult or painful swallowing.

Opportunistic conditions include the following:

- Cancers, especially Kaposi's sarcoma, cervical cancer, or cancers of the immune system known as lymphomas

- Parasitic infections such as *Pneumocystis carinii* pneumonia and toxoplasmosis

- Fungal infections such as candidiasis and histoplasmosis

- Viral infections such as cytomegalovirus (CMV) disease, herpes simplex, hepatitis B, and non-A and non-B hepatitis

Persons who are HIV positive are at a higher risk for tuberculosis and syphilis

Treatment

There is no cure for AIDS; however, certain drugs may slow the virus. Treatment of the HIV/AIDS disease uses three classes of antiretroviral agents. The nucleoside reverse transcriptase inhibitors (NRTIs) interrupt an early stage of the virus replication; an example is AZT. These drugs may slow the spread of HIV in the body and delay the onset of opportunistic infections. Another group of antiretroviral agents is nonnucleoside reverse transcriptase; an example is delavirdine. A third class of anti-HIV drugs, called protease inhibitors, interrupts virus replication at a later stage in its life cycle. Because HIV can become resistant to each class of drugs, combination treatments are necessary to effectively suppress the virus. At the present time these drugs do not cure AIDS and the drugs may have serious side effects. The treatments are very expensive. A number of drugs are available to treat the opportunistic infections, when they occur.

AIDS-Related Complex

AIDS-related complex (ARC) is the term used for the case in which an individual contracts HIV and develops other conditions but not AIDS itself. Symptoms range from chronic diarrhea, to chronic lymphadenopathy, to unexplained weight loss.

Asymptomatic Infection

A small number of peoples (less than 50) initially infected with HIV for 10 or more years have not developed any symptoms. Scientists are trying to determine what factor accounts for the lack of progression of HIV into AIDS.

Measures to Prevent Transmission

The most important methods in the prevention of AIDS are education and training. It is important to understand that it is not who a person is, but rather what the person does that puts a person at risk of contracting the disease. The following measures will help to prevent transmission of the disease.

- Limit the number of sexual contacts.

- Have protected sex. CDC recommends that people use male latex condoms when having oral, anal, or vaginal sex.

- Do not share hypodermic needles or syringes.

- Ensure that soiled articles, materials, and surfaces are cleaned with soap and hot water after incidents involving bleeding.

- Cover an open cut, sore, or wound with a bandage.

- To prevent health care workers from contracting AIDS and other diseases, the CDC has published guidelines called Standard Precautions (see Appendix).

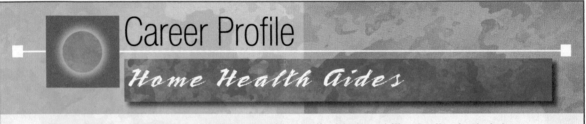

Career Profile

Home Health Aides

Home health aides help people who are elderly, disabled, and ill, who live in their homes instead of in a health care facility.

Home health aides provide housekeeping services, personal care, and emotional support for their clients. Aides may plan meals, shop for food, and cook. Home health aides take vital signs, help get clients in and out of bed, and assist with medication routines. Occasionally, they change nonsterile dressings, use special equipment such as hydraulic lifts, and give massages.

continues

continued

Home health aides also provide psychological support. They assist with toilet training for severely mentally handicapped children or just listen to clients talk about their problems. In home care agencies, aides are supervised by a registered nurse, a physical therapist, or a social worker who assigns them their specific duties.

The federal government has enacted guidelines for home health aides who receive reimbursement from Medicare. Federal law requires home health aides to pass a competency test covering 12 areas. Federal law suggests at least 75 hours of classroom and practical training supervised by a registered nurse. Home health aides who do not receive reimbursement under Medicare provisions may receive on-the-job training.

Job outlook is good and is expected to be one of the fastest growing occupations in the years ahead.

Medical Terminology

aden	glands
-itis	inflammation of
aden/itis	inflammation of the glands
hepato	liver
-megaly	enlargement of
hepato/megaly	enlargement of the liver
hyper	over
-sensitive	sensitive
-ity	condition of
hyper/sensitiv/ity	condition of being oversensitive
immun	not serving disease
immun/ity	condition of not serving disease represents protection against disease
-tion	process of
immuni/za/tion	process of protection against disease
inter	between
-stitial	tissues
inter/stitial	between the body tissues
leuko	white
-penia	deficiency of
leuko/penia	deficiency of white blood cells
lymph	clear white fluid
-oma	tumor
lymph/oma	tumor of the lymph
spleno	spleen

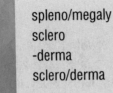

spleno/megaly	enlargement of the spleen
sclero	hard
-derma	skin
sclero/derma	condition in which the skin hardens

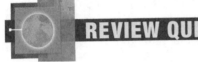

REVIEW QUESTIONS

Select the letter of the choice that best completes the statement.

1. Lymph fluid may also be called:
   a. plasma
   b. blood
   c. interstitial
   d. serum

2. The function of the lymph nodes is to produce:
   a. platelets
   b. lymphocytes
   c. basophils
   d. erythrocytes

3. The name of the vessel through which lymph finally rejoins general circulation is called:
   a. thoracic duct
   b. left lymphatic duct
   c. superior vena cava
   d. right lymphatic duct

4. The organ composed of lymphatic tissue which filters blood and produces white blood cells is called the:
   a. spleen
   b. liver
   c. kidney
   d. stomach

5. The ability of the body to resist disease is known as:
   a. sensitivity
   b. resistance
   c. immunity
   d. noninfection

MATCHING

Match each term in Column I with its correct description in Column II.

Column I	Column II
_____ **1.** natural immunity	a. immunization
_____ **2.** acquired active immunity	b. immune globulin
_____ **3.** acquired passive immunity	c. inherited
_____ **4.** acquired active artificial	d. obtained through mother's milk
_____ **5.** acquired passive artificial	e. have the disease and recover

COMPLETION

Complete the following sentences:

1. A person who is highly sensitive to an allergen is said to be _____.

2. An antigen that causes an allergic response is an _____.

3. A fatal allergic response is _____.

4. A cancer of the lymph nodes is called _____.

5. A mass of lymph tissue in the throat is called _____.

APPLYING THEORY TO PRACTICE

1. A family member is entering school and must have his immunizations complete. Explain to the parent what this means.

2. Your friend says, "I think I have the kissing disease. What is it?" Explain the disease to your friend and how the disease is transmitted and treated.

3. You go to the doctor because you have swollen glands and a temperature of 101°F. The doctor states that the body is fighting an infection which is causing your swollen glands. What does it mean?

4. A woman is complaining of swelling in her left arm after a mastectomy on her left breast. She also had lymph nodes removed for testing. Explain to the patient why the swelling has occurred.

5. Many diseases are being classified as autoimmune. Explain autoimmunity and lupus and other examples of autoimmune diseases.

6. Research the advances that are being made in the treatment of HIV and AIDS. What did you find? What are the limitations in the treatments?

CASE STUDY

Mrs. Jones is a volunteer at a hospice and she is confused about the disease AIDS and is afraid if she comes in contact with a patient's urine or feces she may get the disease. Alycia, the LPN, tries to reassure Mrs. Jones she cannot get AIDS in this manner. The following actions may help Alycia explain the disease to Mrs. Jones.

1. Explain what HIV and AIDS are.

2. Describe the mode of transmission.

3. Explain the diagnostic tests done to check for HIV.

4. Discuss the early and later symptoms.

5. Describe opportunistic infections.

6. Explain what scientists say about casual contact with people infected with HIV.

7. Explain how to prevent HIV/AIDS.

8. Explain why AIDS is such a social and world health concern.

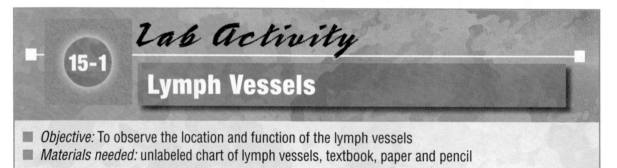

Lab Activity

15-1

Lymph Vessels

- *Objective:* To observe the location and function of the lymph vessels
- *Materials needed:* unlabeled chart of lymph vessels, textbook, paper and pencil

On the unlabeled chart of the lymph vessels, locate the right lymphatic duct and the left lymphatic duct. Compare with the diagram in the textbook. Into what structures do the lymph fluids from the right and left lymphatic empty? Record your answer.

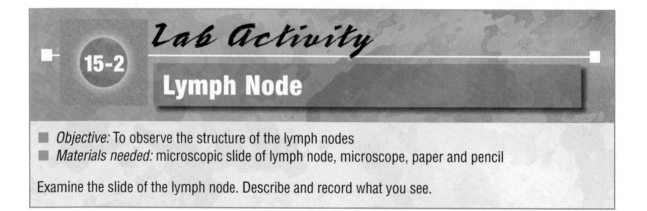

Lab Activity

15-2

Lymph Node

- *Objective:* To observe the structure of the lymph nodes
- *Materials needed:* microscopic slide of lymph node, microscope, paper and pencil

Examine the slide of the lymph node. Describe and record what you see.

Chapter 16

INFECTION CONTROL AND STANDARD PRECAUTIONS

Objectives

- Describe five types of pathogenic microorganisms

- Explain infection

- Describe methods to break the chain of infection

- Discuss normal defense mechanisms

- Describe the stages of infection

- Explain standard precautions

- Define the key words that relate to this chapter

Key Words

agent
airborne
   transmission
bacteria
biological agent
chemical agent
cleansing
compromised host
contact
   transmission
convalescent stage
disinfection
flora
fomite
fungi

host
humoral immunity
illness stage
incubation stage
mode of
   transmission
nosocomial
   infection
pathogenicity
physical agent
portal of entry
portal of exit
prodromal stage
protozoa
reservoir

resident flora
reverse isolation
rickettsia
spore
sterilization
susceptible host
transient flora
vectorborne
   transmission
vehicle
   transmission
virulence
virus

Health care workers are responsible for providing care that utilizes infection control principles to provide a safe environment. This chapter discusses infection control principles as they relate to microorganisms, pathogens, infection and colonization, chain of infection, normal defense mechanisms, stages of the infectious process, and nosocomial infections.

FLORA

Flora are microorganisms that occur or have adapted to live in a specific environment such as the intestine, skin, vagina, and oral cavity. There are two types of flora: resident and transient. **Resident,** or normal, **flora** are always present. They prevent the overgrowth of harmful microorganisms. Only when the balance is upset does disease result. An example is proprioni bacterium found on the skin. **Transient flora** occur in periods of limited duration. An example is *Staphylococcus aureus*. They attach to the skin for a brief time but do not continually live on the skin. Vigorous handwashing with soap and water is an effective means of removing flora.

PATHOGENICITY AND VIRULENCE

Most microorganisms found in the environment do not cause disease or infection, but some do. Disease-producing microorganisms are called pathogens; **pathogenicity** refers to the ability of a microorganism to produce disease. **Virulence** refers to the frequency with which a pathogen causes disease. Factors affecting virulence are the strength of the pathogen to adhere to healthy cells, the ability of the pathogen to damage cells or interfere with the body's normal systems, and the ability of a pathogen to evade the action of the white blood cells. There are five types of pathogenic microorganisms: bacteria, viruses, fungi, protozoa, and rickettsia.

Bacteria

Bacteria are small, one-celled microorganisms that lack a true nucleus or mechanism to provide metabolism. Bacteria need an environment that will provide food for survival. Although most bacteria multiply by simple cell division, some forms of bacteria produce **spores,** a resistant stage that withstands an unfavorable environment. When proper environmental conditions return, spores germinate and form new cells. Spores are resistant to heat, drying, and disinfectants.

Pathogenic bacteria cause a wide range of illnesses including diarrhea, pneumonia, sinusitis, urinary tract infections, and gonorrhea, Figure 16-1.

Viruses

Viruses are organisms that can live only inside cells. They cannot get nourishment or reproduce outside the cell. Viruses contain a core of DNA or RNA surrounded by a protein coating. Some viruses have the ability to create an additional coating called an envelope. This envelope protects the virus from attack by the immune system. Viruses damage the cell they inhabit by blocking the normal protein synthesis and by using the cell's mechanism for metabolism to reproduce themselves.

The same viral infection may cause different symptoms in different individuals. Some viruses will immediately trigger a disease response, while others may remain latent for many years. Viral infections include the common cold, influenza, measles, hepatitis, genital herpes, HIV, and the West Nile virus, Figure 16-2.

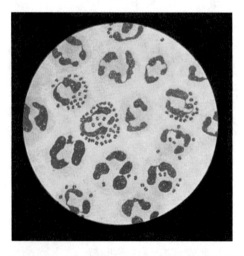

Figure 16-1 *Neisseria gonorrhea (Courtesy of the Centers for Disease Control and Prevention)*

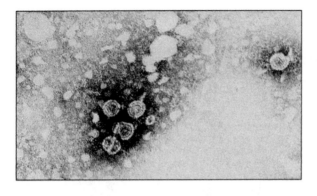

Figure 16-2 *Electron micrograph of hepatitis B virus* *(Courtesy of the Centers for Disease Control and Prevention)*

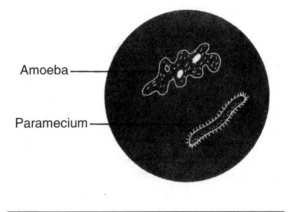

Figure 16-4 *Protozoa*

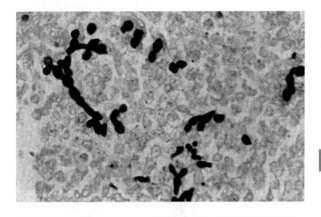

Figure 16-3 *Candida albicans* *(Courtesy of the Centers for Disease Control and Prevention)*

Fungi

Fungi grow in single cells as in yeast or in colonies as in molds, Figure 16-3. Fungi obtain food from living organisms or organic matter. Disease from fungi is found mainly in individuals who are immunologically impaired. Fungi can cause infections of the hair, skin, nails, and mucous membranes. Fungi infections include athlete's foot.

Protozoa

Protozoa are single-celled parasitic organisms with the ability to move, Figure 16-4. Most protozoa obtain their food from dead or decaying organic matter. Infection is spread through ingestion of contaminated food or water or through insect bites. Common infections are malaria, gastroenteritis, and vaginal infections.

Rickettsia

Rickettsia are intercellular parasites that need to be in living cells to reproduce. Infection from rickettsia is spread through the bites of fleas, ticks, mites, and lice. Common infections are Lyme disease, Rocky Mountain spotted fever, and typhus.

CHAIN OF INFECTION

The chain of infection describes the elements of an infectious process. It is an interactive process that involves the agent, host, and environment. This process must include several essential elements or "links in the chain" for the transmission of microorganisms to occur. Figure 16-5 identifies the six essential links. Without the transmission of microorganisms, the infectious process cannot occur. Knowledge about the chain of infection facilitates control or prevention of disease by breaking the links in the chain. This is achieved by altering one or more of the interactive processes of agent, host, or environment.

Agent

An **agent** is an entity that is capable of causing disease. Agents that cause disease may be as follows:

- **Biological agents**—living organisms that invade the host, such as bacteria, virus, fungi, protozoa, and rickettsia

- **Chemical agents**—substances that can interact with the body such as pesticides,

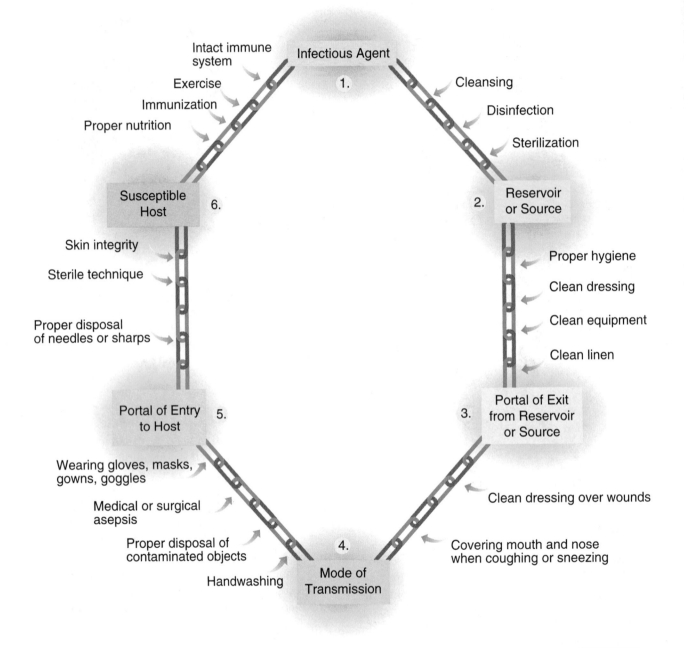

Figure 16-5   *The chain of infection: Preventive measures follow each link of the chain*

food additives, medications, and industrial chemicals

- **Physical agents**—factors in the environment such as heat, light, noise, and radiation

In the chain of infection, the main concern is biological (infectious) agents and their effect on the host.

Reservoir

The **reservoir** is a place where the agent can survive. Colonization and reproduction take place while the agent is in the reservoir. A reservoir that promotes growth of pathogens must contain the proper nutrients (such as oxygen and organic matter), maintain proper temperature, contain moisture, maintain a compatible pH level, and maintain the proper amount of light exposure. The most common reservoirs are humans, animals, environment, and **fomites.** Fomites are objects contaminated with an infectious agent such as instruments or dressings.

Humans and animals can have symptoms of the infectious agents or can be strictly carriers of the agent. Carriers have the infectious agent but are symptom free. The agent can be spread to others in both instances.

Portal of Exit

The **portal of exit** is the route by which an infectious agent leaves the reservoir to be transferred to a susceptible host. The agent leaves the reservoir through body secretions, such as sputum, semen, vaginal secretions, urine, saliva, feces, blood, and draining wounds.

Mode of Transmission

The **mode of transmission** is the process that bridges the gap between the portal of exit of the infectious agent from the reservoir and the portal of entry of the susceptible "new" host. Most infectious agents have a usual mode of transmission; however, some microorganisms may be transmitted by more than one mode, Table 16-1.

- **Contact transmission** involves the physical transfer of an agent from an infected person to an uninfected person through direct contact with the infected person. Contact with the infected person through contaminated secretions is called indirect contact, Figure 16-6. Examples of direct contact are sexually transmitted diseases, colds, and flu.

- **Airborne transmission** occurs when a susceptible person contacts contaminated droplets or dust particles that are suspended in the air, Figure 16-7. The longer the particle is suspended, the greater the chance it will find an available port of entry in the human host. An example of an organism that relies on airborne transmission is measles. Spores of anthrax are also transmitted in an airborne powder form.

Table 16-1 *Modes of Transmission*

MODE	EXAMPLES
Contact	Direct contact of health care provider with client: • Touching • Bathing • Rubbing • Toileting (urine and feces) • Secretions from client Indirect contact with fomites: • Clothing • Bed linens • Dressings • Health care equipment • Instruments used in treatments • Specimen containers used for laboratory analysis • Personal belongings • Personal care equipment • Diagnostic equipment
Airborne	Inhaling microorganisms carried by moisture or dust particles in air: • Coughing • Talking • Sneezing
Vehicle	Contact with contaminated inanimate objects: • Water • Blood • Drugs • Food • Urine
Vectorborne	Contact with contaminated animate hosts: • Animals • Insects

- **Vehicle transmission** occurs when the agent is transferred to a susceptible host by contaminated inanimate objects such as water, food, meat, drugs, and blood, Figure 16-8. An example is salmonellosis transmitted through contaminated food.

- **Vectorborne transmission** occurs when an agent is transferred to a susceptible person host by animate means such as mosquitoes, fleas, ticks, lice, and other animals, Figure 16-9. Lyme disease is an example.

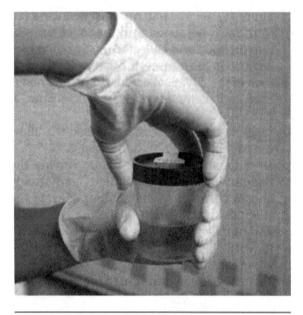

Figure 16-6 *Care must be taken in the handling of bodily fluids to prevent the transfer of infectious agents through contact with secretions.*

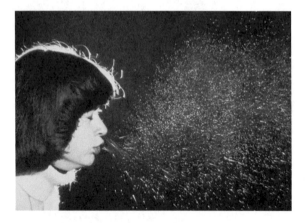

Figure 16-7 *The width of the area that droplet nuclei from a sneeze can encompass* *(Courtesy of Lester V. Bergman/Corbis)*

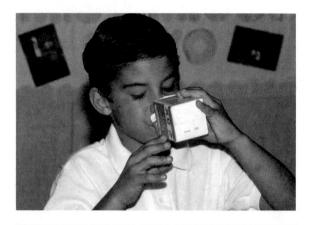

Figure 16-8 *Vehicle transmission can occur through contaminated food such as milk.*

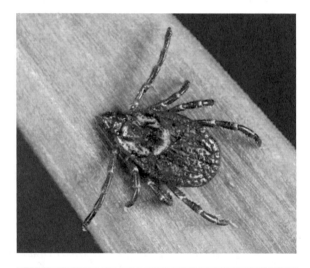

Figure 16-9 *Lyme disease is caused by the bite of a deer tick.* *(Courtesy of the Centers for Disease Control and Prevention Public Health Image Library)*

Portal of Entry

A **portal of entry** is the route by which an infectious agent enters the host. Portals of entry include the following:

- Integumentary system—a break in the skin or mucous membrane
- Respiratory tract—by inhaling contaminated droplets
- Genitourinary tract—through contamination with infected vaginal secretions or semen
- Gastrointestinal tract—by ingesting contaminated food or water
- Circulatory system—through the bite of insects or rodents
- Transplacental—through transfer of a microorganism from mother to fetus via the placenta and umbilical cord

Host

A **host** is a simple or complex organism that can be affected by an agent. As the term is used here, a host is an individual who is at risk of contracting an infectious disease. A **susceptible host** is a person who lacks resistance to an agent and is vulnerable to a disease. A **compromised host** is a person whose normal defense mechanisms are impaired and who is therefore more susceptible to infection.

The following characteristics of the host influence the susceptibility to and severity of infections.

- Age—as a person ages, immunity declines.

- Concurrent disease—the existence of other diseases indicates susceptibility.

- Stress—a person experiencing a compromised emotional state has lower defense mechanisms.

- Immunization/vaccination status—certain people are not fully immunized.

- Lifestyle—practices such as having multiple sex partners, sharing needles, or tobacco/drug use can alter defenses.

- Occupation—Forms of employment involve an increased exposure to pathogenic sources such as needles or chemical agents.

- Nutritional status—people who maintain targeted weight for height and body frame are less prone to illness.

- Heredity—some people are naturally more susceptible to infections than others.

BREAKING THE CHAIN OF INFECTION

Health care workers focus on breaking the chain of infection by applying proper infection control practices to interfere with the spread of microorganisms. Specific strategies can be directed at breaking or blocking the transmission of infection from one link in the chain to the next. A discussion regarding each of the six links follows.

Between Agent and Reservoir

The keys to eliminating infection between agent and reservoir in the chain are cleansing, disinfection,

and sterilization. These tactics serve to prevent the formation of a reservoir and environment within which infectious agents can live and multiply.

- **Cleansing** is the removal of soil or organic matter from equipment used in providing a person care. To reduce the amount of contamination and loosen material on reusable objects, the objects are cleansed prior to sterilization and disinfection. The steps for proper cleansing are as follows:

  1. Rinse the object under cold water, because warm water causes proteins in organic material to coagulate and stick.

  2. Apply detergent and scrub the object under running water with a soft brush.

  3. Rinse the object under warm water.

  4. Dry the object before sterilization.

- **Disinfection** is the elimination of pathogens, except spores, from inanimate objects. Disinfectants are chemical solutions used to clean inanimate objects. Common disinfectants are alcohol and sodium hypochlorite. In the home, Lysol and bleach are common disinfectants.

- **Sterilization** is the total elimination of all microorganisms including spores. Methods of achieving sterilization are moist heat or steam, radiation, chemicals, and ethylene oxide gas. The method of sterilization depends on the type and amount of contamination and the object to be sterilized. Boiling water is not a totally effective sterilization method, because some spores and viruses can survive boiling water; however, boiling water is still the best and most common method of sterilization in the home.

If the reservoir is an already infected individual, that individual may need to be isolated. The individual's infectious condition needs to be vigorously treated to reduce the reservoir of infectious material or eliminate the agent.

Between Reservoir and Portal of Exit

Promoting proper hygiene, maintaining clean dressings and linen, and ensuring the use of clean equipment in a client's care can break the chain between the reservoir and the portal of exit. The aim is to eliminate the reservoir for the microorganism before the pathogen can escape to a susceptible host.

- Proper hygiene. Health care workers must teach the importance of maintaining the cleanliness and integrity of the skin and mucous membranes. Bathing and handwashing are the means of eliminating the potential for infection.

- Clean dressings. An open injury represents a potential reservoir for infectious agents or portal of exit for a pathogen to be transferred to another individual. Dressings on open or oozing wounds must be changed and cleansed regularly.

- Clean linen. Dressing gowns, linens, or towels are catchalls for body secretions. Infectious agents can be transferred from one individual to the next through contact with linens.

- Clean equipment. All equipment used in the care of a client must be cleansed and disinfected after each use. To protect themselves, health care workers may wear gloves and masks when cleaning equipment to avoid being splashed with contaminated waste products or secretions.

Between Portal of Exit and Mode of Transmission

The goal in breaking the chain here is to block the exit of the infectious agent. The health care worker must maintain clean dressings on all injuries or wounds. People should be encouraged to cover the mouth and nose when sneezing or coughing, and the health care worker must do so as well. Gloves must be worn when caring for a person who may have infectious secretions and care must be taken to properly dispose of contaminated articles.

Between Mode of Transmission and Portal of Entry

The goal is to break the chain of infection between the mode of transmission and portal of entry. Health care workers must always wash their hands between care cases which may involve contact with contaminated items. Barrier protection must be worn when care involves contact with body secretions. Gloves, masks, gowns, and goggles are all forms of barrier protection.

Between Portal of Entry and Host

Maintaining skin integrity and using sterile techniques for client contacts are methods of breaking the chain between portal of entry and host. The goal is to prevent the transmission of infection to an uninfected person including the health care worker.

Between Host and Agent

To break the chain between host and agent means eliminating infection before it begins. Proper nutrition, exercise, and immunization allow an individual to maintain an intact immune system, thus preventing infection.

NORMAL DEFENSE MECHANISMS

The individual's immune system serves as the normal defense mechanism against the transmission of infectious agents. A unique feature of the immune system is its ability to recognize which agents are not consistent with the genetic makeup of the host. These agents are called antigens. Antibodies will form to protect the body against the antigens. The immune defenses are categorized as specific and nonspecific.

Nonspecific Immune Defense

The nonspecific immune defense mounts a response to protect the individual from all microorganisms; it is not dependent on prior exposure to the antigens. Nonspecific immune defenses are skin and normal flora; mucous membranes; sneezing, coughing, and tearing reflexes; elimination and acidic environment; and inflammation.

- Skin and normal flora serve as a physical barrier against infectious agents.

- Mucous membranes entrap infectious agents and contain antibodies, lactoferin, and lyozyme which inhibit bacterial growth.

- Sneezing, coughing, and tearing reflexes physically expel mucus and microorganisms with force. Tears continually flush away microorganisms. They also contain bactericides which are bacteria-killing chemicals.

- Elimination and acidic environment prevents microbial growth of pathogenic organisms. These include resident flora of the large intestine, acidity of the urine, and normal vaginal flora. The mechanical process of defecation evacuates the bowel of feces and microorganisms. The flushing action of urination prevents microorganisms from ascending the urinary tract.

- Inflammation is the nonspecific response to cellular injury. Tissue injury releases multiple substances that produce dramatic changes in the injured tissue, Figure 16-10. The intensity of the inflammatory process is usually in proportion to the degree of tissue injury. For a detailed description on inflammation, see Chapter 12.

Specific Immune Defense

The specific immune defense mounts a response which is specific to the invading antigen. This defense is activated by the failure of phagocytes to completely destroy the antigen. This causes the production of T-lymphocytes (T-cells), which regulate the immune response by activating other cells. These sensitized T-cells migrate to the portal of entry or area of injury and release chemical substances called lymphokines. These lymphokines attract other phagocytes and lymphocytes to the area and assist in antigen destruction.

T-cells also stimulate production of B-cells, which differentiate into plasma cells producing antibodies specific to the antigen. The stimulation of B-cells and the production of antibodies are collectively referred to as **humoral immunity.**

The B-cell activation causes formation of memory B-cells. These cells remember the antigen and prepare the host for future antigen invasion. The formation of these antibodies is called acquired immunity. For more information on natural and acquired immunity, see Chapter 15 and Table 15-1.

STAGES OF THE INFECTIOUS PROCESS

Activation of the immune response indicates the occurrence of infection. Infection results from tissue invasion and damage by an infectious agent. There are two types of infectious responses:

- Localized infection, which is limited to a defined area or single organ with symptoms that resemble inflammation (redness, tenderness, and swelling) such as a cold sore

- Systemic infections, which affect the entire body and involve multiple organs such as AIDS

Localized and systemic infections progress through four stages: incubation, prodromal, illness, and convalescence.

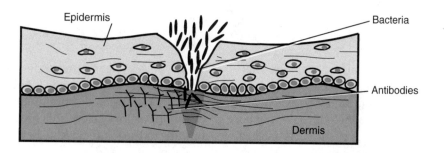

Figure 16-10 *The body's response to inflammation*

Incubation

The **incubation stage** is the time interval between entry of an infectious agent into the host and the onset of symptoms. During this time the infectious agent invades the tissue and begins to multiply to produce an infection; the client is typically infectious to others during this period. The incubation period for chickenpox is 2 to 3 weeks; the infected person is contagious from 5 days before the skin eruptions to no more than 6 days after the eruptions appear.

Prodromal

The **prodromal stage** is the time interval from the onset of nonspecific symptoms until specific symptoms begin to appear. During this period the infectious agent continues to invade and multiply in the host. A client may also be infectious to others during this period.

Illness

The **illness stage** is the time period when the client is manifesting specific signs and symptoms of an infectious process.

Convalescent

The **convalescent stage** is the period of time from the beginning of disappearance of acute symptoms until the client returns to the previous state of health.

NOSOCOMIAL INFECTIONS

A **nosocomial infection** is acquired in a hospital or other health care facility and was not present or incubating at the time of the client's admission. Nosocomial infections are also referred to as hospital-acquired infections. These types of infections typically fall into four categories: urinary tract, surgical wounds, pneumonia, and septicemia.

Nosocomial infections include those that become symptomatic after the client is discharged, as well as infections passed among health care workers. Personnel who fail to follow proper handwashing principles transmit most infections.

Hospitalized clients are at risk for infections, because the environment provides exposure to a variety of virulent organisms to which the client has not typically been exposed. Therefore, the client has not developed resistance to these organisms.

The most common nosocomial infection involves the urinary tract, upper and lower respiratory tract, digestive tract, conjunctiva of the eyes, and skin. Individuals in long-term care facilities often have multiple illnesses, which decrease their resistance to infection.

STANDARD PRECAUTIONS

Standard precautions are guidelines to be used during routine patient care and cleaning duties. They must be used when you expect to have contact with blood, any body fluid except sweat, mucous membranes, and nonintact skin.

Handwashing

Handwashing is the single most effective way to prevent infection.

1. Wash hands after touching blood, body fluids, secretions, excretions, and contaminated items, *regardless if gloves are worn.*

2. Wash hands immediately after removing gloves, between client contacts, and when otherwise indicated to avoid transfer of microorganisms to other clients or the surrounding environment.

3. Use a plain (nonantimicrobial) soap for handwashing.

4. Wash hands for a minimum of 10 seconds.

Gloves

Wear gloves (clean, nonsterile gloves are adequate) when touching blood, body fluids, secretions, excretions, and contaminated items. Put on clean gloves just before touching mucous membranes and nonintact skin. Remove gloves after use and wash hands.

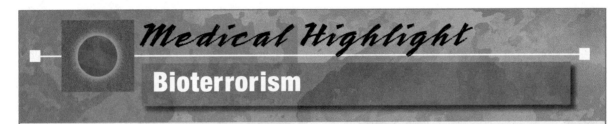

Bioterrorism

The use of biological weapons and efforts to make them more useful as a means of waging war have been recorded numerous times in history. The threat of a biological attack on the United States became a reality as a result of the September 11, 2001, terrorist attack on New York's World Trade Center and the Pentagon in Washington, D.C.

Terrorists could use many disease-causing organisms and even chemical agents. Some of the potential threats include the following:

- Anthrax. The bacterium *Bacillus anthrax* and its spore cause anthrax (see Chapter 17).
- Smallpox. This is a highly contagious viral disease which has been eradicated in the public due to worldwide vaccinations. However, the threat of the virus as a biological weapon remains as long as there are samples of the virus that have been preserved in laboratories. Symptoms include a high fever, fatigue, and aches, followed by a rash. The lesions resemble tiny pus-filled blisters most prominent on the face, arms, and legs. The disease is spread by droplet infection with respiratory secretions. There is no proven treatment for smallpox. The disease is fatal about 30% of the time. If smallpox vaccination is given, the vaccine can lessen the severity of the disease or even prevent it. The United States stopped vaccinating against smallpox about 30 or 40 years ago, because the disease had been mostly eradicated and no longer posed a health threat. The vaccine has been known to cause adverse side effects in some individuals. Due to biological threats, the smallpox vaccination program is subject to change.
- Plague. This highly infectious disease is caused by the bacterium *Yersinia pestis,* which is found in rodents. It is transmitted by fleabites or by eating contaminated animal tissues. Antibiotics can be used to prevent or treat plague.
- Botulism. This muscle paralyzing disease is caused by a toxin made by the bacterium *Clostridium botulinum.* It is among the most lethal weapons known, as it can kill within 24 hours by paralyzing the respiratory muscles. Botulism is normally contracted by consuming improperly canned food that contains the naturally occurring bacteria. The Centers for Disease Control and Prevention and some health departments keep an antidote to botulism in storage.
- Tularemia. This illness usually affects wild animals such as rabbits and squirrels. It is caused by bacterium *Francisella tularensis.* Doctors can use IV antibiotic therapy. Without treatment the disease is fatal less than 5% of the time.
- Viral hemorrhagic fevers. These illnesses are caused by a family of viruses. Whereas some cause relatively mild illnesses, others, such as the Ebola, may be life threatening. Viral hemorrhagic viruses can be transmitted by the body fluids of infected people. Vaccines are available for two-yellow fever and Argentine hemorrhagic fever. In the case of an outbreak of viral hemorrhagic fever it would be necessary to isolate the infected patients.
- Chemical weapons. Examples of chemical weapons include ricin, sarin, mustard gas, chlorine, phosgene, and hydrogen cyanide.

To minimize the effect of a biological or chemical terrorist attack, health care professionals and public health authorities must be aware of the threat and have an increased awareness that such an

continues

continued

attack could occur. The CDC has recommended that antibiotics only be used in situations when exposure to anthrax or other bacterial disease is suspected or confirmed. Unneeded use of antibiotics may lessen their effectiveness. Stockpiling antibiotics for future use will not be necessary. Most antibiotics are effective for only certain organisms and it is impossible to predict which one will be needed.

Widespread vaccination against smallpox and anthrax may be a possibility one day. It is unclear at this time if "gas masks" would help in a biological or chemical attack. For example, anthrax cannot be seen or smelled. Effective mask types must be selected on the basis of the threat involved. There are no universal masks short of a complete space suit approach.

At the present time, government and health officials tell people not to panic but instead to use common sense in times of heightened security. Fear itself is contagious. Be alert for any suspicious activity and report these activities to local authorities. If you come in contact with any type of gas or chemical, cover your nose and mouth and leave the area immediately. Use water to quickly and thoroughly rinse your eyes and any skin that has been exposed to the agent. Remove all contaminated clothing and shower thoroughly, especially skin and hair which received exposure.

Experts say biological and chemical agents are more likely to be used against small groups rather than large populations, in part because these weapons are difficult to control once they are released. For that reason the risk to most Americans is considered low. For updated information on bioterrorism, the following websites may be helpful: www.bt.cdc.gov and www.cdc.gov/ncidod/disease/bioterr.htm.

Mask, Eye Protection, and Face Shield

Wear a mask and eye protection or a face shield to protect mucous membranes of the eyes, nose, and mouth during procedures and client care activities that are likely to generate splashes or sprays of blood, body fluids, secretions, or excretions.

Gown

Wear a clean, nonsterile gown to protect skin and prevent soiling of clothing during procedures and client care activities that are likely to generate splashes or sprays of blood, body fluids, secretions, or excretions, or cause soiling of clothing. Remove a soiled gown promptly and wash hands to avoid transfer of microorganisms to other clients or to the surrounding environment.

Client Care Equipment

Handle used client care equipment soiled with blood, body fluids, secretions, or excretions in a manner that prevents skin and mucous membrane exposures, contamination of clothing, and transfer of microorganisms to other clients and environments. Be certain that reusable equipment is properly cleaned and reprocessed before it is used on another client. Single-use items must be discarded properly.

Linens

Handle, transport, and process used linen soiled with blood, body fluids, secretions, or excretions in a manner that prevents skin and mucous membrane exposures and contamination of clothing, and avoids transfer of microorganisms to other clients and environments.

Occupational Health and Bloodbourne Pathogens

1. Take care to prevent injuries from needles, scalpels, and other sharp instruments or devices when handling these sharp instruments

after procedures, when cleaning used instruments, and when disposing of used needles. *CAUTION:* Never recap used needles or use any technique that involves directing the point of the needle toward any part of the body. Place used disposable syringes, needles, scalpels, and other sharp items in appropriate puncture-resistant containers located as close as practical to the area in which the items were used.

2. Use mouthpieces, resuscitation bags, or other ventilation devices as an alternative to mouth-to-mouth resuscitation methods in areas where there is need for resuscitation.

Client Placement

Place a client who contaminates the environment or who does not assist in maintaining appropriate hygiene or environmental precautions in a private room or other relatively isolated area. See Table 16-2.

ISOLATION

The 1996 CDC guideline eliminated the previous category-specific isolation precautions and condensed the former disease-specific precautions into three sets of precautions based on the route of

Table 16-2 *Examples of Personal Protective Equipment in Common Health Care Worker Tasks*

TASKS	GLOVES	GOWN	GOGGLES/ FACE SHIELD	SURGICAL MASK
Controlling bleeding with squirting blood	Yes	Yes	Yes	Yes
Wiping a wheelchair or shower chair with disinfectant solution	Yes	No	No	No
Emptying a catheter bag	Yes	No	Yes, if facility policy	Yes, if facility policy
Serving a meal tray	No	No	No	No
Giving a back rub to a patient who has intact skin	No	No	No	No
Giving oral care	Yes	No	No	No
Helping the dentist with a procedure	Yes	Yes, if facility policy	Yes	Yes
Cleaning a resident and changing the bed after an episode of diarrhea	Yes	Yes, if facility policy	No	No
Taking an oral temperature	Yes, if facility policy	No	No	No
Taking a rectal temperature	Yes	No	No	No
Taking a blood pressure	No	No	No	No
Cleaning soiled care utensils, such as bedpans	Yes	Yes, if splashing is likely	Yes, if splashing is likely	Yes, if splashing is likely
Shaving a patient with a disposable razor	Yes*	No	No	No
Giving eye care	Yes	No	No	No
Giving special mouth care to an unconscious patient	Yes	No, unless coughing is likely	No, unless coughing is likely	No, unless coughing is likely
Washing a patient's genital area	Yes	No	No	No
Washing the patient's arms and legs when the skin is intact	No	No	No	No

*Because of the high risk of this procedure for contact with blood

transmission: airborne (Figure 16-11), contact (Figure 16-12), or droplet (Figure 16-13). These new transmission-based precautions are to be used *in addition to* the Standard Precautions. Transmission-based precautions are practices designed for clients documented as or suspected of being infected with highly transmissible or epidemiologically important pathogens for which additional precautions beyond the Standard Precautions are required to interrupt transmission in hospitals, Table 16-3.

The transmission-based precautions are also used in the event of suspicious infections and with clients who are immunosuppressed either from disease or chemotherapy. More than one of the transmission-based precautions is used at the same time for clients with certain infections or conditions.

Clients requiring isolation should be placed in a private room with adequate ventilation and should have their own supplies. Personal belongings should be kept to a minimum, and health care providers should use disposable supplies and equipment when possible. All articles leaving the room, such as soiled linen and collected speci-

CONTACT PRECAUTIONS
(In addition to Standard Precautions)

VISITORS: Report to nurse before entering

Patient Placement
Private room, if possible. Cohort if private room is not available.

Gloves
Wear gloves when entering patient room.
Change gloves after having contact with infective material that may contain high concentrations of microorganisms (**fecal** material and **wound drainage**).
Remove gloves before leaving patient room.

Wash
Wash hands with an **antimicrobial** agent immediately after glove removal. After glove removal and handwashing, ensure that hands do not touch potentially contaminated environmental surfaces or items in the patient's room to avoid transfer of microorganisms to other patients or environments.

Gown
Wear gown when **entering** patient room if you anticipate that your clothing will have substantial contact with the patient, environmental surfaces, or items in the patient's room, or if the patient is **incontinent**, or has **diarrhea**, an **ileostomy**, a **colostomy**, or **wound drainage** not contained by a dressing. **Remove** gown before leaving the patient's environment and ensure that clothing does not contact potentially contaminated environmental surfaces to avoid transfer of microorganisms to other patients or environments.

Patient Transport
Limit transport of patient to essential purposes only. During transport, ensure that precautions are maintained to minimize the risk of transmission of microorganisms to other patients and contamination of environmental surfaces and equipment.

Patient-Care Equipment
Dedicate the use of noncritical patient-care equipment to a single patient. If common equipment is used, clean and disinfect between patients.

Figure 16-12 *Contact precautions (From BREVIS Corporation, Salt Lake City, UT. Copyright © 1996 by BREVIS Corporation. Reprinted with permission.)*

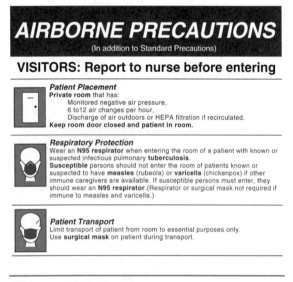

AIRBORNE PRECAUTIONS
(In addition to Standard Precautions)

VISITORS: Report to nurse before entering

Patient Placement
Private room that has:
  Monitored negative air pressure,
  6 to 12 air changes per hour,
  Discharge of air outdoors or HEPA filtration if recirculated.
Keep room door closed and patient in room.

Respiratory Protection
Wear an **N95 respirator** when entering the room of a patient with known or suspected infectious pulmonary **tuberculosis**.
Susceptible persons should not enter the room of patients known or suspected to have **measles** (rubeola) or **varicella** (chickenpox) if other immune caregivers are available. If susceptible persons must enter, they should wear an **N95 respirator**.(Respirator or surgical mask not required if immune to measles and varicella.)

Patient Transport
Limit transport of patient from room to essential purposes only.
Use **surgical mask** on patient during transport.

Figure 16-11 *Airborne precautions (From BREVIS Corporation, Salt Lake City, UT. Copyright © 1996 by BREVIS Corporation. Reprinted with permission.)*

DROPLET PRECAUTIONS
(In addition to Standard Precautions)

VISITORS: Report to nurse before entering

Patient Placement
Private room, if possible. Cohort or maintain spatial separation of **3 feet** from other patients or visitors if private room is not available.

Mask
Wear mask when working within **3 feet** of patient (or upon entering room).

Patient Transport
Limit transport of patient to essential purposes only.
Use **surgical mask** on patient during transport.

Figure 16-13 *Droplet precautions (From BREVIS Corporation, Salt Lake City, UT. Copyright © 1996 by BREVIS Corporation. Reprinted with permission.)*

Table 16-3 *Precautions Related to Type of Disease*

PRECAUTION	TYPE OF DISEASE
Standard Precautions	All clients, regardless of disease or condition
Airborne Precautions	In addition to Standard Precautions, used for clients known to have or suspected of having serious illnesses spread by airborne droplet nuclei, including: • Measles • Varicella • Tuberculosis
Contact Precautions	In addition to Standard Precautions, used for clients known to have or suspected of having serious illnesses easily spread by direct client contact or contact with fomites, including: • Wound infections • Gastrointestinal infections • Respiratory infections • Skin infections including: Herpes simplex Impetigo Major abscesses, cellulitis, or pressure ulcers Pediculosis Scabies Varicella (Zoster) • Viral hemorrhagic infections (Ebola)
Droplet Precautions	In addition to Standard Precautions, used for clients known to have or suspected of having illnesses spread by large particle droplets, including: • Meningitis • Adenovirus • Pneumonia • Influenza • Diphtheria • Mumps • Pertussis • Rubella • Scarlet fever • Parvovirus 19

From Table 1 Synopsis of Types of Precautions and Patients Requiring Precautions [On-line], by Centers for Disease Control and Prevention (CDC)/Hospital Infection Control Practices Advisory Committee (HICPAC), 1997c, Available:www.cdc.gov/ncidod/hip/isolat/isotab_1.htm

mens, should be labeled and either placed in impermeable bags or double bagged.

Reverse isolation, also known as protective isolation, is a barrier protection designed to prevent infection in clients who are severely compromised and highly susceptible to infection. This includes clients who are taking immunosuppressive medications; are receiving chemotherapy or radiation therapy; have diseases such as leukemia, which depress resistance to infectious organisms; and, have extensive burns, dermatitis, or other skin impairments that prevent adequate coverage with dressings.

These clients are at increased risk for infection from their own microorganisms, contact with health care workers whose hands have not been properly washed, and exposure to improperly disinfected and nonsterile items such as air, food, water, and equipment. Responsibilities toward these clients include ensuring that everyone entering the client's room has completed a meticulous handwashing and is properly attired in gown, gloves, and mask; ensuring that the client's environment is as clear of pathogens as possible; and knowing the institutional policy regarding caring for clients requiring reverse isolation.

Medical Terminology

coloniza	group of microorganisms living together
-tion	process of
coloniza/tion	process of microorganisms living together
dis	removal of
-fect	contamination with pathogens
dis/infect/ion	process of removal of pathogenic microorganisms
infect/ion	process of contamination with pathogenic microorganisms
nosocomi	hospital or infirmary
-al	pertaining to
nosocomi/al	pertaining to hospital or infirmary
pathogenic	producing disease
-ity	capable of
pathogenic/ity	capable of producing disease
prodrom	early symptom
prodrom/al	pertaining to early symptoms of disease
steriliz	free from microorganisms
steriliza/tion	process of being free of microorganisms
vir/u/lence	frequency by which pathogens cause disease

REVIEW QUESTIONS

Select the letter of the choice that best completes the statement.

1. The type of microorganisms that are always present, especially on the skin, are called:
   a. transient flora
   b. rickettsia
   c. resident flora
   d. viruses

2. Organisms that can only live inside the cells are called:
   a. flora
   b. bacteria
   c. virus
   d. fungi

3. Infections that are spread by fleas and ticks are caused by:
   a. virus
   b. fungi
   c. protozoa
   d. rickettsia

4. In the chain of infection, colonization and reproduction take place while the agent is in the:
   a. portal of entry link
   b. reservoir link
   c. portal of exit link
   d. transmission link

5. Salmonellosis, a disease caused by contaminated food, is transmitted by:
   a. vehicle transmission
   b. vectorborne transmission
   c. contact transmission
   d. airborne transmission

6. The process used for the total elimination of all microorganisms including spores include all but:
   a. steam
   b. radiation
   c. ethylene gas
   d. alcohol

7. Using clean linen and equipment will help break the chain of infection:
   a. between reservoir and portal of entry
   b. between portal of exit and mode of transmission
   c. between agent and reservoir
   d. between portal of entry and host

8. In an infectious process, the time interval from the onset of nonspecific symptoms until specific symptoms appear is called:
   a. incubation stage
   b. prodromal stage
   c. illness stage
   d. convalescent stage

9. A person is most infectious to other people during the:
   a. incubation stage
   b. prodromal stage
   c. illness stage
   d. convalescent stage

10. The most common endemic nosocomial infection involves all but the:
   a. respiratory system
   b. circulatory system
   c. integumentary system
   d. digestive system

COMPLETION

Complete the following statements.

1. Some forms of bacteria produce resistant forms called _____.

2. Malaria is caused by a group of parasitic organisms known as _____.

3. _____ of disease may have the infectious agent but are symptom free.

4. A _____ host is a person whose normal defense mechanisms are impaired and who is therefore more susceptible to infection.

5. When cleaning medical equipment it first must be rinsed with _____ water.

6. Forms of barrier protection include gloves, masks, gowns, and _____.

7. The stimulation of B-cells and the production of antibodies are collectively referred to as

_____ _____.

8. Memory B-cells form antibodies against a specific antigen. This process is called

_____ _____.

9. Nosocomial infections are referred to as _____ acquired infections.

10. Nosocomial infections are passed among _____ _____

_____.

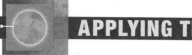

APPLYING THEORY TO PRACTICE

1. Ticks may bite people who live or visit wooded areas. What diseases do the ticks carry? How are the diseases carried by ticks transmitted? Define the term "mode of transmission" and the types involved.

2. Mrs. Gregory, 90 years old, was admitted to the hospital for the repair of a hip fracture. To monitor her urinary output, a Foley catheter was inserted prior to surgery. A few days after surgery, Mrs. Gregory developed a urinary tract infection. What was the probable cause of her infection and how is it related to her hospitalization?

3. Health care workers may be exposed to diseases because of their occupations. List at least five diseases to which a health care worker may be exposed and how they would contract these diseases. Describe methods by which the health care worker may prevent each of these diseases.

4. You are a medical assistant in an HMO. Chris, a 32-year-old mother, comes to the HMO and tells the medical assistant she is very worried. Her son Nicholas, age 7, is going to camp for a 2-week stay. Chris is afraid Nicholas may be exposed to all kinds of infections or disease. Explain to Chris about the normal defense mechanisms the body has and how they will protect her son.

5. Two members of Mike's family have the flu. He is worried about other family members getting the flu. Explain to Mike the chain of infections and what actions he should take to prevent the flu from spreading.

CASE STUDY

Richard is a physician's assistant at a major metropolitan hospital. Since the attacks on the World Trade Center and the Pentagon on September 11, 2001, his hospital has been preparing for a terrorist attack.

1. What are some diseases which can be used by bioterrorists?

2. What symptoms would Richard see in the ER if a patient had been exposed to some of these attacks?

3. What treatments are currently available to combat some of these diseases?

4. Why does the CDC recommend using antibiotics only when exposure to disease is suspected or confirmed?

5. The most contagious effect of bioterrorism is fear. What are some of the actions suggested by health care officials in the event you believe you have been exposed to a chemical type of terrorism?

Chapter 17

RESPIRATORY SYSTEM

Objectives

- Describe the functions of the respiratory system

- Describe the structures and functions of the organs of respiration

- Explain the breathing and respiratory process

- Discuss how breathing is controlled by neural and chemical factors

- Discuss respiratory disorders

- Define the key words that relate to this chapter

Key Words

alveolar sacs
(alveoli)
anthrax
anterior nares
apnea
asbestosis
asthma
atelectasis
bronchiectasis
bronchiole
bronchitis
bronchoscopy
bronchus
cancer of the
larynx
cancer of the lungs
cellular respiration
(oxidation)
chronic obstructive
pulmonary
disease (COPD)
cilia
common cold

coughing
diphtheria
dyspnea
emphysema
epiglottis
eupnea
expiration
expiratory reserve
volume (ERV)
external respiration
functional residual
capacity
glottis
Hering-Brewer
reflex
hiccough
hyperpnea
hyperventilation
influenza
inspiration
inspiratory reserve
volume (IRV)
internal respiration

laryngitis
larynx
mediastinum
medulla oblongata
nasal polyps
nasal septum
olfactory nerve
orthopnea
pertussis
(whooping
cough)
pharyngitis
pharynx
phrenic nerve
pleura
pleural fluid
pleurisy
pneumonia
pneumothorax
pulmonary
embolism
rales

continues

Key Words continued

residual volume	sudden infant	total lung capacity
rhinitis	death syndrome	trachea
silicosis	(SIDS)	tuberculosis
sinus	surfactant	turbinate
sinusitis	tachypnea	vital lung capacity
sneezing	thoracentesis	wheezing
spirometer	tidal volume	yawning

INTRODUCTION TO THE RESPIRATORY SYSTEM

The respiratory system obtains oxygen for use by the millions of body cells and eliminates carbon dioxide and water that is produced in cellular respiration. Oxygen and nutrients stored in the cells combine to produce heat and energy. Oxygen must be in constant supply for the body to survive.

FUNCTIONS OF THE RESPIRATORY SYSTEM

1. Provides the structures for the exchange of oxygen and carbon dioxide in the body through respiration, which is subdivided into external respiration, internal respiration, and cellular respiration. See Figure 17-1.

2. Responsible for the production of sound, the larynx contains the vocal cords. When air is expelled from the lungs it passes over the vocal cords and produces sound.

Respiration

Respiration is the physical and chemical processes by which the body supplies its cells and tissues with the oxygen needed for metabolism and relieves them of the carbon dioxide formed in the energy-producing reactions. Respiration is subdivided into external respiration, which takes place in the lungs, internal respiration, which is between the cells of the body and the blood by way of the fluid bathing the cells, and cellular respiration, which occurs within the cells of the body.

External respiration is also known as breathing, or ventilation. This is the exchange of oxygen and carbon dioxide between the lungs, body, and the outside environment. The breathing process consists of inspiration (inhalation) and expiration (exhalation). On inspiration, air enters the body and is warmed, moistened, and filtered as it passes to the air sacs of the lungs (alveoli). The concentration of oxygen in the alveoli is greater than in the bloodstream. Oxygen diffuses from the area of greater concentration (the alveoli) to an area of lesser concentration (the bloodstream), then into the red blood cells. At the same time, the concentration of carbon dioxide in the blood is greater than in the alveoli, so it diffuses from the blood to the alveoli. Expiration expels the carbon dioxide from the alveoli of the lungs. Some water vapor is also given off in the process.

Internal respiration includes the exchange of carbon dioxide and oxygen between the cells and the lymph surrounding them, plus the oxidative process of energy in the cells. After inspiration, the alveoli are rich with oxygen and transfer the oxygen into the blood. The resulting greater concentration of oxygen in the blood diffuses the oxygen into the tissue cells. At the same time, the cells build up a higher carbon dioxide concentration. The concentration increases to a point that exceeds the level in the blood. This causes the carbon dioxide to diffuse out of the cells and into the blood where it is then carried away to be eliminated.

Deoxygenated blood, produced during internal respiration, carries carbon dioxide in the form of bicarbonate ions (HCO_3^-). These ions are transported by both blood plasma and red blood cells. Exhalation expels carbon dioxide from the red

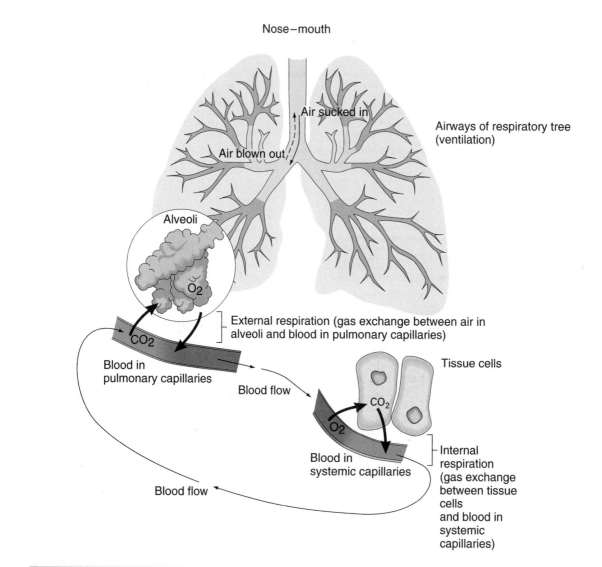

Figure 17-1   *Respiration*

blood cells and the plasma; it is released from the body in the following manner:

$$H_2CO_3 \rightarrow H_2O + CO_2$$

(Bicarbonate ions decompose to form water and carbon dioxide)

Cellular respiration, or **oxidation,** involves the use of oxygen to release energy stored in nutrient molecules such as glucose. This chemical reaction occurs within the cells. Just as wood, when burned (oxidized), gives off energy in the form of heat and light, so too does food give off energy when it is burned, or oxidized in the cells. Much of this energy is released in the form of heat

to maintain body temperature. Some of it, however, is used directly by the cells for such work as contraction of muscle cells. It is also used to carry on other vital processes.

Food, when oxidized, gives off waste products including carbon dioxide and water vapor. These waste products are carried away through the process of internal respiration.

RESPIRATORY ORGANS AND STRUCTURES

Air moves into the lungs through several passageways. The following structures are included: nasal

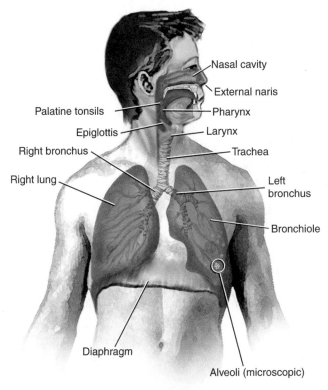

Figure 17-2 *Pathway of external respiration: air enters through the nasal cavity → pharynx → larynx → trachea → bronchial tree → bronchus → bronchiole → alveoli*

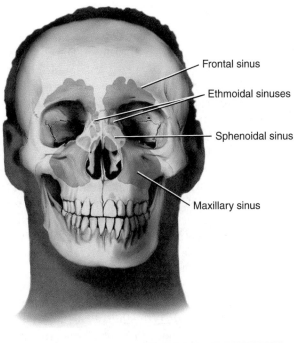

Figure 17-3 *Paranasal sinuses*

cavity, pharynx, larynx, trachea, bronchi, bronchioles, alveoli, lungs, pleura, and mediastinum. See Figure 17-2.

The Nasal Cavity

In humans, air enters the respiratory system through two oval openings in the nose. They are called the nostrils, or **anterior nares.** From here, air enters the nasal cavity, which is divided into a right and left chamber, or smaller cavity, by a partition known as the **nasal septum.** Both cavities are lined with mucous membranes.

Protruding into the nasal cavity are three **turbinate,** or nasal conchae bones. These three scroll-like bones (superior, middle, and inferior concha) divide the large nasal cavity into three narrow passageways. The turbinates increase the

surface area of the nasal cavity causing turbulence in the flowing air. This causes the air to move in various directions before exiting the nasal cavity. As it moves through the nasal cavity, air is being filtered of dust and dirt particles by the mucous membranes lining the conchal and nasal cavity. The air is also moistened by the mucus and warmed by blood vessels which supply the nasal cavity. At the front of the nares are small hairs or **cilia** which entrap and prevent the entry of larger dirt particles. By the time the air reaches the lungs, it has been warmed, moistened, and filtered. Nerve endings providing the sense of smell (**olfactory nerves**) are located in the mucous membrane, in the upper part of the nasal cavity.

The **sinuses,** named frontal, maxillary, sphenoid, and ethmoid, are cavities of the skull filled with air in and around the nasal region, Figure 17-3. Short ducts connect the sinuses with the nasal cavity. Mucous membrane lines the sinuses and helps to warm and moisten air passing through them. The sinuses also give resonance to the voice. The unpleasant voice sound of a nasal cold results from the blockage of sinuses.

The Pharynx

After air leaves the nasal cavity it enters the **pharynx,** commonly known as the throat. The pharynx serves as a common passageway for air and food. It is about 5 inches long and can be subdivided into the nasopharynx, the oropharynx, and laryngopharynx. The nasopharynx lies above and behind the soft palate. The left and right eustachian tubes open directly into the nasopharynx, connecting with each middle ear. Because of this connection, nasopharyngeal inflammation can lead to middle ear infections. The oropharynx is also called the oral part of the mouth; it extends from the soft palate, behind the mouth, to just above the hyoid bone. The laryngopharynx is located below the oropharynx and superior to the larynx. Air travels down the pharynx on its way to the lungs; food travels this route on its way to the stomach.

The **epiglottis** is the flap of cartilage lying behind the tongue and in front of the entrance to the larynx. At rest the epiglottis is upright and allows air to pass through the larynx and to the lungs. During swallowing, it folds back to cover the entrance to the larynx, preventing food and drink from entering the trachea. The larynx draws upward and forward to close the trachea. At the end of each swallow, the epiglottis moves up again, the larynx returns to rest, and the flow of air into the trachea continues. See Figure 17-4.

The Larynx

The **larynx,** or voice box, is a triangular chamber found below the pharynx. The laryngeal walls are composed of nine fibrocartilaginous plates. The largest of these is commonly called the Adams apple. During puberty, the vocal cords become larger in the male. Therefore, the Adams apple is more prominent.

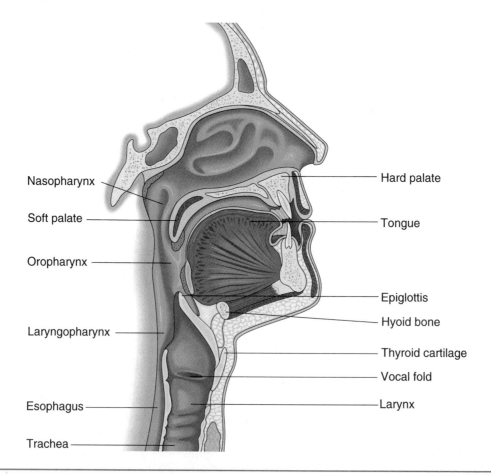

Figure 17-4   *Sagittal section of the face and neck*

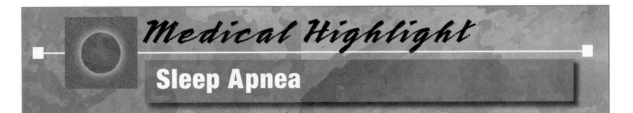

Medical Highlight

Sleep Apnea

Sleep apnea causes excessive daytime sleepiness. According to a Mayo Clinic report, an estimated 18 million Americans have this potentially serious disorder. Signs of sleep apnea include loud snoring, having more than a few breathing pauses during a night's sleep, and daytime drowsiness. There are two kinds of sleep apnea: obstructive sleep apnea and central sleep apnea.

Obstructive sleep apnea is caused by a blockage in the back of the throat preventing air from reaching the lungs. In obstructive sleep apnea, the muscles that normally keep the airway open relax and sag during sleep, causing the tongue and palate to repeatedly block the breathing for about 20 seconds. This lowers the level of oxygen in the blood. The brain senses this decrease and briefly rouses the person from sleep so that the airway can be reopened.

With central sleep apnea, the brain fails to send proper signals to the muscles that keep you breathing adequately. As a result, you may awaken within 20 seconds for lack of air.

In addition to the decline in well-being and the danger associated with major sleep deprivation, sudden drops in blood oxygen levels may increase blood pressure and strain the cardiovascular system. Obstructive sleep apnea is more common in individuals who are overweight, or who consume alcohol, sedatives, or tranquilizers. Evaluation of the condition is done at a sleep center, which involves overnight monitoring of lung, brain, heart activity, breathing patterns, and blood oxygen levels using a test called a polysomnography.

Treatment includes losing weight and sleeping on the side or stomach. For the moderate to severe sleep apnea problem, the doctor may recommend a nasal continuous positive airway pressure (CPAP) machine. Through a mask placed over the nose, a CPAP machine delivers air at a pressure greater than the surrounding air. The pressure increase is just enough to keep the airway passages open.

The larynx is lined with a mucous membrane, continuous from the pharyngeal lining above to the tracheal lining below. Within the larynx are the characteristic vocal cords. There is a space between the vocal cords known as the **glottis.** When air is expelled from the lungs, it passes the vocal cords. This sets off a vibration, creating sound. The action of the lips and tongue on this sound produces speech.

The Trachea

The **trachea,** or windpipe, is a tubelike passageway some 11.2 centimeters (about 4.5 inches) in length. It extends from the larynx, passes in front of the esophagus, and continues to form the two bronchi (one for each lung). The walls of the trachea are composed of alternate bands of membranes, and 15 to 20 C-shaped rings of hyaline cartilage. These C-shaped rings are virtually non-collapsible, keeping the trachea open for the passage of oxygen into the lungs. However, the trachea can be obstructed by large pieces of food, tumorous growths, or the swelling of inflamed lymph nodes in the neck.

The walls of the trachea are lined with both mucous membrane and ciliated epithelium. The function of the mucus is to entrap inhaled dust particles; the cilia then sweep such dust-laden mucus upward to the pharynx. Coughing and expectoration dislodges and eliminates the dust-laden mucus from the pharynx, Figure 17-4.

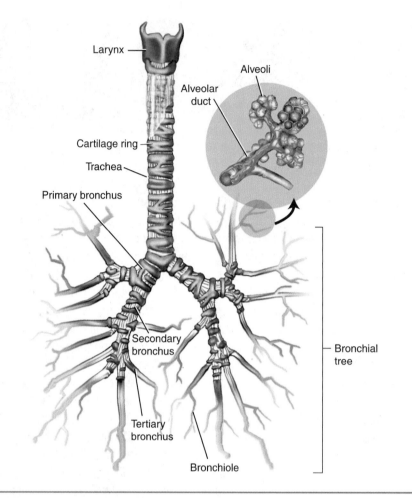

Larynx

Alveoli

Alveolar
duct

Cartilage ring

Trachea

Primary bronchus

Secondary
bronchus

Bronchial
tree

Tertiary
bronchus

Bronchiole

Figure 17-5   *Larynx, trachea, and bronchial tree*

The Bronchi and The Bronchioles

The lower end of the trachea separates into the right **bronchus** and the left bronchus. There is a slight difference between the two bronchi, the right bronchus being somewhat shorter, wider, and more vertical in position.

As the bronchi enter the lung, they subdivide into bronchial tubes and smaller **bronchioles.** The divisions are Y-shaped in form. The two bronchi are similar in structure to the trachea, because their walls are lined with ciliated epithelium and ringed with hyaline cartilage. However, the bronchial tubes and smaller bronchi are ringed with cartilaginous plates instead of incomplete C-shaped rings. The bronchioles lose their cartilaginous plates and fibrous tissue. Their thinner walls are made from smooth muscle and elastic tissue lined with ciliated epithelium. At the

end of each bronchiole is an alveolar duct which ends in a saclike cluster called **alveolar sacs (alveoli)**, Figure 17-5.

The Alveoli

The alveolar sacs consist of many alveoli which have a single layer of epithelial tissue. There are about 500 million alveoli in the adult lung, about three times the amount necessary to sustain life. Each alveolus forming a part of the alveolar sac possesses a globular shape. Their inner surfaces are covered with a lipid material known as **surfactant.** The surfactant helps to stabilize the alveoli, preventing their collapse. Each alveolus is encased by a network of blood capillaries.

It is through the moist walls of both the alveoli and the capillaries that rapid exchange of carbon dioxide and oxygen occurs. In the blood capillaries, carbon dioxide diffuses from the erythrocytes, through the capillary walls, into the alveoli, and is exhaled through the mouth and nose.

The opposite process occurs with oxygen, which diffuses from the alveoli into the capillaries, and from there into the erythrocytes.

The Lungs

The lungs are fairly large, cone-shaped organs filling up the two lateral chambers of the thoracic cavity, Figure 17-6. They are separated from each other by the mediastinum and the heart. The upper part of the lung, underneath the collarbone, is the apex; the broad lower part is the base. Each base is concave, allowing it to fit snugly over the convex part of the diaphragm.

Lung tissue is porous and spongy, due to the alveoli and the tremendous amount of air it contains. If you were to place a specimen of a cow lung into a tankful of water, for example, it would float quite easily.

The right lung is larger and broader than the left because the heart inclines to the left side. The right lung is also shorter due to the diaphragm's upward displacement on the right to accommodate the liver. The right lung is divided by fissures (clefts) into three lobes: superior, middle and inferior.

The left lung is smaller, narrower, and longer than its counterpart. It is subdivided into two lobes: superior and inferior.

The Pleura

The lungs are covered with a thin, moist, slippery membrane of tough endothelial cells, or **pleura**. There are two pleural membranes. The one covering the lungs and dipping between the lobes is the pulmonary, or visceral pleura. Lining the thoracic cavity and the upper surface of the diaphragm is the parietal pleura. Consequently, each lung is enclosed in a double-walled sac. **Pleurisy** is an inflammation of this lining.

The space between the two pleural membranes is the pleural cavity, filled with serous fluid called **pleural fluid.** This fluid is necessary to prevent friction between the two pleural membranes as they rub against each other during each breath.

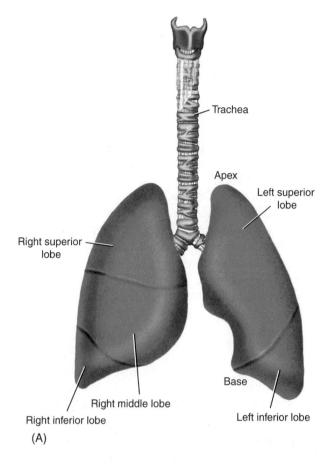

Trachea

Apex

Left superior lobe

Right superior lobe

Right middle lobe

Right inferior lobe

Base

Left inferior lobe

(A)

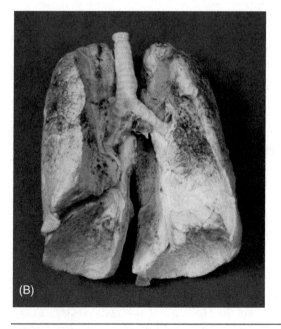

(B)

Figure 17-6   *(A) Structures of the lungs;* *(B) human lungs*   *(Photo courtesy of Oak Ridge National Laboratory, Oak Ridge, TN)*

The pleural cavity may, on occasion, fill up with an enormous quantity of serous fluid. This occurs when there is an inflammation of the pleura. The increased pleural fluid compresses and sometimes even causes parts of the lung to collapse. This makes breathing extremely difficult. To alleviate the pressure, a **thoracentesis** may be performed. This procedure entails the insertion of a hollow, tubelike instrument through the thoracic cavity and into the pleural cavity, to drain the excess fluid.

Another disorder that can affect the pleural cavity is **pneumothorax.** This condition occurs if there is a buildup of air within the pleural cavity on one side of the chest. The excess air increases pressure on the lung, causing it to collapse. Breathing is not possible with a collapsed lung, but the unaffected lung can still continue the breathing process.

The Mediastinum

The **mediastinum,** also called the interpleural space, is situated between the lungs along the median plane of the thorax. It extends from the sternum to the vertebrae. The mediastinum contains the thoracic viscera: the thymus gland, heart, aorta and its branches, pulmonary arteries and veins, superior and inferior vena cava, esophagus, trachea, thoracic duct, lymph nodes, and vessels.

MECHANICS OF BREATHING

Pulmonary ventilation (breathing) of the lungs is due to changes in pressure which occur within the chest cavity. The normal pressure within the pleural space is always negative, less than atmospheric pressure. The negative pressure helps to keep the lungs expanded. The variation in pressure is brought about by cellular respiration and mechanical breathing movements.

THE BREATHING PROCESS

Pulmonary ventilation allows the exchange of oxygen between the alveoli and erythrocyte, and eventually between the erythrocyte and cells.

Inhalation/Inspiration

There are two groups of intercostal muscles: external intercostals and internal intercostals. Their muscle fibers cross each other at an angle of 90 degrees. During inhalation, or **inspiration,** the external intercostals lift the ribs upward and outward, Figure 17-7. This increases the volume of the thoracic cavity. Simultaneously, the sternum rises along with the ribs and the dome-shaped diaphragm contracts and becomes flattened, moving downward. As the diaphragm moves downward, pressure is exerted on the abdominal viscera. This causes the anterior muscles to protrude slightly, increasing the space within the chest cavity in a vertical direction. As a result, there is a decrease in pressure. Since atmospheric pressure is now greater, air rushes in all the way down to the alveoli, resulting in inhalation.

Exhalation/Expiration

In exhalation, or **expiration,** just the opposite takes place. Expiration is a passive process; all the contracted intercostal muscles and diaphragm relax. The ribs move down, the diaphragm moves up. In addition, the surface tension of the fluid lining the alveoli reduces the elasticity of the lung tissue and causes the alveoli to collapse. This action, coupled with the relaxation of contracted, respiratory muscles, relaxes the lungs; the space within the thoracic cavity decreases, thus increasing the internal pressure. Increased pressure forces air from the lungs, resulting in exhalation.

The lungs are extremely elastic. They are able to change capacity as the size of the thoracic cavity is altered. This ability is known as compliance. When lung tissue becomes diseased and fibrotic, the lung's compliance decreases and ventilation decreases.

Respiratory Movements and Frequency of Respiration

The rhythmic movements of the rib cage where air is drawn in and expelled from the lungs makes up the respiratory movements. Inspiration and expiration combined is counted as one respiratory movement. Thus, the normal rate in quiet breathing for an adult is about 14 to 20 breaths per minute. This rate is changeable. The respiratory rate can be in-

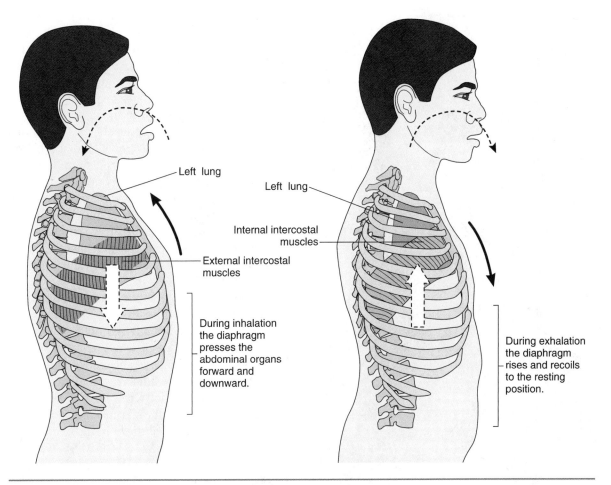

Figure 17-7   *Mechanics of breathing—inhalation and exhalation*

creased by muscular activity, increased body temperatures, and in certain pathological disorders such as hyperthyroidism. It changes with sex, females having the higher rate at 16 to 20 breaths per minute. Age will also change the respiratory rate. For example, at birth the rate is 40 to 60 breaths per minute; at 5 years, 24 to 26 breaths. The body's position also affects the respiration rate. When the body is asleep or prone, the rate is 12 to 14 breaths per minute; in a sitting position, it is 18, and in a standing position, it is 20 to 22 breaths per minute. Emotions play a role in decreasing or increasing the respiratory rate, probably through the hypothalamus and pons. (see Chapter 8).

Other situations that can affect the respiratory rate are:

- **Coughing**—a deep breath is taken followed by a forceful exhalation from the mouth to clear the lower respiratory tract.

- **Hiccoughs** (hiccups)—caused by a spasm of the diaphragm and a spasmodic closure of the glottis. It is believed to be the result of an irritation to the diaphragm or the phrenic nerve.

- **Sneezing**—occurs like a cough except air is forced through the nose to clear the upper respiratory tract.

- **Yawning**—a deep, prolonged breath that fills the lungs, believed to be caused by the need to increase oxygen within the blood.

CONTROL OF BREATHING

The rate of breathing is controlled by neural (nervous) and chemical factors. Although both have the same goal—that of respiratory control—they function independently of one another.

Effects of Aging on The Respiratory System

The lung tissue loses elasticity, the rib cage becomes less flexible, and the muscle strength decreases. The number of functioning alveoli decreases. These factors compromise the oxygen–carbon dioxide exchange, reducing the oxygen content in the blood. The combination of a less efficient heart pump and reduced oxygen cause characteristic signs of activity intolerance.

Breathlessness is the most common physiological response to exercise of a sedentary person. It is estimated that the maximum oxygen consumption rate during stress and moderate exercise can increase nine times for an elderly person. Maximum breathing capacity is diminished by 50%.

Lung capacity exhibits changes also. There is an increase in residual volume and functional residual capacity and a decrease in vital capacity and expiratory airflow.

The presence of respiratory disease tends to be higher in the elderly. The elderly should take the flu vaccine annually and pneumonia vaccine as recommended by their physician.

Neural Factors

The respiratory center is located in the **medulla oblongata** in the brain, Figure 17-8. It is subdivided into two centers: one to regulate inspiration, the other for expiratory control.

The upper part of the medulla contains a grouping of cells that is the seat of the respiratory center. An increase of CO_2 or lack of O_2 in the blood will trigger the respiratory center.

Two neuronal pathways are involved in breathing. One group of motor nerves, called the **phrenic nerves,** leads to the diaphragm and the intercostal muscles. The other nerve pathway carries sensory impulses from the nose, larynx, lungs, skin, and abdominal organs via the vagus nerve in the medulla.

The rhythm of breathing can be changed by stimuli originating within the body's surface membranes. For example, a sudden drenching with cold water can make us gasp, while irritation to the nose or larynx can make us sneeze or cough.

Although the medulla's respiratory center is primarily responsible for respiratory control, it is not the only part of the brain that controls breathing. A lung reflex, called the **Hering-Breuer reflex** (K. Ewald Hering (1834–1918), German physiologist, and Josef Breuer (1842–1925), Austrian physician) is involved in preventing the overstretching of the lungs. When the lungs are inflated, the nerve endings in the walls are stimulated. A nerve message is sent from the lungs to the medulla by way of the vagus nerve, inhibiting inspiration and stimulating expiration. This mechanism prevents overinflation of the lungs, keeping them from being ripped apart like an overinflated balloon.

Chemical Factors

Chemical control of respiration is dependent upon the level of carbon dioxide in the blood. When blood circulates through active tissue, it receives carbon dioxide and other metabolic waste products of cellular respiration. As blood circulates through the respiratory center, the respiratory center senses the increased carbon dioxide in the blood and increases the respiratory rate. For example, a person performing vigorous exercise or physical labor breathes more deeply and quickly to

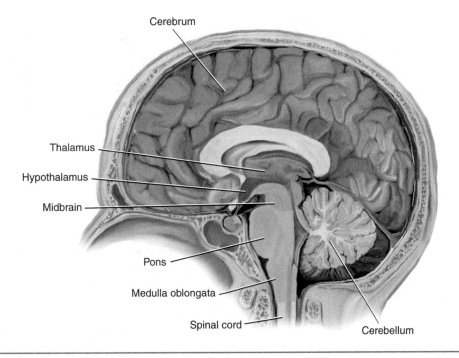

Figure 17-8 *Cross section of the brain—the medulla oblongata is the respiratory center.*

cope with the need for more oxygen and to rid the body of excess carbon dioxide produced.

Other chemical regulators of respiration are the chemoreceptors which are found in carotid arteries and the aorta. These chemoreceptors are sensitive to the amount of the blood oxygen levels. As the arterial blood flows around these carotid and aortic bodies, the chemoreceptors are particularly sensitive to the amount of oxygen present. If oxygen declines to very low levels, impulses are sent from the carotid and aortic bodies to the respiratory center, which will stimulate the rate and depth of respiration. The respiratory center can be affected by drugs such as depressants, barbiturates, and morphine.

LUNG CAPACITY AND VOLUME

Have you ever held your breath for so long that you thought you would burst? To measure how much air you can hold (your lung capacity), use a device called a **spirometer.** A spirometer measures the volume and flow of air during inspiration and expiration. By comparing the reading with the norm for a person's age, height, weight, and sex, it can be determined if any deficiencies exist. Disease processes such as chronic obstructive pulmonary disease (COPD) affect lung capacity, Figure 17-9.

■ **Tidal volume** is the amount of air that moves in and out of the lungs with each breath. The normal amount is about 500 ml.

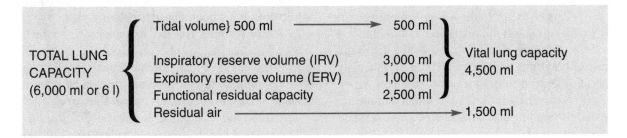

Figure 17-9 *Lung capacity and volume*

▪ **Inspiratory reserve volume (IRV)** is the amount of air you can force a person to take in over and above the tidal volume. The normal amount is 2,100–3,000 ml.

▪ **Expiratory reserve volume (ERV)** is the amount of air you can force a person to exhale over and above the tidal volume. The normal amount is 1,000 ml.

▪ **Vital lung capacity** is the total amount of air involved with tidal volume, inspiratory reserve volume, and expiratory reserve volume. The normal vital capacity is 4,500 ml.

▪ **Residual volume** is the amount of air that cannot be voluntarily expelled in the lungs. It allows for the continuous exchange of gases between breaths. The normal residual volume is 1,500 ml.

▪ **Functional residual capacity** is the sum of the expiratory reserve volume plus the residual volume. The normal amount is 2,500 ml.

▪ **Total lung capacity** includes tidal volume, inspiratory reserve, expiratory reserve, and residual air. The normal amount is 6,000 ml.

TYPES OF RESPIRATION

The health care professional should be aware of the various changes to the respiratory rate and sounds of human respiration. These changes can be alerts to an abnormal respiratory condition in a patient. The following conditions describe various kinds and conditions of respiration.

Apnea is the temporary stoppage of breathing movements.

Dyspnea is difficult, labored, or painful breathing, usually accompanied by discomfort and breathlessness.

Eupnea is normal or easy breathing with the usual quiet inhalations and exhalations.

Hyperpnea is an increase in the depth and rate of breathing accompanied by abnormal exaggeration of respiratory movements.

Orthopnea is difficult or labored breathing when the body is in a horizontal position. It is usually corrected by sitting or standing.

Tachypnea is an abnormally rapid and shallow rate of breathing.

Hyperventilation is a condition that can be caused by disease or stress. Rapid breathing occurs which causes the body to lose carbon dioxide too quickly. The blood level of carbon dioxide is lowered which leads to alkalosis. Symptoms are dizziness and possible fainting. To correct this condition, the person should breathe into a paper bag. The exhaled air contains more carbon dioxide; the air breathed in will have higher levels of carbon dioxide from the paper bag, so this activity will restore the normal blood levels of carbon dioxide.

DISORDERS OF THE RESPIRATORY SYSTEM

The majority of the disorders of the respiratory system involve some defect or problem that prevents outside air from reaching the alveoli. In many cases the cause of the problem is an infection within the upper or lower airway. The problem may also stem from a mechanical obstruction of the airway.

Infectious Causes

The respiratory system is subject to various infections and inflammations caused by bacteria, viruses, and irritants.

The **common cold** is usually caused by a virus that is highly contagious. This infection is responsible for the greatest loss of production hours each year. This respiratory infection spreads quickly through the classroom, factory, or business office. It is often the basis for more serious respiratory disease. It lowers body resistance, making it subject to infection. The direct cause of a cold is usually a virus. Indirect causes include chilling, fatigue, lack of proper food, and not enough sleep. A person who has a cold should stay in bed, drink warm liquids and fruit juice, and eat wholesome, nourishing foods.

Pharyngitis is a red, inflamed throat which may be caused by one of several bacteria or viruses. It also occurs as a result of irritants such as too much smoking or speaking. It is characterized by painful swallowing and extreme dryness of the throat.

Laryngitis is an inflammation of the larynx, or voice box. It is often secondary to other respiratory infections. It can be recognized by the incidence of hoarseness or loss of voice.

Sinusitis is an infection of the mucous membrane which lines the sinus cavities. One or several of the cavities may be infected. Pain and nasal discharge are symptoms of this infection which, if severe, may lead to more serious complications. The sinuses affected can be the ethmoid, frontal, sphenoid, and maxillary sinuses.

Bronchitis is an inflammation of the mucous membrane of the trachea and the bronchial tubes which produces excessive mucus. It may be acute or chronic and often follows infections of the upper respiratory tract. Acute bronchitis can be caused by the spreading of an inflammation from the nasopharynx, or by inhalation of irritating vapors. This condition is characterized by a cough, fever, substernal pain, and **rales** (raspy sound).

Chronic bronchitis usually occurs in middle or old age. Cigarette smoking is the most common cause of chronic bronchitis. Acute bronchitis may become chronic after many episodes. Symptoms include a severe and persistent cough and large amounts of discolored sputum. To be termed "chronic," the cough must last for 3 months and have occurred for 2 consecutive years. Treatment is symptomatic; the patient must stop smoking.

Influenza or "flu" is a viral infection characterized by inflammation of the mucous membrane of the respiratory system. The infection is accompanied by fever, a mucopurulent discharge, muscular pain, and extreme exhaustion. Complications such as bronchopneumonia, neuritis, otitis media (middle ear infection), and pleurisy often follow influenza. Treatment is aimed at the symptoms.

Pneumonia is an infection of the lung. It may be caused by a bacteria or virus. In this condition, the alveoli become filled with a thick fluid called exudate which contains both pus and red blood cells. The symptoms of pneumonia are chest pain, fever, chills, and dyspnea. Treatment may require the administration of oxygen and antibiotics.

Tuberculosis (TB) is an infectious disease of the lungs, caused by the tubercle bacillus, *Mycobacterium tuberculosis*. The organs usually most affected in TB are the lungs; however, the organism may also affect the kidney, bones, and lymphs. In pulmonary TB, lesions called tubercles form within the lung tissue. Symptoms of TB are cough, low grade fever in the afternoon, weight loss, and night sweats. The diagnostic test for TB is the Mantoux test—a skin test which is read within 48 to 72 hours by a health care professional. A positive skin test must be followed by a chest x-ray and sputum sample.

The incidence of TB had been declining because of early detection, treatment with drugs, and patient education. The Centers for Disease Control and Prevention, however, now sees an increase in the number of cases. The reasons for the increase include illegal immigration (illegal immigrants do not go through a screening process for tuberculosis), an increase in the number of homeless and poor, and the spread of AIDS. In addition, there is a new strain of the TB bacteria which is resistant to treatment. People with TB must stay on the drug INH for a long time. Many people stop taking the drug which then leads to drug-resistant organisms. There is concern we will once again see tuberculosis as a widespread infectious disease.

Diphtheria is a very infectious disease caused by the *Corynebacterium diphtheriae bacterium*. As part of the normal immunization process, children receive a vaccine which is effective against diphtheria.

Pertussis (whooping cough) is characterized by severe coughing attacks that end in a "whooping" sound and dyspnea. The widespread use of the pertussis vaccine limits the number of cases in the United States to about 4,000 each year; worldwide pertussis attacks 50 million children.

Anthrax is a disease-causing organism that can create a potential health hazard. The bacterium *Bacillus anthracis* and its spores cause anthrax, Figure 17-10. The inactive microscopic spores normally reside in the soil. In a favorable environment the spores can change into the anthrax bacteria, which produce a toxin than can be fatal to humans and animals.

Anthrax spores are invisible, odorless, and tasteless. The amount needed to make a person ill is smaller than a speck of dust. The disease has three forms.

- *Cutaneous anthrax*, in which spores enter a cut and cause a local infection, Figure 17-11.

- *Intestinal anthrax*, in which the bacteria is ingested from contaminated meat. Symptoms include diarrhea and vomiting of blood.

- *Inhalation anthrax*, which is the most deadly form. If inhaled, anthrax spores convert to the active bacillus and infect the lungs. Initial

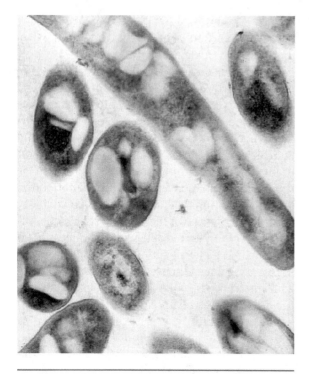

Figure 17-10 *Bacillus anthrax* *(Courtesy of the Centers for Disease Control Public Health Image Library)*

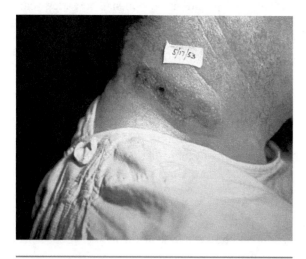

Figure 17-11 *Cutaneous anthrax* *(Courtesy of the Centers for Disease Control Public Health Image Library)*

symptoms may resemble a mild cold or the flu. After several days, the infection progresses to produce a high fever and pneumonia. Once the infection has spread, inhalation anthrax is about 90% fatal.

All three forms of anthrax are generally treatable with antibiotics if treatment begins early. Cutaneous and intestinal anthrax are not usually fatal. With inhalation anthrax, antibiotics must be given at the earliest indication of symptoms to be beneficial. Anthrax is not considered contagious. No form is known to be transmitted from an infected person to another person. People who may have been exposed to anthrax can take antibiotics to prevent the disease. Anthrax can also be prevented with a vaccine. Because of negative side effects, the use of the vaccine is limited.

Noninfectious Causes

Respiratory ailments unrelated to infectious causes sometimes develop in the respiratory system.

Rhinitis is the inflammation of the nasal mucous membrane causing swelling and increased secretions. Various forms include acute rhinitis and allergic rhinitis caused by any allergen (more commonly known as hay fever).

Asthma is a disease in which the airway becomes obstructed due to an inflammatory response to a stimuli. It was previously thought that the obstruction was due primarily to bronchoconstriction. The stimuli may be an allergen or psychological stress. About 5% of the American population have asthma, which is an increase over the past 10 years. The symptoms include difficulty in exhaling, dyspnea, **wheezing** (sound produced by a rush of air through a narrowed passageway), and tightness in the chest. Treatment is with anti-inflammatory drugs. An inhaled bronchodilator may be used as supplemental therapy.

Atelectasis is a condition in which the lungs fail to expand normally due to bronchial occlusion.

Bronchiectasis is the dilation of a bronchus caused by an inflammation, accompanied by heavy pus secretion.

Asbestosis is a respiratory disease caused by inhaling asbestos fibers, which can result in scar tissue (fibrosis) formation inside the lung. Scarred lung tissue does not expand and contract normally. Asbestos fibers were commonly found in construction materials before 1975. Asbestos-related diseases include pleural plaques (calcification), malignant tumors, and pleural effusion. Symptoms include shortness of breath on exertion, cough, tightness in the chest, and chest pain. There is no cure available. Supportive treatment of symptoms include treatment to remove secretions from the lungs, aerosol medication to thin secretions, and oxygen therapy.

Silicosis is caused by breathing dust containing silicon dioxide over a long period of time. The lungs become fibrosed which results in a reduced capacity for expansion. Silicosis is also called chalicosis, lithosis, miner's asthma, or miner's disease.

Nasal polyps are growths that sometimes occur in the sinus cavity and cause an obstruction of the air pathway, Figure 17-12. The polyps may be surgically removed which will correct the condition.

Chronic obstructive pulmonary disease (COPD) is a term that health care professionals use to indicate chronic lung conditions, especially emphysema and chronic bronchitis.

In **emphysema,** the alveoli of the lung become overdilated, lose their elasticity, and cannot rebound. The alveoli may eventually rupture. In

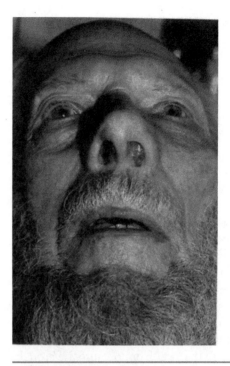

Figure 17-12   *Nasal polyp*

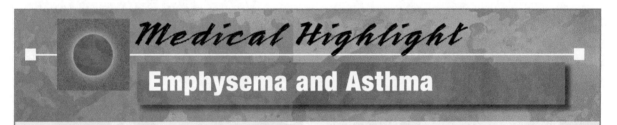

Medical Highlight
Emphysema and Asthma

EMPHYSEMA
Surgery for emphysema is not a cure but a type of treatment to improve quality of life. Lung volume reduction surgery may either involve one lung or both lungs. In surgery about one-third of the damaged lung tissue is removed. The surgeon then sews the rest of the lung(s) back together. By removing some of the expanding lung tissue, the surgeon allows the diaphragm and ribs to shift back toward their original positions prior to lung disease. This surgery is showing some promise in promoting weight gain, greater range of activity, better breathing capacity, and less reliance on oxygen replacement therapy. However, only about two-thirds of patients have shown improvement, and long-term gains are limited.

ACUPUNCTURE FOR ASTHMA
Acupuncture may reduce both the severity and the amount of medication the asthma patient must take, says Dr. Kim Jobst from Oxford University, England. Patients should not stop taking their asthma medication, but there is evidence that acupuncture can be effective in reducing the severity of the disease. Doctors cannot explain exactly how acupuncture is effective, but suggest it may have a relaxing effect on patients. Acupuncture is no longer considered an investigational medical treatment by the FDA. Acupuncture is approved to be used by qualified practitioners. Each state sets the criteria for "qualified practitioner."

this process, air becomes trapped in the alveoli, is difficult to exhale, forced exhalation is required, and there is a reduced exchange of carbon dioxide and oxygen. The patient with emphysema experiences dyspnea which becomes more severe as the disease progresses.

The goal of treatment in COPD is to alleviate the symptoms as much as possible. Persons with COPD need to reduce their exposure to respiratory irritants, stop smoking, prevent infections, and restructure their activity to minimize their need for oxygen.

Cancer of the lungs is caused by a small cell (also known as an oat cell) which spreads rapidly to other organs. This type is found mainly in people who are smokers. The other types of lung cancer are squamous cell or adenocarcinoma, which do not spread as rapidly. Symptoms include cough and weight loss. Diagnosis is made by x-ray and white-light **bronchoscopy.** A small, flexible tube is passed through the mouth or nose into the bronchi and into the lung. The area is flooded with a white light in order to find abnormal tissue; a piece of tissue is then obtained for study. It is important for the heath care worker to know that the throat may be anesthetized for this procedure and that the cough reflex must have returned before the person can have fluid or food. Treatment of the cancer may be surgery, chemotherapy, and/or radiation.

Cancer of the larynx is curable if early detection is made of the disorder. It is found most frequently in men over 50.

Pulmonary embolism occurs when a blood clot (embolism) travels to the lung. This condition may occur after surgery or if a person has been on bed rest. Symptoms include a sudden severe pain in the chest and dyspnea. Diagnosis is confirmed by a lung scan. Treatment includes anticoagulant therapy. To prevent this, early ambulation (or walking) after surgery is important.

Sudden infant death syndrome (SIDS) is also known as "crib death," and usually occurs in infants between 2 weeks and 1 year of age. The infant stops breathing during sleep. The exact cause of SIDS is unknown; however, evidence suggests that there is a disturbance of the respiratory control center in the brain. The National Institute of Child Health and Human Development (NICHD), leader of the "Back to Sleep" campaign, recommends all infants under 1 year of age should be placed on their backs to sleep. Babies should be placed on a firm mattress with no blankets or fluffy bedding underneath and no pillows or stuffed toys. It is also very important to keep the baby from being overheated. If there is any indication that SIDS may occur, the infant is monitored so that an alarm sounds if the infant stops breathing.

Medical Terminology

alveol	tiny cavity
-i	pertaining to
alveol/i	pertaining to tiny cavity
a	without
-pnea	breathing
a/pnea	without breathing
bronch	major branch of windpipe
-itis	inflammation of
bronch/itis	inflammation of major branch of windpipe
-scop	instrument used to examine
-y	pertaining to
bronch/o/scop/y	pertaining to examination of windpipe
dys	difficult

dys/pnea	difficult breathing
emphysem	blowing up with air
-a	pertaining to
emphysem/a	pertaining to blowing up with air
ex	out
-pira	breathe
-tion	process
ex/pira/tion	process of breathing out
in	in
in/spira/tion	process of breathing in
laryng	voicebox
laryng/itis	inflammation of voicebox
pharyng	throat
pharyng/itis	inflammation of the throat
pneumon	lungs, air
-ia	abnormal condition of
pneumon/ia	abnormal condition of the lungs
-thorax	chest
pneumo/thorax	air in the chest cavity
spiro	breath
-meter	instrument used to measure
spiro/meter	instrument used to measure breaths
tachy	fast
tachy/pnea	fast breathing

REVIEW QUESTIONS

Select the letter of the choice that best completes the statement.

1. The exchange of oxygen and carbon dioxide between the body and the air we breathe in is called:
 a. cellular respiration
 b. external respiration
 c. internal respiration
 d. breathing

2. Oxygen moves from an area of higher concentration through a process called:
 a. active transport
 b. osmosis
 c. diffusion
 d. filtration

3. When air travels through the nose it is filtered and:
   a. warmed and moistened
   b. warmed and exchanged for carbon dioxide
   c. cooled and exchanged for carbon dioxide
   d. cooled and moistened

4. The structure responsible for giving tone to the voice is:
   a. nares
   b. nasal septum
   c. glottis
   d. conchae

5. This structure contains 15 to 20 cartilage rings and serves as a passageway for air; it is known as the:
   a. nasopharynx
   b. trachea
   c. pharynx
   d. larynx

6. The structure at the end of the bronchial tree where the exchange between oxygen and carbon dioxide occurs is the:
   a. alveolar ducts
   b. alveoli
   c. bronchiole
   d. bronchial tree

7. Collapse of the lung is called:
   a. pleurisy
   b. pneumonia
   c. pneumothorax
   d. thoracentesis

8. The rate of breathing is affected by which part of the brain?
   a. cerebrum
   b. medulla
   c. cerebellum
   d. frontal lobe

9. Difficult or labored breathing is known as:
   a. eupnea
   b. dyspnea
   c. orthopnea
   d. hyperpnea

10. Pharyngitis is the inflammation of the:
   a. throat
   b. voicebox
   c. windpipe
   d. upper nose

11. An inflammation of the lining of the lung is called:
   a. pneumonia
   b. pleurisy
   c. sinusitis
   d. tuberculosis

12. The vaccine used to protect children against whooping cough is:
   a. MMR
   b. Mantoux
   c. Trepedia/DPT vaccine
   d. Salk

13. Chronic obstructive pulmonary disease means the person has:
   a. asthma
   b. pneumonia
   c. bronchiectasis
   d. emphysema

14. A respiratory disorder with wheezing and dyspnea is known as:
   a. acute bronchitis
   b. atelectasis
   c. asthma
   d. SIDS

15. A respiratory disease that has shown a marked increase in the past few years is:
   a. asthma
   b. cancer of the lung
   c. tuberculosis
   d. COPD

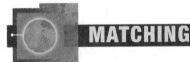

MATCHING

Match each term in Column I with its function or description in Column II.

Column I	Column II
1. respiratory control center	a. opposite of inhalation
2. inspiration and expiration	b. measures of the ability to inspire and expire air
3. vagus nerve	c. complemental air
4. exhalation	d. located in the medulla
5. increased respiratory rate	e. occur from 16 to 24 times a minute
6. diaphragm	f. result of increase in carbon dioxide content of the blood
7. intercostal muscles	g. becomes flattened and moves downward during inhalation
8. tidal air	h. air which cannot be forcibly expelled from the lungs
9. residual volume	i. less than atmospheric pressure
10. pressure in pleural space	j. air inhaled and exhaled during rest
	k. muscles in between the ribs which contract during inhalation
	l. inhibits inspiration and stimulates expiration

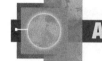

APPLYING THEORY TO PRACTICE

1-A. You are a little molecule of oxygen, floating in the air. Suddenly you feel a whoosh, and you are in this dark tube with little hairs tickling you. Is this that thing called the nose? Trace your journey from there to the alveoli of the lung; you will recognize it when you get there. It looks like a bunch of grapes. Name the structures along the way.

1-B. To go even further, after you arrive at the alveoli, squeeze into the capillary around the alveolus and get to the pulmonary vein. You can now begin a new journey to the left knee; trace that journey. Name the structures and vessels along the way.

2. You have a cold, sinusitis, and you talk funny. What is happening? How do you explain it?

3. Take a breath; now breathe deeper, deeper, deeper. Name the process you have just experienced. Let the breath out; force more and more air out until you gasp. Name the process you have experienced.

4. Tuberculosis is a disease that has been with us for a long time. Scientists believed that the disease was responding to treatment. However, in the past few years there has been an increase in the number of cases of tuberculosis. Explain the reason for this increase.

5. Breathe on a mirror. Note the moisture that appears from the exhaled air. Discuss the fact that carbon dioxide, heat, and water vapor are given off in exhalation.

6. Jog in place. Note the effect of body activity on the rate of breathing. How does exercise change breathing? Why?

7. One of the weapons terrorists may use to instill fear in the population is the release of anthrax spores. Explain the different types of anthrax. Describe the symptoms and treatment. Is the disease contagious?

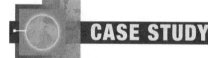

CASE STUDY

Alan has been smoking for the past 20 years and has been experiencing some shortness of breath and a cough. His physician, Dr. Bryan, sees him. The doctor orders a lung capacity test and a chest x-ray.

1. Explain what factors are measured in a lung capacity test.

After the results of the test, Dr. Bryan tells Alan he has COPD in the form of emphysema.

2. Explain COPD and emphysema.

3. Name the organs of external respiration.

4. What structural changes occur with emphysema?

5. What is the principal cause of emphysema?

6. What other body systems are affected by emphysema?

7. Describe the treatment of emphysema.

8. Is there any surgical procedure for emphysema?

9. How does this disease affect a person's lifestyle?

Lab Activity

17-1

Breathing Process

■ *Objective:* To observe the mechanism involved in breathing
■ *Materials needed:* bell jar, Y-tube, two balloons of the same size, rubber stopper to fit top of bell jar, another small rubber stopper, scissors, string, rubber bands, piece of thin rubber sheeting, textbook, paper and pencil

Step 1: Carefully insert a glass Y-tube into the opening of a rubber stopper.

Step 2: Fasten the two balloons to the two arms of the Y-tube. Use string or rubber bands to keep balloons in place.

Step 3: Place the rubber stopper in the bell jar so that the balloons are inside the jar.

Step 4: Using the scissors, carefully cut a piece of rubber sheeting large enough to fit over the bottom of the bell jar.

Step 5: From the center of the rubber sheeting, pinch out a piece of the sheeting but do not pierce it. Attach a small rubber stopper into this area.

Step 6: Take the string and tie it around the rubber stopper so you may now use this place as a handle to grasp the rubber sheeting.

Step 7: Take another piece of string and secure the rubber sheeting to the bottom of the bell jar.

Step 8: Grasp the "handle" and pull down on the rubber sheeting. Observe what is happening to the balloons. Record your observations and describe how it relates to the breathing process.

Step 9: Grasp the "handle" and push up on the rubber sheeting. Observe what is happening to the balloons. Record your observations and describe how it relates to the breathing process.

Step 10: Compare the bell jar apparatus with Figure 17-2 in the textbook. What structure do the bell jar, balloons, top of the Y-tube, branches of the Y-tube, and the rubber sheeting represent?

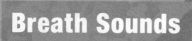

Lab Activity

17-2

Breath Sounds

■ *Objective:* To observe the sounds made during breathing
■ *Materials needed:* stethoscope, alcohol wipes, paper and pencil

This activity is done with a lab partner.

Step 1: Clean the earpieces of the stethoscope with alcohol wipes.

Step 2: Place the diaphragm of the stethoscope on the throat of your lab partner just above the sternum. Listen to the sounds made during inspiration and expiration. Are the sounds similar? Describe and record the sounds you hear.

Step 3: Move the stethoscope down until you no longer hear breath sounds.

Step 4: Place the stethoscope at two different intercostal spaces. Describe and record the sounds you hear.

Step 5: Place the stethoscope on the upper area of the back and listen to the sounds on inspiration and expiration. Describe and record the sounds you hear.

Step 6: Remove the stethoscope and clean the earpieces.

Switch places with your lab partner and repeat steps 2 through 5.

Compare your results.

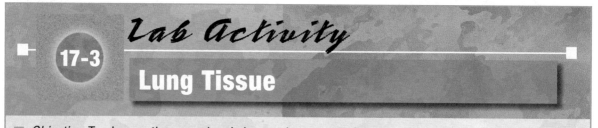

Lab Activity

17-3

Lung Tissue

■ *Objective:* To observe the normal and abnormal structure of the lung tissue
■ *Materials needed:* slides of normal lung tissues, slides of pathological lung tissue showing (1) emphysema and (2) lung cancer, microscope, textbook, paper and pencil

Step 1: Examine the slide of normal lung tissue. Identify, if possible, a bronchiole and alveolus. Draw a sketch of what you see. What is the function of the alveolus?

Step 2: Examine the slide of tissue showing emphysema. Compare the slide to the nor-

mal lung tissue. Describe and record your observations.

Step 3: Examine the slide of cancer tissue. Compare the slide to the normal lung tissue. Describe and record your observations.

DIGESTIVE SYSTEM

Key Words

continues

Key Words continued

parotid glands	pylorospasm	stomach
peptic ulcer	rectum	stomach cancer
periodontal	root	stomatitis
membrane	rugae	taste buds
peristalsis	salivary amylase	transverse colon
peritoneum	sublingual gland	trypsin
peritonitis	submandibular	ulcer
protease	gland	uvula
ptyalin	segmented	vermiform
pulp cavity	movement	appendix
pyloric sphincter	sigmoid colon	villi
pyloric stenosis	steapsin	wisdom teeth

All food which is eaten must be changed into a soluble, absorbable form within the body before it can be used by the cells. This means that certain physical and chemical changes must take place to change the insoluble complex food molecules into simpler soluble ones. These can then be transported by the blood to the cells and be absorbed through the cell membranes. The process of changing complex solid foods into simpler soluble forms which can be absorbed by the body cells is called **digestion.** It is accomplished by the action of various digestive juices containing enzymes. **Enzymes** are chemical substances that promote chemical reactions in living things although they themselves are unaffected by the chemical reactions.

Digestion is performed by the digestive system, which includes the alimentary canal and accessory digestive organs. The **alimentary canal** is also known as the digestive tract or gastrointestinal (GI) tract. The alimentary canal consists of the mouth (oral cavity), pharynx (throat), esophagus (gullet), stomach, small intestine, large intestine (colon), and the anus, Figure 18-1. It is a continuous tube some 30 feet (9 meters) in length, from the mouth to anus.

The accessory organs of digestion are the tongue, teeth, salivary glands, pancreas, liver, and gallbladder.

LAYERS OF THE DIGESTIVE SYSTEM

The walls of the alimentary canal are composed of four layers: (1) the innermost lining, called the mucosa, is made of epithelial cells; (2) the submucosa consists of connective tissue with fibers, blood vessels, and nerve endings; (3) the third layer consists of circular muscle; and (4) the fourth has longitudinal muscle. The mucosa secretes slimy mucus. In some areas, it also produces digestive juices. This slimy mucus lubricates the alimentary canal, aiding in the passage of food. It also insulates the digestive tract from the effects of powerful enzymes while protecting the delicate epithelial cells from abrasive substances within the food.

LINING OF THE DIGESTIVE SYSTEM

The abdominal cavity is lined with a serous membrane called the **peritoneum.** This is a two-layered membrane with the outer side, or parietal, lining the abdominal cavity and the inner side, or visceral, lining covering the outside of each organ in the abdominal cavity. An inflammation of the lining of this cavity caused by disease-producing organisms is called **peritonitis.**

There are two specialized layers of peritoneum. The peritoneum that attaches to the posterior wall of the abdominal cavity is called the **mesentery.** The small intestines are attached to this layer. In the anterior portion of the abdominal cavity a double fold of peritoneum extends down from the greater curvature of the stomach. This hangs over the abdominal organs like a protective apron. This layer contains large amounts of fat and is called the **greater omentum.** The peri-

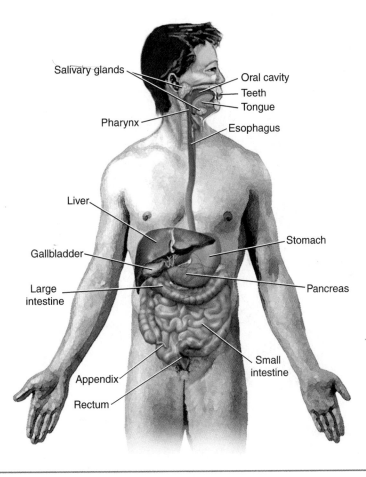

Figure 18-1 *Structures of the digestive system*

toneal structure between the liver and stomach is called the lesser omentum.

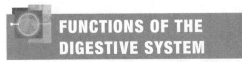

FUNCTIONS OF THE DIGESTIVE SYSTEM

The functions of the digestive system are to change food into forms that the body can use and to eliminate the waste products. These functions are accomplished in four major steps.

1. Break down food physically into smaller pieces

2. Change food chemically by digestive juices into the end products of fat, carbohydrates, and protein

3. To absorb the nutrients into the blood capillaries of the small intestines for use in the body

4. To eliminate the waste products of digestion

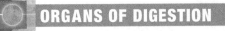

ORGANS OF DIGESTION

There are many organs that contribute to digestion. Each serves a specific function in the process.

Mouth

Food enters the digestive tract through the mouth (oral or **buccal cavity**). The lips (labia) protect the opening to the mouth. The inside of the mouth is covered with a mucous membrane. Its roof consists of a hard and soft palate. The hard palate is hard because it is formed from the maxillary and palatine bones, which are covered by mucous membrane. Behind the hard palate is the soft palate made from a movable mucous membrane fold. The soft palate is an arch-shaped structure, separating the mouth from the nasopharynx. Hanging from the middle of the soft palate is a

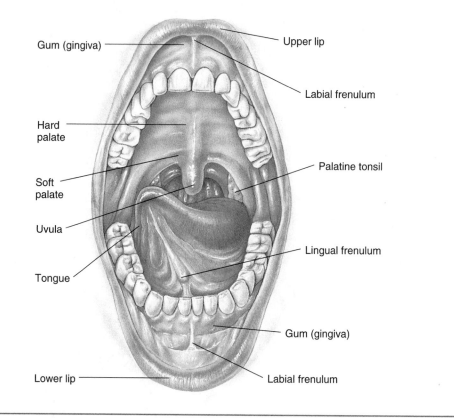

Figure 18-2   *The mouth and its structures*

cone-shaped flap of tissue called the **uvula.** This prevents food from entering the nasal cavity when swallowing, Figure 18-2.

Tongue/Accessory Organ of Digestion

The tongue and its muscles are attached to the floor of the mouth, helping in both chewing and swallowing. The tongue is made from skeletal muscles that lie in many different planes. Because of this, the tongue can be moved in various directions. It is attached to four bones: the hyoid, the mandible, and two temporal bones. On the tongue's epithelial surface are projections called **papillae,** Figure 18-3. There are nerve endings located in many of these papillae forming the sense organs of taste, or **taste buds.** These taste buds respond to bitterness, saltiness, sweetness, and sourness in foods, see Figure 18-3. They are also sensitive to cold, heat, and pressure.

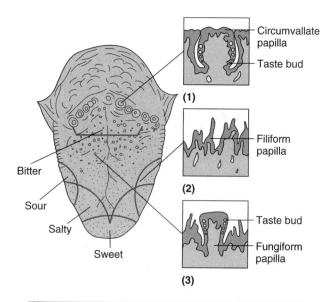

Figure 18-3   *The three types of papillae found on the tongue*

For food to be tasted, it must be in solution. The solution passes through the taste bud openings, stimulating the nerve endings in the taste cells.

The sensation of taste is coupled with the sense of smell. When we experience an odor, it stimulates the olfactory nerve endings in the upper part of the nasal cavity. We may confuse the odor of a food with its flavor when it is simultaneously present in the mouth. A bad cold, with nasal congestion, frequently impedes the ability to taste the flavor of foods, because increased mucus secretions cover the olfactory nerve endings.

Salivary Glands

Saliva is secreted into the oral cavity by three pairs of salivary glands: the parotid, the submandibular, and the sublingual, Figure 18-4. The **parotid salivary glands** are found on both sides of the face, in front and below the ears. They are the largest salivary glands, the ones that become inflamed during an attack of mumps. Chewing, at such times, is painful, because the motion squeezes these tender, inflamed glands. A parotid duct carries its secretion (almost entirely salivary amylase) into the mouth. It opens upon the inner surface of the cheeks, opposite the second molar of the upper jaw.

Below the parotid salivary gland and near the angle of the lower jaw is a **submandibular gland.** This gland is about the size of a walnut and its secretions contain both mucin and ptyalin. The secretions enter the buccal cavity via the submandibular duct at the anterior base of the tongue.

The final pair of salivary glands are the **sublingual glands,** the smallest of the three. They are found under the sides of the tongue. Their secretion consists mainly of mucus and contains no ptyalin.

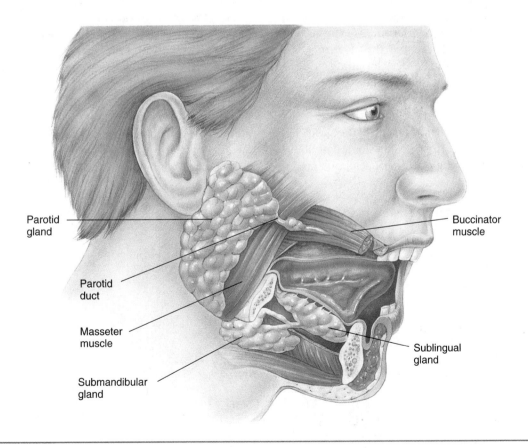

Parotid gland

Parotid duct

Masseter muscle

Submandibular gland

Buccinator muscle

Sublingual gland

Figure 18-4   The salivary glands

TEETH/ACCESSORY ORGAN OF DIGESTION

The **gingivae,** or gums, support and protect the teeth. They are made up of fleshy tissue covered with mucous membrane. This membrane surrounds the narrow portions of the teeth (also called cervix or neck), and covers the structures in the upper and lower jaws.

Food must be thoroughly chewed, or **masticated,** by the teeth. Teeth help break food down into very small morsels, increasing the food's surface area. This activity enables the digestive enzymes to digest the food more efficiently and quickly. During normal growth and development, the human mouth develops two sets of teeth: (1) the deciduous or milk teeth, which are later replaced by (2) the permanent teeth.

Deciduous teeth start to erupt at about 6 months and continue until around 2 years of age. In total, 20 deciduous teeth are cut during the first 2 years. They include four incisors, two canines, and four molars. This relationship is expressed in the dentition formula as shown in Figure 18-5. The **incisors** have sharp edges for biting, the **canines** are pointed for tearing, and the **molars** have ridges, designed for crushing and grinding. There are no premolars among the deciduous teeth. Deciduous teeth may last up to the age of 12.

Permanent teeth begin developing at about the age of 6, pushing out their deciduous predecessors. The last permanent teeth to emerge are the third molars, or **wisdom teeth,** which may appear anywhere from 17 to 25 years of age. In total, the adult mouth develops 32 teeth, 16 in each jaw, Figure 18-5.

The adult mouth has eight premolars, or **bicuspids:** four in the upper and four in the lower jaw. Bicuspids are broad, with two ridges on each crown, and have only two roots. Their design is ideal for grinding food. Figure 18-6 shows the arrangement of the deciduous and permanent teeth.

Structure of a Tooth

Each tooth may be divided into three major parts: the crown, the neck, and the root, Figure 18-7. The **crown** portion is the part of the tooth which is visible; the **neck** is where the tooth enters the gumline; the **root** is embedded in the alveolar processes of the jaw. Helping to anchor the tooth in place is the **periodontal membrane.**

Gum disease or peridontal disease describes bacterial growth and factors that gradually destroy the tissue surrounding and supporting the teeth. Gum disease begins with plaque that can harden into tartar. Tartar can only be removed by professional cleaning. In gingivitis the gums become red, swollen and bleed easily. When gingivitis is untreated it can advance to periodontitis. At this point the inner layer of gum and bone recede

A. The dentition formula for deciduous teeth is:

	Molars	Canine	Incisors	Canine	Molars
Upper jaw	2	1	4	1	2
Lower jaw	2	1	4	1	2

B. The dentition formula for permanent teeth is:

	Molars	Premolars	Canine	Incisors	Canine	Premolars	Molars
Upper jaw	3	2	1	4	1	2	3
Lower jaw	3	2	1	4	1	2	3

Figure 18-5   *Dentition formulas for deciduous and permanent teeth*

(A) PERMANENT TEETH

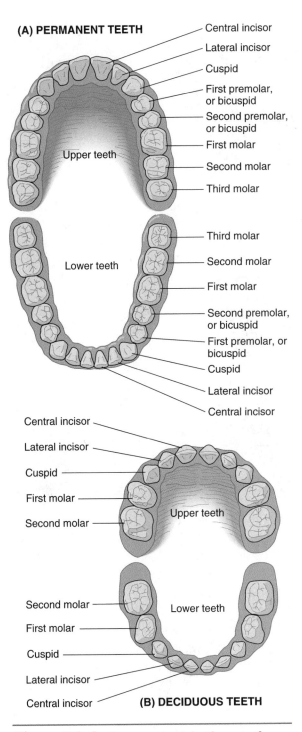

Figure 18-6 *Permanent and deciduous teeth*

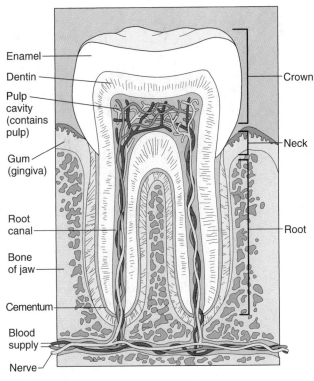

Figure 18-7 *Structure of the tooth*

giene is necessary to prevent tartar formation and periodontitis.

Inside the tooth is the **pulp cavity** which contains the nerves and blood supply. The pulp cavity is surrounded by calcified tissue called **dentin.** In the crown portion the dentin is covered by **enamel.** Enamel is the hardest substance in the body. If the enamel wears down on the surface of the tooth, bacteria may enter and caries or cavities will develop.

ESOPHAGUS

When food is swallowed it enters the upper portion of the esophagus. The **esophagus** is a muscular tube about 25 centimeters (10 inches) long. It begins at the lower end of the pharynx, behind the trachea. It continues downward through the mediastinum, in front of the vertebral column, and passes through the diaphragm. From there the esophagus enters the upper part, or cardiac portion, of the stomach. This point can be located at the end of the sternum, near the level of the xiphoid process.

from the teeth and form pockets which can collect debris and become infected. As the disease progresses there is no longer an anchor for the teeth, they become loose and may fall out. Good oral hy-

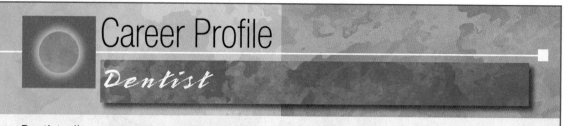

Career Profile

Dentist

Dentists diagnose, prevent, and treat problems of the teeth and tissues of the mouth. They also perform corrective surgery of the gums and supporting bones in gum disease. Dentists extract teeth and make molds and measurements for dentures to replace missing teeth. They may administer anesthetics and write prescriptions for medications. Most dentists are general practitioners. Other dentists may practice in several specialty areas.

Dentists should have good visual memory, excellent judgment of space and shape, and a high degree of manual dexterity. High school students who wish to become dentists should take courses in biology, chemistry, physics, health, and mathematics.

All dentists must be licensed. To qualify for a license, a candidate must graduate from a dental school accredited by the American Dental Association Commission on Dental Accreditation and pass written and practical examinations.

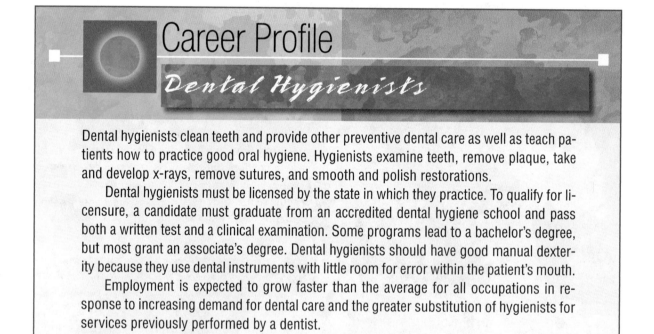

Career Profile

Dental Hygienists

Dental hygienists clean teeth and provide other preventive dental care as well as teach patients how to practice good oral hygiene. Hygienists examine teeth, remove plaque, take and develop x-rays, remove sutures, and smooth and polish restorations.

Dental hygienists must be licensed by the state in which they practice. To qualify for licensure, a candidate must graduate from an accredited dental hygiene school and pass both a written test and a clinical examination. Some programs lead to a bachelor's degree, but most grant an associate's degree. Dental hygienists should have good manual dexterity because they use dental instruments with little room for error within the patient's mouth.

Employment is expected to grow faster than the average for all occupations in response to increasing demand for dental care and the greater substitution of hygienists for services previously performed by a dentist.

The esophageal walls have four layers: the mucosa, submucosa, muscular, and external serous layer. The muscles in the upper third are voluntary and the lower portion is smooth muscle, or involuntary.

STOMACH

The **stomach** is found in the upper part of the abdominal cavity, just to the left of and below the diaphragm. The shape and position are determined

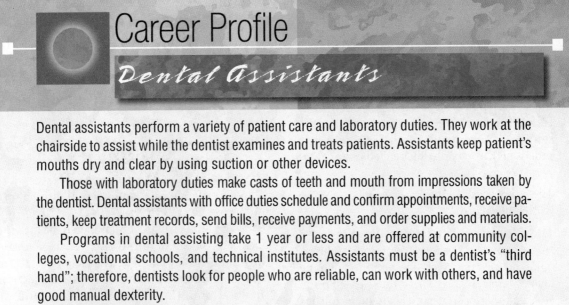

Career Profile

Dental Assistants

Dental assistants perform a variety of patient care and laboratory duties. They work at the chairside to assist while the dentist examines and treats patients. Assistants keep patient's mouths dry and clear by using suction or other devices.

Those with laboratory duties make casts of teeth and mouth from impressions taken by the dentist. Dental assistants with office duties schedule and confirm appointments, receive patients, keep treatment records, send bills, receive payments, and order supplies and materials.

Programs in dental assisting take 1 year or less and are offered at community colleges, vocational schools, and technical institutes. Assistants must be a dentist's "third hand"; therefore, dentists look for people who are reliable, can work with others, and have good manual dexterity.

Employment is good. Population growth and greater retention of natural teeth by middle-aged and older people will fuel the demand for dental services.

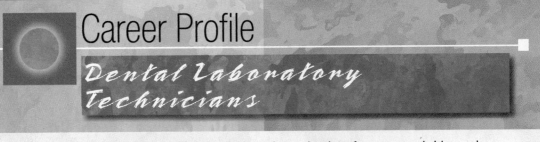

Career Profile

Dental Laboratory Technicians

Dental laboratory technicians fill prescriptions from dentists for crowns, bridges, dentures, and other dental prosthetics.

Training in dental laboratory technology is available through community colleges, vocational schools, and technical institutes. Programs vary in length. A high degree of manual dexterity, good vision, and the ability to recognize very fine color shadings and variations in shape are necessary.

by several factors. These include the amount of food contained within the stomach, the stage of digestion, the position of a person's body, and the pressure exerted upon the stomach from the intestines below.

The stomach is divided into three portions: the upper part or fundus, the middle section called the body or greater curvature, and the lower portion called the pylorus. The opening from the esophagus into the stomach is through a circle of muscle, called the **cardiac sphincter,** which controls passage of food into the stomach. It is called the cardiac sphincter because of its proximity to the heart. Toward the other end of the stomach lies the **pyloric sphincter** valve which regulates entrance of food into the **duodenum** (the first part of the small intestine). Sometimes the pyloric sphincter valve fails to relax in infants. In such cases, food remaining in the stomach does not get completely digested and eventually is vomited. This condition is called **pylorospasm.**

The stomach wall consists of four layers: mucous, submucous, muscular, and serous layers.

1. The mucus coat is the innermost layer. It is a thick layer made up of small gastric glands embedded in connective tissue. When the stomach is not distended with food, the gastric mucosa is thrown into folds called **rugae,** Figure 18-8A.

2. The submucosa coat is made of loose areolar connective tissue.

3. The muscular coat consists of three layers of smooth muscle: the outer, longitudinal layer; a middle, circular layer; and an inner, oblique layer, Figure 18-8A. These muscles help the stomach perform peristalsis which pushes food into the small intestine.

4. The serosa is the thick outer layer covering the stomach. It is continuous with the peritoneum. The serosa and peritoneum meet at certain points, surrounding the organs around the stomach and holding them in a kind of sling.

Gastric Juices

The gastric mucosa contains millions of gastric glands which secrete gastric juice necessary for digestion, Figure 18-8B.

- Enteroendocrine glands secrete gastrin which in turn stimulates cells to produce hydrochloric acid (HCL) and pepsinogen.

- Parietal cells produce HCL acid which converts pepsinogen into pepsin and destroys bacteria and microorganisms that enter the stomach. It is the body's natural sterilizer.

- Parietal cells also produce the intrinsic factor, an element necessary for the absorption of vitamin B_{12}; without it, a condition known as pernicious anemia exists.

- Chief type cells produce pepsinogen which converts to pepsin. The enzyme pepsin breaks down protein into smaller pieces called protease and peptone.

- Mucus cells secrete alkaline mucus which helps neutralize the effects of HCL acid and the other digestive juices.

- Rennin is found in infants and children, but not adults. It prepares milk proteins for digestion by other enzymes.

SMALL INTESTINE

The small intestine has the same four layers as the stomach: the mucosa, submucosa, muscle layer, and serosa, Figure 18-9.

The final preparation of food to be absorbed occurs in the small intestine. This coiled portion of the alimentary canal can be as long as 20 feet. The small intestine is divided into three sections: the duodenum, the **jejunum,** and the **ileum.** The small intestine is held in place by the mesentery. The small intestine lining secretes digestive juices and is covered with villi which absorb the end products of digestion, Figure 18-10.

The first segment of the small intestine is the duodenum. This 12-inch structure curves around the head of the pancreas. A few inches into the duodenum is the ampulla of Vater, which is the site where the pancreatic duct and the common bile duct of the liver enter. The pancreatic duct empties the digestive juices of the pancreas and the common bile duct empties bile from the liver.

The next section of the small intestine is the jejunum, which is about 8 feet long, and the ileum, which is 10 to 12 feet long.

Digestive Juices in the Small Intestines

- Enzymes, secretin, and cholecystokinin stimulate the digestive juices of the pancreas, liver, and gallbladder.

- Pancreatic juices, namely **protease** or **trypsin** which breaks down protein to amino acids, **amylase** or **amylopsin** which breaks down starches to glucose, and **lipase** or **steapsin** which breaks down fats to fatty acids and glycerol. The pancreatic juices also contain sodium bicarbonate which

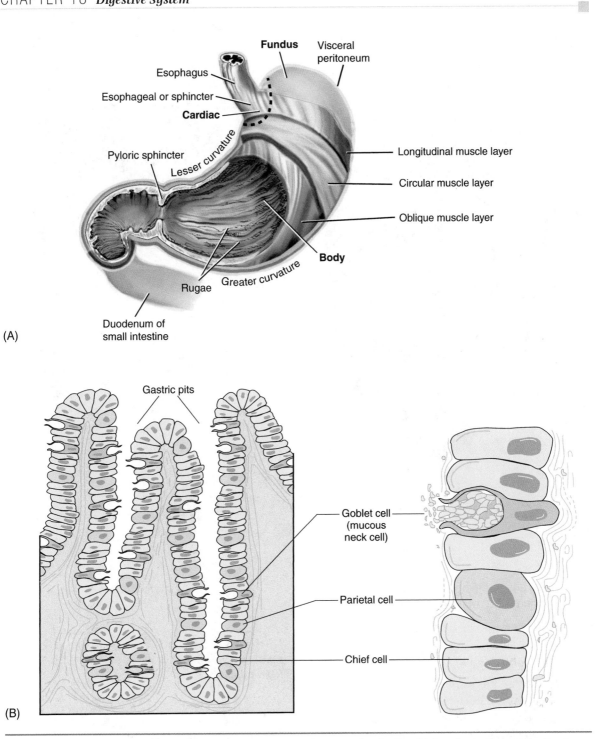

Figure 18-8 *(A) Parts of the stomach; (B) three types of gastric gland cells which make up the gastric glands that line the stomach*

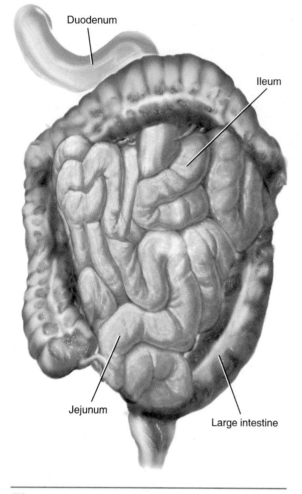

Figure 18-9 *The small intestine*

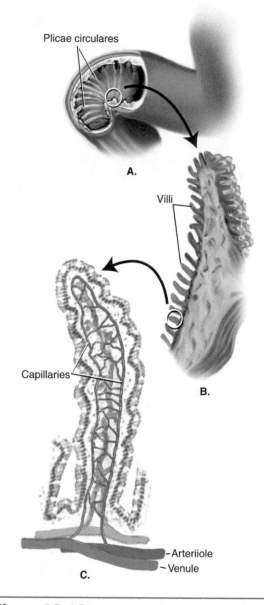

Figure 18-10 *Structures of absorption in the small intestine: (A) plicae circulares; (B) villi; and (C) capillaries*

neutralizes the food content of the stomach which is high in acid.

- **Bile** is necessary to break down or emulsify fat into smaller fat globules to be digested by lipase and steapsin.

- Intestinal juices secreted by the cells of the small intestine—including maltase, lactase, and sucrase—change starch into glucose; peptidase changes protease and peptone into amino acids; and steapsin changes fat into fatty acids and glycerol.

The combined action of pancreatic juice, bile, and intestinal juice completes the process of changing carbohydrates first into starch then into glucose, protein into amino acids, and fats into fatty acids and glycerol, Figure 18-11. The end products of digestion are now ready for absorption. See Table 18-1.

Absorption in the Small Intestine

Absorption is possible because the lining of the small intestine is not smooth. It is covered with millions of tiny projections called **villi.** Each mi-

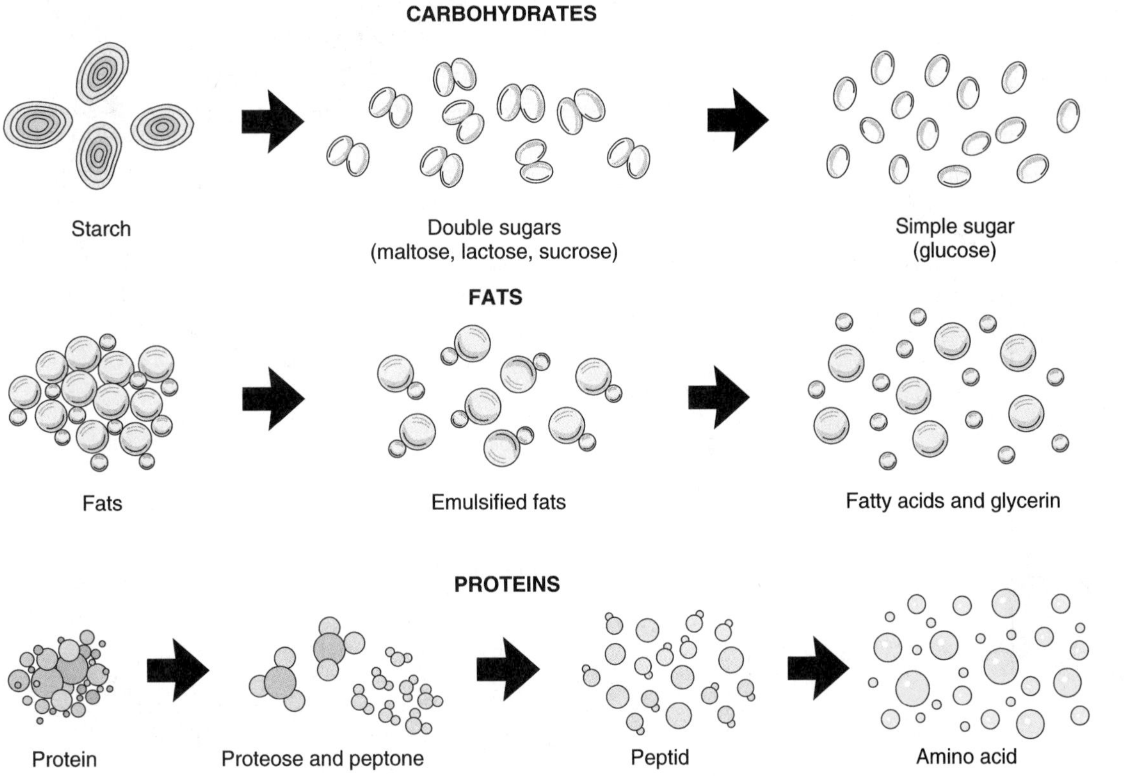

CARBOHYDRATES

Starch → Double sugars (maltose, lactose, sucrose) → Simple sugar (glucose)

FATS

Fats → Emulsified fats → Fatty acids and glycerin

PROTEINS

Protein → Proteose and peptone → Peptid → Amino acid

Figure 18-11 *Phases in the digestion of starch, fat, and protein*

croscopic villus contains a network of blood and lymph capillaries, see Figure 18-10. The digested portion of the food passes through the villi into the bloodstream and on to the body cells. The undigestible portion passes on to the large intestine.

PANCREAS/ACCESSORY ORGAN OF DIGESTION

The pancreas is a feather-shaped organ located behind the stomach, Figure 18-12. It functions both as an exocrine gland, meaning it has a duct that carries away its secretion, and as an endocrine gland, meaning it is ductless and the secretions are emptied directly into the bloodstream. The digestive juices are carried by the pancreatic duct into the duodenum, at the sphincter of Oddi.

LIVER/ACCESSORY ORGAN OF DIGESTION

The **liver** is the largest organ in the body. It is located below the diaphragm, in the upper right quadrant of the abdomen, see Figure 18-12. The portal vein carries the products of digestion from the small intestine to the liver. Some of the liver's many functions are as follows:

- Manufacture bile, a yellow to green fluid, which is necessary for the digestion of fat. About 800 to 1,000 cc of bile is produced daily. Bile contains bile salts, bile pigments (mainly **bilirubin,** which comes from the breakdown of the hemoglobin molecule), cholesterol, phospholipids, and some electrolytes. The **hepatic duct** from the liver joins with the **cystic duct** of the gallbladder

Table 18-1 *Summary of Digestive Enzymes Involved in Human Digestion*

ORGAN	JUICE	GLAND	ENZYME(S)	ACTION	ADDITIONAL FACTS
Mouth	Saliva	Salivary	Amylase found in ptyalin	Starch → Maltose	Physical and chemical hydrolysis Mucous flow starts here and continues throughout digestive tract
Esophagus	Mucus	Mucus	None	Lubrication of food	Peristalsis begins here
Stomach	Gastric juice along with HCl acid	Gastric	Protease, pepsin	Proteins → peptones and proteoses	Gastrin activates the gastric glands HCl supplies an acidic medium and kills bacteria Temporary food storage
Small intestine	Intestinal	Intestinal	Peptiadases	Peptones and proteoses into amino acids	Absorption of end products occurs in small intestine
			Maltase	Maltose → glucose	Villi facilitates absorption
			Lactase	Lactose → glucose and galactose	
			Sucrase	Sucrose → glucose and fructose	
			Lipase	Fats → fatty acids and glycerol	
	Bile	Liver	None	Emulsifies fat	Neutralizes stomach acid
	Pancreatic	Pancreas	Protease (trypsin)	Proteins → peptones and amino acids	Secretin stimulates the flow of pancreatic juice
			Amylase (amylopsin)	Starch → maltose	
			Lipase (steapsin)	Fats → fatty acids and glycerol	
			Nucleases	Nucleic acids (DNA/RNA) nucleotides	

to form the **common bile duct**, which carries the bile to the duodenum. If this duct is blocked, bile may then enter the blood stream causing **jaundice**, which gives the skin and sclera of the eyes a yellow color.

- Produce and store glucose in the form of **glycogen.**

- Detoxify alcohol, drugs, and other harmful substances.

- Manufacture blood proteins such as fibrinogen and prothrombin which are necessary for blood clotting, albumin which is needed for fluid balance in the cells, and globulin which is necessary for immunity.

- Prepare urea, the chief waste product of protein metabolism, from the breakdown of amino acids.

- Store vitamins A, D, and B complex.

- Breaks down hormones no longer useful to the body.

- Removes worn-out red blood cells from circulation and recycles the iron content.

GALLBLADDER/ACCESSORY ORGAN OF DIGESTION

The **gallbladder** is a small green organ in the inferior surface of the liver, see Figure 18-12. It

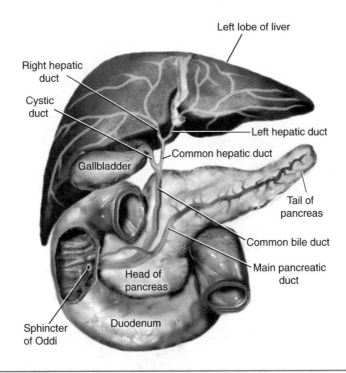

Figure 18-12 *Liver, gallbladder, and pancreas*

stores and concentrates bile when it is not needed by the body. When food high in fat enters the duodenum at the sphincter of Oddi bile is released by the gallbladder through the cystic duct.

LARGE INTESTINE

The ileum empties its intestinal **chyme** (semiliquid food) into the side wall of the large intestine through an opening called the **ileocecal valve.** This valve permits passage of the chyme to the large intestine and prevents the backflow of chyme into the ileum. The large intestine is about 5 feet long and it is approximately 2 inches in diameter. The secretion of the colon mucosa is large amounts of mucus, which lubricates the passage of fecal material. The longitudinal smooth muscle layer is in three bands called tenae coli. The remainder of the colon is gathered to fit these bands giving the colon a puckered appearance. These little puckers or pockets are called haustra providing for more surface area in the colon. The **colon,** as it is also called, frames the abdomen, Figure 18-13.

Cecum and Appendix

Located slightly below the ileocecal valve, in the lower right portion of the abdomen, is a blind pouch called the **cecum.**

To the lower left of the cecum is the **vermiform appendix.** The appendix is a fingerlike projection protruding into the abdominal cavity, see Figure 18-13. It has no digestive function.

Ascending, Transverse, and Descending Colon

The colon continues upward, along the right side of the abdominal cavity, to the underside of the liver (hepatic flexure), forming the **ascending colon.** Then it veers to the left of the abdominal cavity, across the abdominal cavity, to a point below the spleen (splenic flexure), forming the **transverse colon.** The **descending colon** travels down from the splenic flexure on the left side of the abdominal cavity. As the descending colon reaches the left iliac region, it enters the pelvis in

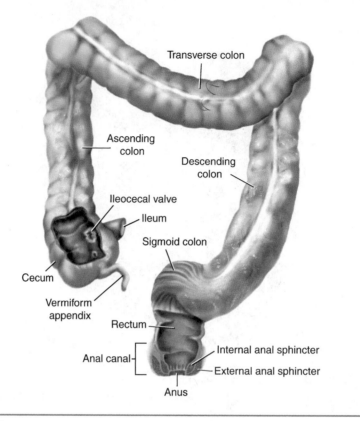

Figure 18-13 *The large intestine*

an S-shaped bend. This section is known as the **sigmoid colon,** which extends some 7 or 8 inches as the **rectum.** The rectum opens into the anus, see Figure 18-13.

Anal Canal

The anal canal is the last portion of the large intestine. Its external opening is the **anus.** The anus is guarded by two anal sphincter muscles. One is an internal sphincter of smooth, involuntary muscle; the other is an external sphincter of striated, voluntary muscle. Both of these remain contracted to close the anal opening until defecation takes place. The mucus membrane lining the anal canal is folded into vertical folds called rectal columns. Within each rectal column is an artery and a vein. The condition leading to inflammation or enlargement of the rectal column veins is known as **hemorrhoids.**

GENERAL OVERVIEW OF DIGESTION

Food enters the gastrointestinal tract via the mouth. In the oral cavity, food is mechanically digested by the cutting, ripping, and grinding action of the teeth. Chemical digestion of carbohydrates is initiated by the secretion of saliva containing a digestive enzyme. Then, the action of the saliva and rolling motion of the tongue turn the food into a soft, pliable ball called a **bolus.** The bolus slides down to the throat (pharynx) to be swallowed. Next it travels through the esophagus into the stomach. Food is pushed along the esophagus by rhythmic, muscular contractions called **peristalsis.** From the stomach, peristaltic contractions continue to push the food into the small intestine. The nervous system stimulates gland activity and peristalsis.

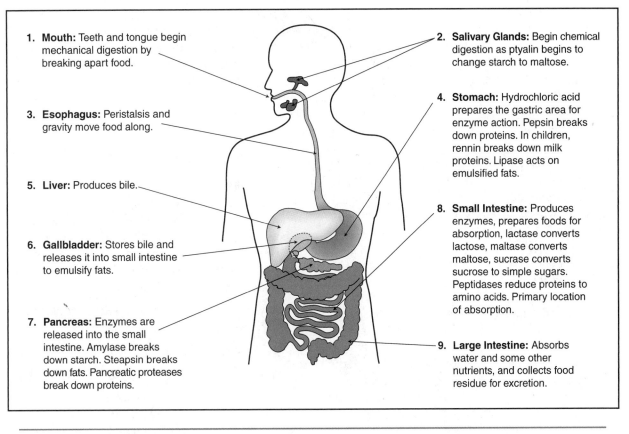

1. **Mouth:** Teeth and tongue begin mechanical digestion by breaking apart food.

2. **Salivary Glands:** Begin chemical digestion as ptyalin begins to change starch to maltose.

3. **Esophagus:** Peristalsis and gravity move food along.

4. **Stomach:** Hydrochloric acid prepares the gastric area for enzyme action. Pepsin breaks down proteins. In children, rennin breaks down milk proteins. Lipase acts on emulsified fats.

5. **Liver:** Produces bile.

6. **Gallbladder:** Stores bile and releases it into small intestine to emulsify fats.

8. **Small Intestine:** Produces enzymes, prepares foods for absorption, lactase converts lactose, maltase converts maltose, sucrase converts sucrose to simple sugars. Peptidases reduce proteins to amino acids. Primary location of absorption.

7. **Pancreas:** Enzymes are released into the small intestine. Amylase breaks down starch. Steapsin breaks down fats. Pancreatic proteases break down proteins.

9. **Large Intestine:** Absorbs water and some other nutrients, and collects food residue for excretion.

Figure 18-14 *Overview of digestion*

Each part of the alimentary canal contributes to the overall digestive process. Protein digestion, for instance, is initiated by the stomach. Then the small intestine starts and finishes fat digestion, and completes the digestion of carbohydrates and proteins. Numerous digestive glands are located in the stomach and small intestine, which secrete digestive juices containing powerful enzymes to chemically digest the food. Due to digestion, insoluble food becomes a soluble fluid substance. This substance is then transported across the small intestinal wall into the bloodstream.

Circulated and absorbed through the blood capillaries into the interstitial fluid and finally into the body cells, the soluble food molecules are utilized for energy, repair, and production of new cells. The remaining undigested substances (**feces**) pass into the large intestine and leave the alimentary canal via the anus, Figure 18-14.

Action in the Mouth

Food is broken down by the teeth and mixed with saliva. Saliva contains **salivary amylase,** also known as **ptyalin,** which converts the starches in carbohydrates into simple sugars. For example, if you place a cracker in your mouth for a few minutes it will have no taste because it is being broken down into glucose. Saliva is affected by the nervous system; just thinking of food will cause your mouth to water or the opposite effect can occur—a dry mouth when you are nervous or frightened.

Action in the Pharynx

Food leaves the mouth and travels to the pharynx. This structure serves as the common passageway for food and air.

Swallowing. Swallowing, or **deglutition,** is a complex process involving the constrictor muscles of the pharynx. It begins as a voluntary process, changing to an involuntary process as the food enters the esophagus. When we swallow, the tip of the tongue arches slightly and moves backward and upward. This action forces the food against the hard palate; simultaneously, the soft palate and the uvula shut off the opening to the nasopharynx. Food is thus prevented from entering the nasopharynx.

In swallowing, the constrictor muscles of the pharynx contract, pushing food into the upper part of the esophagus. At the same time, other pharyngeal muscles raise the larynx causing the epiglottis to cover the trachea (windpipe) to prevent food from entering it. If we talk while eating, the epiglottis may not close and food enters the trachea.

The act of swallowing is voluntary. But, as a bolus of food passes over the posterior part of the tongue and stimulates receptors in the walls of the pharynx, swallowing becomes an involuntary reflex action. With the contraction of the pharyngeal muscles, followed by the contraction of the muscles lining the esophagus, food passes down into the stomach. (When you swallow, place your fingers near the trachea; you can feel the structure move upward.)

Action in the Esophagus

Food is pushed through the esophagus by peristalsis. This action explains why you can swallow even standing on your head; once food enters the esophagus it goes to the stomach and it is not affected by gravity.

Action in the Stomach

When the food reaches the stomach, the cardiac sphincter relaxes and allows food to enter. About 2 to 3 quarts of digestive juices are produced daily which may explain the gurgling noises you hear at times. When food enters, the gastric juices are released and begin to work on proteins. Salivary amylase continues its work in the stomach.

The action of the gastric juices is helped by the churning of the stomach walls. The semiliquid food is called chyme. The chyme leaves the stomach through the pyloric sphincter which acts as a gatekeeper. This action allows a small squirt of

chyme into the duodenum from time to time. Food takes about 2 to 4 hours to leave the stomach. Food moves through the stomach by peristalsis; vomiting is an action which occurs because of reverse peristalsis. The only known substances to be absorbed in the stomach are alcohol and some medications.

Action in the Small Intestine

In the small intestine the process of digestion is completed and absorption occurs. Bile emulsifies fat to prepare it for digestion by pancreatic and intestinal juices. Pancreatic juices neutralize the acidic chyme and completes the digestion of carbohydrates, fats, and proteins. (Refer to Figure 18-11.) The end products of digestion are as follows:

- Carbohydrates are converted to simple sugars such as glucose.

- Proteins are broken down into amino acids.

- Fats are changed into fatty acids and glycerol.

The glucose, amino acids, fatty acids, and glycerol are then absorbed through the villi of the small intestine into the blood and lymph capillaries. The portal vein transports the blood from the small intestine and takes it to the liver where it is distributed to the organs of the body.

The passage of food through the small intestine occurs because of peristalsis and **segmented movement.** Segmented movement is when single segments of the intestine alternate between contraction and relaxation. Because inactive segments exist between active ones, the food is moved forward and backward—it is mixed as well as propelled. It takes about 6 to 8 hours for food to go through the small intestine; undigested foods then reach the ileocecal valve and enter the large intestine.

Action in the Large Intestine

The large intestine is concerned with water absorption, bacterial action, fecal formation, gas formation, and defecation. The purpose of these functions is to regulate the body's water balance while storing and excreting waste products of digestion.

Absorption. The large intestine aids in the regulation of the body's water balance by absorbing large quantities of water back into the bloodstream. The water is drawn from the undigested food and indigestible material (e.g., cellulose) that pass through the colon. The large intestine absorbs vitamins B complex and K.

Bacterial action. A few hours following the birth of an infant, the lining of the colon starts to accumulate bacteria. These bacteria persist throughout the person's lifetime. The bacteria multiply rapidly, to form the bacterial population or flora, of the colon. The intestinal bacteria are harmless (nonpathogenic) to their host. They act upon undigested food remains, turning them into acids, amines, gases, and other waste products. These decomposed products are excreted through the colon. Another benefit of the bacterial action is the synthesis (formation) of moderate amounts of B-complex vitamins and vitamin K (needed for blood clotting).

Gas formation. Most people produce 1 to 3 pints of gas per day and pass it through the rectum (**flatulence**). Gas is produced by swallowed air and the normal breakdown of food. The unpleasant odor of flatulence comes from bacteria in the large intestine, which produces gas-containing sulfur or methane. Swallowed air usually remains in the stomach and is relieved by burping and belching.

Research has not shown why some foods produce gas in one person and not in another or why some people produce methane gas. Some foods that produce gas are beans, vegetables such as broccoli and cabbage, fruit, whole grains, milk and milk products, and foods containing the artificial sweetener sorbitol.

Lactose is the natural sugar found in milk and milk products. Some people have low levels of the enzyme lactase which is necessary to digest lactose. As people age, their level of lactase decreases, which may explain why older people experience discomfort after ingesting milk products.

Diet modification may reduce the amount of gas produced; however, it is important to remember that some of the foods that produce gas provide essential nutrients.

Fecal formation. Initially, the undigested or indigestible material in the colon contains a lot of water and is in a liquid state. Due to water absorption and bacterial action, it is subsequently converted into a semisolid form, called feces.

Feces consist of bacteria, waste products from the blood, acids, amines, inorganic salts, gases, mucus, and cellulose. Amines are waste products of amino acids. The gases are ammonia, carbon dioxide, hydrogen, hydrogen sulfide, and methane. The characteristically foul odor of feces derives from these substances.

Cellulose is the fibrous part of plants that humans are unable to digest. It contributes to the bulk of the feces. This bulk stimulates the muscular activity of the colon, resulting in defecation. Regular defecation (regularity) can be promoted by exercising daily and eating foods containing cellulose such as whole-grain cereals, fruits, and vegetables. These foods supply the necessary bulk to initiate bowel movements.

Defecation. Once approximately every 12 hours the fecal material moves into the lower bowel (lower colon and rectum) by means of a series of long contractions called mass peristalsis. However, frequency of bowel movements in healthy people varies from three movements a day to three a week. When the rectum becomes distended with the accumulation of feces, a **defecation** reflex is triggered. Nerve endings in the rectum are stimulated, and a nerve impulse is transmitted to the spinal cord. From the spinal cord, nerve impulses are sent to the colon, rectum, and internal anal sphincter. This causes the colon and rectal muscles to contract and the internal sphincter to relax, resulting in emptying of the bowels.

For defecation to occur, the external anal sphincter must also be relaxed. The external anal sphincter surrounds and guards the outer opening of the anus and is under conscious control. Due to this control, defecation can be prevented when inconvenient, despite the defecation reflex. However, if this urge is continually ignored, it lessens or disappears totally, resulting in constipation. Temporary relief from constipation may be obtained with the use of laxatives and cathartics. (A laxative is a substance that induces gentle bowel movement; a cathartic stimulates more vigorous movement, which may eventually reduce the bowel's muscle tone.)

Effects of Aging on The Digestive System

Changes most frequently associated with aging are a decrease in the sensory ability of the taste buds and a reduction in the production of saliva. Dry mouth is also a side effect of more than 400 commonly used medicines including drugs for high blood pressure, antidepressants, and antihistamines. In addition, there is sometimes a loss of teeth due to gum disease or decay. These changes lead to a loss of appetite and result in poor nutrition.

There is a slowdown in peristalsis from the esophagus to the colon. It may become more difficult to swallow, digest food, and eliminate the waste products of digestion. This slowdown in peristalsis may also lead to the development of diverticulosis and chronic constipation.

METABOLISM

After digestion and absorption, nutrients are carried by the blood to the cells of the body. Within the cells, nutrients are changed into energy through a complex process called metabolism. During aerobic metabolism, nutrients are combined with oxygen within each cell. This process is known as oxidation. Oxidation ultimately reduces carbohydrates to carbon dioxide and water; proteins are reduced to carbon dioxide, water and nitrogen. Anaerobic metabolism reduces fats without the use of oxygen. The complete oxidation of carbohydrates, proteins and fats is commonly called the Krebs cycle.

As nutrients are oxidized, energy is released. When this released energy is used to build new substances from simpler ones, the process is called anabolism. An example of anabolism is the formation of new body tissues. When released energy is used to reduce substances to simpler ones, the process is called catabolism. This building up and breaking down of substances (metabolism) is a continuous process within the body and requires a continuous supply of nutrients.

Metabolism is governed primarily by the hormones secreted by the thyroid gland. These secretions are *triiodothyronine* (T_3) and *thyroxine* (T_4). When the thyroid gland secretes too much of these hormones, a condition known as hyperthyroidism may result. In such a case, the body metabolizes its food too quickly, and weight is lost. When too little T_4 and T_3 are secreted, the condition hypothyroidism may occur. In this case, the body metabolizes food too slowly and the patient tends to become sluggish and accumulates fat.

COMMON DISORDERS OF THE DIGESTIVE SYSTEM

In times of stress it is not unusual to have "butterflies" in the stomach, nausea, or another type of distress associated with the digestive system. Diseases of the digestive system are responsible for the hospitalization of more people in the United States than any other group of diseases. In recent years, researchers have begun to shed some light on the puzzling aspects of digestive diseases. Diseases once thought to be caused by emotional problems may in fact be caused by viruses interacting with the body's immune system. Some of these diseases are briefly discussed in this section.

Stomatitis is an inflammation of the soft tissues of the mouth cavity. Pain and salivation may occur also.

Gastroesophageal reflux disease (GERD) is a disorder that affects the sphincter muscle connecting

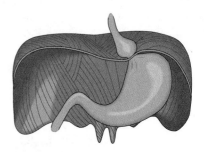

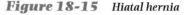

Figure 18-15   *Hiatal hernia*

the esophagus with the stomach. In GERD, the sphincter muscle is weak or relaxes inappropriately allowing the stomach's contents to flow up into the esophagus. This is a common occurrence in people who suffer from hiatal hernia or heartburn.

Hiatal hernia, or rupture, occurs when the stomach protrudes above the diaphragm through the esophagus opening, Figure 18-15. Hiatal hernia is not uncommon in people over the age of 50. Changes in the diet may relieve the symptoms; surgery is not usually required.

Heartburn or acid indigestion results from a backflow of the highly acidic gastric juice into the lower end of the esophagus. This irritates the lining of the esophagus, causing a burning sensation. Heartburn may be experienced on a daily basis by some people and 25% of all pregnant women experience heartburn.

Temporary relief from heartburn can be obtained by doing the following:

- Stop smoking.

- Take nonprescription antacids to provide temporary relief.

- Avoid lying down for 2 to 3 hours after eating.

- Avoid coffee, chocolate, citrus fruits and juices, fried and fatty foods, and tomato products.

Pyloric stenosis is a narrowing of the pyloric sphincter at the lower end of the stomach. It is often found in infants. Projectile vomiting may result; surgery is often necessary.

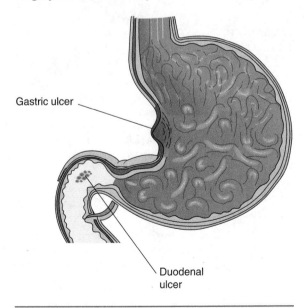

Gastric ulcer

Duodenal ulcer

Figure 18-16   *Peptic ulcer*

Gastritis is an acute or chronic inflammation on the stomach lining.

Gastroenteritis is the inflammation of the mucus membrane lining of the stomach and intestinal tract. A common cause is a virus which causes diarrhea and vomiting for 24 to 36 hours. If this condition persists, dehydration may occur. Treatment is symptomatic.

Enteritis is the inflammation of the intestine that may be caused by a bacterial, viral, or protozoan infection. Enteritis can also be caused by an allergic reaction to certain foods or food poisoning.

An **ulcer** is a sore or lesion that forms in the mucosal lining of the stomach or duodenum where acid and pepsin are present. Ulcers found in the stomach are called gastric ulcers; those in the duodenum are called duodenal ulcers. In general, both types are referred to as **peptic ulcers,** Figure 18-16. Research shows that most ulcers develop as a result of an infection with bacteria called *Helicobacter pylori* (*H. pylori*).

Other factors associated with peptic ulcer include cigarette smoking, intake of food and beverages containing caffeine, alcohol consumption, and physical stress associated with major injuries or illness. Nonsteroidal anti-inflammatory drugs may make the stomach vulnerable to the harmful effects of acid and pepsin.

The most common symptom of an ulcer is a burning pain in the abdomen between the sternum and navel. The pain occurs between meals and in the early hours of the morning. It may be relieved by eating or taking an antacid.

Ulcers are diagnosed by x-ray and testing for the *H. pylori* bacteria. If the cause is *H. pylori*, antibiotics are the treatment. Elimination of the bacteria allows the ulcer to heal and not recur.

Treatment for ulcers from other causes include the use of H_2 blockers. These drugs reduce the amount of acid the stomach produces by blocking **histamine,** a powerful stimulant of acid secretion. Initially, treatment with H_2 blockers lasts about 6 to 8 weeks. However, since this type of ulcer recurs in about 50% to 80% of cases, many people must continue therapy for years.

Additional treatment includes the use of drugs which reduces the stomach's acid production, mucosal protective medications, and lifestyle changes.

Inflammatory bowel disease (IBD) is a disorder that affects about 1 million Americans, according to a Mayo Clinic report. The most frustrating symptom is chronic diarrhea. Crohn's disease and ulcerative colitis are two separate inflammatory diseases, which are considered IBDs.

Medical Highlight

Swallowable Imaging Capsule

In August 2001, the FDA approved a swallowable camera-in-a-capsule that snaps pictures as it travels through the digestive tract. The device offers a more friendly technique for detecting abnormalities in the small intestine. The camera uses wireless technology to beam back colored pictures of the intestines as it winds its way through the digestive tract.

The video "pill," made by the Given Imaging Company, is called M2A Swallowable Imaging. The capsule travels through the body by the natural movement of the digestive tract and is excreted in 8 to 72 hours. The patient is encouraged to walk to help its movement through the system. The camera beams its pictures to an external receiver the patient wears on a waistband. The strength of the signal indicates the capsule's location.

The pill will not replace colonoscopies, because the battery does not last long enough to return images from the large intestine; nor can it be used for anyone known or suspected to have intestinal obstructions, including problems such as fistulas or strictures. People with anemia or unexplained blood in their stool might be candidates for the pill when standard endoscopic exams fail to diagnose the problem.

- Crohn's disease can occur anywhere in the digestive tract. It may occur simultaneously in different locations. Crohn's disease generally penetrates every layer of tissue in the affected area. Patients with Crohn's may have remissions and exacerbations (flare-ups).

- Ulcerative colitis is typically found in the colon and rectum. It usually affects only the innermost lining of the colon and rectum.

The cause of IBD is unknown. The symptoms are similar, chronic diarrhea, vomiting, abdominal cramping, blood in the stool, weight loss, and fatigue. Diagnosis may involve blood tests and examinations of the digestive tract including a possible colonoscopy. Treatment is mainly drug therapy including anti-inflammatory drugs, immune modulators, and antibiotics. Life treatments include diet modification, high fluid intake, and the reduction and management of stress. Surgical treatment may be necessary for about 70% of patients with Crohn's disease and for about 20% of patients with ulcerative colitis.

Appendicitis occurs when the veriform appendix becomes inflamed, Figure 18-17. If it ruptures, the bacteria from the appendix can spread to the peritoneal cavity causing peritonitis.

Hepatitis is an inflammation of the liver. Clinical symptoms are fever, nausea, anorexia, and jaundice. The different strains of viral hepatitis include

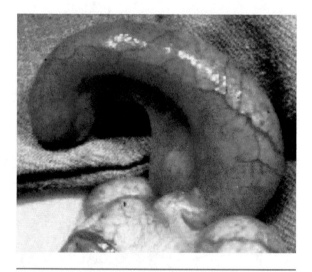

Figure 18-17 *Appendicitis* *(Courtesy of The Division of Pediatric Surgery, Brown Medical School, Providence, RI)*

hepatitis A, B, C, D, and E. Standard Precautions are followed in the care of all hepatitis patients.

- Hepatitis A is caused by the hepatitis A virus (HAV). This viral infection of the liver often spreads through contaminated water or food.

- Hepatitis B is a viral infection caused by the hepatitis B virus (HBV) found only in the blood. It is transmitted by a blood transfusion contaminated with the virus or through the use of inadequately sterilized needles, syringes, or surgical equipment. It is prevalent among drug addicts who use contaminated needles. Treatment is with the drugs interferon and ribavirin. A vaccine is available for hepatitis B and it is recommended for all ages; babies are now receiving the vaccine as part of their regular immunization program.

■ Hepatitis C is a viral infection caused by the hepatitis C virus (HCV). Intravenous drug use is the single biggest risk factor for Hepatitis C. Blood screening procedures have all but ended the transmission of Hepatitis C through contaminated blood. A hepatitis C epidemic has been steadily growing over the past 20 years. It currently affects over 4 million Americans. Most hepatitis C patients are unaware of their infection as they can be symptom free for maybe a decade. The disease can be life threatening; the consequences are a severely damaged liver. A combination of the drugs ribavirin capsules and interferon injections is the standard of care for chronic hepatitis C patients.

■ Hepatitis D virus (HDV) requires coinfection with the B type.

■ Hepatitis E virus (HEV) is transmitted through intestinal excretions.

Cirrhosis is a chronic, progressive inflammatory disease of the liver, characterized by replacement of normal tissue with fibrous connective tissue. Three-fourths of cirrhosis is caused by excessive alcohol consumption. Viral hepatitis may also cause cirrhosis.

Cholecystitis is the inflammation of the gallbladder. This condition may cause blockage of the cystic duct which would inhibit the release of stored bile.

Gallstones or cholelithiasis, are collections of crystallized cholesterol in the gallbladder. These are combined with bile salts and bile pigments. Gallstones can block the bile duct, causing pain and digestive disorders; pain may also occur in the back between the shoulder blades. In such cases, bile cannot flow into the small intestine to help in fat emulsification, digestion, and absorption. Most gallstones are small and may pass with undigested food. However, the larger and obstructive ones must be surgically removed. The gallstones and/or gallbladder may be removed through laparoscopic surgery. This procedure does not require the stomach muscles to be cut, resulting in less pain, quicker healing, and fewer complications.

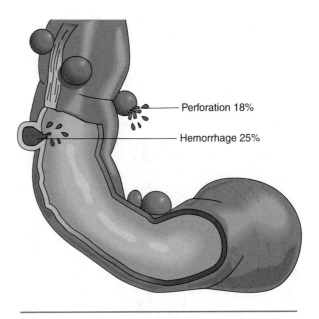

Figure 18-18   *Diverticulosis*

Pancreatitis is the inflammation of the pancreas. The pancreas can become edematous, hemorrhagic, or necrotic. One-third of pancreatitis cases are due to unknown causes. Some may be associated with chronic alcoholism.

Diverticulosis is a condition in which little sacs (diverticula) develop in the wall of the colon, Figure 18-18. The majority of people over the age of 60 in the United States have this condition. Most people have no symptoms and would not know they had diverticulosis unless there was an x-ray or intestinal examination. About 20% of people with this condition may develop **diverticulitis,** which is an inflammation in the wall of the colon. People with this condition must follow a restricted diet.

Diarrhea is characterized by loose, watery, and frequent bowel movements. It may result from irritation of the colon's lining by dysentery bacteria, poor diet, nervousness, toxic substances, or irritants in food. Excessive diarrhea may lead to dehydration and electrolyte imbalance. This can be a life-threatening situation in the very young and the very old.

Chronic **constipation** is when defecation is delayed. The colon absorbs excessive water from the feces rendering them dry and hard. When this occurs, defecation (or evacuation) becomes difficult.

For this reason, suppressing the need to defecate at normal times can lead to constipation. Constipation can also be caused by emotions such as anxiety, fear, or fright. Headaches and other symptoms that frequently accompany constipation result from the distension of the rectum, as opposed to toxins from the feces.

Treatment usually consists of eating proper foods, especially cereals, fruits and vegetables, drinking plenty of fluids, getting enough exercise, setting regular bowel habits, and avoiding tension as much as possible.

Stomach cancer (also called gastric cancer) can develop in any part of the stomach and may spread throughout the stomach and to other organs. Stomach cancer is hard to diagnose. Often there are no symptoms in the early stages and, in many cases, the cancer has spread before it is found.

The initial symptoms of stomach cancer are much like those of other digestive disorders: heartburn, loss of appetite, persistent indigestion, slight nausea, a feeling of bloated discomfort after eating, and occasional mild stomach pain. Later symptoms include traces of blood in the feces, pain, weight loss, and vomiting.

Treatment involves surgical removal of the stomach tumor as soon as possible. Depending on the size and the extent of growth of the tu-mor, part or all of the stomach may have to be removed.

If the cancer has spread, chemotherapy is prescribed. Radiation therapy plays a limited role in the treatment of stomach cancer.

Colon cancer is believed to arise from a polypoid lesion. Early detection is critical. The following procedures are recommended for early detection: After the age of 40, an annual digital rectal examination is prescribed; after the age of 50, a stool slide specimen is obtained, looking for hidden blood (**hemoccult**).

A colon resection may be performed in a patient with colon cancer. Sometimes it may be necessary to perform a **colostomy**. In this procedure, an opening is made through the abdomen into the colon, the cancerous tissue is removed, and the healthy tissue is brought out through the opening onto the skin. A pouch is worn to collect the body's wastes. This procedure causes stress and anxiety. The health care worker must be supportive of a patient with this condition.

Medical Terminology

absorp	being absorbed
-tion	process of
absorp/tion	process of being absorbed
aliment	food
-ary	pertaining to
aliment/ary canal	pertaining to the food canal
appendic	appendix, attachment
-itis	inflammation of
appendic/itis	inflammation of the appendix
cec	blind
-um	presence of
cec/um	presence of a blind pouch
cholecyst	gallbladder
cholecyst/itis	inflammation of the gallbladder
cirrh	reddish, yellowness
-osis	condition of
cirrh/osis	condition of yellowness indicates disease of the liver
colo	colon
-ostomy	opening into
col/ostomy	opening into the colon

degluti	swallowing
degluti/tion	process of swallowing
dia	through
-rrhea	flow or discharge
dia/rrhea	excessive flow through of liquid fecal material
diverticul	offshoot, bypass
-osis	condition of
diverticul/osis	condition of bypass, abnormal outpouching in the intestines
gastro	stomach
-enteri	small intestines
gastro/enter/itis	inflammation of the stomach and small intestines
gingiv	gums
-ae	pertaining to
gingiv/ae	pertaining to the gums
hemo	blood
-occult	hidden
hem/occult	hidden blood
hepat	liver
hepat/itis	inflammation of the liver
intrins	within a body or organ
-ic	relating to
intrins/ic factor	a factor within a body or organ
mastic	chew or gnash
-ate	process of
mastic/ate	process of chewing
peri	around
-dont	teeth
-al	pertaining to
peri/o/dont/al membrane	pertaining to membrane around tooth
-ton/e	strength, stretching
-um	presence of
peri/ton/e/um	a type of serous membrane that is stretched around structures
pylor	gatekeeper to the small intestines
pylor/ic sphincter	muscle that is the gatekeeper to the small intestines
sigm	means an *s*
-oid	resembling
sigm/oid colon	resembling an S shape
stoma	mouth
stoma/titis	inflammation of the mouth

REVIEW QUESTIONS

Select the letter of the choice that best completes the statement.

1. The process of changing complex foods into simpler substances to be absorbed is called:
   a. metabolism
   b. cellular respiration
   c. peristalsis
   d. digestion

2. The walls of the digestive tube that contain mucus are called:
   a. submucosa
   b. mucosa
   c. circular muscle
   d. visceral peritoneum

3. The accessory organs of the alimentary canal are the tongue, teeth, salivary glands, pancreas, liver, and:
   a. stomach
   b. esophagus
   c. gallbladder
   d. colon

4. The taste buds are found on projections called:
   a. papillae
   b. parotid
   c. palatine
   d. pharynx

5. The involuntary muscle action of the alimentary canal is called:
   a. pushing
   b. peristalsis
   c. stenosis
   d. contraction

6. Semiliquid food entering the small intestine is called:
   a. pepsin
   b. ptyalin
   c. chyme
   d. bolus

7. The lining of the abdominal cavity is called:
   a. pleural
   b. peritoneal
   c. submucosa
   d. epithelial

8. The pancreatic enzyme that breaks down starches is called:
   a. trypsin
   b. steapsin
   c. secretion
   d. amylopsin

9. The enzyme that stimulates the liver to produce bile is called:
  a. protease
  b. steapsin
  c. secretin
  d. trypsin

10. Food is absorbed in the small intestine in the:
  a. villi
  b. submucosa
  c. peritoneal lining
  d. colon

MATCHING

Match each of the terms in Column I with its correct description in Column II

Column I	Column II
_____ **1.** papillae	a. substances that promote chemical reactions in living things
_____ **2.** enzyme	b. bleeding gums
_____ **3.** digestion	c. a small soft structure suspended from the soft palate
_____ **4.** teeth	d. gums that protect the teeth
_____ **5.** enamel	e. tract consisting of the mouth, stomach, and intestines
_____ **6.** gingivae	f. aids in chewing and swallowing
_____ **7.** accessory organs and structures of digestion	g. teeth, tongue, salivary glands, pancreas, liver, gallbladder, and appendix
_____ **8.** salivary amylase	h. hardest substance in the body
_____ **9.** uvula	i. projections on the surface of the tongue containing the taste buds
_____ **10.** alimentary canal	j. the process of changing complex solid foods into soluble forms to be absorbed by cells
_____ **11.** cirrhosis	
_____ **12.** gastroenteritis	k. the enzyme manufactured by the salivary glands
_____ **13.** peptic ulcers	l. frequent liquid bowel movements
_____ **14.** hiatal hernia	m. chronic liver disease
_____ **15.** heartburn	n. protrusion of the stomach into the esophagus
_____ **16.** diarrhea	o. viral infection of the liver
_____ **17.** cholecystitis	p. inflammation of the abdominal cavity
_____ **18.** infectious hepatitis	q. obstruction of the hepatic duct
_____ **19.** pyloric stenosis	r. inflammation of the stomach and intestinal lining
_____ **20.** peritonitis	s. inflammation of the gallbladder
	t. narrowing of sphincter in the stomach
	u. cardiospasm
	v. lesions that may result from acid secretion
	w. common symptoms characterized by a burning sensation

TRUE OR FALSE

Read each statement carefully and determine if it is true or false.

T F **1.** The large intestine is called the colon.

T F **2.** The large intestine is 20 feet long and 2 inches wide.

T F **3.** The cecum is located where the small intestine joins the large intestine.

T F **4.** The function of the appendix is unknown.

T F **5.** The large intestine stores and eliminates the waste products of digestion.

T F **6.** Regulation of water balance occurs in the large intestine because its lining absorbs water.

T F **7.** Constipation may be overcome by intensive and long periods of work and exercise.

T F **8.** Bulk foods such as whole-grain cereals, fruits, and vegetables may help avoid constipation.

T F **9.** The rectum is an extension of the descending colon.

T F **10.** The transverse colon lies between the ascending and the descending colon.

LABELING

Label the teeth on the following diagram. (The teeth on the left are deciduous, those on the right are permanent.)

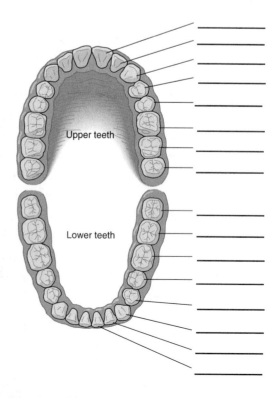

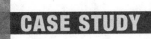

APPLYING THEORY TO PRACTICE

1. You have just eaten a slice of pizza for lunch. In about 12 hours, that slice of pizza will be ready for absorption in the villi of the small intestine. Trace the journey of the pizza, naming all the enzymes involved, where the action takes place, and the end products of carbohydrate, protein, and fat metabolism. Would you consider pizza a good nutritious snack? Explain your answer.

2. Enzymes secreted by the stomach are high in acid content. Explain the reason why the lining of the digestive system does not become ulcerated.

3. Dental checkups make you nervous. Why is it a good health practice to see your dentist at least once a year? Describe the health careers in the dental profession.

4. A pregnant woman comes into the doctor's office and states, "I have so much heartburn, I know my baby will be born with a full head of hair." Explain to her the reasons for heartburn and why her statement is a myth.

5. In the emergency room a woman, age 40, is complaining of a sharp pain between her shoulder blades on the right side. What is this symptomatic of and what type of treatment is necessary for this condition?

6. Your friend states, "All this stress is going to give me an ulcer." Explain to your friend why this is no longer an accurate statement.

CASE STUDY

Kevin, age 40, goes to his HMO to see his physician, Dr. Scotty. He is complaining of general fatigue and loss of appetite, and he notices the whites of his eyes look yellowish. Dr. Scotty orders blood tests for Kevin. The blood tests reveal he has hepatitis C.

1. Explain what hepatitis C is.

2. What is unusual about the appearance of symptoms in hepatitis C?

3. What functions of the liver may be impaired?

4. Are there any other organs of digestion involved with this disease?

5. Are any other body systems affected by hepatitis?

6. Describe hepatitis A and hepatitis B.

7. What is the prognosis for Kevin?

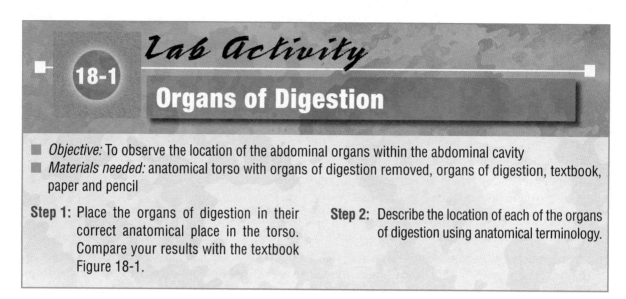

Lab Activity

18-1

Organs of Digestion

■ *Objective:* To observe the location of the abdominal organs within the abdominal cavity
■ *Materials needed:* anatomical torso with organs of digestion removed, organs of digestion, textbook, paper and pencil

Step 1: Place the organs of digestion in their correct anatomical place in the torso. Compare your results with the textbook Figure 18-1.

Step 2: Describe the location of each of the organs of digestion using anatomical terminology.

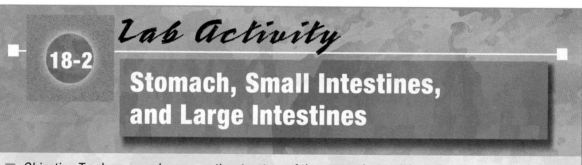

Lab Activity

18-2

Stomach, Small Intestines, and Large Intestines

■ *Objective:* To observe and compare the structure of the stomach, small intestines, and large intestines
■ *Materials needed:* slides of cross sections of stomach, jejunum including villi, colon, microscope, textbook, paper and pencil

Step 1: Identify and describe the mucosa layers and gastric gland cells of the stomach. Compare your observations with Figure 18-8.

Step 2: Sketch and identify the mucosa and villi of the jejunum. Compare your observations with Figure 18-9. Compare with the slides of the mucosa of the stomach. Describe and record the differences.

Step 3: Examine the slide of the mucosa of the colon. Compare with the slide of the jejunum. Describe and record the differences between the colon and jejunum.

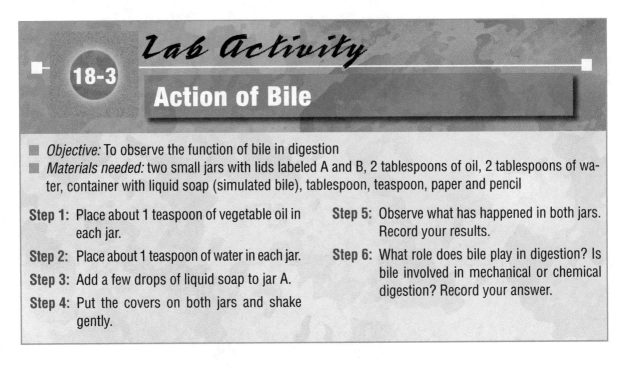

Lab Activity 18-3

Action of Bile

- *Objective:* To observe the function of bile in digestion
- *Materials needed:* two small jars with lids labeled A and B, 2 tablespoons of oil, 2 tablespoons of water, container with liquid soap (simulated bile), tablespoon, teaspoon, paper and pencil

Step 1: Place about 1 teaspoon of vegetable oil in each jar.

Step 2: Place about 1 teaspoon of water in each jar.

Step 3: Add a few drops of liquid soap to jar A.

Step 4: Put the covers on both jars and shake gently.

Step 5: Observe what has happened in both jars. Record your results.

Step 6: What role does bile play in digestion? Is bile involved in mechanical or chemical digestion? Record your answer.

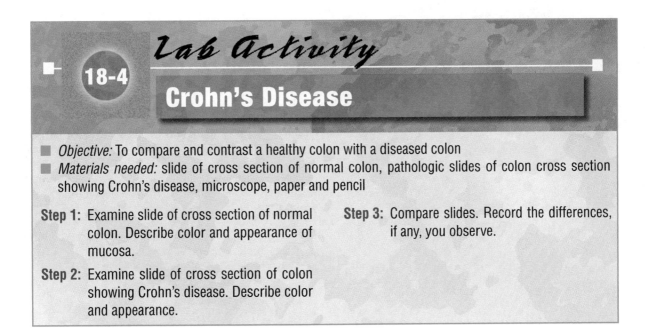

Lab Activity 18-4

Crohn's Disease

- *Objective:* To compare and contrast a healthy colon with a diseased colon
- *Materials needed:* slide of cross section of normal colon, pathologic slides of colon cross section showing Crohn's disease, microscope, paper and pencil

Step 1: Examine slide of cross section of normal colon. Describe color and appearance of mucosa.

Step 2: Examine slide of cross section of colon showing Crohn's disease. Describe color and appearance.

Step 3: Compare slides. Record the differences, if any, you observe.

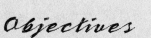

Chapter 19

NUTRITION

Objectives

- Define the term *nutrient*
- Describe the function(s) of the different types of nutrients
- Differentiate between the fat-soluble and water-soluble vitamins
- Describe the concept of Recommended Daily Dietary Allowances
- List the Dietary Guidelines for Americans
- Define the key words that relate to this chapter

Key Words

Adequate
  Intakes (AI)
anorexia nervosa
Basal metabolic
  rate (BMR)
Body mass index
  (BMI)
bulimia
calorie
complete proteins

essential amino
  acids
fiber
HDL
incomplete
  proteins
kilocalorie
LDL
mineral
nutrient

obesity
roughage
Recommended
  Dietary
  Allowances
  (RDA)
trace element
triglycerides
Upper Limits (UL)
vitamin

The pace of an active daily life can at times be hectic and stress filled. This can occasionally cause one to eat "on the run," to "grab a bite" at a fast-food restaurant, or to forget to eat nutritiously.

The food one eats and drinks may or may not be nutritious. For food to be nutritious, it must contain the materials needed by the individual cells for proper cell functioning. These materials or **nutrients** are:

- Water
- Carbohydrates
- Lipids
- Proteins
- Minerals
- Vitamins

WATER

Water is an essential component of all body tissues. It has several important functions in the human body.

- Acts as a solvent for all biochemical reactions.
- Serves as a transport medium for substances.
- Functions as a lubricant for joint movement and the digestive tract.
- Helps control body temperature by evaporation from the pores of the skin.
- Serves as a cushion for body organs, such as the lungs and brain.

Water makes up between 55% and 65% of our total body weight. The body is continually losing water through evaporation, excretion, and respiration. This water loss must be replaced. Drinking 8 (8oz) glasses of water daily helps to replace the water lost through normal daily activity. Most foods we eat also contain some water. Exercise, sweating, vomiting increases the body's need for water. By the time thirst develops the body is already in a state of mild dehydration.

CARBOHYDRATES

Carbohydrates include simple sugars, such as monosaccharides like glucose ($C_6H_{12}O_6$). Depending on the number of simple sugars found in the carbohydrate, they are classified as monosaccharides, disaccharides, or polysaccharides (starch). Only the monosaccharides are small enough to be absorbed and eventually taken into the cells. The other carbohydrates are broken down by digestion into the smallest possible molecular subunits prior to absorption.

Carbohydrates are the main source of energy for the body. Excess carbohydrates are converted into fat and stored in fat tissue. Nutritionists recommend that carbohydrates comprise between 50% and 60% of the daily intake of calories.

A **calorie** is a unit that measures the amount of energy contained within the chemical bonds of different foods. The small calorie is defined as the amount of heat required to raise the temperature of 1 gram of water by 1° Celsius. A **kilocalorie**, or large calorie, is equal to 1,000 small calories. The calorie content of food is determined by measuring the amount of heat released when food is burned. The energy content of fat (9 kilocalories per gram) is slightly more than twice that of carbohydrate (4 kilocalories per gram) or protein (4 kilocalories per gram).

A normal adult usually requires between 1,600 and 3,000 kilocalories a day depending on age, sex, body weight, and degree of physical activity. Newborn infants and young children have higher energy requirements per unit of body weight than adults because of the high energy expenditure of growth. See Table 19-1 for daily recommended energy intakes.

An excess of the wrong foods can cause an overweight condition called obesity. Obesity usually results when we take in more calories than we use. There are carbohydrates that should be avoided or minimized in the daily diet. These foods are candies, cakes, cookies, jams, sugar-coated cereals, and sugary soft drinks. These foods contain large amounts of highly refined carbohydrates as sugar. They supply calories, but little else. Energy obtained from such foods is commonly referred to as "empty calories." Intake of these foods can also contribute to tooth decay. Foods containing starches and cellulose are a healthier source of carbohydrates. These foods, besides providing energy, can also provide needed minerals, roughage, and vitamins. **Roughage** is the indigestible portion of many foods and is necessary to maintain a

Table 19-1 *Median Heights and Weights and Recommended Energy Intake*

CATEGORY	AGE (YEARS) OR CONDITION	WEIGHT (KG)	WEIGHT (LB)	HEIGHT (CM)	HEIGHT (IN)	REE[a] (KCAL/DAY)	MULTIPLES OF REE	PER KG	PER DAY[c]
Infants	0.0–0.5	6	13	60	24	320		108	650
	0.5–1.0	9	20	71	28	500		98	850
Children	1–3	13	29	90	35	740		102	1,300
	4–6	20	44	112	44	950		90	1,800
	7–10	28	62	132	52	1,130		70	2,000
Males	11–14	45	99	157	62	1,440	1.70	55	2,500
	15–18	66	145	176	69	1,760	1.67	45	3,000
	19–24	72	160	177	70	1,780	1.67	40	2,900
	25–50	79	174	176	70	1,800	1.60	37	2,900
	51+	77	170	173	68	1,530	1.50	30	2,300
Females	11–14	46	101	157	62	1,310	1.67	47	2,200
	15–18	55	120	163	64	1,370	1.60	40	2,200
	19–24	58	128	164	65	1,350	1.60	38	2,200
	25–50	63	138	163	64	1,380	1.55	36	2,200
	51+	65	143	160	63	1,280	1.50	30	1,900
Pregnant	1st trimester								+0
	2nd trimester								+300
	3rd trimester								+500
Lactating	1st 6 months								+500
	2nd 6 months								+500

a. Calculation based on FAO equations, then rounded.
b. In the range of light to moderate activity, the coefficient of variation is ± 20%
c. Figure is rounded.
Source: Reprinted with permission from *Recommended Dietary Allowances, 10th Edition,* © 1989 by the National Academy of Sciences. Published by National Academy Press, Washington, D.C.

healthy digestive system. Foods high in roughage are whole-grain breads and cereals, fruits, vegetables, macaroni, rice, and potatoes.

LIPIDS

Lipids are a group of compounds containing fatty acids combined with an alcohol. They can be subdivided into two groups: simple lipids (fats, oils, waxes) and compound lipids (phospholipids, glycolipids, sterols). Like carbohydrates, fats are a source of energy. The same amount of fats can release more than twice as many calories as the same amount of carbohydrate or protein. The human body stores reserves of energy as fat in fat cells. Likewise, any excess carbohydrate and protein in the diet is transformed into fat and stored along with any excess fat.

Fats are an essential nutrient to the maintenance of the human body. Stored fats provide a supply of energy during emergencies such as sickness or during deficient caloric intakes. Fats also cushion the internal organs and serve as an insulation against the cold. Fats are components of the cell membrane, and contribute to the formation of bile and steroid hormones, such as the sex hormones. Fats also contain certain kinds of vitamins called fat-soluble vitamins which are an important part of our daily diet. It is therefore essential to have a diet containing fats without exceeding the body's calorie needs. Total daily dietary fat intake should not exceed 25% to 30% of the daily caloric intake.

Cholesterol is a fat found in animal products such as meat, eggs, cheese, and ice cream. Cholesterol is a white, waxlike substance used to build cells and make hormones. It is also manufactured by the liver. The cholesterol that you eat is not digested. There are no calories in cholesterol, but once in the body it is difficult for the body to get rid of it. Fats and oils in food are called **triglycerides.** Your body turns excess calories into triglycerides which are stored throughout the body as adipose tissue.

Triglycerides and cholesterol must be carried through blood cells by special proteins called lipoprotein: **HDL** and **LDL,** and **VLDL.** The lipoprotein LDL carries fats to the cells; HDL or high-density lipoprotein is sometimes referred to as the "heavenly" or "good" kind because it removes excess cholesterol from cells and carries it back to the liver to be broken down or eliminated.

Over the years, if more cholesterol is carried by the LDL than can be removed by HDL or used up in the cells, it will start to build up inside the artery walls, causing atherosclerosis.

The recommended level of blood cholesterol for people age 40 and over is under 200 mg/dl; any level over 200 mg/dl is considered too high for the long-term health of the heart. See Medical Highlights on page 252.

The two most important steps you can take to lower your blood cholesterol are to reduce your intake of foods high in saturated fat and to lose weight if you are overweight. Fats are defined as follows:

- Saturated fat—oil from animal products that are solid at room temperature, such as butter, cheese, and meat fat

- Polyunsaturated fat—oil from vegetable products, liquid at room temperature, used in moderation lowers blood cholesterol; includes safflower oil and sunflower oil

- Monosaturated fat—oil from other vegetable products, liquid at room temperature, lowers blood cholesterol; includes olive oil and peanut oil

If a label says "cholesterol free" it does not necessarily mean it is good for you. Look carefully—many products with no cholesterol have saturated fats in them.

Foods to substitute for saturated fat include skim milk, low-fat cheese, poultry, margarine, and low-fat ice cream. Some of the foods that help lower cholesterol include garlic, fresh fruit and vegetables, oat bran, wheat bran, and prunes.

PROTEINS

Proteins are structurally more complex than carbohydrates and lipids and contain an amino (NH_2) group. They are synthesized in the cell cytoplasm from constituent molecules called amino acids.

Proteins serve many different functions in the body. Some are enzymes and regulate the rate of chemical reactions; others are important in growth and repair of tissues. When necessary, proteins can also be used as a source of energy. In addition, contractile systems (muscles), hormonal systems, plasma transport systems, clotting, and defense systems (antibodies) are all dependent upon proteins.

The body can synthesize some amino acids, but not all. The amino acids that cannot be made in the body are **essential amino acids.** Proteins that contain all of the essential amino acids are known as **complete proteins.** Sources of such complete proteins are eggs, meat, milk, and milk products. Proteins that do not contain all the essential amino acids are called **incomplete proteins.** Vegetables contain incomplete proteins; however, a varied diet including vegetables will supply all the necessary complete proteins. For example, beans and wheat eaten alone will not provide all of the necessary complete proteins. When eaten together, however, they will complement each other and supply the necessary complete proteins.

Unlike fats, the human body is unable to store excess amino acids. Any unused amino acids are broken down by the liver, and the amino group is excreted as a nitrogenous waste product called urea. The remainder of the amino acid may be burned for immediate energy or stored as fat or glycogen, a polysaccharide.

Protein synthesis cannot occur without all of the essential amino acids present at the same time. Therefore, it is important to include some source of complete protein throughout the various foods we eat during the day. The daily intake of calories from proteins should be no more than 15% to 20%.

Most adults in the United States eat a daily intake of protein in excess of the recommended dietary allowance. This practice puts an extra burden on the liver, and kidney, which must eliminate the urea from the body.

MINERALS AND TRACE ELEMENTS

A **mineral** is a chemical element that is obtained from inorganic compounds in food. Our knowledge of the role of the essential minerals and trace elements is incomplete. Many are notably necessary for normal human growth and maintenance.

Among the most important of these nutrients are sodium, potassium, calcium, iron, phosphorous, and zinc.

Trace elements are present in the body in very small amounts. These include zinc, copper, iodine, cobalt, manganese, selenium, chromium, molybdenum, and fluorine.

The toxic limits of some trace elements are extremely close to the recommended levels. This means that there is a critical difference between toxicity, health, and deficiency. Most of the essential minerals and trace elements are already present in the average normal American diet in sufficient concentrations, and supplementation is only indicated for special conditions of disease, during pregnancy, and old age. However, governmental surveys indicate that females in the United States might be consuming less than optimal daily intakes of calcium and iron.

Age-related osteoporosis is one of the most severely debilitating diseases in the United States. Although the question of whether osteoporosis is a nutritional disorder remains unanswered, there is much convincing evidence that calcium deficiency accelerates the age-related loss of bone. Menopause results in diminished calcium absorption in the intestines. The physiological consequence of reduced estrogen, results in lower bone density in females and requires that proper attention be paid to calcium intake throughout the life cycle (see chapter 6).

Women of child-bearing age have a tendency to have low iron levels because of blood loss during the menstrual flow. Fatigue and iron deficiency anemia in these women can usually be corrected by taking iron supplements. Table 19-2 summarizes the most important minerals and trace elements in the human diet.

VITAMINS

A **vitamin** is defined as a biologically active organic compound, often functioning as a coenzyme, that is necessary for normal health and growth. Most enzymatic activity relies on the presence of coenzymes. A dietary deficiency of a vitamin results in a specific disorder. The term *vitamin* usually implies that the substance is not synthesized within the organism and, as a result, must be obtained from the diet. Vitamins are transported by the circulatory system to all the tissues of the body.

Recent evidence indicates that certain vitamins actually behave like hormones physiologically. For instance, both vitamin D and niacin are synthesized in the human (in inadequate amounts) conferring on them hormonal qualities, since hormones are produced in the body. The fat-soluble vitamins A, D, E, and K are readily stored in the body, and within the cell they demonstrate many similarities to the steroid hormones (estrogen, testosterone, cortisol). The water-soluble vitamins are B_1, B_2, B_3, B_6, B_{12}, pantothenic acid, folic acid, biotin, and vitamin C. An excessive intake of water-soluble vitamins results in increased excretion rather than additional storage.

Certain conditions such as pregnancy, disease, emotional stress, and old age must be considered when determining daily individual vitamin requirements. Table 19–3 summarizes the major vitamins needed in the human diet.

FIBER

Fiber is found only in plant foods such as whole-grain breads, cereals, beans, and peas, and other vegetables and fruits. Eating a variety of fiber-containing plant foods is important for proper bowel function, reducing the symptoms of chronic

Table 19-2 *Summary of Essential Minerals and Trace Elements Needed for Health*

MINERAL	FOOD SOURCES	FUNCTION	DEFICIENCY DISEASES
Calcium	Milk, cheese, dark green vegetables, dried legumes, sardines, shellfish	Bone and tooth formation Blood clotting Nerve transmission	Stunted growth Rickets Osteoporosis Convulsions
Chlorine	Common table salt, seafood, milk, meat, eggs	Formation of gastric juices Acid-base balance	Muscle cramps Mental apathy Poor appetite
Chromium	Fats, vegetable oils, meats, clams, whole-grain cereals	Involved in energy and glucose metabolism	Impaired ability to metabolize glucose
Copper	Drinking water, liver, shellfish whole grains, cherries, legumes, kidney, poultry, oysters, nuts, chocolate	Constituent of enzymes Involved with iron transport	Anemia
Fluorine	Drinking water, tea, coffee, seafood, rice, spinach, onions, lettuce	Maintenance of bone and tooth structure	Higher frequency of tooth decay
Iodine	Marine fish and shellfish, dairy products, many vegetables, iodized salt	Constituent of thyroid hormones	Goiter (enlarged thyroid)
Iron	Liver, lean meats, legumes, whole grains, dark green vegetables, eggs, dark molasses, shrimp, oysters	Constituent of hemoglobin Involved in energy metabolism	Iron-deficiency anemia
Magnesium	Whole grains, green leafy vegetables, nuts, meats, milk, legumes	Involved in energy conversions and enzyme function	Growth failure Behavioral disturbances Weakness Spasms
Phosphorus	Milk, cheese, meat, fish, poultry, whole grains, legumes, nuts	Bone and tooth formation Acid-base balance Involved in energy metabolism	Weakness Demineralization of bone
Potassium	Meats, milk, fruits, legumes, vegetables	Acid-base balance Body water balance Nerve transmission	Muscular weakness Paralysis
Selenium	Fish, poultry, meats, grains, milk, vegetables (depending on amount in soil)	Necessary for vitamin E function	Anemia Deficiency is rare
Sodium	Common table salt, seafood, most other foods except fruit	Acid-base balance Body water balance Nerve transmission	Muscle cramps Mental apathy
Sulfur	Meat, fish, poultry, eggs, milk, cheese, legumes, nuts	Constituent of certain tissue proteins	Related to deficiencies of sulfur-containing amino acids
Zinc	Milk, liver, shellfish, herring, wheat bran	Involved in many enzyme systems Necessary for vitamin A metabolism	Growth failure Lack of sexual maturity Impaired wound healing Poor appetite

Table 19-3 *Summary of Major Vitamins Needed in the Human Diet*

VITAMIN	FOOD SOURCES	FUNCTION	DEFICIENCY DISEASES
A (Fat soluble)	Butter, fortified margarine, green and yellow vegetables, milk, eggs, liver	Night vision Healthy skin Proper growth and repair of body tissues	Night blindness Dry skin Slow growth Poor gums and teeth
B_1 (thiamine) (Water soluble)	Chicken, fish, meat, eggs, enriched bread, whole-grain cereals	Promotes normal appetite and digestion Needed by nervous system	Loss of appetite Nervous disorders Fatigue Severe deficiency causes beriberi
B_2 (riboflavin) (Water soluble)	Cheese, eggs, fish, meat, liver, milk, cereals, enriched bread	Needed in cellular respiration	Eye problems Sores on skin and lips General fatigue
B_3 (niacin) (Water soluble)	Eggs, fish, liver, meat, milk, potatoes, enriched bread	Needed for normal metabolism Growth Proper skin health	Indigestion Diarrhea Headaches Mental disturbances Skin disorders
B_{12} (cyanocobalamin) (Water soluble)	Milk, liver, brain, beef, egg yolk, clams, oysters, sardines, salmon	Red blood cell synthesis Nucleic acid synthesis Nerve cell maintenance	Pernicious anemia Nerve cell malfunction
Folic Acid (Water soluble)	Liver, yeast, green vegetables, peanuts, mushrooms, beef, veal, egg yolk	Nucleic acid synthesis Needed for normal metabolism and growth	Anemia Growth retardation
C (ascorbic acid) (Water soluble)	Citrus fruits, cabbage, green vegetables, tomatoes, potatoes	Needed for maintenance of normal bones, gums, teeth, and blood vessels	Weak bones Sore and bleeding gums Poor teeth Bleeding in skin Painful joints Severe deficiency results in scurvy
D (Fat soluble)	Beef, butter, eggs, milk	Needed for normal bone and teeth development Controls calcium and phosphorus metabolism	Poor bone and teeth structure Soft bones Rickets
E (tocopherol) (Fat soluble)	Margarine, nuts, leafy vegetables, vegetable oils, whole wheat	Used in cell respiration Protects red blood cells from destruction Acts as an anti-oxidant	Anemia in premature infants No known deficiency in adults
K (Fat soluble)	Synthesized by colon bacteria Green leafy vegetables, cereal	Essential for normal blood clotting	Slow blood clotting

constipation, diverticula disease, and hemorrhoids, and may lower the risk of heart diseases and some cancers. However, some of the health benefits associated with a high-fiber diet may come from other components present in these foods, not just from fiber itself. For this reason, fiber is best obtained from foods, rather than a supplement.

Effects of Aging on Nutrition

Many factors affect the diet of the elderly, including chronic disease and societal, economic, physical, and emotional factors. Because most seniors have one or more chronic diseases, the medications they take can interfere with their nutrition. An example is digoxin, a medication good for heart failure, but it suppresses the appetite. Seniors may also lose their taste for meat, a protein that is necessary to build and repair tissue. Arthritis, heart disease, or other ailments make cooking a physical challenge. The loss of a spouse may make an individual not want to bother cooking for one-self. Economic factors influence the choices people make regarding the buying of food.

The new Screening Initiative sponsored by the American Dietetic Association and the American Academy of Family Physicians, which provides thousands of doctors a guide to nutrition concerns regarding chronic illnesses, is making physicians more aware of these problems.

RECOMMENDED DAILY DIETARY ALLOWANCES

Developing universal "minimum daily requirements" that apply to everyone is an extremely difficult task. Nutritional requirements among individuals might vary for several reasons. Malabsorption disorders sometimes require that an individual needs greater than the average daily dosage of certain nutrients. Differences in the microbial environment of the intestine, and genetic factors influencing biochemical reactions, must also be considered. People experiencing psychological or physical stress often require a greater amount of certain nutrients to help the body maintain homeostasis or a relatively constant internal environment.

In recognition of individual variations in nutritional requirements, a table of **Recommended Dietary Allowances (RDA)**, **Adequate Intakes (AI)**, and **Upper Limits (UL)** (see Table 19-4) has been approved by the Food and Nutrition Board, National Academy of Sciences. It contains the daily recommendations for protein, fat-soluble vitamins, water-soluble vitamins, and minerals. The allowances are intended to provide for individual variations among most normal persons as they live in the United States under usual environmental stresses.

Basal Metabolic Rate

The **basal metabolic rate (BMR)** is the measure of the total energy utilized by the body to maintain those body processes necessary for life, the minimum level of heat produced by the body at rest. BMR is the number of calories needed to keep the heart pumping, to keep breathing, and to carry out all activities of daily living.

The purpose in determining the BMR is to calculate basic caloric needs for a person. A way to estimate the BMR is as follows:

For women: $661 + (4.38 \times \text{Weight in pounds}) + (4.33 \times \text{Height in inches}) - (4.7 \times \text{Age}) = \text{BMR}$

For men: $67 + (6.24 \times \text{Weight in pounds}) + (12.7 \times \text{Height in inches}) - (6.9 \times \text{Age}) = \text{BMR}$

Next estimate the total number of calories the body needs per day by multiplying the BMR by the appropriate factor, as shown:

- 1.2 for an inactive person

- 1.3 for a moderately active person (exercises three times per week)

Table 19-4 *Dietary Reference Intakes (DRIs): Recommended Intakes for Individuals Food and Nutrition Board, National Academy of Sciences, Institute of Medicine*

FAT-SOLUBLE VITAMINS

Life Stage Group	Protein (g)	Vitamin A (ug/d)		Vitamin D (ug/d)		Vitamin E (mg/d)		Vitamin K (ug/d)		Vitamin C (mg/d)		Thiamin (mg/d)	
		RDA/AI*	UL	RDA/AI*	UL	RDA/AI*	UL	RDA/AI*	UL	RDA/AI*	UL	RDA/AI*	UL
Infants													
0.0–0.6 mo	13	400*	600	5*	25	4*	ND	2.0*	ND	40*	ND	0.2*	ND
0.7–12 mo	14	500*	600	5*	25	5*	ND	2.5*	ND	50*	ND	0.3*	ND
Children													
1–3 yrs	16	300	600	5*	50	6	200	30*	ND	15	400	0.5	ND
4–8 yrs	24	400	900	5*	50	7	300	55*	ND	25	650	0.6	ND
Males													
9–13 yrs	45	600	1700	5*	50	11	600	60*	ND	45	1200	0.9	ND
14–18 yrs	59	900	2800	5*	50	15	800	75*	ND	75	1800	1.2	ND
19–30 yrs	58	900	3000	5*	50	15	1000	120*	ND	90	2000	1.2	ND
31–50 yrs	63	900	3000	5*	50	15	1000	120*	ND	90	2000	1.2	ND
50–70 yrs	63	900	3000	10*	50	15	1000	120*	ND	90	2000	1.2	ND
70+ yrs	63	900	3000	15*	50	15	1000	120*	ND	90	2000	1.2	ND
Females													
9–13 yrs	46	600	1700	5*	50	11	600	60*	ND	45	1200	0.9	ND
14–18 yrs	44	700	2800	5*	50	15	800	75*	ND	65	1800	1	ND
19–30 yrs	46	700	3000	5*	50	15	1000	90*	ND	75	2000	1.1	ND
31–50 yrs	50	700	3000	5*	50	15	1000	90*	ND	75	2000	1.1	ND
50–70 yrs	50	700	3000	10*	50	15	1000	90*	ND	75	2000	1.1	ND
70+ yrs	50	700	3000	15*	50	15	1000	90*	ND	75	2000	1.1	ND
Pregnant	60	770	3000	5*	50	15	1000	90*	ND	85	2000	1.4	ND
Lactating	65	1300	3000	5*	50	19	1000	90*	ND	120	2000	1.4	ND

(continues)

Table 19-4 (continued)

WATER-SOLUBLE VITAMINS

Life Stage Group	Riboflavin (mg/d) RDA/AL*	UL	Niacin (mg/d) RDA/AL*	UL	Vitamin B$_6$ (mg/d) RDA/AL*	UL	Folate (ug/d) RDA/AL*	UL	Vitamin B$_{12}$ (ug/d) RDA/AL*	UL	Calcium (mg/d) RDA/AL*	UL	Phosphorus (mg/d) RDA/AL*	UL
Infants														
0.0–0.6 mo	0.3*	ND	2*	ND	0.1*	ND	65*	ND	0.4*	ND	210*	ND	100*	ND
0.7–12 mo	0.4*	ND	4*	ND	0.3*	ND	80*	ND	0.5*	ND	270*	ND	275*	ND
Children														
1–3 yrs	0.5	ND	6	10	0.5	30	150	300	0.9	ND	500*	2500	460	3000
4–8 yrs	0.6	ND	8	15	0.6	40	200	400	1.2	ND	800*	2500	500	3000
Males														
9–13 yrs	0.9	ND	12	20	1	60	300	600	1.8	ND	1300*	2500	1250	4000
14–18 yrs	1.3	ND	16	30	1.3	80	400	800	2.4	ND	1300*	2500	1250	4000
19–30 yrs	1.3	ND	16	35	1.3	100	400	1000	2.4	ND	1000*	2500	700	4000
31–50 yrs	1.3	ND	16	35	1.3	100	400	1000	2.4	ND	1000*	2500	700	4000
50–70 yrs	1.3	ND	16	35	1.7	100	400	1000	2.4	ND	1200*	2500	700	4000
70+ yrs	1.3	ND	16	35	1.7	100	400	1000	2.4	ND	1200*	2500	700	3000
Females														
9–13 yrs	0.9	ND	12	20	1	60	300	600	1.8	ND	1300*	2500	1250	4000
14–18 yrs	1	ND	14	30	1.2	80	400	800	2.4	ND	1300*	2500	1250	4000
19–30 yrs	1.1	ND	14	35	1.3	100	400	1000	2.4	ND	1000*	2500	700	4000
31–50 yrs	1.1	ND	14	35	1.3	100	400	1000	2.4	ND	1000*	2500	700	4000
50–70 yrs	1.1	ND	14	35	1.5	100	400	1000	2.4	ND	1200*	2500	700	4000
70+ yrs	1.1	ND	14	35	1.5	100	400	1000	2.4	ND	1200*	2500	700	3000
Pregnant	1.4	ND	18	35	1.9	100	600	1000	2.6	ND	1000*	2500	700	3500
Lactating	1.6	ND	17	35	2	100	500	1000	2.8	ND	1000*	2500	700	4000

(continues)

Table 19-4 *(continued)*

Life Stage Group	MINERALS									
	Magnesium (mg/d)		Iron (mg/d)		Zinc (mg/d)		Iodine (ug/d)		Selenium (ug/d)	
	RDA/AL*	UL	RDA/AL*	UL	RDA/AL*	UL	RDA/AL*	UL	RDA/AL*	UL
Infants										
0.0–0.6 mo	30*	ND	0.27*	40	2*	4	110*	ND	15*	45
0.7–12 mo	75*	ND	11	40	3	5	130*	ND	20*	60
Children										
1–3 yrs	80	65	7	40	3	7	90	200	20	90
4–8 yr	130	110	10	40	5	12	90	300	30	150
Males										
9–13 yrs	240	350	8	40	8	11	120	600	40	280
14–18 yrs	410	350	11	45	11	34	150	900	55	400
19–30 yrs	400	350	8	45	11	40	150	1000	55	400
31–50 yrs	420	350	8	45	11	40	150	1000	55	400
50–70 yrs	420	350	8	45	11	40	150	1000	55	400
70+ yrs	420	350	8	45	11	40	150	1000	55	400
Females										
9–13 yrs	240	350	8	40	8	23	120	600	40	280
14–18 yrs	360	350	15	45	9	34	150	900	55	400
19–30 yrs	310	350	18	45	8	40	150	1100	55	400
31–50 yrs	320	350	18	45	8	40	150	1100	55	400
50–70 yrs	320	350	8	45	8	40	150	1100	55	400
70+ yrs	320	350	8	45	8	40	150	1100	55	400
Pregnant	350	350	27	45	11	40	220	1100	60	400
Lactating	310	350	9	45	12	40	290	1100	70	400

Note: The table is adapted from the DRI reports, see www.nap.edu. It represents Recommended Dietary Allowances (RDAs) in bold type, Adequate Intakes (AIs) in ordinary type followed by an asterisk (*), and Upper Limits (ULs). RDAs and AIs may both be used as goals for individual intake. RDAs are set to meet the needs of almost all (97% to 98%) individuals in a group. For healthy breastfed infants, the AI is the mean intake. The AI for other life stage and gender groups is believed to cover the needs of all individuals in the group, but lack of data prevents being able to specify with confidence the percentage of individuals covered by this intake.

UL = The maximum level of daily nutrient intake that is likely to pose no risk of adverse effects. Unless otherwise specified, the UL represents total intake from food, water, and supplements. Due to lack of suitable data, ULs could not be established for vitamin K, thiamin, riboflavin, vitamin B₁₂, pantothenic acid, biotin, or cartenoids. In absence of ULs, extra caution may be warranted in consuming levels above the recommended intakes.

ND = Not determinable due to lack of data of adverse effects in this age group and concern with regard to lack of ability to handle excess amounts. Source of intake should be from food only to prevent high levels of intake.

Sources: Dietary Reference Intakes for Calcium, Phosphorus, Magnesium, Vitamin D, and Fluoride (1997); Dietary Reference Intakes for Thiamin, Riboflavin, Niacin, Vitamin B6, Folate, Vitamin B12, Pantothenic Acid, Biotin, and Choline (1998); Dietary Reference Intakes for Vitamin C, Vitamin E, Selenium, and Carotenoids (2000); and Dietary Reference Intakes for Vitamin A, Vitamin K, Arsenic, Boron, Chromium, Copper, Iodine, Iron, Manganese, Molybdenum, Nickel, Silicon, Vanadium, and Zinc (2001). These reports may be accessed via www.nap.edu. Reprinted with permission of the National Academy of Sciences, courtesy of the National Academy Press, Washington, DC.

Career Profile
Dietitians and Nutritionists

Dietitians and nutritionists plan nutrition programs and supervise the preparation and serving of meals. They help prevent and treat illnesses by promoting healthy eating habits, scientifically evaluating client's diets, and suggesting modification such as reduced fat and sugar for those who are overweight.

Dietitians run food service systems for institutions such as hospitals and schools, and also promote sound eating habits through education and research.

Popular interest in nutrition has led to opportunities in food manufacturing, advertising, and marketing where dietitians analyze foods, prepare literature for distribution, or report on such issues as the nutritional content of recipes, dietary fiber, or vitamin supplements.

The basic education requirement is a bachelor's degree with a major in dietetics, food and nutrition, food service systems management, or a related area. The Commission on Dietetic Registration of the American Dietetic Association (ADA) awards the Registered Dietitian credential to those who pass a certification exam after completing their academic education and supervised experience.

Expectation of employment is expected to grow about as fast as the average for all occupations.

- 1.7 for a very active person
- 1.9 for an extremely active person (e.g., runner, swimmer)

This method is one way to measure the number of calories burned each day. If the metabolic rate is lower than the calories supplied by food the excess calories are converted to fats and weight increases. If all the food calories are burned, weight is maintained. Burning more calories than supplied by the diet results in weight loss.

DIETARY GUIDELINES FOR AMERICANS

The U.S. Department of Agriculture published the Food Guide Pyramid of six food groups in 1992 Figure 19-1. The recommended groups and amounts are as follows:

Bread, cereal, and pasta— 6 to 11 servings

Vegetables— 3 to 5 servings

Fruit— 2 to 4 servings

Milk, yogurt, and cheese— 2 to 3 servings

Meat, poultry, fish, dry beans, eggs, and nuts— 2 to 3 servings

Fats, oils, sweets— use sparingly

The importance of consuming a diet of a variety of foods to provide the essential nutrients at a caloric level to maintain desirable body weight is emphasized. The guidelines were revised in 2000. The following specific guidelines are advocated by the committee to help prevent the most prevalent and devastating diseases in our society: diabetes, cancer, hypertension, and heart disease.

- Aim for a healthy weight.
- Be physically active each day.
- Let the Food Guide Pyramid guide your food choices.
- Choose a variety of grains daily, especially whole grains.

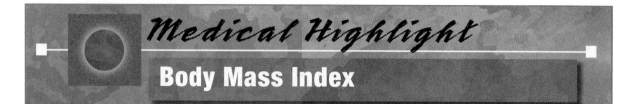

Body Mass Index

Obesity is a major health concern for the American people. Of Americans, 61% are overweight or obese. Obesity has direct links to serious illnesses such as Type II diabetes, high blood pressure, coronary artery disease, and stroke. The liver makes more triglycerides and less HDL. There is an increased risk of gallstones and sleep apnea. It is not uncommon for overweight adults to experience physiological stress, reduced income, and discrimination.

Researchers have found that body fat, instead of body weight, is a better predictor of health.

Body mass index (BMI) relates your body weight with health risks of being overweight. A method to determine BMI is as follows:

1. Multiply weight in pounds × 0.45 (e.g., 140 lb × 0.45 = 63).
2. Multiply height in inches by 0.025 (e.g., 65 inches × 0.025 = 1.625).
3. Square the answer from step 2 (e.g., 1.625 × 1.625 = 2.64).
4. Divide the answer from step 1 by the answer from step 3 (e.g., 63/2.64 = 23.86).

Generally a healthy BMI ranges from 19 to 25.

Source: Medical Essay on Weight Control, supplement to Mayo Clinic Health Letter from USDA Center for Nutrition, Policy and Promotion (March 2000)

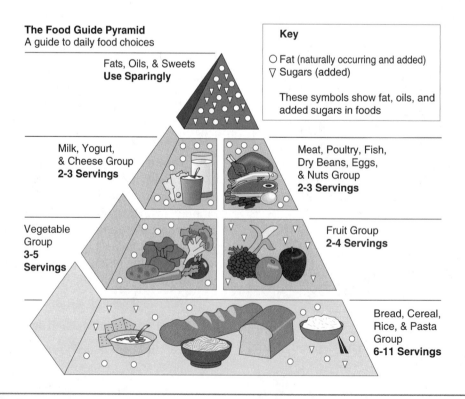

Figure 19-1 *Food Guide Pyramid*

- Choose a variety of fruits and vegetables daily.

- Keep food safe to eat.

- Choose a diet that is low in saturated fat and cholesterol, and moderate in total fat.

- Choose and prepare foods with less salt.

- If you drink alcoholic beverages, do so in moderation.

NUTRITION LABELING

In May 1994, the FDA mandated nutrition labeling for most foods offered for sale and regulated by the FDA, Figure 19-2. The nutrition label is required to include information on total calories and on amounts of calories from fat, cholesterol, sodium, total carbohydrates, dietary fiber, sugars, protein, vitamin A, vitamin C, calcium, and iron—in that order. The information on the package is to represent the packaged product prior to consumer preparation.

This final rule establishes a standard format for nutrition information on food labels consisting of the following:

1. Quantitative amount per serving of each nutrient except vitamins and minerals

2. Amount of each nutrient as a percent of the Daily Value for a 2,000-calorie diet

3. Footnote with reference values for selected nutrients based on 2,000- and 2,500-calorie diets

4. Caloric conversion information

FOOD POISONING

According to the National Institute of Health, food borne germs cause 76 million illnesses every year in the United States. In most cases, symptoms of food poisoning resemble intestinal flu and last a few hours to several days. Microscopic organisms can grow undetected in food because they do not produce an odor, or a difference in color or texture. These microbes can be prevented from comtaminating food by proper storing and handling. The single most important thing is thorough hand washing before handling food. Scrub your hands with soap and water for at least 20 seconds after handling raw meat, fish or poultry. Clean all cooking surfaces and utensils properly. For food safety thoroughly cook all

Nutrition Facts

Serving Size: 1/2 Cup
Servings Per Container: 4

Amount Per Serving	
Calories 100 Calories from Fat 30	
	% Daily Value*
Total Fat 3g	**5%**
Saturated Fat 0g	**0%**
Cholesterol 0mg	**0%**
Sodium 340mg	**14%**
Total Carbohydrate 15g	**5%**
Dietary Fiber 1g	**4%**
Sugars 0g	
Protein 2g	

Vitamin A 0% • Vitamin C 0%
Calcium   0% • Iron   2%

*Percent Daily Values are based on a 2,000 calorie diet. Your daily values may be higher or lower depending on your calorie needs:

	Calories	2,000	2,500
Total Fat	Less than	65g	80g
Sat Fat	Less than	20g	25g
Cholesterol	Less than	300mg	300mg
Sodium	Less than	2,400mg	2,400mg
Total Carbohydrate		300g	375g
Dietary Fiber		25g	30g

Calories per gram:
Fat 9 • Carbohydrate 4 • Protein 4

Ingredients: Flour, Water, Yeast Vegetable Oil, Salt, Artificial Flavor and Color.

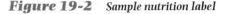

Figure 19-2   *Sample nutrition label*

meat, poultry, eggs and shellfish. Don't leave food at room temperature for over two hours. Refrigerate food below 40 degrees F. This will help to stop the growth of most organisms that cause illness. Observe "sell by" and "use by" dates on label.

EATING DISORDERS

Obesity is one of the most common "nutritional diseases" in our society. An obese person is one who contains excess body fat and who weighs 15% more than the optimum body weight for gender, height, and bone structure.

Being obese can affect physical and mental health. Heart disease, high blood pressure, and noninsulin dependent diabetes mellitus are more common in significantly overweight people than in those closer to ideal body weight.

Because most cases of obesity are due to an excessive intake of calories in proportion to expenditure, a daily reduction of caloric intake along with an increase in exercise are recommended for most overweight individuals.

Anorexia nervosa is a complex eating disorder mostly seen in young women. In true anorexia nervosa, there is no real loss of appetite, but rather a refusal to eat because of a distorted body image and a fear of weight gain.

The criteria for diagnosis of anorexia nervosa are identified by the American Psychiatric Association as follows:

1. Intense fear of becoming obese that does not diminish as weight loss progresses

2. Disturbance of body image, such as claiming to feel fat even when emaciated

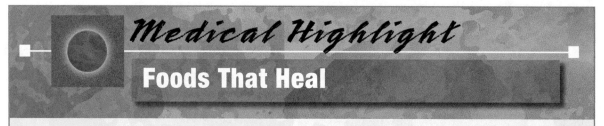

Medical Highlight

Foods That Heal

How many people have family recipes that cure colds, hay fever, asthma, and arthritis? Today scientists are looking at antioxidants, nutrients found in plant foods (such as vitamin C, carotenoids, vitamin E, and certain minerals), because of their potentially beneficial role in reducing the risk of cancer and certain other chronic diseases. Most of this research is in its earliest stages, but experts agree that certain food in moderation seem to boost healing.

Some foods believed to have healing power include:

- Barley—The soluble fiber in barley may be just as effective as oat bran in lowering cholesterol.[1]

- Carrots—Beta carotene, a chemical found in carrots which offers an edge against cancer, may also protect against heart disease.

- Cheese—Identified in dental research as a food that fights, rather than creates, cavities. Tooth-friendly cheeses include cheddar, Monterey Jack, Edam, Gouda, Roquefort, mozzarella, and Stilton.

- Chili peppers—Eating chili peppers helps with a stuffed-up nose. The eye-watering, nose-running properties of peppers are good for people suffering from bronchitis, sinusitis, and colds.[2]

- Garlic—An all-around healing food; it lowers blood pressure and cholesterol levels and fights infection.

- Persimmons—A more powerful source of vitamin C than oranges, one persimmon is equal to 218 mg of vitamin C; one orange is equal to 70 mg of vitamin C.

- Prunes—Contain 60% of a fiber known as pectin which is known to reduce cholesterol. They are also high in iron, potassium, and beta carotene.

- Dried beans—Help to lower cholesterol.

- Fish oil—Contains omega-3, a fatty acid currently being tested to help with inflammation from arthritis. Effective types of fish include mackerel, salmon, bluefish, oysters, mussels, crabs, and clams.

- Spinach and collard greens—Have two specific compounds which may be protective against the leading causes of irreversible blindness in older people, a condition known as age-related macular degeneration.[3]

[1] Based on research conducted at Montana University. [2] Based on research conducted by Dr. Irwin Zen at UCLA. [3] Based on research reported in the Journal of the AMA.

3. Weight loss of at least 25% of the original body weight

4. Refusal to maintain body weight over a minimal normal weight for age and height

5. No known physical illness that would account for the weight loss

6. Amenorrhea, or the cessation of menstruation

Bulimia is an eating disorder associated with fear of weight gain. It is characterized by episodic binge eating followed by purging behavior such as self-induced vomiting and laxative abuse. Bulimic patients are most often women somewhat older than those with anorexia nervosa. In some instances, a young woman alternates between the two disorders.

The treatment of anorexia nervosa and bulimia is difficult and lengthy. The goals are restitution of normal nutrition and resolution of the underlying psychological problems. Early intervention is essential; the starvation associated with anorexia can cause irreversible tissue damage and the purging associated with bulimia can cause homeostatic imbalances that lead to cardiac irregularities and, in extreme cases, death.

Medical Terminology

BMI	body mass index
BMR	basal metabolic rate
HDL	high-density lipoprotein
LDL	low-density lipoprotein
micro	millionth
gram	unit of measurement of mass metric system
micro/gram	one-millionth of a gram
milli	thousand
milligram	one-thousandth of a gram

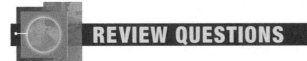

REVIEW QUESTIONS

Select the letter of the choice that best completes the statement.

1. Materials needed by the individual cells for proper cell function are:
   a. proteases
   b. enzymes
   c. amylases
   d. nutrients

2. A gram of fat contains:
   a. 9 calories
   b. 4 calories
   c. 5 calories
   d. 7 calories

3. The main source of energy for the body is provided by:
   a. fats
   b. carbohydrates
   c. proteins
   d. water

4. To build and repair body tissue you need:
   a. fats
   b. carbohydrates
   c. proteins
   d. water

5. The most common bone disease is:
   a. osteomyelitis
   b. fracture
   c. osteoporosis
   d. bone cancer

6. The minerals necessary to build bone and teeth are:
   a. iodine and calcium
   b. calcium and potassium
   c. calcium and phosphorus
   d. fluorine and calcium

7. Iodine is required for the formation of the:
   a. adrenal hormone
   b. thyroid hormone
   c. parathyroid hormone
   d. pituitary hormone

8. A vitamin needed to prevent night blindness is:
   a. vitamin A
   b. vitamin K
   c. vitamin C
   d. vitamin D

9. The vitamin essential for blood clotting is:
   a. vitamin A
   b. vitamin K
   c. vitamin C
   d. vitamin D

10. A food that has been identified to help lower cholesterol is:
   a. cheddar cheese
   b. garlic
   c. white bread
   d. broccoli

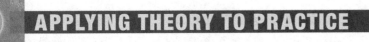

APPLYING THEORY TO PRACTICE

1. The USDA changed from the basic four food groups to the six group pyramid plan, the model for Recommended Dietary Allowances. Compare your daily diet with the food pyramid plan. Should you consider changing your diet to meet these requirements?

2. Plan a 3-day meal plan including between-meal snacks that will meet both recommended calorie intake and dietary allowances for yourself. Adjust this diet to meet the needs of a 12-year-old male, height 62 inches. Adjust this diet to meet the needs of a 70-year-old female, height 60 inches.

3. A patient has anemia. The doctor requests that you assist the patient in establishing a menu plan that will assist in the formation of red blood cells.

4. Nutritionists recommend 50% to 60% of carbohydrates daily in a 2,000-calorie diet. What proportion of the diet would 60% be? How many calories would be in carbohydrates?

5. A physician orders a diet of 20 gm of protein, 300 gm of carbohydrate, and 80 gm of fat. What are the total calories, and how much caloric value is there in protein, carbohydrates, and fat? Calculate the percentage of protein, carbohydrates, and fat.

CASE STUDY

Lauren S. is a 60-year-old woman who weighs 200 pounds and is 5'5" in height. She has been recently diagnosed with Type II diabetes. Her physician states it is necessary for her to lose weight and sends her to see Jodi, the HMO nutritionist. Jodi first discusses with Lauren what makes up a balanced diet. In addition, Jodi will help Lauren determine her BMR and her caloric needs to reach and maintain a healthy weight.

1. Discuss the role of carbohydrates, fats, and proteins in the diet.

2. What is the importance of healthy cholesterol and triglyceride blood levels?

3. Explain the Food Guide Pyramid.

4. How many servings of each type of food are allowed according to the Food Guide Pyramid?

5. What is the recommended weight for Lauren according to weight and height scales?

6. Explain the term "Recommended Dietary Allowances."

7. What is Lauren's BMR? What factors influence the BMR?

8. Researchers state that BMI is a better indicator of health; Jodi should help Lauren determine her BMI.

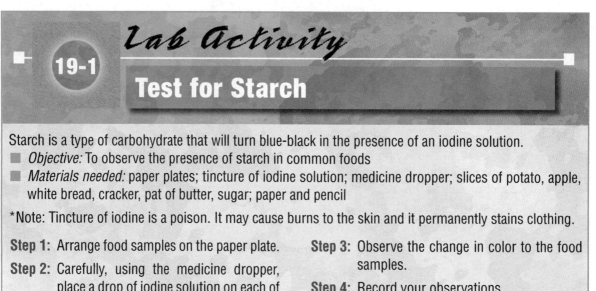

Lab Activity

19-1 Test for Starch

Starch is a type of carbohydrate that will turn blue-black in the presence of an iodine solution.
- *Objective:* To observe the presence of starch in common foods
- *Materials needed:* paper plates; tincture of iodine solution; medicine dropper; slices of potato, apple, white bread, cracker, pat of butter, sugar; paper and pencil

*Note: Tincture of iodine is a poison. It may cause burns to the skin and it permanently stains clothing.

Step 1: Arrange food samples on the paper plate.

Step 2: Carefully, using the medicine dropper, place a drop of iodine solution on each of the food samples.

Step 3: Observe the change in color to the food samples.

Step 4: Record your observations.

Step 5: Which food samples contain starch? Record your answer.

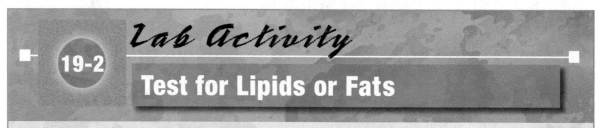

Lab Activity

19-2 Test for Lipids or Fats

Fats will leave brown paper greasy.
- *Objective:* To observe the presence of fat in common foods
- *Materials needed:* brown paper, slice of raw potato, teaspoon of cooking oil, butter, corn kernels, bean seeds, a light source, paper and pencil

Step 1: Place a few drops of cooking oil on brown paper. Hold the paper up to a light and look through the spot. Record your observations.

Step 2: Repeat the process with the butter, bean seeds, raw potato, and corn kernels by rubbing these foods onto the brown paper. Hold the paper up to the light.

Step 3: Record your observations.

Step 4: Which food samples contain lipids or fats? Record your answer.

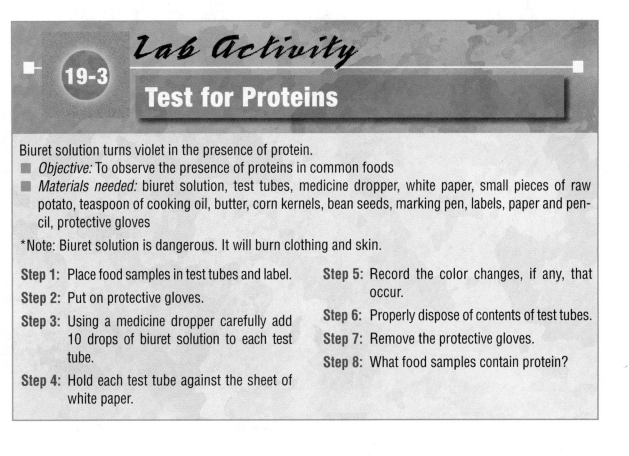

Lab Activity

19-3

Test for Proteins

Biuret solution turns violet in the presence of protein.

■ *Objective:* To observe the presence of proteins in common foods

■ *Materials needed:* biuret solution, test tubes, medicine dropper, white paper, small pieces of raw potato, teaspoon of cooking oil, butter, corn kernels, bean seeds, marking pen, labels, paper and pencil, protective gloves

*Note: Biuret solution is dangerous. It will burn clothing and skin.

Step 1: Place food samples in test tubes and label.

Step 2: Put on protective gloves.

Step 3: Using a medicine dropper carefully add 10 drops of biuret solution to each test tube.

Step 4: Hold each test tube against the sheet of white paper.

Step 5: Record the color changes, if any, that occur.

Step 6: Properly dispose of contents of test tubes.

Step 7: Remove the protective gloves.

Step 8: What food samples contain protein?

Chapter 20

URINARY/EXCRETORY SYSTEM

Objectives

- Explain the function of the excretory organs

- Describe the structure and function of the organs in the urinary system

- Explain how the kidneys regulate water balance

- List and describe some common disorders of the urinary system

- Define the key words that relate to this chapter

Key Words

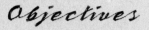

acute kidney failure
acute glomerulon-ephritis
afferent arteriole
aldosterone
anuria
Bowman's capsule
calyces
chronic renal failure
chronic glomer-ulonephritis
collecting tubule
cortex
cystitis
dialysis
dialyzer
distal convoluted tubule
dysuria
efferent arteriole
extracorporeal shockware

lithotripsy (ESWL)
filtrate
fistula
glomerulonephritis
glomerulus
graft
hematuria
hemodialysis
hilum
hydronephrosis
incontinence
kidney
kidney stones (renal calculi)
loop of Henle
medulla
nephron
neurogenic bladder
nocturia
oliguria

osmoreceptor
peritoneal dialysis
proximal convoluted tubule
polyuria
pyelonephritis
pyuria
renal column
renal fascia
renal papilla
renal pelvis
renal pyramid
renin
retroperitoneal
threshold
uremia
ureter
urethra
urinalysis
urinary bladder
urinary meatus

URINARY SYSTEM

Food is transformed through the process of digestion, absorption, and metabolism. The blood and lymph transport products of digestion to the tissues. After the cells of the tissues have used the food and oxygen needed for growth and repair, the waste products formed must be taken away and excreted from the body. The blood and lymph transport the cellular waste to the excretory organs. The excretory organs eliminate the metabolic wastes and undigested food residue.

The excretory organs through which elimination takes place include the kidneys, skin, intestines, and lungs. The lungs, serve an excretory function in that they give off carbon dioxide and water vapor during exhalation. The urinary system functions largely as an excretory agent of nitrogenous wastes, salts, and water, while the skin excretes dissolved wastes present in perspiration, mostly dissolved salts. The indigestible residue, water, and bacteria are excreted by the intestines. The excretion of waste products is described and summarized in Table 20-1.

The urinary system performs the main part of the excretory function in the body, Figure 20-1. The most important excretory organs are the **kidneys.** If the kidneys fail to function properly, toxic wastes start to accumulate in the body. Toxic wastes accumulating in the cells cause them to "suffocate" and literally poison themselves.

The urinary system consists of two kidneys (that form the urine), two ureters, a bladder, and a urethra. Each kidney has a long, tubular ureter that carries urine to the urinary bladder. This is a temporary storage sac for urine, from which urine is excreted through the urethra.

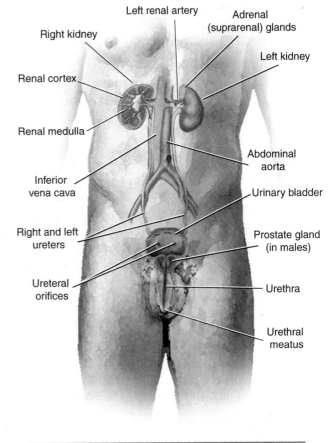

Figure 20-1   *Structures of the urinary system*

FUNCTIONS OF THE URINARY SYSTEM

1. Excretion, which is the process of removing nitrogenous waste material, certain salts, and excess water from the blood

Table 20-1 Elimination of Waste Products		
ORGAN	**PRODUCT OF EXCRETION**	**PROCESS OF ELIMINATION**
Lungs	carbon dioxide and water vapor	exhalation
Kidneys	nitrogenous wastes and salts dissolved in water to form urine	urination
Skin	dissolved salts	perspiration
Intestines	solid wastes and water	defecation

2. Aid in maintaining acid-base balance by evaluating elements in the blood and selectively reabsorbing water and other substances to maintain the pH balance

3. Secretion of waste products in the form of urine

4. Elimination of urine from the bladder where it is stored

KIDNEYS

The kidneys are bean-shaped organs resting high against the dorsal wall of the abdominal cavity; they lie on either side of the vertebral column, between the peritoneum and the back muscles. Because the kidneys are located behind the peritoneum, they are said to be **retroperitoneal.** They are positioned between the twelfth thoracic and the third lumbar vertebrae. The right kidney is situated slightly lower than the left due to the large area occupied by the liver.

Each kidney and its blood vessels is enclosed within a mass of fat tissue called the adipose capsule. In turn, each kidney and adipose capsule is covered by a tough, fibrous tissue called the **renal fascia.**

There is an indentation along the concave medial border of the kidney called the **hilum.** The hilum is a passageway for the lymph vessels, nerves, renal artery and vein, and the ureter. At the hilum the fibrous capsule continues downward, forming the outer layer of the ureter. Cutting the kidney in half lengthwise reveals its internal structure. The upper end of each ureter flares into a funnel-shaped structure known as the **renal pelvis,** Figure 20-2.

The kidneys have the potential to work harder than they actually do. Under ordinary circumstances, only a portion of the nephron (the functional unit of the kidney) is used. Should one kidney not function, or have to be removed, more nephrons and tubules open up in the second kidney to assume the work of the nonfunctioning or missing kidney.

Medulla and Cortex

The kidney is divided into two layers: an outer, granular layer called the **cortex,** and an inner,

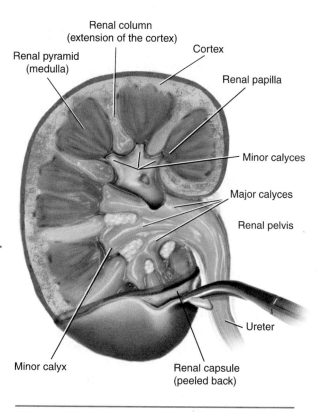

Figure 20-2 *Structures of the kidney*

striated layer, the **medulla.** The medulla is red and consists of radially striated cones called the **renal pyramids.** The base of each renal pyramid faces the cortex, while its apex (**renal papilla**) empties into cuplike cavities called **calyces.** These, in turn, empty into the renal pelvis.

The cortex is reddish brown, and consists of millions of microscopic functional units of the kidney called nephrons. Cortical tissue is interspersed between renal pyramids, separating and supporting them. These interpyramidal cortical supports are the **renal columns.** The renal columns and the renal pyramids alternate with one another, see Figure 20-2.

NEPHRON

The **nephron** is the basic structural and functional unit of the kidney. Most of the nephron is located within the cortex, with only a small, tubular portion in the medulla. Each kidney has over 1 million nephrons which altogether comprise 140 miles of filters and tubes.

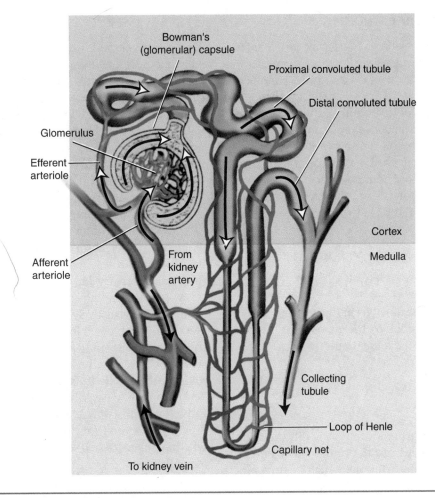

Bowman's
(glomerular) capsule

Proximal convoluted tubule

Distal convoluted tubule

Glomerulus

Efferent
arteriole

Afferent
arteriole

From
kidney
artery

Cortex

Medulla

Collecting
tubule

Loop of Henle

Capillary net

To kidney vein

Figure 20-3   *Structure of the nephron*

A nephron begins with the **afferent arteriole,** which carries blood from the renal artery. The afferent arteriole enters a double-walled hollow capsule, the **Bowman's capsule** (named for Sir William Bowman [1816–1892], English anatomist). Within the capsule the afferent arteriole finely divides, forming a knotty ball called the **glomerulus,** which contains some 50 separate capillaries. The combination of the Bowman's capsule and the glomerulus is known as the renal corpuscle. The Bowman's capsule sends off a highly convoluted (twisted) tubular branch referred to as the **proximal convoluted tubule.**

The proximal convoluted tubule descends into the medulla to form the **loop of Henle.** In Figure 20-3, observe that the loop of Henle has a straight descending limb, a loop, and a straight as-

cending limb. When the ascending limb of Henle's loop returns to the cortex, it turns into the **distal convoluted tubule.** Eventually this convoluted tubule opens into a larger, straight vessel known as the **collecting tubule.** Several distal convoluted tubules join to form this single straight collection tubule. The collecting tubule empties into the renal pelvis, then into the ureter.

As Figure 20-3 shows, the walls of the renal tubules are surrounded by capillaries. After the afferent arteriole branches out to form the glomerulus, it leaves the Bowman's capsule as the **efferent arteriole.** The efferent arteriole branches to form the peritubular capillaries surrounding the renal tubules. All of these capillaries eventually join together to form a small branch of the renal vein which carries blood from the kidney.

The Path of the Formation of Urine

Blood enters the afferent arteriole → passes through the glomerulus → to Bowman's capsule → now it becomes filtrate (blood minus the red blood cells and plasma proteins) → continues through the proximal convoluted tubule → to the loop of Henle → to the distal convoluted tubule → to the collecting tubule (at this time about 99% of the filtrate has been reabsorbed) → approximately 1 ml of urine is formed per minute → the 1 ml of urine goes to the renal pelvis → to the ureter → to the bladder → to the urethra → to the urinary meatus.

URINE FORMATION IN THE NEPHRON

The kidney nephrons form urine by three processes: (1) filtration by the glomerulus, (2) reabsorption within the renal tubules, and (3) secretion by the tubular cells.

Filtration

The first step in urine formation is filtration. In this process, blood from the renal artery enters the smaller afferent arteriole, which in turn enters the even smaller capillaries of the glomerulus. As the blood from the renal artery travels this course, the blood vessels grow narrower and narrower. This results in an increase in blood pressure. In most of the capillaries throughout the body, blood pressure is about 25 mm/Hg; in the glomerulus, it is between 60 and 90 mm/Hg.

This high blood pressure forces a plasmalike fluid to filter from the blood in the glomerulus into the Bowman's capsule. This fluid is called the **filtrate.** It consists of water, glucose, amino acids, some salts, and urea. The filtrate does not contain plasma proteins or red blood cells because they are too large to pass through the pores of the capillary membrane. The Bowman's capsule filters out 125 ml of fluid from the blood in a single minute. In 1 hour, 7,500 ml of filtrate leave the blood; this amounts to some 180 l in a 24-hour period.

As the nephric filtrate continues along the tubules, 99% of this fluid is reabsorbed back into the bloodstream; therefore, only 1.0 to 1.5 l (1,000 to 1,500 ml) of urine are excreted per day.

Reabsorption

This process includes the reabsorption of useful substances from the filtrate within the renal tubules into the capillaries around the tubules (peritubular capillaries). These include water, glucose, amino acids, vitamins, bicarbonate ions (HCO_3^-), and the chloride salts of calcium, magnesium, sodium, and potassium. Reabsorption starts in the proximal convoluted tubules; it continues through the Henle's loop, the distal convoluted tubules, and the collecting tubules.

The proximal tubules reabsorb approximately 80% of the water filtered out of the blood in the glomeruli. Water absorbed through the proximal tubules constitutes obligatory water absorption (amount necessary for cell function). Simultaneously, glucose, amino acids, vitamins, and some sodium ions are actively transported back into the blood. However, when levels exceed normal limits, the selective cells lining the tubules no longer reabsorb substances such as glucose but allow it to remain in the tubule to be eliminated in the urine. The term used to describe the limit of reabsorption is the **threshold.** Passing this level is referred to as "spilling over the threshold." For example, people who have diabetes spill sugar frequently and therefore sugar can be found in their urine (glycosuria). Another example is, when a person is taking medications the tubules will only reabsorb a certain amount of the drug; therefore, the medication may have to be taken every 4 to 6 hours to maintain a therapeutic dosage of the drug in the blood.

In the distal convoluted tubules about 10% to 15% of water is reabsorbed into the bloodstream, depending on the needs of the body. This type of water absorption is called optional reabsorption. It is controlled by the antidiuretic hormone (ADH) and aldosterone. ADH and aldosterone help maintain balance of body fluids, Figure 20-4.

Secretion

The process of secretion is the opposite of reabsorption. Some substances are actively secreted into the tubules. Secretion transports substances from the blood in the peritubular capillaries into the urine in the distal and collecting tubules. Substances secreted into the urine include ammonia creatinine, hydrogen ions (H^+), potassium ions (K^+), and some

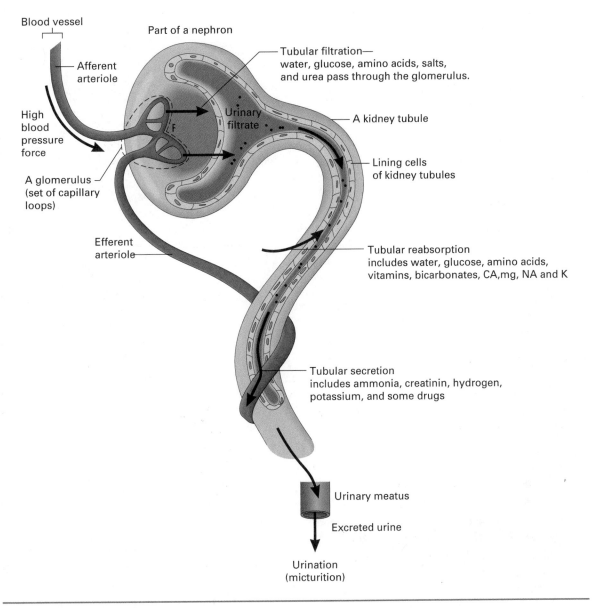

Figure 20-4 *Processes and structures of the nephron*

drugs. The electrolytes are selectively secreted to maintain the body's acid-base balance.

Urinary Output

The amount of urinary output is between 1,000 and 2,000 ml/24 hours with an average of 1,500 ml per day. Volume will vary with diet, fluid intake, temperature, and physical activity. Another factor regulating secretion is the amount of solutes in the filtrate. Again considering the diabetic, when there

is an increase in the amount of glucose, it spills over into the urine, thus increasing the urine volume eliminated that day because more fluid is allowed to pass through to dilute the glucose content.

Urinalysis, an examination of the urine, can determine the presence of blood cells, bacteria, acidity level, specific gravity (weight), and physical characteristics such as color, clarity, and odor. A urinalysis is the most common noninvasive diagnostic test done. See Figure 20-5 for a lab report which shows normal values for a routine urinalysis.

PHYSICAL EXAMINATION:

Appearance ___CLEAR, STRAW-COLORED___

pH ___4.5 TO 7.5 (RANGE)___   Specific Gravity ___1.010 TO 1.025 (RANGE)___

CHEMICAL ANALYSIS:

Albumin (protein) ___NONE TO TRACE___   Urobilinogen ___NEG.___

Sugar (glucose, dextrose) ___NONE___   Porphyrins ___NEG.___

Ketones (acetone) ___NONE___   PKU ___NEG.___

Bilirubin ___NONE___   Occult Blood ___NEG.___

MICROSCOPIC EXAMINATION:

Cells: Epithelial ___FEW___

WBCs ___0 TO 4___

RBCs ___FEW TO OCCASIONAL___

Casts: Hyaline ___NEG.___

Epithelial ___NEG.___

Blood ___NEG.___   (EA) 6/30/xx

Crystals: ___FEW___

Other: ___NEG.___

Figure 20-5   *Lab report showing normal values for a routine urinalysis*

URETERS

Urine passes from the kidneys out of the collecting tubules into the renal pelvis, down the ureter, into the urinary bladder. There are two **ureters** (one from each kidney) carrying urine from the kidneys to the urinary bladder. They are long, narrow tubes, less than 1/4 inch wide and 10 to 12 inches long. Mucous membrane lines both renal pelves and the ureters. Beneath the mucous membrane lining of the ureters are smooth muscle fibers. When these muscles contract, peristalsis is initiated, pushing urine down the ureter into the urinary bladder.

URINARY BLADDER

The **urinary bladder,** a hollow muscular organ made of elastic fibers and involuntary muscle,

acts like a reservoir. It stores the urine until about 1 pint (500 ml) is accumulated. The bladder then becomes uncomfortable and must be emptied. Emptying the bladder, or voiding, takes place by muscular contractions of the bladder which are involuntary, although they can be controlled to some extent through the nervous system. Contraction of the bladder muscles forces the urine through a narrow canal, the **urethra,** which extends to the outside opening, the **urinary meatus.**

CONTROL OF URINARY SECRETION

The control of the secretions of urine is under both chemical and nervous control.

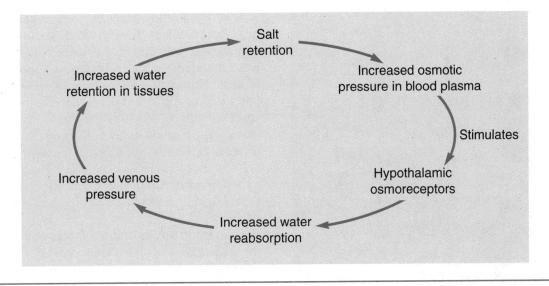

Figure 20-6 *Effects of salt retention on water retention in tissues*

Chemical Control

The reabsorption of water in the distal convoluted kidney tubules and the collecting ducts is influenced by ADH, which helps to increase the size of the cell membrane pores in the epithelial cells of the distal tubule and collecting ducts by increasing their permeability to water. The secretion and regulation of the ADH is under the control of the hypothalamus. In the hypothalamus, highly sensitive receptor cells, called **osmoreceptors,** are sensitive to the osmotic pressure of blood plasma. An increase in the osmotic blood pressure due to salt retention causes an increase in ADH secretion. This will inhibit normal urine formation, and water may also be held in the tissues. Figure 20-6 shows the effect of salt retention on human tissues.

There are other hormones involved in the reabsorption process. **Aldosterone** secreted by the adrenal cortex promotes the excretion of potassium and hydrogen ions and the reabsorption of sodium ions; chloride ions and water are also absorbed. As the blood passes through the glomerulus to Bowman's capsule, specialized cells are able to detect a drop in blood pressure. A hormone called **renin** is released by the kidneys into the bloodstream. Renin stimulates the release of aldosterone by the adrenal cortex and constricts the blood vessels. In the absence of aldosterone, sodium and water are excreted in large amounts, and potassium is retained. Any dysfunction to the

adrenal cortex produces pronounced changes in the salt and water content of body fluids.

Diuretics increase urinary output by inhibiting the reabsorption of water. Alcohol and caffeine are examples of common diuretics. Alcohol inhibits the secretion of ADH from the pituitary gland. This increases urinary output and may cause dehydration. (This explains why after drinking alcohol the night before you may wake up feeling "parched" and dried out.) Caffeine increases the loss of sodium ion, thus increasing the loss of water.

Nervous Control

The nervous control of urine secretion is accomplished directly through the action of nerve impulses on the blood vessels leading to the kidney and on those within the kidney leading to the glomeruli. Indirect nerve control is achieved through the stimulation of certain endocrine glands, whose hormonal secretions will control urinary secretion.

DISORDERS OF THE URINARY SYSTEM

Acute kidney failure may be sudden in onset. Causes may be nephritis (inflammation of the nephron), shock, injury, bleeding, sudden heart

Effects of Aging on The Urinary System

With advancing age, the kidneys shrink due to a loss of nephrons within the cortical region of the kidney. There is also evidence of collapsing glomeruli and sclerotic changes in the larger renal blood vessels. The end result is a decrease in renal blood flow. This change in flow compromises the ability of the kidney to eliminate unwanted substances from the blood-stream. There is also a decline in the glomerular filtration rate. Decrease in this rate means that, for drugs excreted by the kidney, the dose of drugs needs to be adjusted to compensate for the age-related decrease in kidney function. If adjustments are not made, there is an age-related risk for drug overdose. Other functions such as glucose resorption also decrease in the aged with the resulting problem of hyperglycemia.

There is a loss of muscle tone in the urinary bladder, which frequently causes nocturia (frequent nighttime urination). Weakening of the bladder and the sphincters reduces the ability to maintain continence. Urinary incontinence, the involuntary loss of urine, is frequently observed in the elderly.

failure, or poisoning. The symptoms of acute kidney failure include **oliguria,** which is scanty or diminished production of the urine, or **anuria,** which is absence of urine formation. Suppression of urine formation is dangerous; unless anuria is relieved, **uremia** will develop. Uremia is a toxic condition which occurs when the blood retains urinary waste products. Symptoms resulting from uremia are headaches, dyspnea, nausea, vomiting, and in extreme cases, coma and death.

Chronic renal failure is the condition where there is a gradual loss of function of the nephrons.

Glomerulonephritis is an inflammation of the glomerulus of the nephron. The filtration process is affected. Plasma proteins are filtered through and protein is found in the urine as albumin (albuminuria). In addition, red blood cells are present (**hematuria**).

Acute glomerulonephritis occurs in some children about 1 to 3 weeks after a bacterial infection, usually a strep throat. The illness is treated with antibiotics and recovery takes place.

Chronic glomerulonephritis occurs when the filtration membrane may be permanently affected. There is diminished function of the kidney, which may result in kidney failure.

Hydronephrosis occurs when the renal pelvis and calyces become distended due to an accumulation of fluid, Figure 20-7. The urine backs up because of a blockage in the ureter or pressure on the outside of the ureter, which may narrow the passageway. The blockage may be caused by a kidney stone. Other conditions which may cause hydronephrosis are pregnancy or an enlarged prostate gland, which causes pressure on the ureters or bladder. The treatment for this condition is the removal of the obstruction.

Pyelonephritis is the inflammation of the kidney tissue and the renal pelvis. This condition generally results from an infection that has spread from the ureters. One of the symptoms is **pyuria,** the presence of pus in the urine. The course of treatment includes the administration of antibiotics.

Kidney stones or **renal calculi** are stones formed in the kidney. Some materials contained in urine are only slightly soluble in water. Therefore, when stagnation occurs, the microscopic crystals of calcium phosphate, along with uric acid and other substances, may clump together to form kid-

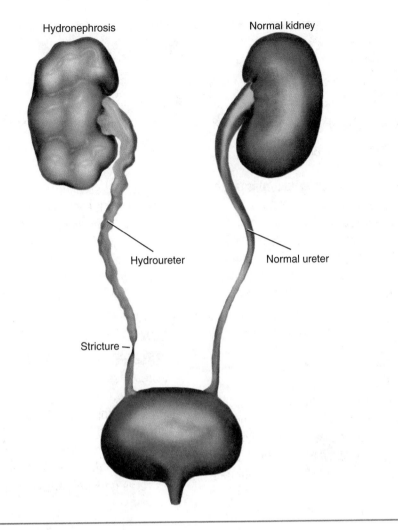

Hydronephrosis

Normal kidney

Hydroureter

Normal ureter

Stricture —

Figure 20-7   *Hydronephrosis*

ney stones. These kidney stones slowly grow in diameter. They eventually fill the renal pelvis and obstruct urine flow in the ureter. Usually, the first symptom of a kidney stone is extreme pain, which occurs suddenly in the kidney area or lower abdomen and moves to the groin. Other symptoms include nausea and vomiting, burning, frequent urge to void, chills, fever, and weakness. There may also be hematuria. Diagnosis is made by symptoms, ultrasound, and x-rays such as intravenous pyelogram (IVP) and kidney, ureter, and bladder (KUB). Treatment includes an increase in fluids which will increase urinary output. This may help to flush out the stone. Medications are given to help to dissolve the stone. If this is not successful, a urethroscope, or lithotripsy, may be done. (See Medical Highlight).

Cystitis is the inflammation of the mucous membrane lining of the urinary bladder. The most common cause of cystitis is from the bacteria *E. coli* which is normally found in the rectum or from urethritis which usually leads to painful urination (**dysuria**) or frequent urination (**polyuria**). This condition is more common in the female. The length of the female urethra is about 1.25 to 2 inches. Organisms can easily enter the urethra from the outside of the body. The treatment of cystitis involves antibiotics and urinary antiseptics with increased fluids. The patient should be taught proper wiping techniques after urination. The patient with cystitis must be reminded to complete the prescribed amount of medication to prevent reinfection.

Medical Highlight
Kidney Stone Removal

EXTRACORPOREAL SHOCKWAVE LITHOTRIPSY

A surgical procedure called **extracorporeal shockwave lithotripsy (ESWL)** may be done to remove kidney stones located high in the ureters or the renal pelvis. ESWL uses shockwaves created outside the body to travel through the skin and body tissues until the waves hit the dense stones. The stones become sandlike and are passed through the urinary tract. There are several devices used. One device positions the patient in the water bath while the shockwaves are transmitted. Most devices use either x-ray or ultrasound to help the surgeon locate the stone during the treatment.

This procedure can be done on an outpatient basis. Recovery time is short and most people resume normal activities in a few days. Some complications may occur such as hematuria, bruising, and minor discomfort on the back or abdomen. In addition, the shattered stone fragments may cause discomfort as they pass through the urinary tract.

PERCUTANEOUS NEPHROLITHOTOMY

In the procedure called percutaneous nephrolithotomy, the surgeon makes a tiny hole in the patient's back and creates a tunnel directly into the kidney. Using an instrument called a nephroscope, the surgeon locates and removes the stones. For larger stones, an ultrasonic energy probe may be needed to break the stone into smaller pieces. One advantage of this procedure over ESWL is that the surgeon removes the stone fragments instead of relying on their natural passage from the kidney.

URETEROSCOPIC STONE REMOVAL

Ureteroscopic stone removal is done for mid and lower stones. A surgeon passes a small fiber optic instrument called a urethroscope through the urethra and bladder into the ureter. The surgeon then locates the stone and either removes it with a cagelike device or shatters it with a special instrument that produces a form of shockwave.

Incontinence is also known as involuntary micturition (urination). Here, an individual loses voluntary control over urination. Incontinence occurs in babies prior to toilet training, since they lack control over the external sphincter muscle of the urethra. Thus, urination occurs when the bladder fills. Similarly, a person who has suffered a stroke or whose spinal cord has been severed may have no bladder control. In these conditions a patient may require an indwelling catheter. This is a tube inserted into the neck of the bladder through the urethra. It directs the urine into a sterile urinary drainage bag.

Neurogenic bladder is a condition caused by damaged nerves that control the urinary bladder. This results in dysuria, the inability to empty the bladder completely, and incontinence.

Dialysis

Dialysis is the type of treatment used for kidney failure. Dialysis involves the passage of blood through a device which has a semipermeable membrane to rid the blood of harmful wastes, extra salt, and water. Dialysis devices serve as a substitute kidney. The two forms of dialysis are hemodialysis and peritoneal dialysis.

Hemodialysis is a process for purifying blood by passing it through thin membranes and exposing it to a solution which continually circulates around the membrane. The solution is called a dialysate. Substances in the blood pass through the membranes into the lesser concentrated dialysate in response to the laws of diffusion. The part of the unit that actually substitutes for the

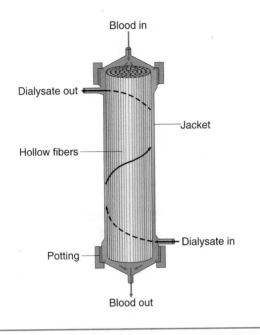

Blood in

Dialysate out

Jacket

Hollow fibers

Dialysate in

Potting

Blood out

Figure 20-8 *A dialyzer*

kidney is a glass tube called a **dialyzer,** which is filled with thousands of minute hollow fibers attached firmly at both ends, Figure 20-8. Blood from the client flows through the fibers, which are surrounded by circulating dialysate. The dialysate

is individualized for each patient to provide the appropriate levels of sodium, bicarbonate, and other substances. These cross the membrane and enter the blood. At the same time, extra water and waste products leave the blood to enter the dialysate.

The client is connected to the dialysis unit by means of needles and tubing that take blood from the client to the machine and return it to the client. A **fistula** (opening between an artery and a vein) or a **graft** (vein inserted between the artery and a vein) is surgically constructed to provide a site for inserting the needles. Artificial veins may last from 3 to 5 years. Most clients are assigned to a dialysis center for periodic treatment; however, treatment can also be done in the home if the client and family are willing to assume responsibility. It is usually done two to three times a week and each treatment lasts from 2 to 4 hours. To avoid side effects, the client is advised to follow special diet instructions and take medications as prescribed.

Peritoneal dialysis uses the client's own peritoneal lining instead of a dialyzer to filter the blood. A cleansing solution called the dialysate travels through a catheter implanted into the abdomen. Fluid, wastes, electrolytes, and chemicals pass from tiny blood vessels in the peritoneal

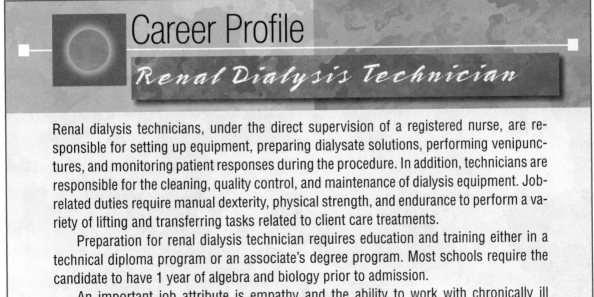

Career Profile

Renal Dialysis Technician

Renal dialysis technicians, under the direct supervision of a registered nurse, are responsible for setting up equipment, preparing dialysate solutions, performing venipunctures, and monitoring patient responses during the procedure. In addition, technicians are responsible for the cleaning, quality control, and maintenance of dialysis equipment. Job-related duties require manual dexterity, physical strength, and endurance to perform a variety of lifting and transferring tasks related to client care treatments.

Preparation for renal dialysis technician requires education and training either in a technical diploma program or an associate's degree program. Most schools require the candidate to have 1 year of algebra and biology prior to admission.

An important job attribute is empathy and the ability to work with chronically ill clients, and to work efficiently and accurately under pressure.

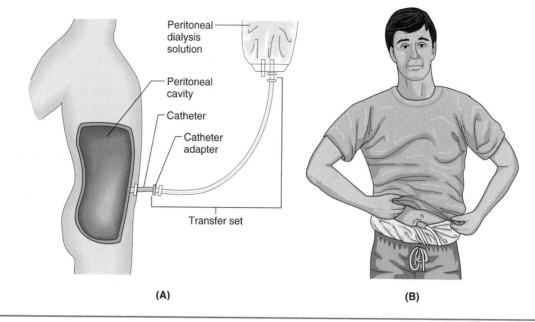

(A)

(B)

Figure 20-9 *Peritoneal dialysis*

membrane into the dialysate. After several hours, the dialysate is drained from the abdomen, taking the wastes from the blood with it. The abdomen is filled with fresh dialysate and the cleaning procedure begins again. The most common type of peritoneal dialysis is continuous ambulatory peritoneal dialysis (CAPD). The dialysate stays in the abdomen for 4 to 6 hours. The process of draining the dialysate and replacing it with fresh solution takes about 30 minutes. Most people change the solution four times a day, Figure 20-9.

Automated peritoneal dialysis, a type of peritoneal dialysis which can be done at night while the patient is asleep, takes 6 to 8 hours.

The main complication of peritoneal dialysis is peritonitis, an inflammation of the peritoneal lining.

Kidney Transplants

Kidney transplants are done in cases of prolonged chronic debilitating diseases and renal failure involving both kidneys. Usually the client has been on dialysis for a long period of time waiting for a compatible organ. The transplant requires a donor organ from an individual who has a similar immune system to prevent rejection. Blood and other cellular material must match to ensure the greatest potential for success in a transplant. The client is usually in a state of relatively poor physical condition due to the effects of the extended illness. This status plus the tendency of the body to reject a "substance" that is foreign and not of the same cellular structure sometimes results in the organ not surviving in the new host. The use of drugs to control the body's natural defensive mechanism of rejection increases the rate of success.

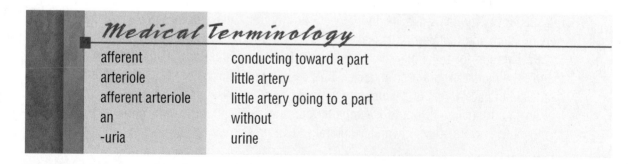

Medical Terminology

afferent	conducting toward a part
arteriole	little artery
afferent arteriole	little artery going to a part
an	without
-uria	urine

an/uria	without urine
cyst	bladder
-itis	inflammation of
cyst/itis	inflammation of the bladder
dia	across or through
-lysis	breaking down
dia/lysis	breaking down through a semipermeable membrane
dys	painful
dys/uria	painful urination
efferent	conducting outward from a part
efferent arteriole	little artery going away from a part
filtr	filter
-ate	relating to
filtr/ate	fluid passing through a filter
glomerulo	resembles a little ball of yarn
-nephr	kidney
glomerulo/ nephr/itis	inflammation of the glomeruli of the kidney
hema	blood
hemat/uria	blood in the urine
hemo/dia/lysis	blood breaking down through a semipermeable membrane
hydro	water
-osis	abnormal condition of
hydro/nephr/osis	abnormal condition of water on the kidney
olig	scanty
olig/uria	scanty urine
pyelo	renal pelvis
pyelo/nephr/itis	inflammation of the renal pelvis of the kidney
ren	kidney
-al	relating to
ren/al	relating to the kidney
ur	urine
-emia	blood condition
ur/emia	accumulation in the blood of the normal constituents of urine
urin/ana/lysis	breaking down parts of urine to study

REVIEW QUESTIONS

Select the letter of choice that best completes the statement.

1. The kidneys are responsible for excreting:
   a. carbon dioxide and water
   b. solid wastes and water
   c. nitrogenous wastes and water
   d. perspiration

2. In addition to kidneys, the organ(s) responsible for excretion of carbon dioxide and water is:
   a. lungs
   b. kidneys
   c. skin
   d. large intestine

3. The kidneys are located in which area?
   a. abdominal
   b. pelvic
   c. peritoneal
   d. retroperitoneal

4. A ball of capillaries is called the:
   a. Bowman's capsule
   b. cortex
   c. glomerulus
   d. medulla

5. The process of plasmalike fluid passing through the glomerulus to Bowman's capsule is called:
   a. filtration
   b. reabsorption
   c. secretion
   d. excretion

6. The hormone ADH affects reabsorption in the:
   a. glomerulus
   b. proximal convoluted tubule
   c. loop of Henle
   d. distal convoluted tubule

7. The pathway of urine formation is:
   a. kidney, ureter, urethra, bladder
   b. ureter, pelvis, urethra, bladder
   c. kidney, urethra, bladder, ureter
   d. kidney, ureter, bladder, urethra

8. The average normal daily urinary output is:
   a. 600 ml
   b. 1,200 ml
   c. 1,500 ml
   d. 2,400 ml

9. Inflammation of the urinary bladder is called:
   a. nephritis
   b. cystitis
   c. pyelitis
   d. urethritis

10. Involuntary urination is known as:
   a. polyuria
   b. anuria
   c. incontinence
   d. frequency

COMPLETION

If laboratory facilities and supervision are available, obtain and examine several specimens of fresh normal urine.

1. What is the color of the specimen?

2. Is it clear or cloudy?

3. Is the urine acid, alkaline, or neutral? To test, dip blue litmus paper into the urine. If acid is present, it will turn red. Dip in red litmus paper. If urine is alkaline, it will turn the paper blue. If neither paper changes color, the urine is neutral.

4. What is the specific gravity of a specimen? To test, use a urinometer.

5. Using Acetest reagent tablets, examine the urine for acetone. Have the results and your interpretation checked by the instructor.

Place the reagent tablet on a clean white sheet of paper. Place a drop of urine on the tablet. In 30 seconds, compare the resulting color with the color chart enclosed with the tablets. Record the result on the chart.

6. Using Clinitest tablets and/or Clinistix reagent strips, test for sugar. Have the results and your interpretation checked by the instructor.

Clinitest tablets: Place five drops of urine and ten drops of water in a test tube. Add the Clinitest tablet. Observe the reaction. Then shake the test tube and compare the color of the solution with the color scale enclosed with the tablets. Record the result.

Clinistix reagent strips: Dip the test end of the Clinistix in the urine and remove it. (Avoid contact with fingers or other objects because misleading results may occur.) If the moistened end turns blue, the result is positive. When sugar is present, the blue color will appear in less than 1 minute. Record the result.

MATCHING

Match each term in Column I with its description in Column II.

Column I	Column II

_____ **1.** nephron   a. tubes that connect the kidneys with the bladder

_____ **2.** glomerulus   b. mass of capillaries

_____ **3.** bladder   c. structure that absorbs filtrate from the capillary mass

_____ **4.** urethra   d. one of millions of tiny filtering units

_____ **5.** ureter   e. returns blood to the inferior vena cava

_____ **6.** ADH   f. hormone which regulates water reabsorption

_____ **7.** collecting tubules   g. contraction of bladder muscles

_____ **8.** Bowman's capsule   h. canal which opens to the outside of the body

_____ **9.** kidney   i. primarily acts as a reservoir

_____ **10.** renal vein   j. allow urine to drain into the renal pelvis

_____ **11.** anuria   k. bean-shaped organ

_____ **12.** dysuria   l. scanty urine

_____ **13.** pyuria   m. blood in the urine

_____ **14.** hematuria   n. no urine

_____ **15.** oliguria   o. pus in the urine

_____ **16.** carbon dioxide   p. painful urination

_____ **17.** calculi   q. helps regulate body temperature

_____ **18.** urine   r. blood retains urinary waste products

_____ **19.** cystitis   s. stones in the kidneys

_____ **20.** uremia   t. waste product eliminated through the lungs

                                u. inflammation of the mucous membranes lining the bladder

                                v. water and nitrogenous wastes

APPLYING THEORY TO PRACTICE

1. The amount of daily water loss is approximately 1,500 to 1,800 ml through urinary output, 500 ml through the skin, and 500 ml through respiration. Keep a log for 24 hours. Measure your liquid intake and urinary output. Answer the question, "Are you taking in enough fluid to maintain your body in good fluid balance?"

2. You have just run a mile and sweated profusely. When you urinate you notice there is only a small amount and it is concentrated. Explain what has happened.

3. Your doctor has prescribed for you an antibiotic. The instructions say to take it every 6 hours. Why is it necessary to maintain this over 24 hours?

4. A client comes to the emergency health center complaining of a severe back pain. After an examination and history, the diagnosis is kidney stones. The client inquires, "How did I get stones in my kidney?" Explain the cause and treatment.

5. In kidney failure, dialysis may be necessary. Define dialysis. What type do you think would be best for a vision-impaired 70-year-old client? What type do you think would be best for a mother with children ages 2, 6, and 10?

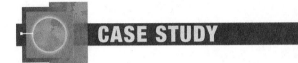

CASE STUDY

Ken James comes to the doctor's office with a complaint of severe back pain. The pain is located on the right side lateral to vertebrae and superior to the buttocks. The doctor orders an IVP for Ken. Meghan, the nurse clinician, explains to him the preparation for the IVP test.

1. Explain the process of the IVP test.

2. Describe the location of the back pain.

3. Explain the functions of the kidney.

After the test is done, the doctor reports that Ken has a stone in the renal pelvis of his right kidney. The physician schedules an appointment for Ken to have the stone removed.

4. Name the parts of the kidney and their function.

5. What other body systems do diseases of the kidney affect?

6. There is more than one procedure to remove kidney stones. Which procedure do you think will be scheduled for Ken?

7. Explain the types of procedures for kidney stone removal.

8. Ken inquires if he will have this problem in the future. What will the doctor tell him?

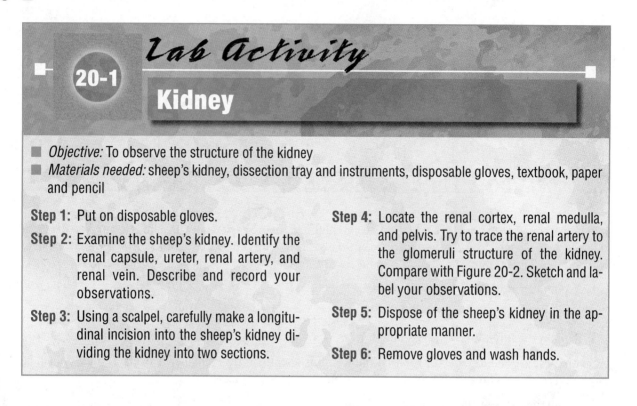

Lab Activity

20-1

Kidney

- *Objective:* To observe the structure of the kidney
- *Materials needed:* sheep's kidney, dissection tray and instruments, disposable gloves, textbook, paper and pencil

Step 1: Put on disposable gloves.

Step 2: Examine the sheep's kidney. Identify the renal capsule, ureter, renal artery, and renal vein. Describe and record your observations.

Step 3: Using a scalpel, carefully make a longitudinal incision into the sheep's kidney dividing the kidney into two sections.

Step 4: Locate the renal cortex, renal medulla, and pelvis. Try to trace the renal artery to the glomeruli structure of the kidney. Compare with Figure 20-2. Sketch and label your observations.

Step 5: Dispose of the sheep's kidney in the appropriate manner.

Step 6: Remove gloves and wash hands.

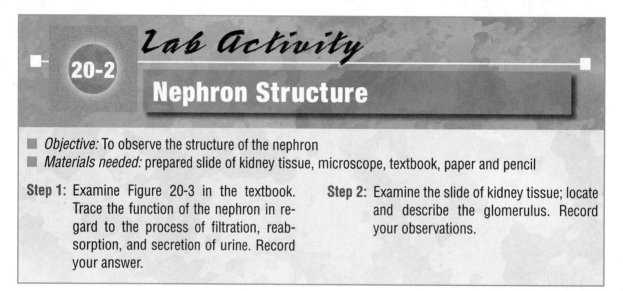

Lab Activity

20-2

Nephron Structure

- *Objective:* To observe the structure of the nephron
- *Materials needed:* prepared slide of kidney tissue, microscope, textbook, paper and pencil

Step 1: Examine Figure 20-3 in the textbook. Trace the function of the nephron in regard to the process of filtration, reabsorption, and secretion of urine. Record your answer.

Step 2: Examine the slide of kidney tissue; locate and describe the glomerulus. Record your observations.

REPRODUCTIVE SYSTEM

Objectives

- Compare somatic cell division (mitosis) with germ cell division (meiosis)

- Explain the process of fertilization

- Identify the organs of the female reproductive system and explain their functions

- Explain menopause and the changes that occur during this time

- Describe the stages and changes that occur during the menstrual cycle

- Identify the organs of the male reproductive system and explain their functions

- List some common disorders of the reproductive system

- Define the key words that relate to this chapter

Key Words

amenorrhea
areola
artificial
    insemination
Bartholin's glands
benign prostatic
    hypertrophy
    (BPH)
breast
bulbourethral
    gland (Cowper's
    gland)
cervix
chlamydia
circumcision
clitoris
coitus
corona radiata
corpus luteum
cryptorchidism
ductus deferens
dysmenorrhea
ectopic pregnancy
ejaculatory duct
endometriosis

endometrium
epididymis
epididymitis
episiotomy
estrogen
fallopian tube
    (oviduct)
fertilization
fibroid tumors
fimbriae
foreskin
fundus
gamete (germ cell)
genital herpes
genital warts
glans penis
gonorrhea
graafian follicle
hymen
hysterectomy
impotence
in vitro fertiliza-
    tion (IVF)
infertility
labia minora

labia majora
laparoscope
laparoscopy
lumpectomy
mammogram
mastectomy
meiosis
menarche
menopause
menstrual cycle
menstruation
mons pubis
myometrium
oogenesis
orchitis
ova
ovary
oviduct
ovulation
Papanicolaou
    (Pap) smear
pelvic
    inflammatory
    disease (PID)
continues

419

Key Words continued

penile shaft	scrotum	toxic shock
penis	seminal vesicle	syndrome
perineum	seminiferous	trichomoniasis
premenstrual	tubule	uterus
syndrome (PMS)	spermatogenesis	vagina
progesterone	spermatozoa	vas deferens
prostate gland	sterile	vestibule
prostatectomy	syphilis	vulva
prostatitis	testes	yeast infection
puberty	testosterone	zygote
salpingitis		

All living organisms, whether unicellular or multicellular, small or large, must reproduce in order to continue their species. Humans and most multicellular animals reproduce new members of their species by sexual reproduction.

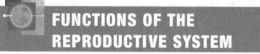

FUNCTIONS OF THE REPRODUCTIVE SYSTEM

1. Has the necessary organs capable of accomplishing reproduction, the creation of a new individual

2. Manufacture hormones necessary for the development of the reproductive organs and secondary sex characteristics

   - Females—estrogen and progesterone

   - Males—testosterone

Specialized sex cells or **germ cells (gametes)** must be produced by the gonads of both male and female sex organs before sexual reproduction can take place. The female gonads, called the ovaries, produce egg cells (ova). The male gonads, the testes, produce sperm. Normal cell division is known as mitosis. In the formation of the germ cells, a special process of cell division occurs called **meiosis.** In the female, the specific meiotic process is called **oogenesis;** in the male, **spermatogenesis.**

In humans, the somatic (body) cells, including skin, fat, muscle, nerve, and bone cells, contain 46 chromosomes in the nucleus. Forty-four of these are autosomes (nonsex chromosomes). The remaining two are sex chromosomes. Each chromosome has a partner of the same size and shape so that they can be paired, Figure 21-1. In the female, the somatic cells contain 22 pairs of autosomes, and a single pair of sex chromosomes (both are X chromosomes). In the male, the combination is also 22 autosomal pairs and a single pair of sex chromosomes. However, the male sex chromosomal pair consists of an X and Y chromosome.

Oogenesis and spermatogenesis reduce the chromosome number of 46 to 23 in the gametes or germ cells. All multicellular organisms start from the fusion of two gametes: the sperm (spermatozoon) from the male, and the ovum from the female. Figure 21-2 shows the structure of a spermatozoon and an ovum.

FERTILIZATION

During sexual intercourse, or **coitus,** sperm from the testes is deposited into the female vagina, Figure 21-3. Spermatozoa entering the female reproductive tract live for only a day or two at the most, though they may remain in the tract up to 2 weeks before degenerating. Approximately 100 million spermatozoa are contained in 1 ml (1 cc) of ejaculated seminal fluid. They are fairly uniform in shape and size. If the count is less than 20 million per milliliter, the male is considered to be **sterile.** These millions of sperm cells swim toward the ovum that has been released from the ovary. The large quantity of sperm is necessary because a great number are destroyed before they even approach the ovum. Many die from the acidity of the secretions in the male urethra or the vagina. Some cannot withstand the high temper-

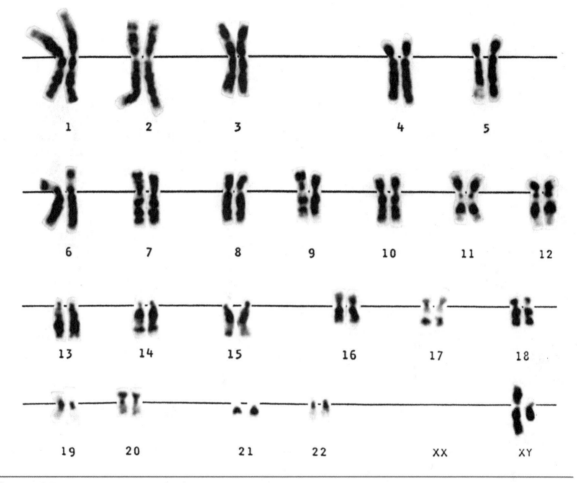

Figure 21-1   *Karyotype of human from a male somatic cell. A karyotype is the arrangement of chromosome pairs according to shape and size.*

ature of the female abdomen, while others lack the propulsion ability to progress from the vagina to the upper uterine (fallopian) tube.

For a sperm to penetrate and fertilize an ovum, the **corona radiata** must first be penetrated. This is the layer of epithelial cells surrounding the zona pellucida, see Figure 21-2. Eventually, only one sperm cell penetrates and fertilizes an ovum. To accomplish this successfully, the sperm head produces an enzyme called hyaluronidase. Hyaluronidase acts upon hyaluronic acid, a chemical substance that holds together the epithelial cells of the corona radiata. As a result of the action of the hyaluronidase, the epithelial cells fall away from the ovum. This exposes an area of the plasma membrane for sperm penetration. Figure 21-3 illustrates the route of the ovum and the sperm.

True **fertilization** (conception) occurs when the sperm nucleus combines with the egg nucleus to form a fertilized egg cell, or **zygote.** The type of fertilization that occurs in humans is referred to as internal fertilization; fertilization takes place within the female's body.

Fertilization restores the full complement of 46 chromosomes possessed by every human cell, each parent contributing one chromosome to each of the 23 pairs.

Deoxyribonucleic acid (DNA) is found in the chromosomes. It contains the genetic code that is replicated and passed on to each cell as the zygote divides and redivides to form the embry. The early process whereby the zygote repeats divides to form an early embryo is known as cleavage. After early cleavage, actual em

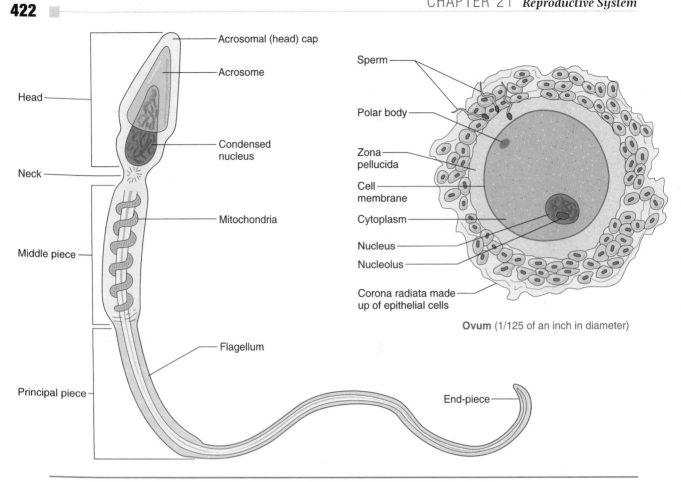

Head

Neck

Middle piece

Principal piece

Acrosomal (head) cap

Acrosome

Condensed nucleus

Mitochondria

Flagellum

End-piece

Sperm

Polar body

Zona pellucida

Cell membrane

Cytoplasm

Nucleus

Nucleolus

Corona radiata made up of epithelial cells

Ovum (1/125 of an inch in diameter)

Figure 21-2   *Structures of the human sperm and ovum*

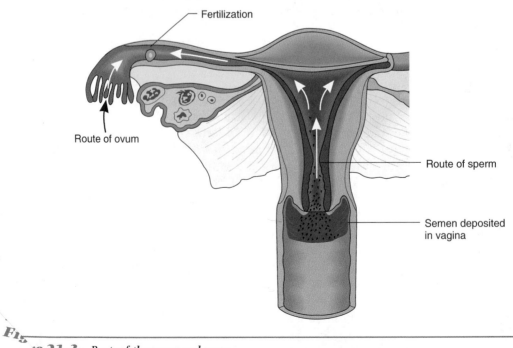

Fertilization

Route of ovum

Route of sperm

Semen deposited in vagina

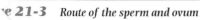

Figure 21-3   *Route of the sperm and ovum*

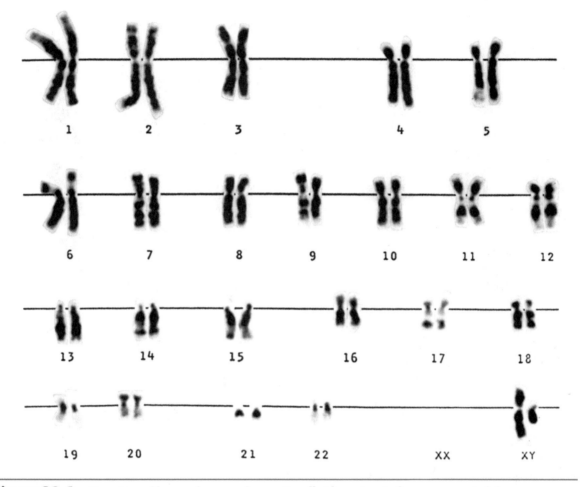

Figure 21-1 *Karyotype of human from a male somatic cell. A karyotype is the arrangement of chromosome pairs according to shape and size.*

ature of the female abdomen, while others lack the propulsion ability to progress from the vagina to the upper uterine (fallopian) tube.

For a sperm to penetrate and fertilize an ovum, the **corona radiata** must first be penetrated. This is the layer of epithelial cells surrounding the zona pellucida, see Figure 21-2. Eventually, only one sperm cell penetrates and fertilizes an ovum. To accomplish this successfully, the sperm head produces an enzyme called hyaluronidase. Hyaluronidase acts upon hyaluronic acid, a chemical substance that holds together the epithelial cells of the corona radiata. As a result of the action of the hyaluronidase, the epithelial cells fall away from the ovum. This exposes an area of the plasma membrane for sperm penetration. Figure 21-3 illustrates the route of the ovum and the sperm.

True **fertilization** (conception) occurs when the sperm nucleus combines with the egg nucleus to form a fertilized egg cell, or **zygote.** The type of fertilization that occurs in humans is referred to as internal fertilization; fertilization takes place within the female's body.

Fertilization restores the full complement of 46 chromosomes possessed by every human cell, each parent contributing one chromosome to each of the 23 pairs.

Deoxyribonucleic acid (DNA) is found in the chromosomes. It contains the genetic code that is replicated and passed on to each cell as the zygote divides and redivides to form the embryo. The early process whereby the zygote repeatedly divides to form an early embryo is known as cleavage. After early cleavage, actual embryonic

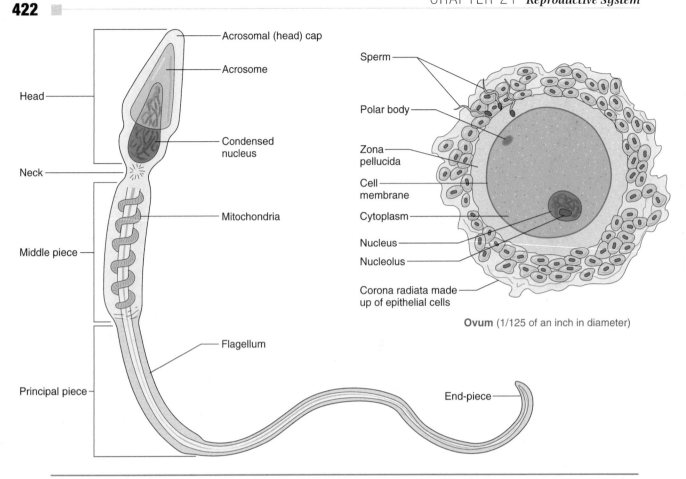

Figure 21-2   *Structures of the human sperm and ovum*

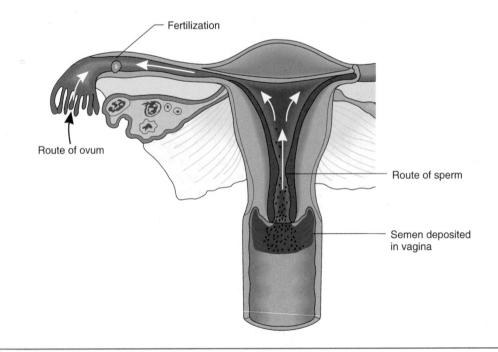

Figure 21-3   *Route of the sperm and ovum*

development occurs until the fetus is completely formed.

All of the inherited traits possessed by the offspring are established at the time of fertilization. This is a point to remember when working with parents. A young mother-to-be may hope that her baby will be a girl with curly hair, or a prospective father may insist that he wants a son. The health care provider can assure them that the sex, and physical characteristics such as eye color and curly hair, are determined at the time of fertilization. The sex chromosomes of the male parent determine the sex of the child but other characteristics are a combination of both parents.

FETAL DEVELOPMENT

If fertilization occurs, the zygote travels down the fallopian tube and is implanted in the endometrial wall of the uterus. The zygote rapidly grows into an embryo and then a fetus, see Figures 21-4 and 21-5.

Fetal development is a 9-month process as outlined in Table 21-1.

DIFFERENTIATION OF REPRODUCTIVE ORGANS

Reproductive organs are the only organs in the human body that differ between the male and female and yet there is still a significant similarity. This likeness results from the fact that female and male organs develop from the same group of embryonic cells. For approximately 2 months, the embryo develops without a sexual identity. Then the influence of the X or Y chromosome begins to make a difference.

The gonads (sexual organs) of the female begin to evolve at about the tenth or eleventh week of pregnancy. The ovaries of the female embryo develop from the same type of tissue as the testes of the male embryo. However, the testes evolve from the medulla of the gonad while the ovary

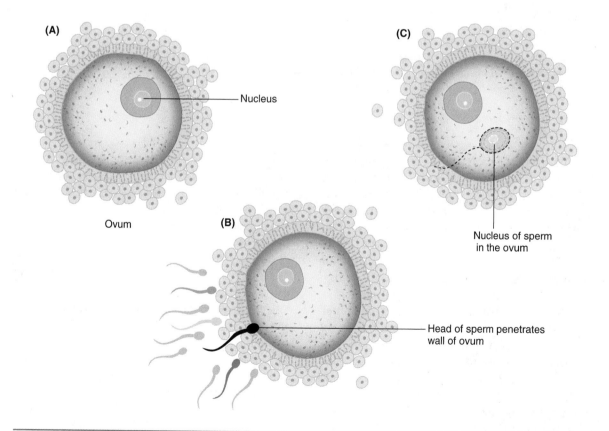

Figure 21-4   *Fertilization*

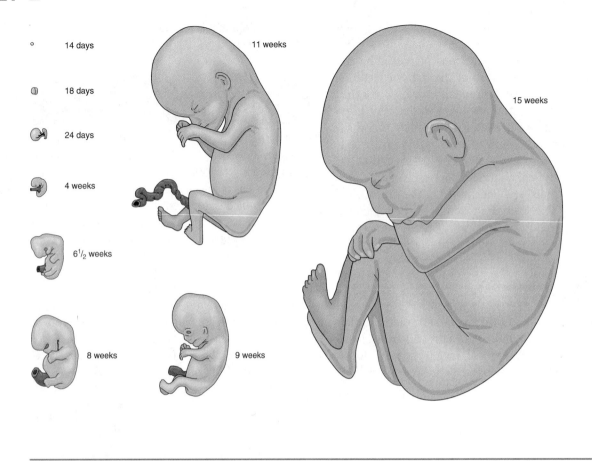

Figure 21-5   *Growth of an embryo into a fetus once fertilization has occurred*

develops from the cortex of the gonad. Figure 21-6 illustrates how the undifferentiated external genitalia develop into fully differentiated structures. In the male, the tubercle becomes the **glans penis,** the folds become the **penile shaft,** and the swelling develops into the **scrotum.** In the female, the tubercle becomes the **clitoris,** the folds the **labia minora,** and the swelling the **labia majora.** Internally there is also a differentiation from initially similar structures. The embryonic muellerian ducts degenerate and the wolffian ducts become the **epididymis, vas deferens,** and the **ejaculatory duct** in the male. In the female, the wolffian ducts degenerate and the muellerian ducts develop into the **fallopian tubes,** the **uterus,** and the upper portion of the vagina. It is believed that the presence of the testes in the male is the differentiating factor in the development.

Without the androgens (male hormones) from the testes, a female will develop. With the androgens, a male develops. Another substance called the muellerian inhibitor works in partnership with the androgen to produce the sex differentiation.

ORGANS OF REPRODUCTION

The function of the reproductive system is to provide for continuity of the species. In the human, the female reproductive system is composed of two ovaries, two fallopian tubes, the uterus, and the vagina. The male reproductive system is made up of two testes, seminal ducts, glands, and the penis. The principal male organs are located outside the body in contrast to the female organs which are largely located within the body.

Table 21-1 Fetal Development

TIME PERIOD	PHASES OF FETAL DEVELOPMENT	DEVELOPMENT
Ovulation	Phase 1	Fertilization occurs, zygote forms
1–5 days after ovulation	Phase 2	The zygote now begins to divide. When cell division reaches about 16 cells, the zygote becomes a morula (mulberry shaped). Three to 5 days after fertilization the morula leaves the fallopian tube and enters the uterine cavity.
4–6 days after ovulation	Phase 3	Cell division continues and a cavity known as the blastocele forms in the center of the morula. The entire structure is now called a blastocyst. The presence of the blastocyst indicates that two cell types are forming; the embryoblast (inner cell mass on the inside of the blastocele), and the trophoblast (the cells on the outside of the blastocele).
5–6 days after ovulation	Phase 4	The trophoblast cells secrete an enzyme, which erodes the epithelial uterine lining and creates an implantation site for the blastocyst. This new implantation site becomes swollen with new capillaries.
7–12 days after ovulation	Phase 5	Implantation is complete and the placental circulation begins. The top layers of cells will become the embryo and amniotic cavity; the lower cells will become the yolk stalk.
13–28 days after ovulation	Phase 6	Chorionic villi "fingers" in the forming of the placenta now anchor the site to the uterine wall. By the end of this phase the embryo is attached by a connecting stalk (which later will become part of the umbilical cord) to the developing placenta. A narrow line of cells appears on the embryonic disc marking the beginning of gastrulation (the process that gives rise to all three layers of the embryo—the ectoderm, mesoderm, and endoderm). See Table 21-2. The embryo is about 1/10 inch long, the heart is forming, and the eyes begin to develop. The heart begins to beat on about day 24. Foundation of the brain, spinal cord, and nervous system is laid. Muscles are developing. Arms and legs are budding.
At the end of 2 months	Phase 7	The embryo is about 1 inch long, veins are visible, and the heart has divided into two chambers. Brain has human proportions, blood flows in fetus veins, skeleton is formed, and reflex responses have begun.
At the end of 3 months	Phase 8	The fetus is 2.5–3 inches long and has begun swallowing and kicking. All organs and muscles are formed.
At the end of 4 months	Phase 9	The fetus is covered with a layer of thick hair called lanugo. The heartbeat can be heard; the mother may feel the baby's first movements.
At the end of 5 months	Phase 10	A protective covering called vernix caseosa begins to form on the baby's skin. By the end of this month the baby will be nearly 8 inches long and weigh almost 1 pound.
At the end of 6 months	Phase 11	Eyebrows and eyelids are visible. Baby's lungs are filled with amniotic fluid and the baby has started breathing motions. The mother's voice is heard and recognized.
At the end of 7 months	Phase 12	The baby weighs about 3.5 pounds and is 12 inches long. The body is well formed. Fingernails cover the fingertips. A baby born at this age can live outside the uterus.
At the end of 8 months	Phase 13	The baby is gaining about 0.5 pound per week, and layers of fat are piling on. The baby is normally turned head down in preparation for birth.
At the end of 9 months	Phase 14	The baby is 6–9 pounds and measures 19–22 inches. As the area becomes more crowded, movement may be limited. The baby and/or placenta triggers labor and birth occurs.

Table 21-2 Embryonic Germ Layers

ECTODERM-WILL FORM	MESODERM-WILL FORM	ENDODERM-WILL FORM
Skin, hair, nails, lens of the eye, lining of the internal and external ear, nose sinuses, mouth, anus, tooth enamel, pituitary gland, mammary glands, and all parts of the nervous system	Muscles, bones, lymphatic tissue, spleen, blood cells, heart, lungs, and reproductive and excretory systems	Lining of the lungs, tongue, tonsils, urethra, associated glands, bladder, and digestive tract

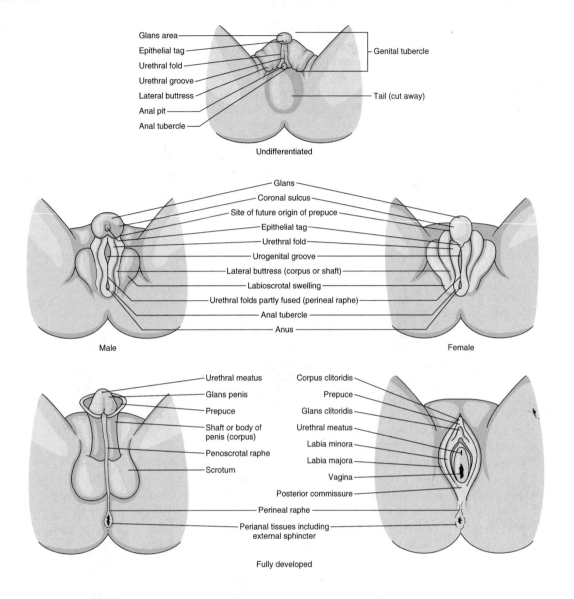

Figure 21-6 *Development of undifferentiated external genitalia into fully differentiated structures*

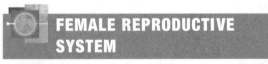

FEMALE REPRODUCTIVE SYSTEM

Placement of the female reproductive organs in the pelvic cavity are shown in Figure 21-7. As shown in Figure 21-8, the female reproductive system consists of two ovaries, two fallopian tubes, the uterus, and the vagina. Accessory organs are the breasts.

Ovaries

The **ovaries** are the primary sex organs of the female. They are located on either side of the pelvis, lateral to the uterus, in the lower part of the abdominal cavity. Each ovary is about the shape and size of a large almond, measuring about 3 cm long and from 1.5 to 3 cm wide. An ovarian ligament, a short

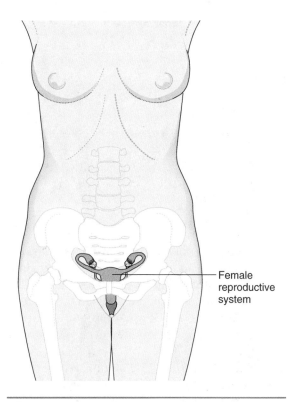

Figure 21-7 *Placement of the female reproductive system in the lower pelvic cavity*

fibrous cord within the broad ligament, attaches each ovary to the upper lateral part of the uterus.

Ovaries perform two functions. They produce the female germ cells, or **ova**, and the female sex hormones, **estrogen** and **progesterone**. Table 21-3 outlines the functions of the female sex hormones.

Each ovary contains thousands of microscopic hollow sacs called **graafian follicles** in varying stages of development. An ovum slowly develops inside each follicle. The process of development from an immature ova to a functional and mature ova inside the graafian follicle is called maturation. In addition, the graafian follicle produces the hormone estrogen.

Usually a single follicle matures every 28 days through the reproductive years of a woman. The reproductive years begin at the time of **puberty** and the **menarche** (initial menstrual discharge of blood).

Occasionally two or more follicles may mature, releasing more than one ovum. As the follicle enlarges, it migrates to the outside surface of the ovary and breaks open, releasing the ovum from the ovary. This process is called **ovulation**; it occurs about 2 weeks before the menstrual period begins. The time of ovulation may vary depending on emotional and physical health, state of mind, and age. During a woman's reproductive years, she produces about 400 ova.

The ovum consists of cytoplasm and some yolk. This yolk is the initial food source for the

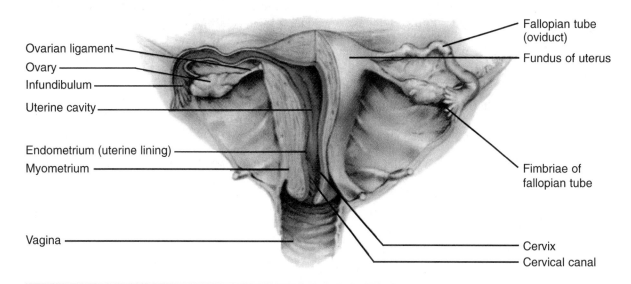

Figure 21-8 *Structures of the female reproductive system*

Table 21-3 *Functions of Estrogen and Progesterone*

HORMONE	FUNCTION

Estrogen	1. Affects the development of the fallopian tubes, ovaries, uterus, and the vagina.
	2. Produces secondary sex characteristics:
	    broadening of the pelvis, making the outlet broad and oval to permit childbirth
	    the epiphysis (growth plate) becomes bone and growth ceases
	    development of softer and smoother skin
	    development of pubic and axillary hair
	    deposits of fat in the breasts and development of the duct system
	    deposits of fat in the buttocks and thighs
	    sexual desire
	3. Prepares the uterus for the fertilized egg.

Progesterone	1. Develops excretory portion of mammary glands. 2. Thickens the uterine lining so it can receive the developing embryo egg. 3. Decreases uterine contractions during pregnancy.

growth of the early embryo. After ovulation, the ovum travels down one of the fallopian tubes, or oviducts. Fertilization of the ovum takes place only in the outer third of the oviduct. The time of fertilization is limited to a day or two following ovulation. Following fertilization, the zygote (fertilized egg) travels to the well-prepared uterus and implants itself in the wall of the endometrium (uterus lining).

The development of the follicle and release of the ovum occur under the influence of two hormones of the pituitary gland; the follicle-stimulating hormone (FSH) and the luteinizing hormone (LH). FSH also promotes the secretion of estrogen by the ovary.

Following ovulation the ruptured follicle enlarges, takes on a yellow fatty substance, and becomes the **corpus luteum** (yellow body). The corpus luteum secretes progesterone, which maintains the growth of the uterine lining. If the egg is not fertilized, the corpus luteum degenerates, progesterone production stops, and the thickened glandular endometrium sloughs off (see The Menstrual Cycle).

Fallopian Tubes

The fallopian tubes, or **oviducts,** about 10 cm (4 inches) long, are not attached to the ovaries, Figure 21-8. The outer end of each oviduct curves over the top edge of each ovary and opens into the abdominal cavity. This portion of the oviduct,

nearest the ovary, is the infundibulum. Since the infundibulum is not attached directly to the ovary, it is possible for an ovum to accidentally slip into the abdominal cavity and be fertilized there. If the fertilized egg implants in the fallopian tube instead of the uterus it is called an **ectopic pregnancy.** An ectopic pregnancy can also occur outside the uterine cavity.

The area of the infundibulum over the ovary is surrounded by a number of fringelike folds called **fimbriae.** Each oviduct is lined with mucous membrane, smooth muscle, and ciliated epithelium. The combined action of the peristaltic contractions of the smooth muscles and the beating of the cilia helps to propel the ova down the oviduct into the uterus. Conception (fertilization) takes place in the outer third of the fallopian tube.

Uterus

The uterus is a hollow, thick-walled, pear-shaped, and highly muscular organ. The nongravid (nonpregnant) uterus measures about 7.5 cm in length, 5 cm wide, and 2.75 cm thick. This is about 3 inches long, 2 inches wide, and about 1 inch thick. The uterus lies behind the urinary bladder and in front of the rectum. The uterine cavity is extremely small and narrow. During pregnancy, however, the uterine cavity greatly expands to accommodate the growing embryo and a large amount of fluid.

The uterus is divided into three parts: (1) the **fundus,** the bulging, rounded upper part above the entrance of the two oviducts into the uterus; (2) the body, or middle portion; and (3) the **cervix,** or cylindrical, lower narrow portion that extends into the vagina, see Figure 21-8. There is a short, cervical canal that extends from the lower uterine cavity (internal orifice, or os of the uterus) to the external os at the end of the cervix. The uterine wall is comprised of three layers.

1. The outer serous layer, or the visceral peritoneum

2. An extremely thick, smooth, muscular middle layer, the **myometrium**

3. An inner mucous layer, the **endometrium**

The endometrium, which lines the oviducts and the vagina, is also lined with ciliated epithelial cells, numerous uterine glands, and many capillaries.

During development of the embryo-fetus, the uterus gradually rises until the top part is high in the abdominal cavity, pushing on the diaphragm. This may cause the expectant mother some difficulty in breathing during the late stages of pregnancy.

Vagina

The **vagina** is the short canal that extends from the cervix of the uterus to the vulva. The vagina consists of smooth muscle with a mucous membrane lining. This type of muscle tissue allows the vaginal canal to accommodate the penis during sexual intercourse; it also permits a baby to pass through the vaginal canal during the birthing process. A membrane called the **hymen** may be found at or near the entrance to the vagina. The hymen has some openings that allow for the flow of blood during menstruation. During the first act of sexual intercourse, the openings in the hymen are enlarged and there may be slight bleeding, Figures 21-9 and 21-10.

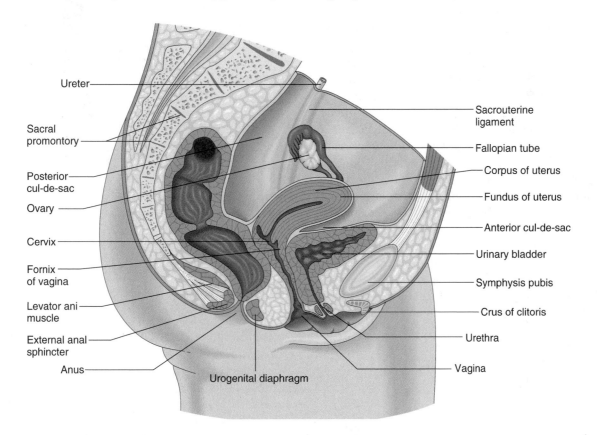

Figure 21-9 Structures of the female reproductive system

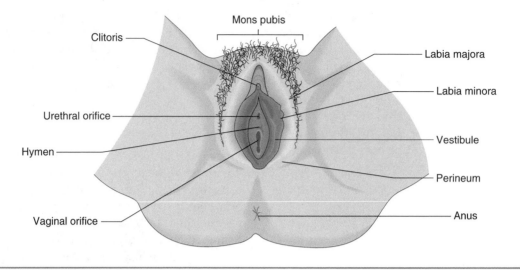

Figure 21-10 *External female genitalia*

External Female Genitalia

The external female genitalia or **vulva** contains the external organs of the reproductive area, see Figure 21-10. The large pad of fat that is covered with coarse hair on the mature female and overlies the symphysis pubis is known as **mons pubis.** The area surrounding the openings of the urethra and vagina is called the **vestibule.** The urethra opening is superior to the vagina. Above the urethral opening is a small structure called the clitoris which contains many nerve endings. When stimulated, the highly sensitive clitoris provides sexual pleasure for the female. After the clitoris is properly stimulated, the vagina is fully lubricated and ready for full insertion of the penis.

The vagina is surrounded by folds of skin called the labia minora and the labia majora. At the entrance to the vagina are the **Bartholin's glands** which produce mucus.

The **perineum** is the area between the vaginal opening and the rectum. The perineal area consists of muscles that form a sphincter for the vestibule. In childbirth, an incision called an **episiotomy** may be made from the vagina into the perineal area to facilitate childbirth.

Breasts

The **breasts** are accessory organs to the female reproductive system, Figure 21-11. They consist of

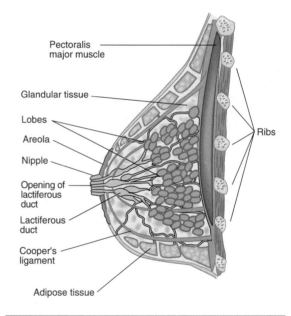

Figure 21-11 *Sagittal section of the female breast*

numerous lobes arranged in a circular formation. Clusters of secreting cells surround tiny ducts. A single duct extends from each lobe to an opening in the nipple. The **areola,** the darker area which surrounds the nipple, changes to a brownish color during pregnancy. Prolactin from the anterior lobe of the pituitary gland stimulates the mammary glands to secrete milk following childbirth.

THE MENSTRUAL CYCLE

In females, a mature egg develops and is ovulated from one of the two ovaries about once every 28 days, through a complex series of actions between the pituitary and the ovary. Before the mature egg is released from the ovary, a series of events occurs to thicken the uterine lining (endometrium). This is necessary to receive and hold a fertilized egg for embryonic development. If the egg is not fertilized, the endometrium starts to break down. Eventually the old unfertilized egg and the degenerated endometrium are discharged out of the female reproductive tract (**menstruation**). The cycle then starts all over again with the development of another ovum and the buildup of the endometrium.

This cycle is called the **menstrual cycle.** The menstrual cycle starts at puberty. It can start as early as 9 years of age to as late as 17 years of age. Generally, the age range is between 12 and 15. The changes that occur during the menstrual cycle involve hormones from the pituitary gland and the ovaries.

The menstrual cycle is divided into four stages: the follicle stage, the ovulation stage, the corpus luteum stage, and the menstruation stage. See Figure 21-12 for a diagram of the menstrual cycle.

Stages of the Menstrual Cycle

Follicle Stage. Follicle-stimulating hormone (FSH) is secreted from the anterior lobe of the pituitary gland on day 5 of the menstrual cycle. FSH is then circulated to an ovary via the bloodstream. When FSH reaches an ovary, it will stimulate several follicles; however, only one matures. As the one follicle grows in size, an egg cell also begins to mature inside the follicle, Figure 21-13. As the follicle grows in size, it fills with a fluid containing estrogen. The estrogen stimulates the endometrium to thicken with mucus and a rich supply of blood vessels. These changes to the endometrium prepare the uterus for the implantation of an embryo. The follicle stage lasts about 10 days.

Ovulation Stage. When the concentration of estrogen in the female bloodstream reaches a high level, it causes the pituitary gland to stop FSH se-

cretion. As this occurs, the luteinizing hormone (LH) is secreted by the pituitary gland. At this point, there are three different hormones circulating in the female bloodstream—estrogen, FSH, and LH. Each hormone is present in different concentrations. Around day 14 of the menstrual cycle, this hormonal combination somehow stimulates the mature follicle to break. When the follicle ruptures, a mature egg cell is released; this event is called ovulation.

Corpus Luteum Stage, or Luteal Phase. After ovulation, LH stimulates the cells of the ruptured follicle to divide quickly. This mass of reddish-yellow cells is called the corpus luteum. The corpus luteum, in turn, secretes a hormone called progesterone. Progesterone helps to maintain the continued growth and thickening of the endometrium, so if an embryo happens to be implanted into the uterine lining, the pregnancy can be maintained. That is why progesterone is often called the "pregnancy hormone." Progesterone also prevents the formation of new ovarian follicles by inhibiting the release of FSH. The corpus luteum stage lasts about 14 days.

Menstruation Stage. If fertilization does not occur and an embryo is not implanted in the uterus, the progesterone reaches a level in the bloodstream that inhibits further LH secretion. With decreased LH secretion, the corpus luteum breaks down causing a decrease in progesterone secretion as well. As the progesterone level decreases, the lining of the endometrium becomes progressively thinner and eventually breaks down. The extra layers of the endometrium, the unfertilized egg, and a small quantity of blood that comes from the ruptured capillaries as the endometrium peels away from the uterus are discharged from the female's body through the vagina. This causes the characteristic menstrual blood flow, and the menstruation stage starts around day 28 of the cycle. The menstruation stage lasts about 4 days. While menstruation is occurring, the estrogen level in the bloodstream is decreasing. The anterior lobe of the pituitary gland is now stimulated to secrete FSH, consequently a new follicle starts to grow and the menstrual cycle starts again.

The relationship between the pituitary gland hormones and the ovarian hormones is one of

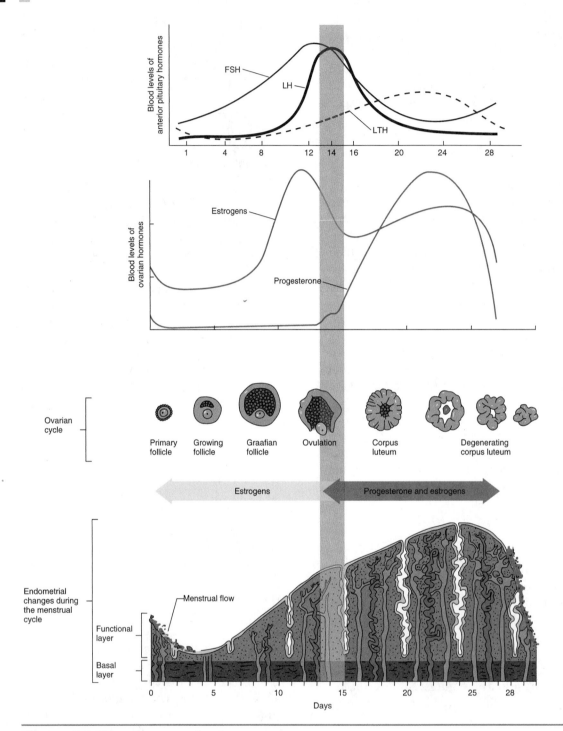

Figure 21-12 *The menstrual cycle*

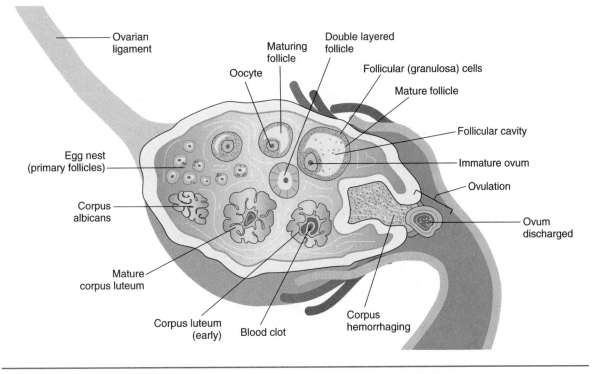

Figure 21-13 *An ovary showing the development of an ovum in a graafian follicle*

feedback. That means pituitary hormones control the functioning of the ovaries; in turn, the ovaries secrete hormones that control pituitary functioning. This is another example of the automatic regulation of many of the body's processes.

 MENOPAUSE

Menopause or "change in life" is the time in a female's life when the monthly menstrual cycle comes to an end. It frequently occurs between ages 45 and 55. Menopause signals the end of follicle growth and ovulation; consequently, it means the end of childbearing. However, a normal sex drive usually remains.

The menopausal female will experience the following anatomical changes.

1. Atrophy of the internal reproductive structures: uterus, fallopian tubes, and ovaries

2. Atrophy of the external genitalia

3. Vagina becomes conical shaped

4. Atrophy of the vaginal mucous membranes

5. Reduction of the secretory activity of the glands associated with the reproductive organs

These changes do not occur overnight, they happen gradually over a period of years. There are also pronounced physiological changes which may occur. These are "hot flashes," dizziness, headaches, rheumatic pains in joints, sweating, and susceptibility to fatigue. Depending on the female going through menopause, sometimes these physiological changes are also accompanied by psychic changes. These include abnormal fears, depression, excessive irritability, and a tendency to worry. Many of these physiological and psychic symptoms can be alleviated by the careful administration of female hormones.

Menopause can be induced prematurely (artificial menopause) by removal of ovarian tissue.

MALE REPRODUCTIVE SYSTEM

The male reproductive organs, Figure 21-14, consist of the following structures.

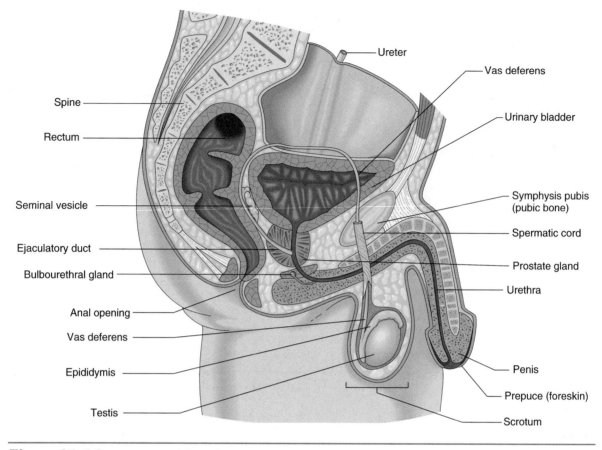

Figure 21-14 *Structures of the male reproductive system*

1. The two testes produce the male gametes, **spermatozoa,** and the male sex hormone **testosterone.** They are suspended from the body wall by a spermatic cord and encased in a pouch called the scrotum.

2. A system of ducts carries the sperm cells out of the testes through the epididymis, two seminal ducts (ductus deferens or vas deferens), two ejaculatory ducts, and the urethra.

3. Accessory glands include the two seminal vesicles, two bulbourethral glands, and a prostate gland. These glands add a viscous fluid to the sperm cells to form seminal fluid.

4. The penis is a copulatory structure that will transfer sperm cells to the female reproductive system.

Testes and Epididymis

The two **testes** are the primary male reproductive organs, Figure 21-15. They are found in a pouch lying outside the male body called the scrotum. Each testis is about the size and shape of a small egg, approximately 4 cm long, 2.5 cm wide, and 2 cm thick. The testes are attached to an overlying structure called the epididymis. A fibrous tissue called the tunica albuginea covers the testes and sends incomplete partitions into the body of each testes. Each one of these partitions is called a lobule, and each testes contains 250 lobules.

Each testicular lobule contains one to four minute and highly convoluted (twisted) **seminiferous tubules.** FSH stimulates the production of

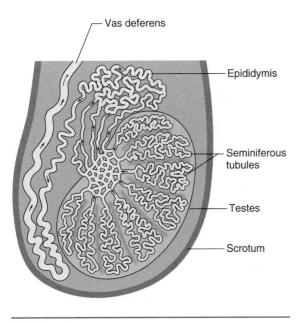

- Vas deferens
- Epididymis
- Seminiferous tubules
- Testes
- Scrotum

Figure 21-15   *Structure of the testis*

Descent of the Testes

In the embryo, the testes are formed and developed in the abdominal wall slightly below the kidneys. During the last 3 months of fetal development, the testes will migrate downward through the ventral abdominal wall into the scrotum. In its descent, each testis carries with it the ductus deferens, blood and lymphatic vessels, and autonomic nerve fibers. These structures and their fibrous tissue covering form the spermatic cord.

Occasionally, as in premature babies, the testes will not descend. If the testes do not descend, this condition is known as **cryptorchidism.** (If one testis does not descend, it is called unilateral cryptorchidism. For two testes, it is called bilateral cryptorchidism.) If the testes stay inside the abdomen after puberty, spermatogenesis will be affected. The increased body temperature will destroy any sperm cells. A simple surgical procedure done before puberty can correct this condition.

Scrotum

The scrotum is an external sac that contains the testes.

Ductus Deferens, Seminal Vesicles, and Ejaculatory Ducts

The right and left **ductus deferens** (vas deferens) are continuations of the epididymides. The ductus deferens has a dual function. It serves as a storage site for sperm cells and as the excretory duct of the testis. Each ductus runs from the epididymis up through the inguinal canal. It then runs downward and backward to the side of the urinary bladder. It then curves around the ureter and goes down to meet with the seminal vesicle duct on the posterior side of the bladder.

The **seminal vesicles** are two highly convoluted membranous tubes. A duct leads away from a seminal vesicle that joins to the ductus deferens to form the ejaculatory duct on either side. The seminal vesicles produce secretions which help to nourish and protect the sperm on its journey up the female reproductive system. At the

sperm in the cells that line the tubules. As the sperm develop, they are released into the tubules. In males, mature sperm formation requires about 74 days. The function begins at about age 12 and the first mature sperm are ejaculated at about age 14. All of the seminiferous tubules intertwine and join to form a small meshlike network of tubules called the rete testis. The rete testis unite to form the epididymis. The seminiferous tubules are supported by a type of tissue called interstitial tissue. The interstitial cells lining the interstitial tissue produce the male hormone testosterone. Testosterone is secreted in relatively steady amounts during the adult life of the male. Testosterone stimulates the growth and development of the male reproductive organs, underlies the sex drive, and is responsible for the secondary sex characteristics. These include the deepening of the voice, growth of hair (beard and body hair especially in the axillary and pubic area), increase in muscle mass, and thickening of the bones of the skeletal system.

The epididymides connect the testes with the ductus deferens and help in the final development of the sperm cells.

precise moment of ejaculation, the seminal fluid is added to the sperm cells as they leave the ejaculatory ducts.

The ejaculatory ducts are short and very narrow. They begin where the ductus deferens and the seminal vesicle duct join. They then descend into the prostate gland to join with the urethra, into which they discharge their contents. See Figure 21-14.

Penis

The external organs are the scrotum and the penis. Internally, the scrotum is divided into two sacs each containing a testis, epididymis, and lower part of the vas deferens. The **penis** contains erectile tissue that becomes enlarged and rigid during intercourse. Loose-fitting skin, called the **foreskin** or **prepuce,** covers the end of the penis. The foreskin can be removed in a simple operation known as **circumcision.**

Prostate Gland

The **prostate gland** is located in front of the rectum and just under the urinary bladder, and it surrounds the opening of the bladder leading into the urethra. It surrounds the beginning portion of the urethra that is called the prostatic urethra. The prostate gland is about the shape and size of a chestnut. It is covered by a dense fibrous capsule and contains glandular tissue surrounded by fibromuscular tissue that contracts during ejaculation. The contraction of the prostate gland closes off the prostatic urethra during ejaculation preventing the passage of urine through the urethra. This contraction of the muscular tissue also aids in the expulsion of semen during an ejaculation. The prostate gland secretes a thin, milky alkaline fluid that enhances sperm motility. It also gives semen its characteristic strong musky odor. Fluid in the ductus deferens is very acidic, and the female vaginal secretions are also quite acidic. Therefore, the alkaline prostatic fluid probably neutralizes the acidic semen and vaginal secretions. This enhances the viability and motility of the sperm cells.

Bulbourethral Glands

The **bulbourethral glands,** also known as **Cowper's glands,** are located on either side of the urethra below the prostate gland. They add an alkaline secretion to the semen that helps the sperm to live longer within the acid medium of the female reproductive tract.

Erection and Ejaculation

The urethra extends down the length of the penis, opening at the urinary meatus of the glans. The urethra serves two purposes: to empty urine from the bladder and to expel semen. Sexual intercourse becomes possible due to the columns of erectile tissue in the penis. When a male is sexually aroused, nerve impulses cause the erectile tissue to engorge with blood which makes the erectile tissue increase in size and become firm. Blood entering the dilated arteries squeezes the veins against the penile structures prohibiting venous return.

Once stimulation of the glans results in maximum stimulation of the seminal vesicles, impulses are sent to the ejaculatory center and orgasm occurs. Orgasm is the result of muscular contractions from the vas deferens, ejaculatory ducs, and prostate glands. Secretions stored in these structures along with the sperm are forcibly expelled through the urethra after which the engorgement gradually subsides.

Impotence

Impotence is the inability to have or sustain an erection during intercourse. Primary impotence refers to the client who has never had an erection. Secondary impotence refers to the client who is currently impotent but has had erections in the past. Transient periods of impotence are not considered a dysfunction and probably occur in half the adult male population between the ages of 40 and 70; the incidence increases with age.

The majority of impotence involves organic causes. Psychological factors such as anxiety and stress can also be causes of impotence.

The type of therapy chosen depends on the specific cause of the dysfunction. Treatment may be sexual therapy if the cause is thought to be related to psychological factors. At the present time, penile implants, injection therapy, and oral medications are being used to treat impotence.

CONTRACEPTION

Some religious and ethnic groups oppose birth control and this text does not ignore that issue. This subject matter is presented factually, from a clinical viewpoint, as information required for practice as a health care worker. As the word implies, *contraception* is literally "against" conception. One choice in contraception is abstinence. Abstinence is the voluntary restraint of sexual intercourse. Abstinence is a positive, healthy choice many people make. Several reasons may be given to avoid pregnancy.

- Avoid health risks to the woman. A woman in poor health may not survive a pregnancy.

- Spacing pregnancies. Some women are very fertile and could conceive every year or less. The infant death rate is reported to be 50% higher at 1-year intervals than at 2 or more years.

- Avoid having babies with birth defects. Some women have chromosome defects or are genetic disease carriers (or married to carriers) and choose not to risk pregnancy.

- Delay pregnancy early in marriage to allow a time for adjustment to avoid additional stress in the new relationship and establish a strong marriage.

- Limiting family size. It is sometimes a personal decision and other times a reality of limited resources.

- Avoid pregnancy among unmarried couples. Single parenthood is difficult.

- Curbing population growth. The concern over worldwide food supply and supportive environment prompts some to promote contraception.

Several methods to prevent conception and their relative percentage of effectiveness are listed in Table 21-4. Selection is usually made by the woman or couple in consultation with a doctor. The cost, ease of use, degree of effectiveness, and likelihood of side effects must be taken into consideration when selecting a method.

INFERTILITY

Infertility is when conception does not occur. Some causes of infertility may be damage to fallopian tubes, a low sperm count, hormonal imbalance, and other disorders.

Infertility Treatments

- Fertility drugs such as clomid and pergonal promote ovulation by stimulating the hormones from the pituitary to prepare an egg or several eggs for ovulation each month. This method is successful for some women.

- **Artificial insemination** occurs when a concentrated dose of sperm is placed in the woman's uterus or fallopian tube by means of a catheter.

- Surgery may be used if blocked tubes, endometriosis, fibroids, genetic defects, or ovarian cysts are implicated in fertility problems. A **laparoscopy** is the direct visualization of the abdominal cavity through a tube (**laparoscope**) placed through a small incision (usually into the navel). The instrument is like a miniature telescope with a fiber optic system which brings light into the abdomen. Carbon dioxide gas is put into the abdomen through a special needle inserted below the navel. This gas helps to separate the organs inside the abdominal cavity making it easier to see the internal organs, and the gas is removed at the end of the procedure. The laparoscope may also be fitted with miniature surgical devices to enable the physician to correct any abnormal conditions.

- Assisted reproductive techniques such as fertility drugs and other conventional treatment

Table 21-4 Different Methods of Preventing Conception

% EFFECTIVE	METHOD	DESCRIPTION/COMMENTS
100%	Abstinence	Refraining from sexual intercourse; absolutely most effective.
100%	Sterilization	Tubal/ligation (cutting of the fallopian tubes) in the female. The cut ends can be sewn back in opposite directions or cauterized. The surgical procedure is done through a laparoscope inserted into the abdomen. The procedure is considered permanent. A vasectomy in the male, with the ends being sewn in opposite directions. The surgery is performed through a small incision at the base of the scrotum. Vasectomies are usually not reversible; however, in some instances, reconstructive surgery has been successful, especially in cases of shorter duration; sperm production is usually significantly decreased in time. Usually a second marriage and the desire for another child prompt the attempt. The method is relatively expensive.
95%–99%	Birth control pills	Many different kinds are available. They are a combination of hormones that prevent ovulation; no ovum, therefore no pregnancy. Failure occurs when pills are not taken as prescribed. Side effects can be prohibitive for some women. Available only by prescription and requires regular visits to a physician. Cost is a factor to consider.
93%–99%	IUD	The intrauterine device is a small piece of plastic or coiled material inserted into the uterus to prevent implantation of a fertilized egg, presumably by providing irritation to the endometrium. Failure can occur if the device is expelled and during the first few months after being inserted. Initial insertion costs involved, and cost of removal. Side effects bother some women.
90%–99%	Diaphragm	A thin piece of dome-shaped rubber with a firm ring, which is inserted into the vagina to cover the cervix and provide a barrier to sperm. It is most effective when used in combination with a contraceptive cream placed into the dome before inserting. Failure usually results from improper insertion, a defect in the rubber, such as a hole, failure to insert before any penile penetration, or failure to maintain in place at least 6 hours following intercourse. Initial cost to examine and fit and purchase. No side effects. Requires cleaning and inspection after each use.
85%–97%	Condom	A thin sheath of rubber or latex that fits over an erect penis to catch the semen. A properly used condom is very effective. It must be unrolled onto an erect penis *before* any penetration occurs. It is important to leave about 1/2" of free air space at the tip (unless the condom is constructed with a tip) to catch the semen; otherwise, the force of the ejaculation may burst the condom. It must also remain in place throughout intercourse. After ejaculation has occurred, care must be taken to withdraw with the condom in place. It may require grasping with the fingers. This is the only contraceptive that also provides a level of protection against sexually transmitted diseases. It is relatively inexpensive, easy to use, and readily available. Remember, only a latex condom is also effective against the AIDS virus.
70%–75%	Spermicides	Contraceptive foams, jellies, and creams with *sperm-killing* ingredients, inserted by applicator, deep into the vagina before intercourse. It must remain for at least 6 to 8 hours afterward. Each application is good for only one act of intercourse. They should not be relied on alone as an effective contraceptive. Combined with diaphragm or condom, they are effective. Few side effects (some report allergic reactions), easily used, and readily available. Must not be confused with lubricants such as K-Y or Lubafax, which contain NO spermicide.
?%	Douching	Absolutely not reliable. It only takes a couple of minutes for sperm to enter the cervix. In all reality, douching cannot be accomplished quickly enough. In fact, it may even assist sperm toward the cervix.
70%–80%	Withdrawal	This method has been practiced since ancient times. It simply requires that the penis be withdrawn and ejaculation occur outside the vagina. It is not very effective because some sperm are deposited in the vagina before ejaculation occurs. In addition, the man may not be able to withdraw in time. It requires a lot of concentration to control. It is also not advised because it may lead to a sexual dysfunction if practiced for a prolonged period of time.
65%–85%	Rhythm	Is the practice of abstinence during an 8-day period from day 10 to 17 of the menstrual cycle when conception is theoretically possible. The method works fairly well for women who are extremely regular in their cycles and couples who can practice strong self-control. However, it requires a careful assessment of at least 6 months of cycles to establish ovulation days. If cycles vary in length, the period of abstinence must be increased to cover the longest possible period of time.

options are combined with high-tech procedures such as egg extraction to treat low sperm count problems or fallopian or ovulation problems. These procedures are quite costly and all couples undertaking them should have counseling regarding risk factors, the possibility of multiple births, and the success rate.

1. **In vitro fertilization (IVF)**—After taking fertility drugs, mature eggs, as determined by ultrasound and hormonal blood levels, are removed from the ovaries using a needle inserted through the vaginal wall or by laparoscopy. The eggs are then combined with the sperm. When an egg is fertilized (zygote) and it reaches the four or eight cell stage, the zygote is transferred to the uterus of the female.

2. Gamete intrafallopian transfer (GIFT)—This procedure is similar to IVF with the exception that the eggs are combined with the sperm and are placed into the fallopian tubes of the woman using a laparoscope.

3. Zygote intrafallopian transfer—This procedure is similar to GIFT except technicians monitor the eggs carefully to be certain they are fertilized before placing them in the fallopian tubes.

4. Donor eggs and embryos—In this case the woman may use a donor's egg and her partner's sperm or use both egg and sperm donors. The woman must take a fertility drug to prepare her uterus for the implantation of the zygote. After the donor egg and sperm are fertilized in the laboratory, the procedure is similar to IVF.

DISORDERS OF THE REPRODUCTIVE SYSTEM

Female Reproductive Disorders

Amenorrhea is a term used to define absence of the menstrual cycle. This is normal if the female is pregnant. Psychological factors, anorexia, and hormonal imbalance are other causes of this condition.

Premenstrual syndrome (PMS) is a group of symptoms which are exhibited just prior to the

Effects of Aging on The Reproductive System

Menopause begins between the ages of 45 and 50; this beginning denotes the end of menstruation and the childbearing period. Estrogen and progesterone production markedly declines, but androgen production continues which maintains the libido (sex drive) aspects of sexuality. These changes also produce physical changes such as narrowing of the vaginal opening, loss of tissue elasticity, and a decrease in vaginal secretions. There are atrophic changes in the uterus, vagina, external genitalia, and breasts. There may be a decline in sexual activity.

For the male, the changes occur at a more gradual pace, varying from person to person. Phases of the sexual response in males are slower, obtaining and maintaining an erection becomes more difficult, and impotence may result. The prostate gland increases in size, testes decrease, sperm level decreases, testosterone level decreases, and the viscosity of seminal fluid diminishes.

Age-related physical changes experienced by both sexes do not prevent sexual function, and they do not alter the pleasure of sex or inhibit desire. It is important to note that medication regimens typically used by the aged are common causes of sexual dysfunction.

menstrual cycle, caused by water retention in the body tissue. Irritability, nervousness, mood swings, and weight gain are some of the symptoms which are seen. PMS is no longer considered just a myth and is treated with medication and diet to reduce water retention.

Dysmenorrhea is a term used to describe painful menstruation. Dysmenorrhea is characterized by cramps, which may be caused by excessive production of an inflammatory substance such as prostaglandin. Aspirinlike substances which block the action of prostaglandin are helpful.

Endometriosis, a word that comes from endometrium, is a disease that affects women during their reproductive years. In this condition, endometrial tissue is found outside the uterus. It is found around the ovaries and other organs in the abdominopelvic cavity.

Every month, like the lining of the uterus, the tissue responds to hormonal changes. The tissue gets bigger, breaks down, and causes bleeding. Endometrial tissue outside the uterus allows no way for the blood to leave the body. The result is internal bleeding, inflammation of the surrounding areas, and formation of scar tissue. This condition causes pain before and during menstruation, during or after sexual activity, infertility, and heavy or irregular bleeding. The cause is unknown, but different theories exist. One theory is that during menstruation some of the tissue backs up through the fallopian tubes, implants in the abdomen, and grows. Some experts believe it is related to an autoimmune problem. Others suggest that endometrial tissue is distributed from the uterus to other parts of the body through the lymph system.

Diagnosis is made by laparoscopy. By moving the laparoscope around the abdomen, the surgeon can check the condition of the organs and see the endometrial implants if they are present. The surgeon can also remove endometrial tissue through this method. In addition to laparoscopic surgery, another treatment is the use of hormonal drugs to stop ovulation and force endometriosis into remission during the time of treatment. Menopause generally ends the activity of mild or moderate endometriosis.

Fibroid tumors are usually benign growths which occur in the uterine wall. Fibroids may enlarge to cause pressure on other organs or may cause excessive bleeding. To treat fibroids, a **hysterectomy** (removal of the uterus) may be done.

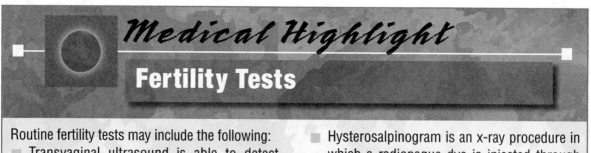

Medical Highlight
Fertility Tests

Routine fertility tests may include the following:
■ Transvaginal ultrasound is able to detect ovulation and the release of ova. This procedure is also able to assess the thickness of the endometrium.
■ Lab tests for semen testing.
■ Cervical mucous tests to see that sperm can penetrate and survive in the cervical mucus.
■ Hormone tests to measure the levels of LH, FSH, estradiol, and progesterone. In addition, other tests may include TSH, free testosterone, and prolactin hormone levels.

■ Hysterosalpinogram is an x-ray procedure in which a radiopaque dye is injected through the cervix into the uterus and fallopian tubes. The dye appears white on the x-ray and allows the radiologist to check for abnormalities.
■ Hysteroscopy is when a fiber optic light is inserted through the cervix into the uterus to check for abnormalities.
■ Laparoscopy may be done to check the reproductive organs.

Breast tumors are either benign or malignant. Benign tumors are usually fluid-filled cysts which enlarge during the premenstrual cycle. Women are taught to do periodic breast examinations to detect any developing lumps. Breast examinations are done by palpating the breasts in a circular fashion. Any suspected lump should be reported to the doctor immediately.

Breast cancer or malignant tumor is the most common cancer in women. Early detection and treatment is vital to one's survival. Surgical treatment consists of a **lumpectomy** (removal of tumor only) or **mastectomy** (removal of the breast). Other types of treatments include radiation and chemotherapy (anticancer drugs). Benefits are associated with all types of treatment; the patient and physician select the most appropriate treatment. **Mammogram** is a special type of x-ray which can detect tumors of the breast before they can be palpated. This test is recommended on an annual basis for all women over the age of 40.

Endometrial cancer is the most common type of uterine cancer. It usually affects women after menopause. Women are instructed to immediately report to their physician any vaginal bleeding which occurs after menopause. Hysterectomy and irradiation are the usual types of treatment.

Ovarian cancer is a leading cause of cancer death in women. It usually occurs between the ages of 40 and 65. Early diagnosis is difficult and treatment is aggressive surgery to remove all reproductive organs.

Cervical cancer is frequently seen in women between the ages of 30 and 50. The test to detect cancer of the cervix is called the **Papanicolaou (Pap) smear,** where a sample of cell scrapings is taken from the cervix and cervical canal for microscopic study. Once a female is sexually active, this test should be done on an annual basis. Early detection and treatment are vital to a good prognosis.

Infections of Female Reproductive Organs

Pelvic inflammatory disease (PID) may be due to infections which occur in the reproductive organs and spread to the fallopian tubes and peritoneal cavity. This disease may also be secondary to another infection such as gonorrhea. The inflammation causes pain, high temperature, and possible scarring of the fallopian tubes. Treatment consists of medications such as antibiotics and analgesics.

Salpingitis is an inflammation of the fallopian tubes which may result in permanent damage.

Toxic shock syndrome is a bacterial infection caused by a staphylococcus organism. Symptoms are fever, rash, and hypotension which may result in shock. The patient is treated with antibiotics.

Vaginal **yeast infections** are generally caused by an organism called *Candida albincans*. This fungus is part of the body's natural organisms. A problem arises when the environment of the vagina is altered. A yeast infection develops when the vagina becomes less acidic. This change results in an overgrowth of candida organisms, causing an infection.

Symptoms include itching, burning, and redness in the vagina and vulva. There may also be an odorless, thick, white discharge (leukorrhea) resembling cottage cheese. Treatment with an antibiotic (for another illness) which alters the normal bacteria of the vagina may cause a yeast infection to occur. Yeast infections are more common in people with diabetes, pregnant women, and those with other causes of hormonal changes. Treatment is the use of a fungicidal agent that destroys the organism. This may be used as a vaginal cream or vaginal insert.

Male Reproductive Disorders

Epididymitis is a painful swelling in the groin and scrotum due to infection of the epididymis. This is treated with antibiotic therapy.

Orchitis is an inflammation of the testes. It may be a complication of mumps, flu, or another infection. Symptoms are swelling of the scrotum, fever, and pain. This disease is treated with antibiotic therapy, pain relievers, and cold compresses.

Prostatitis is an infection of the prostate gland. The prostate gland lies below the urinary bladder and the prostatic urethra passes through the gland. Urinary symptoms are often the first indication there is a prostatic problem. The patient will complain of difficulty in urination. Treatment with antibiotic is effective.

Benign prostatic hypertrophy (BPH) indicates an enlarged prostate. The prostate gland continues to grow during most of a man's life; the enlargement usually does not cause problems until late in life. More than half of men in their 60s and as many as 90% in their 70s have some symptoms of BPH. As the prostate enlarges, the capsule around the prostate does not, which causes the prostate to press up against the urethra like a clamp around a tube. The bladder becomes thick and irritable. Then the bladder begins to contract even when it contains only small amounts of urine, causing frequent urination. As the bladder weakens it loses the ability to empty itself and urine remains in the bladder. The narrowing of the urethra may cause retention of urine and an infection may occur.

Diagnosis is made by rectal exam, ultrasound, and cystoscopy. A cystoscopy is a flexible tube with lens and a light system which is inserted into the urethra. This enables the physician to see the inside of the urethra and the bladder.

Treatment may depend on the extent of the symptoms. At the present time a prostatectomy is the usual treatment.

Prostate cancer is the most common cancer in males over the age of 50. Males over the age of 40 should start to have annual rectal examinations which can detect enlargement of the prostate. A prostate-specific antigen blood screening test (PSA test) detects an abnormal substance released by cancer cells. Symptoms include frequency of urination, dysuria (painful urination), urgency, nocturia (night voiding), and in some cases hematuria (blood in the urine). The most common treatment is a **prostatectomy** (removal of the prostate gland). This procedure is called a transurethral resection of the prostate (TURP). An instrument is inserted into the penis and resects or cuts away the prostate gland which is then removed through the penis. There is no abdominal incision made and recovery time is short.

SEXUALLY TRANSMITTED DISEASE

Sexually transmitted diseases (STDs), also known as venereal diseases, are transmitted through the exchange of body fluids such as semen, vaginal fluid, and blood. STDs can be serious, painful, and cause long-term complications including sterility, chronic infection, scarring of the fallopian tubes, ectopic pregnancy, cancer, and death. The most common of these diseases are chlamydia, genital herpes, genital warts, and trichomoniasis vaginalis.

Most of these diseases have no symptoms. Symptoms, if present, include the following:

▪ In females, an unusual discharge from the vagina, pain in the pelvic area, burning or itching around the vagina, unusual bleeding, and vaginal pain during intercourse

▪ In males, a discharge from the penis

▪ In both females and males, sores or blisters near the mouth or genitalia, burning and pain during urination or a bowel movement, flulike symptoms, and swelling in the groin area

The client who is at a physician's office or a health care center to be checked for an STD may feel some embarrassment. It is critical that the health care worker treat the person in a nonjudgmental manner, because every day that the disease is untreated it causes more severe health problems. Some STDs are diagnosed by physical examination; others require blood or other laboratory tests. For bacterial diseases such as gonorrhea, chlamydia, and syphilis, treatment is with antibiotics. Viral infections usually cannot be cured but the symptoms can be relieved.

Protection from STDs includes abstinence and practicing safe sexual behavior. Abstinence is the voluntary refraining from sexual activity. Abstinence is a positive, healthy choice many people make. Safe sex means using condoms and looking for any signs of venereal disease *before* sexual activity occurs. Once a person is aware of the disease, he or she must notify their sexual partner(s) so he or she can also be checked for the disease. It is often necessary for previous sexual partners to also be notified. All sexually transmitted diseases need to be treated. A high incidence of STDs is leading to an increase in sterility in young females. See Chapter 15 for a discussion on HIV/AIDS.

Chlamydia is caused by the *Chlamydia trachomatis* organism and is the most common cur-

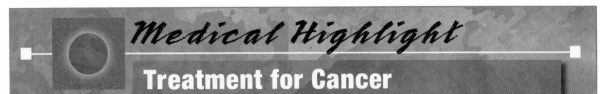

Medical Highlight

Treatment for Cancer

BENIGN PROSTATIC HYPERTROPHY

A number of recent studies have questioned the need for early treatment for benign prostatic hypertrophy (BPH) when the prostate gland is just mildly enlarged. These studies report that early treatment may not be needed because the symptoms of BPH clear up without any treatment in as many as one-third of all mild cases. Instead of immediate treatment the study suggests regular checkups to watch for early problems. If the condition poses a threat to the health or is a major inconvenience, treatment is then recommended.

Some researchers are exploring the use of laser surgery to vaporize obstructing prostate tissue. Early studies suggest that this method may be as effective as conventional surgery.

PROSTATE CANCER

Since the advent of the prostate screening antigen blood test to detect prostate cancer, there has been an increase in the number of people with

positive results. This has led to more discussion on the type of treatment. In some patients the antigen level did not rise over a period of time; therefore, the question remains as to whether surgical removal should be done immediately or a "wait and see" period should occur.

The best therapy should be determined by the physician and then decided based on the individual circumstance of each case. In some cases, surgery is the best choice; however, radiation also has been effective in reducing the tumor. Radiation is performed on an outpatient basis and given daily over a period of 6 to 7 weeks. In cases when there has been extensive spread of the cancer, hormonal therapy is the method of treatment.

Hormonal therapy works by depriving the tumor cells of testosterone used for the maintenance and growth of the malignant cells. The treatment puts the cancer in remission and relieves pain.

Note: Early detection is still the key to fighting prostate cancer.

---

able sexually transmitted disease in the United States. It is the major cause of nongonococcal urethritis, bacterial vaginitis, and pelvic inflammatory disease. Eighty percent of women and 25% of men have no symptoms. If symptoms appear, they may be abnormal genital discharge and burning with urination. A screening test called a DNA probe assay may be done for this disease. It examines secretion from the cervix, urethra, or rectum. Treatment is with antibiotics; however, immunity does not develop after being infected.

Genital warts, or human papillomavirus, is another common sexually transmitted disease. The wart can appear on the shaft of the penis or on the vagina. It is usually asymptomatic. In

many cases the warts are not visible to the naked eye. In other cases they look like small, hard, round spots resembling a cauliflower. Although genital warts are usually painless, they become sore, itchy, and may burn if hit, rubbed, or irritated. Diagnosis is made primarily by examination. Treatment involves the use of an acid to destroy wart tissue or cryosurgery. Cryosurgery uses liquid nitrogen which is placed on the wart and a small area of the surrounding skin. The liquid nitrogen freezes the skin causing ice crystals which results in the sloughing off of the wart.

Gonorrhea is a bacterial infection caused by *Neisseria gonorrhoeae*. The symptoms in the male may be painful urination and the discharge of pus from the penis. In the female, the early stages of the disease may be asymptomatic (no symptoms). This disease is treated with antibiotic therapy. There is a problem with some strains of the organism which have become resistant to the usual treatment.

Complications may occur if the inflammation spreads to the epididymis of the male or the fallopian tube of the female. The tubes may become scarred and blocked, which will result in sterility. In addition, if a pregnant woman contracts the disease and it is untreated, her baby may be born with gonorrheal eye infection.

Genital herpes is a viral infection that is sexually transmitted. The herpes lesion may cause a burning sensation and small blisterlike areas may appear in the genitalia. Other symptoms may be painful irritation and discomfort while sitting or standing. Herpes symptoms may simply disappear after 2 weeks; however the symptoms may continue to reappear throughout the lifetime of the individual. Females who are diagnosed with herpes must consult with their physician whether to have a Cesarean section to prevent herpes infection of the newborn during childbirth.

Syphilis is a potentially life-threatening STD, caused by the bacteria *Treponema pallidum.* In the early stages of syphilis, a genital sore called a chancre develops shortly after infection and eventually disappears on its own. If the disease is not treated it can progress on its own over years. A transient rash may appear; eventually there is serious involvement of the vertebrae, brain, and heart resulting in meningitis, lack of coordination, and stroke. The full course of the disease can take years. Penicillin is the most effective treatment for syphilis.

Trichomoniasis vaginalis is a STD caused by infection with the protozoan *Trichomonas vaginalis.* It causes vaginitis—inflammation of the vagina causing burning, itching, and discomfort. In men, trichomoniasis may cause similar problems in the urethra, called urethritis. Treatment is usually with a single dose of antibiotics.

HUMAN GROWTH AND DEVELOPMENT

Even though individuals differ greatly, each person passes through certain stages of growth and development from birth to death. As a person passes through these stages, four main types of growth and development occur: physical, mental, emotional, and social. Physical growth and development refer to changes occurring in the body, body systems, and organs. Mental growth and development relates to changes occurring in the mind and the ability to solve problems and make judgments. Emotional growth and development relates to the ability to deal with feelings. Social growth and development relates to changes in the way a person interacts with other people.

Tasks must be mastered at each stage of development before a person can progress to the next stage. Tasks build upon one another progressing from the simple to the complex. The rate at which an individual progresses through each stage varies. These stages are generally grouped by age: infancy, toddler, pre-school, school-age, adolescence, young adult, middle adult, and older adult.

Infancy

Infancy lasts from birth to one year. This is the time in which the most dramatic changes in growth and development occur. Weight generally triples from birth to one year and height usually increases by 29 to 30 inches. The muscular and nervous systems undergo rapid change in this stage. Teeth develop and eye sight improves. The other senses become more defined. Mental development also occurs rapidly through the increasing of verbal skills. Emotional development begins at this stage and events occurring at this age related to emotions can have a strong impact on emotional behavior in adulthood. Social development occurs in the infant's ability to recognize others and respond to familiar people.

Toddler

The toddler stage is from 1 to 3 years of age. At this age the child is very mobile. Physical growth progresses at a slower pace. Coordination is becoming fine-tuned allowing the child to walk, run, and climb. Mental development continues to progress rapidly. The toddler learns to use more words, remembers details, and begins to understand basic concepts. Emotional development also progresses rapidly. The toddler begins to become self aware and more independent. Social development shows the toddler progressing from being self-centered to socializing more with other adults and children.

Preschool

The preschool stage is from 3 to 5 years of age. Motor development continues and the child is able to write and use utensils. Children also begin to achieve control over their bladder and bowels. Mental development continues as the preschooler begins to ask more questions about his or her surroundings and make decisions based upon logic. Emotional development progresses and the child may become frustrated as he or she tries to do more than within his or her ability. Children at this stage understand right from wrong. Social develop allows the child to begin to interact and trust others.

School-age

The school-age child is from 6 to 12 years of age. Physical development is slow but steady. Weight gain averages 5 to 7 pounds per year and height usually increases 2 to 3 inches per year. Physical activities and game playing become more complex as muscular coordination is well-developed at this age. The primary teeth are lost and the permanent teeth erupt. Sexual maturity may begin. Mental development increases rapidly as a great deal of time at this stage is spent in school. Speech, reading, and writing skills develop and school-age children are able to solve more complex problems. Children at this stage begin to understand more abstract concepts such as honesty and values. Emotional development continues, allowing children greater independence and the development of their own personalities. Social activities change from wanting to do things on one's own to wanting to be involved in group activities.

Adolescence

Adolescence spans the ages of 12 to 20 years of age. In early adolescence a growth spurt may occur and muscle coordination may not grow at the same rate. This may make the adolescent awkward. The most obvious changes are those related to puberty. Secondary sex organs and sexual characteristics become more prominent. Mental development involves increasing knowledge and sharpening skills. Adolescents make decisions and learn responsibility for their actions. Emotional development is often in conflict as adolescents try to establish their own identities and yet feel uncertain and insecure. This age group responds to peer pressure. Social development sees this age group spending more time with friends and less time with family. Many problems can develop at this stage including eating disorders and substance abuse.

Early Adulthood

Early adulthood spans the ages of 20 to 40 years old. Physical development at this stage is complete. This is the prime time for childbearing. Mental development continues as education is furthered and careers are chosen. Emotional development revolves around preserving the stability founded earlier in life as stresses increase in one's life. Social development usually involves moving away from one's peer groups and developing relationships with others that share similar goals and interests.

Middle Adulthood

Middle Adulthood is from 40 to 65 years of age. Physical changes begin involving aging such as graying hair, formation of wrinkles, loss of hearing and vision, and weight gain. Mental ability can continue to increase; decision-making and problem-solving are done with more confidence. Emotionally, middle adulthood is usually a period of contentment and satisfaction. Socially, family relationships decline and work relationships grow.

Older Adulthood

Older adulthood ranges from 65 and up. Physical development begins to decline and body systems are usually affected. Mental abilities may vary and in some may also begin to decline. Emotional abilities vary as well and are related to the individual's ability to cope with stress and loss. Social adjustment is often required due to retirement, loss of loved ones, and physical limitations.

Medical Terminology

a	without
-men	monthly
-rrhea	flow or discharge
a/men/o/rrhea	without a monthly flow
circumcis	cutting around
-ion	process of
circumcis/ion	process of cutting around
clitor	gatekeeper
-is	presence of
clitor/is	presence of a gatekeeper
coit	sexual intercourse
-us	presence of
coit/us	presence of sexual intercourse
crypt	hidden
-orchid	testes
-ism	abnormal condition of
crypt/orchid/ism	abnormal condition of hidden testes, undescended testicles
dys	painful
dys/men/o/rrhea	painful monthly flow
ectopic	out of place
ectopic pregnancy	a pregnancy that occurs outside the uterus
endo	within
-metr/i/	uterus
-um	presence of
endo/metri/um	pertaining to the lining within the uterus
episi	vulva
-otomy	incision into
episi/otomy	incision into the vulva
hyster	uterus
-ectomy	removal of
hyster/ectomy	removal of the uterus
leuko	white
leuko/rrhea	white discharge
mammo	breast
-gram	x-ray record
mammo/gram	x-ray record of the breasts
mast	breasts

mast/ectomy	removal of the breast
myo	muscle
myo/metri/um	presence of uterine muscle
o/o	egg
-genesis	development
o/o/genesis	development of ova-egg
ovul/a/	releasing a little egg
-tion	process of
ovul/a/tion	process of releasing a little egg
prostat	prostate gland
prostat/ectomy	removal of prostate gland
salping	fallopian tube
-itis	inflammation of
salping/itis	inflammation of the fallopian tube
spermato	seed
spermato/genesis	production of seed

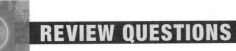

REVIEW QUESTIONS

Select the letter of choice that best completes the statement.

1. One of the male hormones is:
   a. progesterone
   b. luteinizing hormone
   c. follicle-stimulating hormone
   d. testosterone

2. Ovulation usually occurs:
   a. the day before the menstrual period begins
   b. 1 week before the menstrual period begins
   c. 3 weeks before the menstrual period begins
   d. 2 weeks before the menstrual period begins

3. The ovaries contain:
   a. 30 graafian follicles
   b. thousands of graafian follicles
   c. hundreds of graafian follicles
   d. 6 graafian follicles

4. The development of the follicle and release of the ovum are under the influence of:
   a. the follicle-stimulating hormone and the luteinizing hormone
   b. estrogen and corpus luteum
   c. progesterone and the follicle-stimulating hormone
   d. estrogen and the luteinizing hormone

5. Which one of the following statements is *not* correct?
   a. The fallopian tubes are about 4 inches long.
   b. The fallopian tubes serve as ducts for the ovum on its way to the uterus.
   c. The fallopian tubes are also called oviducts.
   d. The fallopian tubes are attached to the ovaries.

MATCHING

Match each term in Column I with its correct description in Column II.

Column I	Column II
_____ **1.** scrotum	a. secondary sex characteristics
_____ **2.** testosterone	b. external sac which holds the testes
_____ **3.** facial and pubic hair	c. excreted from the pituitary gland
_____ **4.** epididymis and penis	d. formed in the seminiferous tubules
_____ **5.** spermatozoa	e. male gamete
	f. secondary reproductive organs
	g. male hormone produced in the testes

COMPLETION

Fill in the blanks.

1. Painful or difficulty in menstruation is known as _____.

2. Amenorrhea is normal when a person is _____.

3. Gonorrhea is a sexually transmitted disease. The male complains of _____ and the female complains of _____.

4. The test done to detect breast tumors is called _____.

5. Sterility results from inflammation of the fallopian tube which can be caused by _____ and _____.

6. A group of symptoms which occur before the menstrual cycle is called _____.

7. The onset of ovulation is known as _____ and the cessation of ovulation is known as _____.

8. A sexually transmitted disease which has small blisterlike areas is known as _____.

9. An enlarged prostate may cause problems with _____.

10. The best methods of preventing sexually transmitted diseases are _____ and _____.

APPLYING THEORY TO PRACTICE

1. A young pregnant woman comes into the doctor's office and states, "I told my husband I will give him a son, because in my family I was the only girl and I have four brothers." Is this a valid statement? Explain to the expectant mother how the sex of the newborn is determined.

2. If a man has a sperm count of 16 million, he would be considered sterile. Fertilization only requires the union of one egg and one sperm; why then are so many sperm necessary for fertilization to occur?

3. You are asked to describe the fertilization process. Explain how the sperm travels from the testes and arrives at the fallopian tube in time to meet the ova.

4. You are invited to a middle school to address 11- to 14-year-old adolescents and discuss puberty. Plan a program to describe how females are affected by estrogen and progesterone and how males are affected by testosterone.

5. A 50-year-old female patient tells you it has gotten very hot in the waiting room and requests that you put on the air conditioner. The temperature outdoors is 30°F. She further states that the doctor told her about changes which usually occur at mid-life. Explain to the patient the physiological and psychological changes which are attributed to menopause.

6. Sexually transmitted disease is a major health concern especially in the teenage population. This condition can lead to pelvic inflammatory disease and sterility. Describe at least three sexually transmitted diseases; explain their symptoms and treatment.

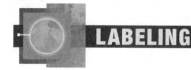

LABELING

Label the structures of the male reproductive system on the following diagram.

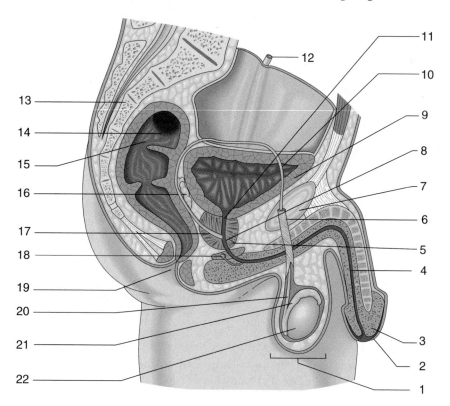

1. _____

2. _____

3. _____

4. _____

5. _____

6. _____

7. _____

8. _____

9. _____

10. _____

11. _____

12. _____

13. _____

14. _____

15. _____

16. _____

17. _____

18. _____

19. _____

20. _____

21. _____

22. _____

CASE STUDY

Jenna, a 25 year-old female, went into premature labor two months before her due date. In the hospital Jenna was very anxious about the health of her baby.

1. Have all of the baby's organs fully developed after seven months?

2. Can the baby safely live outside the uterus after seven months?

3. At what stage of embryological development does the brain and spinal cord begin to develop?

4. At what stage of embryological development does the skeletal system develop?

5. Are there any birth defects related to premature delivery?

6. List the developmental process for each of the nine months of pregnancy.

Lab Activity

21-1

Organs of the Reproductive System

- *Objective:* To observe the location and difference between the male and female reproductive organs
- *Materials needed:* charts of female reproductive organs and male reproductive organs, textbook, paper and pencil

Step 1: Locate and identify the female reproductive organs on the anatomical charts. Describe and record their locations and functions.

Step 2: Locate and identify the male reproductive organs on the anatomical charts. Describe and record their locations and functions.

Step 3: Compare the organs and functions of the female and male reproductive organs. What are their similarities? Record your answer. Compare your answer with the textbook.

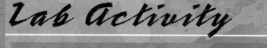

21-2 *Lab Activity*
Examination of an Ovary

■ *Objective:* To observe the structure of the ovaries
■ *Materials needed:* cross-section slide of ovarian tissue, microscope, textbook, paper and pencil

Step 1: Identify and describe a mature graafian follicle with an oocyte, and a maturing graafian follicle. Compare with Figure 21-13. Record your descriptions. What do the cells of the graafian follicle produce? Record your answer.

Step 2: Identify and describe a corpus luteum. Compare with Figure 21-13. Record your observations. What do the cells of the corpus luteum produce?

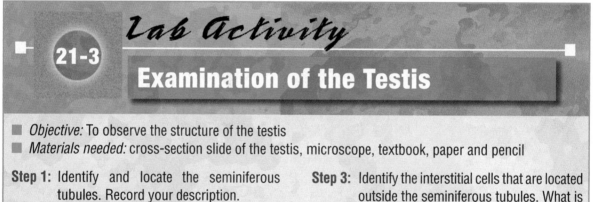

21-3 *Lab Activity*
Examination of the Testis

■ *Objective:* To observe the structure of the testis
■ *Materials needed:* cross-section slide of the testis, microscope, textbook, paper and pencil

Step 1: Identify and locate the seminiferous tubules. Record your description.

Step 2: Observe the cells in the middle of the tubule wall of the seminiferous tubule. Observe the spermatocytes. Record your description.

Step 3: Identify the interstitial cells that are located outside the seminiferous tubules. What is their function? Record your answer.

Chapter

22

GENETICS AND GENETICALLY LINKED DISEASES

Objectives

- Define mutation

- Differentiate between the two basic types of mutations

- Name three human genetic disorders and describe the cause and symptoms of each

- Explain genetic counseling

- Define the key words that relate to this chapter

Key Words

amniocentesis
chorionic villi
   sampling
chromosomal
   mutation
congenital disorder
cystic fibrosis
Duchenne's
   muscular
   dystrophy
gene
gene mutation

genetic counseling
genetic disorder
genetics
hemophilia
Huntington's
   disease
interferon
lethal gene
mutagenic agent
mutation
phenylketonuria
   (PKU)

recombinant DNA
sickle cell anemia
somatic cell
   mutation
Tay-Sachs disease
thalassemia
   (Cooley's
   anemia)
trisomy 21 or
   Down syndrome
   (mongolism)

GENETICS

In sexual reproduction, a new individual is created from the union of the sperm cell and the egg cell. This process is called fertilization. Contained in the nucleus of each gamete are structures called chromosomes. The chromosomes contain DNA (deoxyribonucleic acid), the hereditary material referred to in Chapter 2. The DNA is packaged in small functional units found along the length of a chromosome, called **genes.** A gene is an area of DNA that carries information for the cellular synthesis of a specific protein. These genes are transmitted to the zygote, and will then control the development and characteristics of the embryo as it grows and matures. Eventually, due to the combined influence of all of the genes on all of the chromosomes, a new individual is formed. The new individual possesses all the necessary characteristics or traits needed for survival. Additionally, because the genes come from two parents, the offspring resembles both parents in some ways; however, it is also different from each parent. It has, for instance, all the characteristics of its species. Concurrently, it possesses its own unique traits that set it apart from all other members of its species.

Genetics is the branch of biology that studies how the genes are transmitted from parents to offspring. Occasionally, a gene or chromosome is changed, or mutated, and this mutated gene or chromosome is inherited by the offspring. The inheritance of such a mutated gene or chromosome will cause the appearance of a new and different trait, called a **mutation.** Sometimes the mutation is beneficial or harmless to an organism. Most inherited mutated genes are not beneficial. Still, it must be emphasized that mutations in the genetic material are responsible for biological evolution on this planet.

In June 2000, scientists completed the first working draft of the human genome. With this information, medical researchers can identify sites where mutations can occur. For additional information, see the section in Chapter 3 on genetic engineering, cloning, and stem cell research.

TYPES OF MUTATIONS

There are two types of mutations. One type is called a **gene mutation.** When this mutation occurs, a new or altered gene is produced to replace a normal preexisting gene. The other type is a **chromosomal mutation.** This mutation involves a change in the number of chromosomes found in the nucleus or a change in the structure of a whole chromosome.

Somatic Cell Mutation

Gene mutations occur occasionally at random in all cells of the human body. For instance, skin cells often undergo mutation as an individual ages. Mutations that occur in individual body (somatic) cells will not be transmitted to the offspring. This specific type of mutation is called a **somatic cell mutation.** A somatic cell mutation is not likely to affect other cells or the function of the organism as a whole. As an example, a single cell may lose the ability to make a certain protein and die without having an impact on the total organism.

Gametic Cell Mutation

Mutations that occur in the nucleus of the gametes (sperm and egg cell) will be passed on to the next generation. If either a gene or chromosomal mutation is present in a gamete at the moment of fertilization, all the cells of the embryo and the developed organism will have the mutation in at least half of their DNA.

LETHAL GENES

Inherited mutations are generally negative happenings to the individual. At times, they might even result in the formation of lethal genes. A **lethal gene** is a gene that results in death.

The time at which lethal genes exert their deadly influence varies. Some genes interfere with mitosis of the zygote and life ends before the zygote divides. Some lethal genes interfere with implantation of the fertilized egg in the uterus. Death would occur so early that a woman would never know that conception had even occurred. A lethal gene that prevents normal formation of the heart or normal blood production causes death at about 3 weeks after fertilization because this is the time when circulating blood becomes vital for continued existence. Others may kill at various times during development, depending on the time their products become vital for survival. Other lethal genes causing neonatal deaths involve abnormalities of the lungs and shifts in the circulatory system which must channel blood from the heart to the lungs instead of to the umbilical cord.

Some lethal genes do not exert their effects until later in life. Tay-Sachs disease causes death several years after birth. Duchenne's muscular dystrophy causes death in the teens and early childhood. Huntington's disease usually brings about death at about 40 to 50 years of age.

It is estimated that each person carries two or three different recessive lethal genes. Two similar recessive genes must be present in an individual for the gene to be expressed. Because of the numerous kinds of lethal genes, one's chance of marrying someone with even one matching lethal gene is small. Statistically, should this happen, the lethal gene would be expressed in only one-fourth of the offspring.

When close relatives marry, the chance of the offspring inheriting two similar lethal genes increases. Persons with a common ancestry are more likely to share many genes than nonrelatives. As a result, spontaneous abortions, stillbirths, and neonatal deaths are higher among progeny of people sharing similar gene pools.

HUMAN GENETIC DISORDERS

Some diseases caused by gene mutations in humans are phenylketonuria (PKU), sickle cell anemia, Tay-Sachs disease, Duchenne's muscular dystrophy, Huntington's disease, cystic fibrosis, thalassemia, and hemophilia.

It is important to note that there is a difference between genetic disorders and congenital disorders. A hereditary or **genetic disorder** is caused by a variation in the genetic pattern; a **congenital disorder** is something which evolves during fetal development and is not related to genetic malfunction.

Phenylketonuria

Phenylketonuria (PKU) is a human metabolic disorder caused by an enzyme deficiency. The individual with the trait cannot break down the amino acid phenylalanine and, consequently, there is a buildup of this substance in the body. Excess phenylalanine disrupts the normal development of the brain. If a child born with the defect eats proteins containing phenylalanine during childhood, mental retardation results. A newborn infant is tested for this defect, and, if the test is positive, a phenylalanine-restricted diet is prescribed. In most cases, this diet can be liberalized as the child grows older and brain development and maturation are completed.

Sickle Cell Anemia

Sickle cell anemia is a blood disorder common in individuals of African descent. It is caused by a gene mutation resulting in an abnormal hemoglobin molecule in a red blood cell, Figure 22-1. Especially in times of low oxygen availability, the shape of a red blood cell changes from that of a biconcave disc to a crescent shape. This is referred to as sickling. The sickle shape causes the cells to clump together, thus clogging small blood vessels and capillaries. Since a sickle cell has an abnormal hemoglobin (the pigment that combines with oxygen), it also carries less oxygen to the tissues, resulting in fatigue and listlessness. Breakage of these cells is also very common, as their membranes are excessively fragile. Figure 22-2 shows tissue damage and physiological effects caused by sickle cell anemia.

Tay-Sachs Disease

Tay-Sachs disease is a genetic disorder caused by a mutation resulting in a deficiency of a lysosomal enzyme. The missing enzyme functions in breaking down lipid molecules in the brain. Without the enzyme, lipids accumulate in the brain cells and

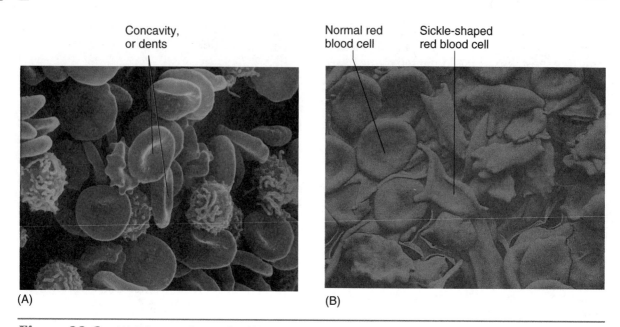

Figure 22-1   *(A) Side view of normal red blood cells, which have a concavity (or dent) on the two sides; (B) sickle-shaped (cresent-shaped) red blood cells*

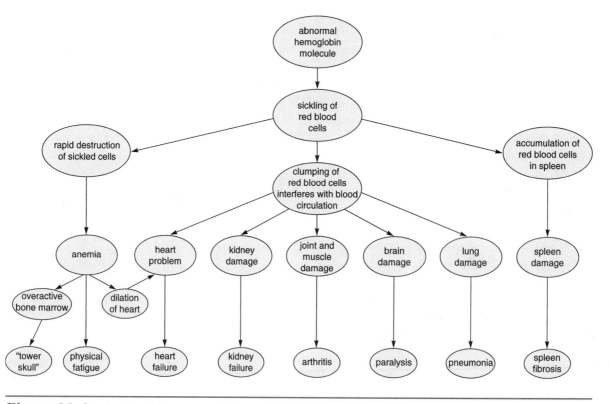

Figure 22-2   *A series of damages and effects caused by sickle cell anemia*

destroy them. This results in severe mental and motor deterioration leading to death several years after birth. This disorder is found most frequently among Jewish people of central and Eastern European ancestry.

Duchenne's Muscular Dystrophy

In **Duchenne's muscular dystrophy,** the muscles suffer a loss of protein and the contractile fibers are eventually replaced by fat and connective tissue, rendering skeletal muscle useless. As the weakening process of the disease continues, the teen or young adult is confined to a wheelchair. In many cases, the victim dies before the age of 20 from respiratory or heart failure.

Huntington's Disease

Huntington's disease is characterized by the degeneration of the central nervous system, which ultimately results in abnormal movements and mental deterioration. In this disorder, the product of an abnormal gene interferes with normal metabolism in nerve tissue.

Cystic Fibrosis

Cystic fibrosis is a disease of the exocrine gland. The lining of the digestive tract, the ducts of the pancreas, and the respiratory tract produce thick mucus which blocks the passageways. The blockage of the respiratory passages causes chronic bronchitis and pneumonia. Pulmonary therapy consists of a procedure called "cupping and clapping," which helps to dislodge the thick mucus from the respiratory tract. These treatments have helped to prolong the life span of patients with cystic fibrosis. Science has discovered the gene that transmits this disease and may soon be able to treat and prevent this illness. The involvement of the lungs is why this is one of the most fatal hereditary disorders.

Thalassemia

Thalassemia (Cooley's anemia) is a blood disease found among people of Mediterranean descent. Symptoms are the same as those associated with any anemia; there is also enlargement of the spleen and possible congestive heart disease. This disease is treated with blood transfusions to replace the defective hemoglobin molecules.

Hemophilia

Hemophilia is a sex-linked genetic disorder which means it is only transmitted on the X chromosome. In this disease the person is unable to produce the factor VIII which is necessary for blood clotting. Persistent bleeding may occur as a result of an injury or spontaneously. Treatment consists of giving the person factor VIII.

Chromosomal Aberrations

Some mutations are caused by chromosomal aberrations. Some involve entire chromosomes and others involve parts of chromosomes. During meiosis (the cell division occurring during the formation of the gametes), a pair of chromosomes may adhere to each other and not pull apart at metaphase. As a result of this nondisjunction, duplicate chromosomes go to one daughter cell and none of this type of chromosome to the other. Nondisjunction of certain chromosomes referred to as sex chromosomes causes various abnormalities of sexual development such as Turner's syndrome in females and Klinefelter's syndrome in males.

One of the most common chromosomal abnormalities involves an extra chromosome designated as chromosome 21. In fact, this disorder is referred to as **trisomy 21** or **Down syndrome (mongolism).** The risk of bearing a child with Down syndrome significantly increases with the age of the mother. Many physicians therefore recommend amniocentesis for all women who become pregnant after age 35. Cells from the amniotic fluid will show trisomy 21 (as well as other chromosomal defects) if present. If a serious defect is detected, prospective parents have the option of therapeutic abortion.

Mutagenic Agents

Although most gene or chromosomal mutations occur spontaneously, the rate or speed of mutations can be increased. This happens when a cell, a group of cells, or an entire organism is exposed to certain chemicals or radiations. Agents that speed up the occurrence of mutations are called **mutagenic agents.** Mutagenic agents can be radiations such as cosmic rays, ultraviolet rays from the sun, x-rays, and radiation from radioactive elements. Some mutagenic chemicals are benzene, formaldehyde, phenol, and nitrous acid.

In recent times, the accelerated use of various chemical and physical agents with mutagenic properties has caused concern among some geneticists who fear possible significant alterations to genes and chromosomes that will be passed onto future generations. The increased use of ionizing radiation in medical diagnosis and the problem of the disposal of nuclear waste from reactors are examples. Certain chemical pollutants in the environment, such as herbicides and insecticides, are also suspect as causing genetic defects.

Because people are being exposed to more and more new substances, and because changes in genes are irreversible, caution should be the rule with regard to any unnecessary exposure to those suspected of being mutagens.

GENETIC COUNSELING

Genetic counseling involves talking to parents or prospective parents about the possibility of genetic disorders.

People who may be especially interested in genetic counseling or testing include the following:

- Those who think they have a birth defect or genetic disorder

- Women who are pregnant after age 34

- Couples who have had one child born with a genetic defect

- Women who have had two or more miscarriages or whose babies died in infancy

- Couples who need information about genetic disorders that occur frequently in their ethnic group

- Couples who are first cousins or other blood relatives

The counseling team usually is made up of members of the health care team, a genealogist, a nurse, laboratory personnel, and social service professionals. In genetic counseling a family history is obtained which is called a pedigree. Any and all facts which pertain to the parents or prospective parents and family members are considered. After careful analysis a genotype is determined; this analysis will be able to predict the possibility of a genetic disorder.

The prospective parents are made aware of what diagnostic tests are available during pregnancy which may indicate a problem. **Chorionic villi sampling** is a test which may be done as early as 8 to 10 weeks into the pregnancy. A sample of fetal cells is removed from the fetal side of the placenta and is examined. **Amniocentesis** is withdrawal of amniotic fluid during week 16 of pregnancy. An examination of the fluid is able to pick up as many as 200 possible genetic disorders. Prior to performing an amniocentesis, a sonogram is done to determine where the fetal structures are located so as to prevent any problems.

Genetic counseling helps prospective parents make informed decisions regarding having children.

GENETIC ENGINEERING

Recent advances in the methods of gene transfer from the cell of one species to another offer exciting possibilities for the treatment of genetic deficiencies. Human insulin, human growth hormone, and human **interferons** (proteins that interfere with virus replication) are now being produced using the sophisticated technology of **recombinant DNA.** We can isolate a desired gene (to correct for a defective one) and grow millions of copies of it in the cells of bacteria and yeast which in turn produce the gene product on a commercial scale.

Some scientists even envision a time when we will have the ability to introduce copies of normal genes into humans whose genes are defective, thus alleviating a large segment of human suffering.

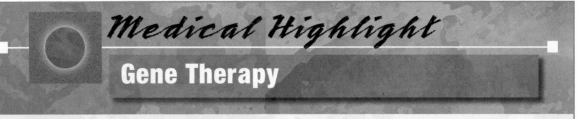
Gene therapy is a procedure that treats a disorder by replacing a faulty gene. It continues to offer much hope for the future treatment of a variety of clinical conditions. Gene therapy is being applied to many different genetic diseases both congenital (since birth) and acquired. The earliest applications of gene therapy were based on the principle that a disease is caused by a faulty gene and if such a gene can be replaced with a "correct" version, the disease might be controlled, prevented, or cured. However, most diseases involve multiple genetic factors. Until the precise involvement of different genes in the disease process and the proteins they encode are established, gene therapy is most likely to be clinically effective as a preventative or curative treatment for single-cell defects such as cystic fibrosis. Scientists have already identified which genes cause muscular dystrophy, some types of mental retardation, certain types of deafness, and many others.

Many people are concerned about ethics and possible misuse of gene therapy. The federal government and national review panels strictly regulate all human gene therapy trials in the United States.

Gene therapy may provide the answers to many health problems. There is a vast amount of research being done at this time. Health care workers must stay informed on new breakthroughs in gene therapy and stay current with the progress being made, which could help individuals with a variety of illnesses.

Medical Terminology

amnio	amnion
-centesis	surgical puncture
amnio/centesis	surgical puncture of the amnion
congenit	dating from birth
-al	pertaining to
congenit/al	pertaining to birth
chromo	colored
-some	body
muta	basic alteration
-tion	process of
chromo/some	
muta/tion	process of basic alteration in the hereditary material
genet	producing protein, i.e., DNA
-ics	pertaining to
genet/ics	pertaining to producing protein (DNA)
hemo	bleeding
-phil	attraction for
-ia	abnormal condition of
hemo/phil/ia	abnormal attraction for bleeding

REVIEW QUESTIONS

Select the letter of the choice that best completes the statement.

1. The branch of science that deals with how human traits are passed down is called:
   a. genetic engineering
   b. biology
   c. genetics
   d. genetic counseling

2. When a change takes place in a gene, what has occurred?
   a. mutation
   b. lethal gene
   c. congenital defect
   d. mutant

3. A deficiency in breaking down fat molecules is characteristic of:
   a. sickle cell
   b. Tay-Sachs
   c. PKU
   d. Down syndrome

4. An extra chromosome can cause a defect known as trisomy 21 or:
   a. Cooley's anemia
   b. Huntington's disease
   c. Down syndrome
   d. PKU

5. A disease that produces thick mucus is called:
   a. PKU
   b. sickle cell
   c. Huntington's disease
   d. cystic fibrosis

APPLYING THEORY TO PRACTICE

1. A friend tells you she has been advised to have an amniocentesis; she is 16 weeks pregnant. The thought of having someone stick a needle in her belly and what may happen to her baby is frightening. Explain the test to her.

2. PKU is a genetic disorder which can be detected in the nursery. Explain the disease and the special dietary restrictions.

3. Sickle cell anemia trait can be diagnosed with a simple blood test. People are afraid to have this test done. List some of the factors which influence people's opinions regarding this test.

4. You are going to participate in a debate on the issue of genetic engineering. One side must present legal, scientific, and moral issues for the limited use of this science; the other side will support unrestricted use of the technology.

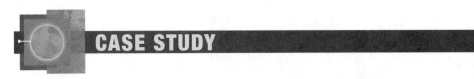

CASE STUDY

A couple comes into the family counseling center and want information on genetic counseling. They are thinking of starting a family but the wife has a family history of Tay-Sach's disease. Kieran is a genetic counselor and will explain the services available at the center. Kieran's discussion will include genetic mutation; tests that may be done during pregnancy and advances which are being made in genetic therapy.

APPENDIX

THE SCIENTIFIC METHOD

The scientific method of inquiry is based on three main concepts: observation, experimentation, and the development of theories or natural laws. The first step in the scientific method is the actual observation and recording of facts. Much of the work of a scientist involves observation and the collection of data. This helps scientists to gain as much information as they can about the anatomy and physiology they are studying and then record that information in an organized way. Observation also involves conducting experiments. Experiments are controlled observations that help to answer questions about what scientists are trying to discover. The next step in the scientific method is the formulation of a theory that might explain how or why the physiology that is being studied is occurring. This is also called a hypothesis, which is an explanation that is supported by a set of facts. This final step in the scientific process is the formulation of a natural law that explains the physiology that is being studied. The formulation of a natural or a physical law helps to explain how certain aspects of anatomy operate and, more importantly, how they can be used to make predictions. Scientists often use observations they have made in the past to make inferences about what might occur in the future. An inference is a prediction or conclusion that is made about a future event based on previous scientific observations. The scientific method is a formal and organized procedure that scientists around the world use to make accurate investigations of anatomy.

SCIENTIFIC EXPERIMENTS

One of the most important aspects of the scientific method is experimentation. An experiment allows scientists to prove or disprove a hypothesis. Experiments are also an important way for students of science to learn about anatomy and gain knowledge by actually practicing science. Conducting experiments also follows an organized pattern, which includes stating the purpose of the experiment, creating a hypothesis, writing out step-by-step procedures, collecting and analyzing data, and formulating a conclusion. All experiments begin by stating the purpose for performing the experiment. The purpose explains exactly what you are trying to determine in your experiment. For example, if you wanted to know at what temperature water boiled, you could determine it by performing a simple experiment. Your purpose is simple: to discover the exact temperature at which water boils.

The next step in experimentation is formulating a hypothesis that might explain your experiment. A hypothesis is an explanation of how or why the phenomenon you are studying is occurring. A hypothesis is usually based on any previous knowledge you have about what you are studying. Using the boiling water example, you may already have an idea at what temperature water boils, so your hypothesis would state this. Or if you have no idea about the boiling temperature of water, you may state in your hypothesis that you believe water always boils at the same temperature, which you are trying to discover.

Writing out the procedures that you took to perform your experiment is another important aspect of experimentation. This allows other scientists or students to understand how the experiment is to be conducted. The procedure is also important because it allows for your experiment to be recreated by other scientists. A procedure is just a step-by-step explanation of what you did to conduct your experiment. It also may include special safety concerns and specific materials or instruments required to conduct your experiment. For example, if you are trying to determine the temperature of boiling water, you must take special precautions to prevent yourself from being burned by the water.

Collecting and recording data from your experiment is the next step in experimentation. Data collection is a precise way of making accurate observations during your experiment. Often experiments are conducted more than once to collect more than one set of data, which allows for more accuracy. For this portion of your experiment, you may choose to record the temperature of the water every 30 seconds until it boils and then repeat that experiment again to gain a more accurate result. You must also consider what units of measurement you will use to record your data. In most scientific experiments the metric system is used, the temperature is often recorded in degrees Celsius. Calculating the results of your experiment involves the analyzation and organization of the data you have collected. Creating a graph or chart to analyze your data often is an effective way to organize your results. A graph is a way to visually display numbers and data that you have collected during an experiment. Graphs are an important tool in the scientific method because they can reveal trends that are occurring in your data.

The final portion of an experiment is stating a conclusion. The conclusion of your experiment should summarize the results of your experiment, which will either support or disprove your hypothesis. If your experiment revealed that the boiling point of water was 100° Celsius, then this should be stated in your conclusion. Carefully conducting an experiment in an organized way ensures that scientific discovery can be well documented and recreated.

LABORATORY SAFETY

Safety should be the number one priority for all individuals working in a laboratory setting. Laboratory hazards may be physical, chemical, or biological.

Physical hazards can be encountered due to equipment and surroundings such as electricity, fire, equipment, and glass. All electrical equipment must be grounded and kept in good working order. Wires should not be frayed or exposed in any way. Electrical circuits should not be overloaded. Electrical equipment must be disconnected when not in use or when being repaired. If open flames are in use, care must be taken to avoid wearing loose clothing. Long hair should also be tied back to avoid coming in contact with the open flame. Flammable chemicals should be stored in a flameproof cabinet. The correct type of fire extinguisher should be readily available and fire blankets should be available in the event that clothing catches fire. Escape routes in the event of a fire should be well-posted and practiced often. Laboratory equipment must only be used as directed by the manufacturer. Only glassware free of chips and cracks should be used. Broken glass should be cleaned up with a dust pan and broom—not bare hands. Glass should be discarded only in containers designated for glass disposal.

Chemicals may be flammable, toxic (poisonous), caustic (causes severe burns), corrosive, carcinogenic (cancer causing), or mutagenic (causing genetic abnormalities). All chemicals must be labeled with hazard information. Material Safety Data Sheets (MSDS) must be available for all chemicals present in a laboratory setting. The MSDS provides information on the hazards of the substance, the personal protective equipment needed when handling the substance, and the body organs that could be affected by exposure to the substance. When working with chemicals, goggles, gloves, an apron, and sometimes a face shield should be worn. Jewelry should not be worn when working in a laboratory. Any chemicals that emit vapors should be used with a fume hood. A safety shower and eye wash should be readily available if chemicals are spilled on the skin or clothing.

Standard precautions are guidelines implemented to protect an individual from biological hazards such as blood and bodily fluids. There should be an exposure control plan in place for any work area where exposure to biological hazards exist.

General principles when working in a laboratory include:

1. No horseplay.
2. No eating, drinking, chewing gum, or applying of cosmetics in the work area.
3. Wear a lab apron or coat with closed toe shoes.
4. Pin up or tie back long hair.
5. Do not wear jewelry.
6. Use gloves when handling chemicals.
7. Clean and disinfect the work area before and after use.
8. Wash hands before and after any procedure.
9. Wear goggles, safety glasses, or a face shield when working with chemicals.
10. Wipe up spills promptly using the appropriate procedure for the type of spill encountered.
11. Use a mask when working with chemicals that give off fumes.
12. Follow manufacturer's instructions for using equipment.
13. Report broken or frayed electrical cords or equipment damage.
14. Do not use bare hands to pick up broken glass.
15. Report accidents immediately.

Environmental Concerns

Environmental concerns are two-fold. Environmental factors can impact the result of experiments and this must be accounted for. Also the environment itself can be impacted by the experiments that are being conducted and should be protected to the best of one's ability.

Temperature, humidity, and atmospheric pressure are just a few of the environmental conditions that can impact the results in experiments. Often it is necessary to control these factors to the best of one's ability while conducting experiments to achieve consistent and accurate results.

People are often concerned with the impact research and experimentation has on the environment. To minimize any adverse impact on the environment all proper safety and disposal measures should be implemented. Chemicals should be stored in proper containers and labeled appropriately. Equipment and tools used should be stored, cleaned, and maintained according to manufacturer's recommendations. All materials used should be disposed of in proper waste containers and removed as appropriate for the type of materials being used.

Use of Resources

Before beginning any lab work, you should gather all the resources you will need to conduct your experiments. Determine the equipment and tools you will need to use for the experiment. Gather all the supplies you will need to use to conduct the experiment. Taking the time to thoroughly think through what you will need and how you will need it will improve the accuracy and efficiency in conducting experiments.

Conservation of Resources

To minimize the resources you will need to conduct experiments, work with a lab partner. This will allow you to share the resources needed. A lab partner will also be able to provide checks and balances to ensure the work is done in an efficient and safe manner. Each pair should have specific roles they are to fulfill when conducting the experiment. All safety measures and proper use of and disposal of resources should be implemented by both partners.

Disposal of Resources

All chemicals should be disposed of according to regulations. Some chemicals can be safely poured down a drain and diluted with adequate amounts of water. However, many chemicals require disposal by specially trained toxic waste personnel.

GLOSSARY

A

abdomen (ab'-do-mun): portion of body lying between thorax and pelvis

abdominal cavity (ab-dom'-in-nul kav'-ih-tee): the area of the body that contains the stomach, liver, gallbladder, pancreas, spleen, small intestine, appendix, and part of the large intestine

abdominal hernia (ab-dom'-i-nul hur'-nee-uh): abnormal protrusion of an organ, or part of an organ, through abdominal wall

abdominopelvic cavity (ab-do'-man-o-pel'-vic kav'-ih-tee): area below diaphragm, with no separation between the abdomen and pelvis

abduction (ab-duck'-shun): movement away from midline or axis of body; opposite of adduction

abscess (ab'-sess): pus-filled cavity

absorption (ub-sorp'-shun): passing of a substance into body fluids and tissues

acetylcholine (as'-e-til-ko-len): chemical released when a nerve impulse is transmitted

acid (as'-id): chemical compound that ionizes to form hydrogen ions (H+) in aqueous solution

acne vulgaris (ak'-ne vul-gayr'-us): chronic disorder of sebaceous gland

acquired immunity (a-kwir'-ed im-yu'-net-e): immunity as a result of exposure to a disease

acquired immunodeficiency syndrome (AIDS) (ah-kwired' im"-yoo-noh-dih-fish'-en-see sin'-drome [aydz]): a fatal disease causing suppression of the immune system

acromegaly (ak'-ro-meg'a-le): excess of growth hormone in adults, overdevelopment of bones of hand, face, feet

action potential (ak'-shan po-ten'-shal): the electric change occurring across the membrane of a nerve or muscle cell during transmission of a nerve impulse

active acquired immunity (ack'-tiv a-kwir'-ed im-yu'-net-e): two types—natural and artificial acquired immunity

active transport (ack'-tiv tranz'-port): process by which solute molecules are transported across a membrane against a concentration gradient, from an area of low concentration to one of high concentration

acute glomerulonephritis (ah-kyoot' glah-mer"-yoo-loh-neh-freye'-tis): inflammation of the glomerulus of the nephron due to bacterial infection

acute kidney failure (ah-kyoot' kid'-nee fail'-yoor): sudden loss of kidney function

Addison's disease (ad'-e-sen di-zez): hypofunction of adrenal gland

adduction (a-duck'-shun): movement of part of body or limb toward the midline of body; opposite of abduction

adenitis (ad'-n-i'-tis): inflammation of a lymph gland

adenoids (ad'-e-noydz): pair of glands composed of lymphoid tissue, found in nasopharynx; also called *pharyngeal tonsils*

adenosine triphosphate (ATP) (a-den'-o-seen try-fos'-fate): chemical compound consisting of one molecule of adenine, one of ribose, and three of phosphoric acid

adequate intake (AI) (a'-deh-quit in'-tayk): the minimum amount of a vitamin or mineral recommended to be taken in

adipose tissue (ad'-i-pose tish'-yoo): fatty or fatlike

adrenal gland (a-dre'-nal gland): endocrine gland that sits on top of kidney; consists of cortex and medulla

adrenalin (ah-dren'-ih-lin): a powerful cardiac stimulant

adrenocorticotropic hormone (ACTH) (ad-ree"-noh-cor"-tih-coh-trop'-ick hor'-mone): a hormone that stimulates the growth and secretion of the adrenal cortex

afferent arteriole (af'-ur-unt ahr-teer'-ee-ole): takes blood from the renal artery to the Bowman's capsule of kidney

afferent neuron (af'-ur-unt new'-ron): a nerve that carries nerve impulses from the periphery to the central nervous system; also known as *sensory neuron*

agent (ay'-jent): entity capable of causing disease

agranulocyte (ay-gran'-yoo-lo-site): nongranular, white blood cell; known as *agranular leukocyte*

airborne transmission (air'-born trans-mish'-un): transfer of an agent to a susceptible host through droplet nuclei or dust particles suspended in the air

albumin (al-bew'-min): plasma protein, maintains osmotic pressure

albuminuria (al-bew'-mi-new'-ree-uh): excess of albumin protein in urine

aldosterone (al-dos'-ta-ron'): hormone secreted by the adrenal cortex, regulates salt and water balance in the kidney

alimentary canal (al"-i-men'-tuh-ree kuh-nal'): entire digestive tube from mouth (ingestion) to anus (excretion)

alkali (al'-kuh-li'): a substance when dissolved in water ionizes into negatively charged hydroxide (OH) ions and positively charged ions of a metal

allergen (al'-er-jen): substance causes an allergic reaction

alopecia (al'-e-pe'-she): loss of hair, baldness

alveolar sacs (al-vee'-oh-lar sacks): air cells found in the lung; also known as alveoli

alveoli (al-vee'-o-li): air cells found in the lung

Alzheimer's disease (alts'-hi'-merz di-zez): progressive disease with degeneration of nerve endings in the cortex of the brain

amblyopia (am'-ble-o'-pe-a): dimness of vision

amenorrhea (a-men"-o-ree'-uh): absence of menstruation

amino acid (a-me'-no as'id): small molecular units that make up protein molecules

amniocentesis (am'ne-o-sen-te'-sis): withdrawal of amniotic fluid for testing

amphiarthrosis (am-phi-är-thro'-sis): partially moveable joint, e.g., symphyis pubis

amylase (am'-e-layz): enzyme that converts starch or glycogen to glucose

amylopsin (am'-e-lop'-sin): pancreatic amylase

anabolism (anab'-o-lizm): building up of complex materials in metabolism

analgesic (an'-el-je'-zik): drug that reduces pain

anaphase (an'-e-fayz'): phase four in mitosis

anaphylactic shock (an-a-fa-lac'-tic shok): or anaphylaxis; severe and sometimes fatal allergic reaction

anaphylaxis (an-ah-fih-lack'-sis): a severe allergic reaction

anatomical position (an-a-tom'-i-kel pō-zish'-un): body standing erect, face forward, arms at side, and palms forward

anatomy (a-nat'-a-me): the study of the structure of an organism

androgen (an'-dro-jen): male hormones

anemia (uh-nee'-mee-uh): blood disorder characterized by reduction in red blood cells or hemoglobin

aneurysm (an'-you-rism): a widening, or sac, formed by dilation of a blood vessel

angina pectoris (anji'-nuh peck'-to-ris): severe chest pain caused by lack of blood supply to heart

angioplasty (an'-je-o-plas-te): balloon surgery to open blocked blood vessels

anorexia nervosa (an"-o-rek'-see-uh nur-vo'-suh): an illness in which a person refuses to eat

antagonist (an-tag'-a-nist): a muscle whose action opposes the action of another muscle

anterior (an-teer'-ee-ur): front or ventral

anterior chamber (an-teer'-ee-ur chame'-bur): space between cornea and iris

anterior nares (an-teer'-ee-or nairz): external portion of the nostril

anterior pituitary lobe (an-teer'-ee-or pih-too'-ih-tair-ee lobe): area of the pituitary gland that is responsible for the secretion of growth hormones

anthrax (an'-thrax): a disease-causing organism that affects the respiratory system

antibody (an'-tih-bod"-ee): substance produced by the body, that inactivates a specific foreign substance which has entered the body

anticoagulant (an"-tih-ko-ag'-yoo-lunt): chemical substance that prevents or slows blood clotting (e.g., heparin)

anticonvulsant (an"-tih-kun-vul'-sunt): therapeutic agent that stops or prevents convulsions

antidiuretic hormone (an"-tih-dye-yoo-ret'-ik hor'-mone): hormone secreted by the posterior pituitary gland, which prevents or suppresses urine excretion (ADH)

antigen (an'-tih-jin): substance stimulating formation of antibodies against itself

antiprothrombin (an"-tih-pro-throm'-bin): chemical substance that directly or indirectly reduces or retards action of prothrombin (such as heparin)

antithromboplastin (an"-tih-throm-bo-plas'-tin): chemical substance inhibiting clot-accelerating effect of thromboplastins

anuria (a-noor'-e-a): absence of urine

anus (ay'-nus): outlet from rectum

anvil (an'-vil): middle ear bone, or ossicle, in a chain of three ossicles of the middle ear

aorta (ay-or'-tuh): largest artery in body, rising from left ventricle of the heart

aortic semilunar valve (ay-or'-tik sem"-ee-loo-nur valv): made up of three half-moon-shaped cups, located between junction of aorta and left ventricle of heart

apex (ay'-peks): top of object; point or extremity of a cone

aphasia (a-fay'-zhuh): loss of ability to speak, may be accompanied by loss of verbal comprehension

aplastic anemia (a-plas'-tik uh-nee'-mee-uh): anemia caused by a suppression of the bone marrow

apnea (ap'-nee-uh): temporary stoppage of breathing movements

aponeurosis (ap"-o-new-ro'-sis): flattened sheet of white, fibrous connective tissue; serves as attachment for flat muscles, or as sheet enclosing/binding muscle groups

appendicitis (a-pen"-di-si'-tis): inflammation of the appendix

appendicular skeleton (ap"-en-dik'-yoo-lur skel'-uh-tun): part of skeleton consisting of pectoral and pelvic girdles, and limbs

aqueous humor (a'-kwe-as hyoo'-mar): watery fluid found in anterior chamber of the eye

arachnoid (uh-rak'-noyd): weblike middle membrane of meninges

areola (a-ree-o'-luh): pigmented ring around nipple; any small space in tissue

areolar tissue (a-ree-o-lar tish'-yoo): a type of connective tissue that surrounds various organs and supports both nerve and blood vessels

arrector pili muscle (ah-reck'-tor pill-eye' muss'-ul): a smooth muscle on the side of each hair follicle; when cold, it stimulates the skin to pucker around the hair

arrhythmia (a-rith'-mee-uh): absence of a normal rhythm in heartbeat

arteriole (ahr-teer'-ee-ole): small branch of artery

arteriosclerosis (ahr-teer"-ee-o-skleh-ro'-sis): hardening of arteries, resulting in thickening of walls and loss of elasticity

artery (ahr'-tur-ee): blood vessel which carries blood away from heart

arthritis (ahr-thry'-tis): inflammation of a joint

articular cartilage (ar-tik'-ye-lar kar'-ta-lij): thin layer of cartilage over the ends of long bones

artificial acquired immunity (ar'-ta-fish'-el a-kwir-ed im-yu-net-e): immunity from injection of vaccine, antigen, or toxoid

artificial insemination (ar'-ta-fish'-el in-sem'-a-na'-shun): procedure in which semen is placed in vagina by means of cannula or syringe

asbestosis (as"-beh-stoh'-sis): a respiratory disease caused by inhaling asbestos fibers

ascending colon (ay-sen'-ding koh'-lun): portion of the colon that travels up the right side of the abdominal cavity

ascites (a-si'-teez): accumulation of fluid in the peritoneal cavity

associative neuron (a-so'-she-a'-tiv noor'-on): carries messages from sensory neuron to motor neuron

asthma (az'-ma): airways obstructed because of inflammatory reaction to a stimulus

astigmatism (a-stig'-ma-tiz'-em): irregular curvature of cornea or lens

atelectasis (a-te-lec'-ta-sis): lungs fail to expand normally

atherosclerosis (ath"-er-o-scle-ro'-sis): hardening of arteries due to deposits of fatlike material in lining of the arteries

athlete's foot (ath'-leets foot): fungal infection of the foot

atlas (at'-lus): first cervical vertebra; articulates with axis and occipital skull bone

atom (at-om): smallest piece of an element

atrioventricular (AV) node (ay"-tree-o-ven-trik'-yoo-lur node): small mass of interwoven conducting tissue

atrioventricular bundle (ay"-tree-oh-ven-trik'-yoo-lar bun'-dl): conducting fibers in the septum; also known as the bundle of His

atrium (ay'-tree-um): upper chamber of heart

atrophy (a'-truh-fee): wasting away of tissue

auricle (aw'-ri-kul): (1) pinna, or ear flap of external ear; (2) atrium of the heart

autoimmune disorder (aw"-toh-ih'-myoon dis-or'-der): a condition that causes destruction of the body's own tissues

autoimmunity (aw"-to-im-yu'-net-e): action of antibodies against one's own body

autonomic nervous system (aw"-tuh-nom'-ik nur'vus sis'-tum): collection of nerves, ganglia, and plexuses through which visceral organs, heart, blood vessels, glands, and smooth (involuntary) muscles receive their innervation

avascular (a-vas'-ku-lar): without blood vessels

axial skeleton (ack'see-ul skel'-e-tun): skeleton of head and trunk

axilla (ak-sil'-uh): armpit

axillary node (ack'-sih-lair-ee node): lymph nodes found under the arms and near the breast

axis (ack'-sis): (1) imaginary line passing through center of the body; (2) second cervical vertebra

axon (acks'-on): nerve cell structure which carries impulses away from cell body to dendrites

B

bacteria (bak-teer"-ee-ah): an agent capable of causing disease or infection

bactericidal (bak-teer"-i-sigh'-dul): bacterial destruction

ball-and-socket joint (bol and sok'-it joynt): diarthroses joint allows the greatest freedom of movement

balloon surgery (ball-oon' sur'-jer-ee): *see* angioplasty

Bartholin's gland (bar-thol'-inz gland): mucous glands at opening of vagina

basal cell carcinoma (bay'-sal sel kahr"-si-noh'-muh): most common and least malignant type of skin cancer

basal metabolic rate (BMR) (bay'-sal met-ah-bol'-ick rate): the measure of the total energy utilized by the body to maintain the body processes necessary for life

base (bays): (1) lowest part of a body; (2) main ingredient of a substance; (3) chemical compound yielding hydroxyl ions (OH^-) in an aqueous solution which will react with acid to form a salt and water

basophil (bay'-suh-fil): leukocyte cell, substance, or tissue that shows an attraction for basic dyes

Bell's palsy (Belz pol'-zee): disorder that affects the facial nerve

belly (bel'-ee): the central part of a muscle

benign prostatic hypertrophy (BPH) (bih'-nine pross'-sta-tic high"-per-troh'-fee): an enlarged prostate

benign (be-nine'): nonmalignant

biceps (bye'-seps): muscle on front part of upper arm

bicuspid (bye-kus'-pid): having two cusps

bicuspid (mitral) valve (bye-kus'-pid [my'-trul] valv): atrioventricular valve of left side of heart

bile (biyl): substance produced by liver, emulsifies fat

bilirubin (bil'-ee-roo'-bin): one of two pigments that determines the color of bile; reddish in color

biochemistry (bye-o-kem'-is-tree): study of chemical reactions of living things

biological agent (beye-oh-lodge'-ih-kahl ay'-jent): living organism that invades a host, causing disease

biology (bye-ol'-ah-jee): the study of all forms of life

biopsy (bye'-op-see): excision of a piece of tissue from a living body for diagnostic study

blind spot (blind' spot'): *see* optic disc

blood-brain barrier (blud brayn bar'-ee-ur): substance cannot penetrate the brain tissue

B-lymphocyte (bee lim'-foh-site): cells synthesized in the bone marrow

body mass index (BMI) (bah'-dee mass in'-dex): a measurement of the amount of body fat in an individual

boil (boyl): bacterial infection of sebaceous gland

bolus (boh'-lus): rounded mass; food prepared by mouth for swallowing

Bowman's capsule (boh-manz kap'-sel): double-walled capsule around the glomerulus of nephron

brachial artery (bray"-kee-ul ar'-ter-ee): artery located at the crook of the elbow along the inner biceps muscle

bradycardia (brad"-ee-cahr'-dee-uh): abnormally slow heartbeat, less than 60 beats per minute

brainstem (brayn'-stem): portion of brain other than cerebral hemispheres and cerebellum

brain tumor (brayn too'-mer): area of abnormal cell growth within the brain

breast (brest): mammary gland in front of the chest, secretes milk after childbirth

bronchiectasis (bran"-kee-ek'-tah-sis): chronic dilatation of the bronchial tubes

bronchiole (bran'-kee-ole): one of small subdivisions of a bronchus

bronchitis (bran-kiy'-tis): inflammation of the bronchial tubes

bronchoscopy (bran-kas'-koh-pee): tubular instrument with light to inspect the interior of the bronchial tubes

bronchus (bran'-kus): one of two primary branches of trachea

buccal cavity (buk'-ul kav'-i-tee): mouth cavity bounded by the inner surface of the cheek

buffer (buf'-er): a compound that maintains the chemical balance in a living organism

bulbourethral gland (bul"-bo-yoo-re'-thral gland): located on either side of urethra in male, adds alkaline substance to semen

bulimia (bul-ee'-mee-a): episodic binge eating

bundle of His (bun'-dl of hiz): *see* atrioventricular bundle

burn (burn): a result of destruction of the skin by fire, boiling water, steam, sun, chemicals or electricity, classified as: first degree, only epidermal layer affected; second degree, epidermis and some dermis is affected, third degree, complete destruction of epidermis, dermis and subcutaneous layers

bursa sacs (bur'-suh sax): small sac interposed between parts that move on one another

bursitis (bur-sigh'-tis): inflammation of a bursa

C

calcaneus (kal-kay'-nee-us): heel bone

calcify (kal'-si-fiy): to deposit mineral salts

calcitonin (kal-si-to'-nin): hormone secreted by thyroid gland that controls calcium ion concentration in body

calorie (kal'-or-ee): a unit that measures the amount of energy

calyx (kay'-liks): cup-shaped part of the renal pelvis

cancer (kan'-sir): a malignant tumor

cancer of the larynx (kan'-sir of the lar'-inks): abnormal cell growth in the larynx

cancer of the lungs (kan'-sir of the lungs): abnormal cell growth in the lungs

canine (kay'-nine): sharp teeth of mammals, between incisors and premolars

capillary (kap'-i-lair-ee): microscopic blood vessel which connects arterioles with venules

carbohydrate (kar"-boh-high'-drayt): an organic compound of carbon, hydrogen, and oxygen as sugar or starch

carbon monoxide (CO) poisoning (kar'-bun mun-ock'-side poy'-zun-ing): a condition in which an odorless gas combines rapidly with hemoglobin and crowds out oxygen

cardiac (kahr'-dee-ak): relating to the heart

cardiac arrest (kahr'-dee-ak uh-rest'): syndrome resulting from failure of heart as a pump

cardiac catheterization (kahr'-dee-ak cath"-eh-ter-ih-zay'-shun): a diagnostic test in which a catheter is inserted into the femoral artery or vein and fed up into the heart

cardiac muscle (kahr'-dee-ak mus'-ul): muscle of the heart

cardiac output (kahr'-dee-ak owt'-put): the total volume of blood ejected from the heart per minute

cardiac sphincter (kahr'-dee-ak sfink'-tur): circular muscle fibers around cardiac end of esophagus

cardiac stents (kahr'-dee-ak stents): device inserted into an artery to open a clog or plaque buildup

cardiopulmonary circulation (kahr"-dee-oh-pull'-mon-air-ee sir"-cue-lay'-shun): the system of carrying blood from the heart to the lungs and back

cardiopulmonary resuscitation (CPR) (kahr"-dee-oh-puhl'-mun-nair-ee ree-sus"-i-tay'-shun): prevention of asphyxial death by artificial respiration

cardiotonic (kar"-dee-oh-ton'-ic): drug to slow and strengthen the heart

caries (kair'-eez): decay of tooth or bone

carotid (kah-ro'-tid): artery supplies blood to the neck and head

carpal (kahr'-pul): bones of the wrist

carpal tunnel syndrome (kahr'-pul tun'-ul sin'-drome): a condition that affects the median nerve and the flexor tendons that attach to the bones of the wrist

cartilage (kahr'-ti-lidj): white, semiopaque, nonvascular connective tissue

catabolism (ca-tab'-oh-lizm): the breaking down and changing of complex materials with the release of energy—process in metabolism

cataract (kat'-uh-rakt): condition in which the eye lens becomes opaque

caudal (kod'-el): refers to direction, near the tail end of the body

cecum (see'-kum): pouch at the proximal end of the large intestine

cell (sel): basic unit of structure and function of all living things

cell membrane (sel mem'-brayn): structure which encloses the cell

cellular respiration (sel'-yu-lar res'-pa-ra'-shun) or oxidation: use of oxygen to release energy from the cell

central nervous system (sen'-trall nur'-vus sis'-tem): consists of the structures of the brain and spinal cord

centrioles (sen'-tree-olz): two cylindrical organelles found near the nucleus in a tiny body called the centrosome; they are perpendicular to each other

centrosome (sen'-tro-sohm): tiny area near the nucleus of an animal cell; it contains two cylindrical structures called centrioles

cerebellum (ser-eh-bell'-um): structure of the brain behind the pons and below the cerebrum

cerebral aqueduct (ser-ee'-bral ack'-wheh-dukt): a narrow canal connecting the third and fourth ventricles of the brain

cerebral cortex (ser-ee'-bral cor'-tex): a layer of gray matter covering the upper and lower surfaces of the cerebrum

cerebral hemorrhage (ser-ee'-bral hem'-ar-ij): bleeding from blood vessels in brain

cerebral palsy (ser-ee'-bral pall'-zee): a disturbance in voluntary muscle action due to brain damage

cerebral vascular accident (CVA) (ser'-ee-bral vas'-cular ak'-su-dent) or stroke: sudden interruption of blood flow to brain

cerebral ventricles (ser-ee'-bral ven'-trick-uls): four lined cavities within the brain filled with cerebrospinal fluid

cerebrospinal fluid (ser"-ee-broh-speye'-nal floo'-id): a substance that forms within the four brain ventricles from the blood vessels of the choroid plexus; this serves as a shock absorber protecting the brain and spinal cord

cerebrum (ser'-ee-brum): the largest part of the brain

cerumen (see-roo'-men): ear wax

cervical vertebrae (sur'-vi-kul vur'-tuh-bray): first seven bones of the spinal column

cervix (sur'-viks): narrow end of the uterus

chemical agent (kem'-ih-kul ay'-jent): substance that interacts with a host, causing disease

chemistry (kem'-is-tree): study of structure of matter, composition of substances, their properties, and their chemical reactions

chlamydia (klah-mid'-ee-uh): a sexually transmitted disease caused by the *Chalmydia trachomatis* organism

cholecystitis (kol"-ah-sis-ti'-tis): inflammation of the gallbladder

cholesterol (koh-les'-tur-ol): a steroid normally synthesized in the liver and also ingested in egg yolks, animal fats, and tissues

chorionic villi sampling (kor"-ee-on'-ick vill'-eye sam'-pling): a test done early in pregnancy to detect genetic problems

choroid coat (koh'-royd coht): the middle layer of the eye

choroid plexus (koh'-royd plek'-sis): the network of blood vessels of the pia mater

chromatid (kroh'-muh-tid): each strand of a replicable chromosome

chromatin (kroh'-mah-ten): DNA and protein material in a loose and diffuse state; during mitosis chromatin condenses to form the chromosomes

chromosomal mutation (kroh"-muh-soh"-mul mew-tay'-shun): a mutation that involves change in the number of chromosomes in the organism's nucleus or a change in the structure of a whole chromosome

chromosome (kroh'-muh-sohm): nuclear material that determines hereditary characteristics

chronic glomerulonephritis (kron'-ik glah-mer"-yoo-loh-neh-freye'-tis): diminished function of the kidney due to damage to the filtration membrane

chronic obstructive pulmonary disease (COPD) (kron'-ik ub-struk'-tiv pul'-mun-ar-ee di-zeez'): chronic lung condition such as emphysema or bronchitis

chronic renal failure (kron'-ik ree'-nal fail'-yor): gradual loss of function of the nephrons

chyme (kime): food which has undergone gastric digestion

cicatrix (sik'-a-triks): scar tissue

cilia (sil'-ee-uh): tiny lashlike processes of protoplasm

ciliary body (sil'-ee-air"-ee bah'-dee): ligaments that suspend the eye

circumcision (sur"-kum-si'-shun): removal of the foreskin of the penis

circumduction (sur"-kum-duk'-shun): circular movement at a joint

cirrhosis (sa-ro'-sis): chronic, progressive inflammatory disease of the liver characterized by the formation of fibrous connective tissue

claudication (klo"-di-kay'-shun): pain in legs or buttocks when walking

clavicle (kla'-vi-kul): collar bone

cleansing (clen'-zing'): removal of soil or organic material from instruments and equipment used in providing client care

clean wound (kleen woond): a wound in which infection is not present

clitoris (kli-tor'-is): small structure over female urethra; has many nerve endings

cloning (kloh'-ning): duplication of biological material

clotting time (clot'-ing time): the time it takes for blood to clot

coagulation (ko-ag"-yu-lay'-shun): process of blood clotting

coccyx (kok'-siks): tailbone

cochlea (kock'-lee-uh): spiral cavity of the internal ear containing the organ of Corti

cochlear duct (kock'-lee-ur dukt): an endolymph-filled triangular canal containing the spiral organ of Corti

coenzyme (coh-en'-zime): a nonprotein part

coitus (ko-oi'-tus): act of intercourse

collagen (kol'-uh-jen): fibrous protein occurring in bone and cartilage

collecting tubule (ko-lek'-ting too'-byool): structure in nephron which collects urine from distal convoluted tubule

colon (ko'-lun): known as the large intestine about 5 feet in length and 2 inches in diameter; divided into ascending, transverse, descending, and sigmoid colon

colon cancer (ko'-lun kan'-sir): abnormal cell growth in the colon

colostomy (ko-los'-tah-mee): artificial opening from the colon onto the surface of the skin

common bile duct (kah'-mun biyl dukt): formed by the union of the hepatic duct and cystic duct which brings bile to the duodenum

common carotid artery (kah'-mun cah-rot'-id ar'-ter-ee): artery found in the neck

common cold (kom'-mon cold): highly contagious virus

comparative anatomy (kum-'par-ah-tiv ah-nat'-oh-mee): the study of structures and functions of the human body in comparison with the structures and functions of other animal species

complete proteins (kum-pleet' pro'-teenz): proteins that contain all the essential amino acids; they enable an animal to grow and carry on fundamental life activities

compound (kom'-pownd): elements combined in definite proportion by weight to form new substance

compromised host (kom'-proh-mized host): person whose normal defense mechanisms are impaired and who is therefore susceptible to infection

conduction defect (kon-duk'-shun de'-fekt): a defect in the electrical impulse system of the heart muscle

cones (cohnz): structures of the eye responsible for colored vision

congenital disorder (kun-jen'-i-tul dis'-or-der): present at birth

congenital heart defect (kun-jen'-i-tul hart dee'-fect): a malformation of the heart during fetal development

congestive heart failure (kon-jes'-tive hart fayl'-yer): heart failure with edema of lower extremities

conjunctivitis (kon-junk"-tih-veye'-tis): an inflammation of the conjunctival membranes in the front of the eye

connective tissue (ka-nek'-tiv tish'-yoo): cells whose intercellular secretions (matrix) support and connect the organs and tissues of the body

constipation (kon"-stih-pay'-shun): difficulty or lack of defecation

contact transmission (kon'-tact trans-mish'-un): physical transfer of an agent from an infected person to a host through direct contact with that person, indirect contact with an infected person through a fomite, or close contact with contaminated secretions

contractibility (kon-track"-tih-bill'-ih-tee): the ability to shorten and reduce the distance between the parts

convalescent stage (kon"-vah-less'-ent stayj): time period in which acute symptoms of an infection begin to disappear until the client returns to the previous state of health

Cooley's anemia (koo'-leez a-nee'-mee-uh), or thallesemia minor: anemia caused by defect in hemoglobin formation

cornea (kor'-nee-uh): a circular area in the very front of the sclerotic coat

corona radiata (kor-oh'-nah ra-dee-ay'-tah): layer of epithelial cells around ova

coronal plane (kor'-en-l plane): frontal plane at a right angle to the sagittal plane, divides the body into anterior and posterior

coronary (kor'-o-nair"-ee): referring to the blood vessels of the heart

coronary artery (kor'-o-nair"-ee ar'-ter-ee): the first branch of the aorta

coronary artery disease (CAD) (kor'-o-nair"-ee ar'-ter-ee dih-seez'): a condition in which the arteries are narrowed, affecting the supply of oxygen and nutrients supplied to heart muscle

coronary bypass (kor'-o-nair"-ee biy'-pas): a shunt to go around area of blockage in the coronary arteries, to provide blood supply to myocardium

coronary circulation (kor'-o-nair"-ee sur"-kyu-la'-shun): brings blood from aorta to myocardium and back to right atrium

coronary sinus (kor'-o-nair"-ee siy'-nus): pocket in posterior of right atrium into which the coronary vein empties

corpus callosum (kor'-pus cal-oh'-sum): a wide band of axonal fibers that holds together the middle region of the two brain hemispheres

corpus luteum (kor'-pus lut'-ee-um): yellow body formed from ruptured graafian follicle and produces progesterone

cortex (kor'-teks): outer part of an internal organ

coughing (kof'-ing): deep breath followed by forceful exhalation from mouth

Cowper's gland (cow'-purz gland): see bulbourethral gland

cranial (kray'-nee-al): refers to the brain or direction toward the head of the body

cranial cavity (kray'-nee-al kav'-ih-tee): area of the body containing the brain

cranial nerves (kray'-nee-al nurvz): twelve pairs of nerves that begin in the brain and transmit messages to various parts of the face and head to stimulate various functions

cretinism (kree'-tin-izm): congenital and chronic condition due to the lack of thyroid hormone

crosseye (cross'-eye): *see* strabismus

crown (krown): pertains to part of tooth that is visible

cryosurgery (cry'-oh-sir-jer-ee): the destruction of tissue by freezing, using liquid nitrogen

cryptorchidism (krip-tor-kih'-dizm): failure of testes to descend into the scrotal sac

Cushing's syndrome (koosh'-ings sin'-drome): disorder of hyperfunction of adrenal cortex

cutaneous (kew-tay'-nee-us): pertaining to the skin

cyanosis (si"-uh-noh'-sis): bluish color of the skin due to insufficient oxygen in the blood

cystic duct (sis'-tik dukt): duct from gallbladder to common bile duct

cystic fibrosis (sis'-tik feye-broh'-sis): a disease of the exocrine gland

cystitis (sis-ti'-tis): inflammation of the mucous membrane of the urinary bladder

cytology (sigh'-tol'-uh-jee): study of cells

cytoplasm (sigh'-toh-plazm): protoplasm of the cell body, excluding the nucleus

cytoskeleton (sigh'-to-skel'-ah-tin): internal framework of the cell consisting of microtubules, intermediate filaments, and microfilaments

D

deciduous (de-sid'-yoo-us): temporary teeth usually lost by 6 years of age

decubitus ulcer (dee-kyoo'-bih-tus ul'-sir): a deterioration of the skin due to constant pressure on the area

deep (deep): term used to describe damage to an organ within the body

defecation (def'"-eh-kay'-shun): elimination of waste material from the rectum

defibrillator (de-fib'-rul-ay-tor): an electrical device used to discharge an electrical current to shock the pacemaker of the heart back to a normal rhythm

deltoid (del'-toyd): triangular-shaped muscle which covers the shoulder prominence; used for intramuscular injections in adults

dementia (de-men'-sha): loss in at least two areas of complex behavior

dendrite (den'-drite): nerve cell process that carries nervous impulses toward the cell body

dentin (den'-tin): main part of the tooth located under the enamel

deoxygenate (dee-ock'-si-jen-ate): process of removing oxygen from a compound

deoxyribonucleic acid (DNA) (dee-ok"-see-ri-boh-nu-klay'-ik as-id): a nucleic acid containing the elements of carbon, hydrogen, oxygen, nitrogen, and phosphorous; genetic material

dermatitis (dur"-muh-tiy'-tus): inflammation of the skin

dermatology (dur"-mah-tol'-ah-jee): study of the physiology and pathology of the skin

dermis (dur'-mis): true skin; lying immediately beneath the epidermis

descending colon (dee'-send-ing koh'-lun): portion of the colon that travels down from the splenic flexure on the left side of the abdomen

detached retina (dee'-tachd ret'-ih-nah): the vitreous fluid contracts as it ages, pulling on the retina and causing a tear

developmental anatomy (dee'-vell-op-men"-tl ah-nat'-oh-mee): study of the growth and development of an organism during its lifetime

deviated nasal septum (dee'-vee-ay-ted nay'-zl sep'-tum): a condition in which there is a bend in the cartilage structure of the septum

diabetes insipidus (dye"-a-bee-teez in-sip'-ah-dus): decrease of ADH of pituitary causing excessive loss of water

diabetes mellitus (dye"-a-bee-teez ma-liy'-tus): pancreas is unable to produce insulin or is unable to produce enough insulin for the cells to use glucose

dialysis (dye-al'-i-sis): the separation of smaller molecules from larger molecules in a solution by selective diffusion through a semipermeable membrane

dialyzer (dye'-al-i-zer): a device to perform dialysis; a kidney machine

diapedesis (dye"-ih-peh'-dee'-sis): passage of blood cells through unruptured vessel wall into tissues

diaphysis (dye-af'-i-sis): shaft of long bone

diarrhea (dye"-ah-ree'-uh): excessive elimination of watery feces

diarthrosis (dye-ar-throh'-sis): moveable joints, e.g., elbow, knee

diastole (dye-as'-tuh-lee): dilation state of the heart; the rest between systoles

diastolic blood pressure (deye-ah-stoll'-ick blud preh'-shur): pressure measured when the ventricles are relaxed

diencephalon (dye"-en-sef'-ah-lon): posterior part of the brain; contains the thalamus, hypothalamus, and pituitary gland

diffusion (dif-yu'-szen): molecules move from higher concentration to lower concentration

digestion (dye-jes'-chun): the complex process of the breaking down of food to be utilized by the body

dilator muscle (dye'-la-tor mus'-ul): a muscle that opens or closes an orifice

diphtheria (dif-theer'-i-uh): infectious disease of respiratory system; rarely seen because of DPT vaccine

diplopia (di-ploh'-pee-uh): double vision

disaccharide (dye-sak'-a-ride): double sugar

disinfection (dis-in-feck'-shun): elimination of pathogens, with the exception of spores, from inanimate objects

dislocation (dis"-loh-kay'-shun): displacement of one or more bones of a joint or organ from original position

distal (dis'-tul): farthest from point of origin of a structure; opposite of proximal

distal convoluted tubule (dis'-tall con-voh-loo'-ted too'-byool): tubular process that ascends to the cortex from the loop of Henle

diuretic (dye-yoo-re'-tik): drug to reduce the amount of fluid in the body

diverticulitis (dye-vur-tik"-yoo-leye'-tis): inflammation of the wall of the colon

diverticulosis (dye-vur-tik"-yul-o'-sis): numerous diverticula in the colon

dorsal (dor'-sul): pertaining to the back

dorsal cavity (dor'-sul kav'-eh-tee): posterior cavity of the body that houses the brain and spinal column

dorsalis pedis artery (dor-sal'-is pee'-dis ar'-ter-ee): artery located at the ankle joint

Down syndrome (down sin'-drome): a disorder characterized by the presence of an extra chromosome; also known as trisomy 21

Duchenne's muscular dystrophy (doo-shenz' mus'-kyoo-lar dis'-troh-fee): a disorder in which muscles suffer from a loss of protein and the contractile fibers are replaced with fat and connective tissue, rendering skeletal muscle useless

ductus arteriosus (duk'-tus ar-teer'-ee-oh-sus): fetal structure which permits blood to flow from pulmonary artery to aorta

ductus deferens or **vas deferens** (duk'-tus def'-uh-renz or vas def'-uh-renz): the part of the duct system of the testes which runs from the epididymis to the ejaculatory duct

duodenum (dew"-o-dee'-num): first part of small intestine, beginning at pylorus

dura mater (dew'-ruh may'-tur): fibrous membrane forming outermost covering of brain and spinal cord

dwarfism (dworf'-izm): caused by hypofunction of growth hormone; growth of long bone is decreased

dysmenorrhea (dis-men"-o-ree'-uh): difficult or painful menstruation

dysphasia (dis-fa'-zya): impairment of speech and verbal comprehension

dyspnea (disp-nee'-uh): labored breathing or difficult breathing

dysuria (dis-yoor'-ee-a): painful urination

E

ectopic (ek-top'-ik): in an abnormal position; said of an extrauterine pregnancy or cardiac beats

ectopic pregnancy (eck-top'-ik preg'-nan-see): implantation of a fertilized egg outside of the uterus

eczema (ek'-se-mah): acute or chronic noncontagious inflammation of the skin

edema (eh-dee'-muh): excessive fluid in tissues

effector (ee-feck'-tor): the responding organs

efferent arteriole (ef'-er-ant ar-teer'-ee-ul): carries blood from glomerulus

efferent neuron *see* motor neuron

ejaculatory ducts (e-jak'-yoo-luh-tor"-ee dukts): short and narrow ducts that begin where the ductus deferens and the seminal duct join

elasticity (e-las'-tis-i-tee): capable of returning to original form after being compressed or stretched

elastin (ee'-las-tin): elasticlike fibers found in connective tissue

electrocardiogram (ECG or EKG) (e-lek"-tro-kar'-dee-o-gram): device used to measure the electric conduction system of the heart

electrolytes (e-lek'-tro-lights): electrically charged particles that help determine fluid and acid-base balance

electromyograph (EMG) (e-lek"-troh-miy'-oh-graf): device used to measure electrical muscle activity

element (el'-e-ment): made up of like atoms; substance that can neither be created nor destroyed

embolism (em'-bo-lizm): obstruction of a blood vessel by a circulating blood clot, fat globule, air bubble, or piece of tissue

embryo (em'-bree-oh): the human young up to the first 3 months after conception; the young of any organism in early development stage

embryology (em-bree-ol'-u-jee): study of the formation of an organism from fertilized egg to birth

emphysema (em-fi-see'-muh): lung disorder in which inspired air becomes trapped and is difficult to expire

enamel (e-nam'-ul): hard calcium substance which covers the teeth

encephalitis (en-sef-u-liy'-tis): inflammation of the brain

endocarditis (en"-doh-car-deye'-tis): an inflammation of the membrane that lines the heart and covers the valves

endocardium (en"-do-kahr'-dee-um): membrane lining interior of heart

endocrine gland (en'-doh-krihn gland): organized groups of tissues that use materials from blood and lymph to make new compounds called hormones

endocrinology (en"-doh-krah-nol'-u-jee): study of the physiology and pathology of the hormonal system

endometriosis (en"-doh-mee-tree-o'-sis): the presence of endometrium which is normally confined to the uterine cavity in other areas of the pelvic cavity

endometrium (en"-doh-mee-tree-um): mucous membrane lining uterus

endoplasmic reticulum (en-do-plas'-mic re-tik'-u-lum): transport system of the cell; can be smooth or rough

endosteum (en-dos'-tee-um): lining of the medullary cavity in the long bone

energy (en'-er-jee): ability to do work

enteritis (en-ter-i'-tis): inflammation of the small intestine

enzyme (en'-zime): organic catalyst that initiates and accelerates a chemical reaction

eosinophil (ee"-o-sin'-uh-fil): white blood cell whose granules stain red with eosin or other acid dyes

epidermis (ep"-i-dur'-mis): outermost layer of skin

epididymis (ep"-i-did'-i-mis): portion of the seminal duct lying posterior to the testes; connected by the efferent ductulis of each testis

epididymitis (ep"-i-did'-i-miy-tis): inflammation of epididymis

epigastric (ep-i-gas'-trik) upper region of the abdominal cavity, located just below the sternum

epiglottis (ep-i-glot'-is): elastic cartilage which prevents food from entering the trachea

epilepsy (ep-ul-ep'-see): seizure disorder

epinephrine (ep"-i-nef'-rin): adrenalin; secretion of the adrenal medulla, which prepares the body for energetic action

epiphysis (ee-pif'-ah-sis): the end of the long bone

episiotomy (e-peez-e-ot'-um-ee): a surgical incision into the perineum

epithelial tissue (e-pi-thee'-lee-al tish'-yoo): protects the body by covering external and internal surfaces

equilibrium (ee-kwuh-lib'-ree-um): a state of balance

ergonomics (er-ga-nom'-iks): the application of biology and engineering to the relationship between the worker and their environment; also called biotechnology

erythroblastosis fetalis (e-rith"-ra-blast-o'-sus fe-tal'-es): hemolytic disease of the newborn

erythrocyte (e-rith'-ro-sight): red blood cell

erythropoiesis (e-rith"-ro-poy-ee'-sis): formation or development of red blood cells

esophagus (e-sof'-uh-gus): a muscular tube; takes food from pharynx to the stomach

essential amino acids (e-sen'-chul a'-mee'-noh as'-ids): amino acids that are necessary for normal growth and development and are not made in the human body

estrogen (es'-tra-jen): secretion of the ovary, female hormone

ethmoid (eth'-moyd): bone of the cranium located between the eyes

eupnea (yoop'-nee-uh): normal or easy breathing with usual quiet inhalations and exhalations

eustachian tube (yoo-sta'-shen tube): passageway from throat to middle ear, equalizes pressure

excitability (ek-sih'-tah-bil'-eh-tee): ability to respond to stimuli

exocrine gland (ecks'-oh-krihn gland): secretions from these glands must go through a duct

exophthalmos (ek"-sof-thal'-mus): abnormal protrusion of the eyes

expiration (ek"-spir-ay'-shun): act of breathing forth or expelling air from lungs

expiratory reserve volume (ERV) (eks-peye'-rah-tor"-ee ree-serve' vol'-yoom): amount of air you can force a person to exhale over and above the tidal volume

extensibility (ex-tense'-a-bill"-ih-tee): the ability to lengthen (stretch) and increase the distance between two parts

extension (ek-sten'-shun): act of increasing the angle between two bones

external (ek-ster'-nul): superficial at or near the surface of the skin

external respiration (ek-ster'-nul res-pih-ray'-shun): breathing; act of inspiration and expiration

extracellular fluid (ek-stra-sel'-u-lar floo'-id): fluid outside the cell

extracorporeal shockwave lithotripsy (ESWL): (ek-stra-kor"-por-ee-al shock'-wave lith-o-trip'-see): a procedure used to reduce kidney stones to sand to enable them to pass through the urinary tract

extrinsic muscle (ecks-trin'-sic muss'-ul): muscles responsible for moving the eye within the orbital socket

F

fallopian tube (fa-lo'-pee-un tewb): uterine tube or oviduct which carries egg from ovary to uterus

farsightedness (far'-sigh-ted-ness): *see* hyperopia

fasciae (fay'-shuh): band or sheet of fibrous membranes covering or binding and supporting muscles

fat (fat): sometimes called triglyceride; organic compound of carbon, hydrogen, and oxygen; made of glycerol and fatty acids

feces (fee'-seez): waste material from the digestive system

femoral artery (fem'-or-al ar'-ter-ee): artery located in the groin area

femoral nerve (fem'-or-al nurv): found in the lumbar plexus; it stimulates the hip and leg

femur (fee'-mur): thighbone

fertilization (fur-til-ah-zay'-shun): the process of the union of the egg and sperm

fetal circulation (fet'-ul ser-kyul-a'-shun): brings blood to the fetus

fetus (fee'-tus): the human young from the third month of the intrauterine period until birth

fiber (fiy'-ber): compound found in plant foods

fibrillation (fi-bre-lay'-shun): heart muscle fibers contract at random without coordination

fibrin (fih'-brin): an insoluble protein necessary for the clotting of blood

fibrinogen (fih'-brin'-o-jen): a protein which is converted into fibrin by the action of thrombin

fibroid tumor (fye'-broyd too'-mer): a benign tumor of smooth muscle especially in the uterus

fibromyalgia (fi-broh-mi-al'-gee-uh): chronic muscle pain

fibula (fib'-yoo-luh): slender bone at outer edge of the lower leg

filtrate (fill'-trayt): plasmalike fluid filtered from the blood in the glomerulus into the Bowman's capsule

filtration (fil-tray'-shun): movement of water and particles across a semipermeable membrane by a mechanical force such as blood pressure

fimbrae (fim'-bray): fringelike projections that fall over the ovary

first degree burn *see* burns

fissures (fish'-urz): the deep furrows within the brain matter

fistula (fis'-choo-luh): an abnormal duct from an abscess, cavity, or hollow organ to the body surface or to another hollow organ

flatfeet (flat-feet): weakening of the leg muscles that support the arch of the foot; also called talipes

flatulence (flach'-uh-lenz): the presence of excessive gas in the digestive tract

flexion (fleks'-ee-on): the act of bending a limb or decreasing the angle between two bones

flora (floor'-ah): microorganisms that occur or have adapted to live in a specific environment

follicle-stimulating hormone (FSH) (fol'-i-kul stim'-yoo-lay-ting hor'-mone): an adenohypophyseal hormone which stimulates follicular growth in the ovary

fomite (foh'-mih-tee): objects contaminated with an infectious agent

fontanel (fon"-tuh-nel'): unossified areas in the infant skull; soft spot

foramen (fo-ray'-men): an opening in a bone

foramen ovale (fo-ray'-men o-val'): an opening in the septum between the right and left atrium of the fetus

foreskin (for'-skin): loose-fitting skin around the end of the penis

fourth ventricle (forth ven'-trick-ul): a structure of the brain situated below the third ventricle, in front of the cerebellum, and behind the pons and medulla oblongata

fovea centralis (foh'-vee-ah cen-tral'-is): structure of the eye that contains the cones for color vision

fracture (frak'-chur): a break in a bone

frontal (frunt'-el): pertaining to the forehead

frontal lobe (frunt'-el lobe): in cerebral cortex, controls the motor function

functional residual capacity (funk'-shun-al rih-zid'-u-al cah-pa'-sih-tee): the sum of the expiratory reserve volume plus the residual volume

fundus (fun'-dus): part farthest from opening of an organ

fungi (fun'-guy): grow in single cells or in colonies

G

gallbladder (gol'-blad-er): a small pear-shaped organ under the right lobe of the liver; it stores bile

gallstones (gol'-stonz): crystallized cholesterol which forms in the gallbladder

gamete (gam'-eet): a mature reproductive cell

gamma globulin (gam'-uh glob'-ye-lin): fractionated part of globulin used to treat infectious diseases

ganglion (gang'-glee-un): a mass of nerve cell bodies outside the central nervous system

gangrene (gang-green'): death of body tissue due to insufficient blood supply

gastric (gas'-trik): pertaining to the stomach

gastric glands (gas'-trik glands): glands lining stomach

gastric mucosa (gas'-trik myoo-coh'-sah): lines the stomach

gastritis (gas-tri'-tis): inflammation of the stomach

gastroenteritis (gas-troh-en"-tur-i'-tis): inflammation of stomach and small intestines

gastroesophageal reflux disease (GERD) (gas-tro-ee-sof'-u-jeel re'-fluks dis-eez'): stomach contents flow back into the esophagus

gene (jene): part of the chromosome that transmits a specific hereditary trait

gene mutation (jene myoo-tay'-shun): production of a new or altered gene

genetic counseling (jeh-neh'-tick cown'-sel-ing): discussions about the possibility of genetic disorders with prospective parents

genetic disorder (jeh-neh'-tick dis-or'-der): a disorder caused by variation in the genetic pattern

genetic engineering (jeh-neh'-tick en-jih-neer'-ing): the ability to snip, rearrange, edit, or program DNA

genetics (je-net'-iks): the branch of biology that studies the science of heredity and the difference and similarities between parents and offspring

genital herpes (jen'-i-tul hur'-peez): a sexually transmitted recurrent disease caused by a virus

genital warts (jen'-i-tul wortz): or human papillomavirus; sexually transmitted disease

genitals (jen-i-tuls): reproductive organs, also called genitalia

germ cell (jerm cell): *see* gamete

gestation (jes-tay'-shun): development period of the human young from conception to birth

gigantism (ji-gan'-tizm): hypersecretion of the growth hormone, overgrowth of long bones

gingiva (jin'-jeh-vae): gums

glans penis (glanz pe'-nis): the head or tip of the penis

glaucoma (gloh-koh'-muh): increase in interocular eye pressure

gliding joint (glid'-ing joynt): the nearly flat surfaces of the bone glide across each other, e.g., vertebra

globin (glo'-bin): protein molecule of hemoglobin

globulin (glob'-yeh-len): plasma protein made in liver, helps in synthesis of antibodies

glomerulonephritis (gla-mer-yul-o-ne-fri'-tis): an inflammation of the glomerulus of the kidney

glomerulus (gla-mer'-yah-lus): part of the nephron, tuft of capillaries situated within Bowman's capsule

glottis (glot'-is): space within the vocal cords of the larynx

glucagon (gloo'-kah-gon): a hormone that stimulates the liver to change glycogen into glucose

glucocorticoid (gloo-koh-kor'-ti-koyd): hormones of the adrenal cortex, namely cortisone and cortisol

glucose (gloo'-kos): a monosaccharide or simple sugar; the principal blood sugar

gluteal (gloo'-tee-ul): pertaining to the area near the buttocks

glycogen (glye'-kuh-jin): polysaccharide formed and stored largely in the liver

goiter (goy'-ter): enlargement of the thyroid gland

Golgi apparatus (gol'-jee ap-ah-ra'-tus): a membranous network that resembles a stack of pancakes; it stores and packages secretions to be secreted by the cell

gonads (goh'-nads): sex glands (ovaries or testes)

gonorrhea (gon-eh-ree'-uh): an infectious disease of the genitourinary tract caused by gonococcus, transmitted mainly by sexual contact

gout (gowt): increase in uric acid crystals in bloodstream which are deposited in joint cavities, especially the great toe

graafian follicle (graf'-ee-an fol'-e-kel): a follicle in the ovary which stores the immature ova

graft (graft): to transplant tissue into a body part to replace damaged tissue

granulation (gran"-yoo-lay'-shun): tiny red granules that are visible in the base of a healing wound; consists of newly formed capillaries and fibroblasts

granulocyte (gran'-ye-loh-site): granular white blood cell

greater omentum (grat'-er o-men'-tum): double fold of peritoneum which hangs down over the abdominal organs like an apron

gross anatomy (grohs' ah-nat'-oh-mee): study of large and easily observable structures of an organism

growth hormone (GH) (growth hor'-mone): hormone responsible for growth and development; also known as somatotropin

gyri (ji'-ree): convolutions in the brain

H

hair follicle (hayr fol'-i-kul): in-pocketing of the epidermis which holds the hair root

hammer (ha'-mer): a tiny bone found in the middle ear; also known as the malleous

heart block (hart blok): interruption of the SA node message to the AV node, there is a lack of coordination between the atria and the ventricles

heart failure (hart fayl'-yur): heart ventricles do not contract effectively

heartburn (hart'-burn): a burning sensation in the esophagus and stomach

hematoma (hee"-muh-toh'-muh): localized clotted mass of blood formed in an organ, tissue, or space

hematuria (hee"-muh-toh'-ee-ah): blood in the urine

hemiplegia (hem"-i-plee'-jee-uh): paralysis of one side of the body

hemoccult (heem'-o-kult): hidden blood

hemodialysis (heem"-oh-di-al'-i-sis): a procedure for removing waste products in the circulating blood of patients with kidney failure

hemoglobin (heem'-uh-gloh-bin): oxygen-carrying pigment of the blood

hemolysis (heem-ol'-ah-sis): the bursting of red blood cells

hemophilia (heem"-oh-fil'-ee-uh): sex-linked, hereditary bleeding disorder occurring only in males but transmitted by females; characterized by a prolonged clotting time and abnormal bleeding

hemorrhoids (hem-uh-roydz): enlarged and varicose condition of the veins in the lower part of the anus or rectum and the tissues of the anus

heparin (hep'-uh-rin): substance obtained from the liver, which slows blood clotting

hepatic duct (he-pat'-ik dukt): structure from the liver to the common bile duct; carries bile

hepatic vein (he-pat'-ik vayn): vein which drains blood from liver into inferior vena cava

hepatitis (hep-ah-tit'-is): inflammation of the liver

Hering-Brewer reflex (heir'-ing brew'-er ree'-flex): a reflex that prevents overstretching of the lungs

hernia (hur'-nee-uh): protrusion of a part of an organ through abnormal opening

herpes (hur'-peez): a contagious viral infection in which small blisters appear

herpes zoster (hur'-peez zos'-ter): *see* shingles

hiatal hernia (high-ay'-tal her'-nee-ah): disorder that occurs when the stomach pushes through the diaphragm

hiccough (hik'-up): spasm of diaphragm and spasmodic closure of glottis

high density lipoprotein (HDL) (high den'-si-tee li'-poh-proh-teen): removes excess cholesterol from walls of the artery

hilum (high'-lem): indentation along the medial border of the kidney

hinge joint (hinj joynt): a joint that moves in one direction or plane

histamine (his'-tah-mihn): a substance that increases gastric secretions

histology (his-tol'-uh-jee): microscopic study of living tissues

hives (hivz): *see* urticaria

Hodgkin's disease (hoj'-kinz di-zeez'): specific type of cancer of the lymph nodes

homeostasis (ho-me-oh-stay'-ses): state of balance

hormone (hor'-mone): chemical secretion, usually from an endocrine gland

host (host): simple or complex organism that can be affected by an agent

human immunodeficiency virus (HIV) (hyoo'-men im"-yoo-noh-dih-fish'-en-see veye'-rus): the causative agent of AIDS

humerus (hyoo'-mor-us): the bone of the upper arm

humoral immunity (hyoo'-mor-al ih-myoo'-nih-tee): type of immunity donated by antibodies

Huntington's disease (hunt'-ing-tunz di-zeez'): genetic disorder characterized by degeneration of the central nervous system

hyaline (hi'-a-line): type of cartilage that forms the skeleton of the embryo

hydrocephalus (hi-dro-sef'-a-lus): increase in the volume of cerebral spinal fluid within the cerebral ventricles, may occur in fetal development

hydronephrosis (high-droh-nef-roh'-sis): renal pelvis and calyces become distended due to the accumulation of fluid

hydroxide (high-drock'-side): one atom of hydrogen and one atom of oxygen

hymen (high'-men): membrane at the opening of the vagina

hyoid (high'-oyd): bone between root of the tongue and larynx, supporting tongue and giving attachment to several muscles

hyperglycemia (high-per-gligh-see'-mee-ya): high concentration of glucose in the blood

hyperopia (high"-per-oh'-pee-uh): farsightedness

hyperpnea (high-per-nee-uh): increase in the depth and rate of breathing accompanied by abnormal exaggeration of respiratory movements

hypersensitivity (high-per-sen-sah-tiv'-i-tee): an abnormal response to a drug or allergen

hypertension (high-per-ten'-shun): abnormally high blood pressure

hyperthermia (high"-per-ther'-mee-uh): a condition in which the body temperature rises above normal

hyperthyroidism (high"-per-thigh'-royd-izm): condition of overactivity of the thyroid gland

hypertonic solution (high"-per-ton'-ick soh-loo'-shun): a solution in which water molecules are moving out of a cell, causing it to shrink

hypertrophy (high-per'-tro-fee): an increase in the size of the muscle cell

hyperventilation (high-per-ven-til-ay'-shun): rapid breathing, rapid loss of carbon dioxide; sometimes causes dizziness or fainting

hypogastric (high-poh-gas'-trik): lower region of the abdominal area

hypoglycemia (high"-poh-gliy-see'-mee-ya): low concentration of glucose in the blood

hypotension (high"-poh-ten'-shun): reduced or abnormally low blood pressure

hypothalamus (high"-poh-thal'-a-mus): part of the diencephalon, lies below the thalamus

hypothermia (high"-poh-ther'-mee-uh): a condition in which the body temperature drops below normal

hypothyroidism (high"-poh-thigh'-royd-izm): condition of underactivity of the thyroid gland

hypotonic solution (high"-poh-ton'-ick soh-loo'-shun): a solution in which water molecules are moving into the cell, causing it to swell

hysterectomy (his"-tur-ek'-tuh-mee): partial or total surgical removal of the uterus

I

ileocecal valve (il'-ee-oh-see'-cal valv): an opening in the sidewall of the large intestine

ileum (il'-ee-um): the lower part of the small intestine, extending from the jejunum to the large intestine

illness stage (ill'-ness stayj): time period when the client is manifesting specific signs and symptoms of an infectious agent

immunity (im-yoo'-neh-tee): ability to resist a disease

immunization (im-yoo-nah-zay'-shun): process of increasing resistance to disease

immunoglobulin (im"-yoo-noh-glob'-ya-lin): protein that acts like an antibody

impetigo (im-peh-tay'-goh): acute and contagious skin disease

impotence (im'-peh-tens): inability to sustain an erection

in vitro fertilization (IVF) (in vee'-tro fer"-til-ih-zay'-shun): a process of fertilization outside the living organism

incisor (in-sigh'-zur): cutting tooth; one of four front teeth of either jaw

incomplete proteins (in"-kum-pleet' pro'-teens): proteins that lack some or most of the essential amino acids

incontinence (in-con'-tin-ence): loss of self-control, especially of urine, feces, or semen

incubation stage (in"-kyoo-bay'-shun stayj): time interval between the entry of an infectious agent in the host and the onset of symptoms

incus (ing'-kus): the middle ear bone, also called the anvil

infectious mononucleosis (in-fek'-shus mon"-oh-nuk-lee-oh'-sis): contagious disease caused by Epstein-Barr virus, sometimes called the "kissing disease"

inferior (in-feer'-ee-er): below another or lower

inferior concha (in-feer'-ee-er kon'-cha): bones that make up sidewalls of the nasal cavity

infertility (in-fer-til'-ah-tee): incapable of reproduction

inflammation (in"-flah-may'-shun): occurs when tissues are subjected to chemical or physical trauma (cut or heat); invasion by pathogenic microorganisms can cause inflammation; pain, heat, redness, and swelling occur

inflammatory bowel disease (in-flam'-ah-tor-ee bow'-l dih-seez'): a disorder affecting the digestive system characterized by chronic diarrhea

influenza (in-floo-en'-zah): inflammation of the mucous membrane of the respiratory tract

inguinal hernia (ing'-gwi-nul hur-nee-uh): located in the groin

insertion (in-sir'-shun): part of a muscle that is attached to a movable part

inspiration (in"-spih-ray'-shun): drawing in of air; inhalation

inspiratory reserve volume (IRV) (in-spir'-ah-tor"-ee ree-surv' vol'-yoom): amount of air you can force a person to take in over and above tidal volume

insulin (in'-sah-lin): hormone produced by the pancreas necessary for glucose metabolism

integument (in-teg'-yoo-munt): covering, especially the skin

integumentary system (in-teg'-yoo-men'-tair-ee sis'-tum): all organs and structures that make up the skin

intercostal muscles (in-tur-kos'-tul mus'-uls): muscles found between adjacent ribs

interferon (in-tur-fear'-on): proteins that interfere with virus replication

internal (in-ter'-nul): term used to describe damage to an organ within the body

internal respiration (in-ter'-nul res-pir-ay'-shun): the exchange of carbon dioxide and oxygen between the cells and the lymph surrounding them, plus the oxidative process of energy in the cells

interneuron (in-ter-neur'-on): *see* associative neuron

interphase (in'-ter-faz): the resting phase in the process of mitosis

interstitial cell–stimulating hormone (ICSH) (in-ter-stish'-al sell stih'-myoo-lay-ting hor'-mone): a hormone that stimulates the growth of the graafian follicle and the production of estrogen in females and the production of sperm in males

interstitial fluid (in-tur-stish'-al floo'-id): another name for lymph fluid

interstitial tissue (in"-tur-stish'-ul tish'-ew): intercellular connective tissue

interventricular foramen (in-ter-ven-trick'-yoo-lar for-ay'-men): the area that connects the third ventricle of the brain to the two lateral ventricles

intestinal mucosa (in-tes'-tin-ul myoo-coh'-sah): lines the small and large intestines

intracellular fluid (in-tra-sel'-ya-ler flu'-id): fluid within the cell

intramuscular (in"-truh-mus'-kew-lur): into the muscle

intrinsic muscle (in-trin'-sick muss'-ul): muscles that help the iris control the amount of light entering the pupil

in-vitro fertilization (IVF) (in-vee'-tro fer"-til-ih-zay'-shun): a process of fertilization outside the living organism

ion (eye'-on): an electrically charged atom

ionize (eye'-oh-nize): production of positively charged hydrogen ions and negatively charged ions of another substance

iris (i'-ris): colored muscular layer surrounding the pupil of the eye

iron-deficiency anemia (eye'-ron dih-fish'-en-see ah-nee'-mee-uh): a condition resulting from lack of adequate amounts of iron in the diet

irritability (ir"-ih-tuh-bil'-ih-tee): ability to react to a stimulus; excitability

islets of Langerhans (i'-letz of lang'-er-hanz): specialized cells in pancreas which produce insulin

isometric (i-soh-meh'-trik): tension in muscle increases but muscle does not shorten

isotonic solution (eye-soh-tahn'-ik soh-loo'-shun): a solution in which movement of water molecules into and out of a cell are the same

isotonic (i-soh-ton'-ik): muscle contracts and shortens

isotope (i'-soh-tope): atoms of a specific element which have the same number of protons but a different number of neutrons

J

jaundice (jon'-dis): yellowish color

jejunum (je-joo'-num): section of small intestine between duodenum and ileum

joint (joynt): place where two bones meet

K

keratin (ker'-uh-tin): chemical belonging to albuminoid or scleroprotein group found in horny tissue, hair, nails

kidney (kid'-nee): organ of the urinary system that functions to rid the body of nitrogenous wastes

kidney stones (kid'-nee stonz): clumping together of calcium phosphate crystals, uric acid, and other substances in the kidneys

kilocalorie (kill'-oh-cal-or-ee): a large calorie; equal to 1,000 calories

kinetic energy (ki-neh'-tik en'-er-jee): work resulting in motion

kyphosis (ki-fose'-is): hunchback, humped curvature in spinal column

L

labia majora (lay'-bee-uh may-jor'-uh): the folds of skin that lie on either side of the vaginal opening

labia minora (lay'-bee-uh meye-nor'-ah): the folds of skin that lie just inside of the vaginal opening

lacrimal (lak'-ri-mul): pertaining to tears

laparoscope (lap'-ah-roh-scope): instrument used to view the internal abdominal organs during a laparoscopy

laparoscopy (lap'-ah-roh-coh-pee): a minor surgical procedure done under anesthesia to visualize the abdominal organs

laryngitis (lar-in-geye'-tis): an inflammation of the larynx or voicebox

larynx (lar'-inks): voicebox, found between trachea and base of tongue; contain the vocal cords

lateral (lat'-ur-ul): toward the side

lateral ventricles *see* cerebral ventricles

left lymphatic duct (left lim-fat'-ick dukt): the lymphatic duct that receives lymph from the left side of the body; also called thoracic duct

left ventricle (left ven'-trick-ul): one of the lower chambers of the heart

lens (lenz): crystal structure for refraction of light rays

lethal gene (lee'-thal jeen): a gene that results in death

leukemia (loo-kee'-mee-uh): a cancerous condition in which there is a great increase in the number of white blood cells

leukocyte (lew'-ko-sight): white blood cell

leukocytosis (lew"-ko-sigh-tow'-sis): an increase in the white blood cell count, above 10,000 cells per cubic millimeter (mm^3)

leukopenia (lew"-ko-pee'-nee-uh): a decrease in the normal number of white blood cells (leukocytes)

life function (life funk'-shun): a series of highly organized and related activities which help living organisms to live, grow, and maintain themselves

ligament (lig'-uh-ment): a band of fibrous tissue connecting bones or supporting organs

lingual (ling'-gwal): tonsils found at the back of the tongue

lipase (lip'-ase): enzyme that changes fats into fatty acids and glycerol

lipid (lip'-id): fatty compound

lithotripsy (lith-oh-trip'-see): *see* extracorpeal shockwave lithotripsy (ESWL)

liver (liv'-ur): large organ of the digestive system, located in upper right quadrant of the abdominal cavity

loop of Henle (loop of hen'-lee): proximal convoluted tubule descends into the medulla forming the loop of Henle

lordosis (lor-do'-sis): forward curvature of lumbar region of spine

low density lipoprotein (LDL) (low den'-sih-tee lip-oh-proh'-teen): lipoprotein that carries fat to the cells

lubb dupp sound (lub dup sownd): sounds made by the heart valves when they close

lumbar (lum'-bahr): vertebrae bones between the posterior thorax and sacral vertebrae

lumbar puncture (lum'-bahr punk'-chur): removal of cerebrospinal fluid for diagnostic purposes by insertion of a needle between the third and fourth lumbar vertebrae

lumbar vertebrae (lum'-bahr vur'-te-bray): five vertebrae associated with lower part of back

lumpectomy (lump-eck'-toh-mee): surgical removal of an abnormal cellular growth

lupus (loo'-pus): a chronic inflammatory autoimmune disease

luteinizing hormone (LH) (loo'-ten-eye-zing hor'-mone): hormone that stimulates ovulation and the production of progesterone in females

lymph (limf): watery fluid in the lymphatic vessels

lymph nodes (limf node): structures that produce lymphocytes and filter out harmful bacteria

lymph vessels (limf ves'-ulz): structures that transport excess tissue fluid back into the circulatory system

lymphadenitis (lim-fa"-den-i'-tis): inflammation of the lymph nodes

lymphatic system (lim-fat'-ik sis'-tum): system of vessels and nodes supplemental to blood circulatory system, carrying lymph

lymphocyte (lim'-foh-sight): a type of white blood cell

lysosome (lye"-so-sohm): cytoplasmic organelle containing digestive enzymes

M

macular degeneration (mak'-yu-ler de-jen"-er-ay'-shun): thinning of retinal layer of eye or leakage may develop under retina disturbing sharp central vision

malignant melanoma (mah-lig'-nant mel-ih-noh'-mah): a type of tumor that develops in the pigmented cells of the skin called melanocytes

malleus (mal'-ee-us): largest of three middle ear bones; also called the hammer

mammogram (mam'-e-gram): an x-ray of the breast

mandible (man'-dih-bul): lower jawbone

mastectomy (mas-tek'-ta-mee): removal of a breast

masticate (mas"-ti-kayt): chew

mastication (mas"-ti-kay'-shun): process of chewing

matrix (may'-tricks): the nailbed

matter (mat'-ur): anything that has weight and occupies space

maxilla (mak-sil'-a): bone of the upper jaw

medial (mee'-dee-ul): toward midline of body

mediastinum (mee"-dee-as'-tih-num): intrapleural space separating the sternum in front and the vertebral column behind

medulla (mah-dul'-uh): inner portion of an organ

medulla oblongata (mah-dul'-uh ob'-lon-gah'-tuh): part of the brainstem, contains the nuclei for vital functions

medullary canal (med'-ul-er-ee cuh-nal'): center of the shaft of long bone

meiosis (mi-yo'-sis): cell division of gamete or cells; there is a reduction in the number of chromosomes

melanin (mel'-a-nin): pigment that gives color to hair, skin, and eyes

melanocytes (mel-ahn'-oh-sites): cells that make the protein melanin to protect against ultraviolet rays

melatonin (mel-eh-toh'-nin): hormone produced by the pineal gland

membrane (mem'-brayn): a thin layer of tissue that covers a surface or divides an organ

membrane excitability (mem'-brayn ex-cite-a-bil'-ih-tee): ability of nerves to carry impulses by creating electric charges

memory (mem'-eh-ree): process by which we store information we have learned

menarche (me-nahr'-kee): time when menstruation begins

Meniere's disease (man-arz' di-zeez'): condition affecting semicircular canals of inner ear

meninges (men-en'-jez): any of three linings enclosing the brain and spinal cord

meningitis (men-in-geye'-tis): inflammation of the lining of the brain and spinal cord

menopause (men'-o-pawz): physiologic termination of menstruation, generally between 50 and 55 years

menstrual cycle (men'-stroo-ul sigh'-kul): recurring series of changes that take place in the ovaries, uterus, and accessory sexual structures during menstruation

menstruation (men"-stroo-ay'-shun): monthly shedding of endometrial lining if ova is not fertilized

mesentery (mez'-en-ter-ee): peritoneum attached to posterior wall of the abdominal cavity

metabolism (me-tab'-oh-lizm): sum total of processes of digestion, absorption, and the resulting release of energy

metacarpal (met"-uh-kahrp-al): bones of wrist

metaphase (met'-uh-faze): phase three in the process of mitosis; nuclear membrane disappears

metastasis (me-tas'-tuh-sis): transfer of malignant cells from an original site to a distant one through the circulatory system or lymph vessels

metatarsal (met"-uh-tahr'-sal): sole of foot, forms the arch

microscopic anatomy (my'-kroh-skah'-pick ah-nat'-oh-mee): study of small tissues, organs, and cells that cannot be seen with the naked eye

midsagittal plane (mid-saj'-eh-tel plane): an imaginary line dividing the body into equal right and left halves

mineral (min'-ur-ul): an inorganic, solid chemical compound found in nature

mineralocorticoids (min'-ur-ul-o-cort'-ih-coydz): hormones of the adrenal cortex, namely aldosterone

miotic (mye-ot'-ik): pertaining to or causing contraction of the pupil

mitochondria (miy-toh-kon'-dree-a): organelle that supplies energy to the cell

mitosis (migh-toe'-sis): cell division involving two distinct processes: (1) mitosis, the exact duplication of the nucleus to form two identical nuclei; (2) cytoplasmic division, after nuclear division, the cytoplasm is divided into two approximately equal parts

mitral valve prolapse (miy'-tral valv proh'-laps): valve between the left atrium and the left ventricle does not close properly

mixed nerve (mikst nurv): nerve composed of both afferent (sensory) fibers and efferent (motor) fibers

mode of transmission (mode of trans-mish'-un): process that bridges the gap between the portal of exit of the infectious agent from the reservoir or source, and the portal of entry of the susceptible host

molar (moh'-lar): teeth designed for crushing and tearing

molecule (mol'-uh-kyool): the smallest unit of the compound that still has the properties of the compound

mongolism (mon-go-lism): *see* Down syndrome

monocyte (mon'-oh-sight): large mononuclear leukocyte with deeply indented nucleus, slate gray cytoplasm, and fine bluish granulations

monosaccharide (mon"-oh-sack'-uh-ride): simple sugar; glucose

mons pubis (monz pyoo'-bihs): fatty tissue overlying the genital region; usually covered by coarse hair

morphology (mor-fol'-ah-jee): study of the shape of an organism

motor nerve (moh'-ter nurv): nerve fibers consisting of both sensory and motor fibers; also known as the efferent nerve

motor neuron (moh'-ter neur'-on): or efferent neuron, carries messages from brain and spinal cord to muscles and glands

motor unit (moh'-ter u'-nit): a motor nerve plus all the muscle fibers it stimulates

mucosa (mew-koh'-suh): mucous membrane

mucous membrane (myoo'-cuhs mem'-brayn): type of tissue that lines surfaces and spaces that lead to the outside of the body

multicellular (mul-ti-sel'-u-lar): many-celled

multiple sclerosis (MS) (mul'-tih-pul skle-roh'-sis): chronic inflammatory disease in which the immune cells attack the myelin sheath of a nerve

murmur (mur'-mer): gurgling or hissing sound from heart valves failing to close properly

muscle fatigue (mus'-ul fah-teeg'): caused by an accumulation of lactic acid in the muscle

muscle spasm (mus'-ul spa'-zum): sustained muscle contraction

muscle tissue (mus'-ul tish'-yoo): contains cell material that has the ability to contract and move the body

muscle tone (mus'-ul tone): muscles always in a state of partial contraction

muscular dystrophy (mus'-kew-ler dis'-tre-fee): muscle disease in which the muscle cells deteriorate

mutagenic agent (mew"-tuh-jen'-ik ay'-junt): any substance causing a genetic mutation

mutation (mew-tay'-shun): the appearance of a new and different organic trait caused by the inheritance of a mutated gene or chromosome

myalgia (migh-al'-juh): muscular pain

myasthenia gravis (migh-es-the'-nee-a gra'vis): disease in which there is abnormal weakness and eventual paralysis of muscles

myelin (migh'-e-lin): a lipoid substance found in the sheath around nerve fibers

myelin sheath (migh'-e-lin sheeth): layers of cell membrane that wrap nerve fibers, providing electrical insulation and increasing the velocity of impulse transmission

myeloblast (migh'-eh-loh-blast): cells that synthesize granulocytes in bone marrow

myocardial infarction (migh"-o-kahr-dee-ahl in-fark'-shun): a heart attack caused by a blockage of blood flow to the heart muscle

myocarditis (migh"-o-kahr-dye'-tis): inflammation of muscular tissue of heart

myocardium (migh"-o-kahr'-de-um): muscle of the heart

myometrium (migh"-o-mee'-tree-um): uterine muscular structure

myopia (migh-o'-pee-uh): nearsightedness

myringotomy (mir-en-got'-oh-mee): opening into the tympanic membrane

myxedema (mik-se-de'-ma): hypofunction of the thyroid gland, swelling around nose and lips

N

nasal (nay'-zul): nose

nasal cavity (nay'-zul kav'-ih-tee): one of the pair of cavities between the anterior nares and the nasopharynx

nasal polyps (nay'-zul pol'-ips): growth that occurs in sinus cavity

nasal septum (nay'-zul sep'-tum): partition between the two nasal cavities

natural acquired immunity (na'-chur-al a-kwi'-erd i-mu'-ni-tee): immunity which is the result of having the disease and recovering

natural immunity (na'-chur-al i-mu'-ni-tee): immunity with which a person is born

nearsightedness (near'-sigh-ted-ness): *see* myopia

neck of tooth (nek of tooth): that part of tooth at gum line

negative feedback (neg'-uh-tiv feed'-bak): return of part of the output to the source or beginning; this leads to an adjustment in the system; may occur in hormonal or nervous control systems

neoplasm (nee'-o-plaz-em): a tumor; can be benign or malignant

nephron (nef'-ron): unit of structure of kidney, contains glomerulus, Bowman's capsule, proximal distal tubule, loop of Henle, and distal tubule

nervous tissue (nur'-vus tish'-yoo): contains cells that react to stimuli and conduct an impulse

neuralgia (noo-ral'-ja): severe, stabbing pain along the pathway of a nerve

neuritis (noo-rih'-tis): inflammation of a nerve

neurogenic bladder (noor-o-jen'-ik blad'-ur): condition caused by damaged nerves that control the bladder

neuroglia (noo-rog'-lee-ah): network of cells that insulate, support, and protect the nerves of the central nervous system

neurology (noo-rol'-ah-jee): study of the physiology and pathology of the nervous system

neuromuscular junction (noor-ih-mus'-kya-lur junk'-shun): point between the motor nerve axon and the muscle cell membrane

neuron (new'-ron): nerve cell, including its processes

neutralization (noo-tral-ah-zay'-shun): an acid and a base combine to form a salt and water

neutrophil (noo'-troh-fil): many-lobed white blood cell phagoytizes bacteria, sometimes called "polys"

nocturia (nock-too'-ree-uh): excessive urination during the night

norepinephrine (nor-ep"-ih-nef'-rin): hormone that acts as a vasoconstrictor

nosocomial infection (nos"-oh-koh'-mee-ahl in-feck'-shun): infection that is acquired in the hospital or other health care facility and was not present or incubating at the time of the client's admission

nuclear membrane (noo'-klee-er mem'-brayn): double-layered membrane that surrounds the nucleus

nucleic acid (noo-klay'-ik as'-id): organic compound containing carbon, hydrogen, oxygen, nitrogen, and phosphorous (i.e., DNA, RNA)

nucleolus (new-klee-uh'-lus): small spherical structure within cell nucleus

nucleoplasm (new'-klee-o-plazm): protoplasm of the nucleus, also called nuclear sap or karyolymph

nucleus (new'-klee-us): core or center of a cell containing large quantities of DNA

nutrient (new'-tree-unt): affording nutrition

nystagmus (ni-stag'-mis): rapid involuntary movement of the eyeball

O

obesity (oh-bee'-sih-tee): increase of body weight due to fat accumulation of 10% to 20% above normal range for the specific age, height, and sex

occipital (ok-cip'-ih-tahl): bone that forms the base of the skull and contains the foramen magnum

occipital lobe (ok-cip'-ih-tel lobe): part of the cerebrum that houses the visual area

olecranon process (oh-lek'-ruh-non pro'-ses): large projection at upper extremity of ulna

olfactory (ol-fak'-tur-ee): pertaining to the sense of smell

olfactory nerve (ol-fak'-tur-ee nurv): nerves that supply the nasal mucosa

oliguria (ol-ig-yoo'-ree-ah): diminished production of urine

oogenesis (o"-oh-jen'-e-sis): process of origin, growth, and formation of ovum in ovary during preparation for fertilization

ophthalmic (of-thal'-mik): referring to the eyes

optic disc (op'-tick disk): an area of the eye devoid of visual reception; also known as the blind spot

oral cavity (or'-el ca'-vi-tee): encloses the teeth and tongue

orbital cavity (or'-bi-tel ca'-vih-tee): contains the eye and its external structures

orchitis (or-ki'-tis): inflammation of testis

organ (or'-gan): group of tissues organized according to structure and function

organelle (or-guh-nel'): microscopic specialized structure within the cell having a special function or capacity

organ of Corti (or'-gan of kor'-tee): hearing organ

organ system (or'-gan sis'-tem): organs that are grouped together because more than one is needed to perform a function

organic catalyst (or-gan'-ick kat'-ah-list): a substance that affects the rate of speed of a chemical reaction without itself being changed

organic compound (or-gan'-ik kom'-pownd): compound that contains the element carbon

origin (or'-eh-jin): part of the skeletal muscle that is attached to the fixed part of the bone

oropharynx (or"-o-fayr'-inks): oral pharynx, found below level of lower border of soft palate and above larynx

orthopnea (or"-thup'-nee-uh): difficult or labored breathing

osmoreceptor (oz"-moh-ree-sep'-tur): structures found in the hypothalamus; sensitive to changes in the osmotic blood pressure and control the release of the antidiuretic hormone (ADH)

osmosis (oz-moh'-sis): passage of fluid through a membrane

osmotic pressure (oz-mot'-ik presh'-ur): pressure developed when two solutions of different concentrations of the solute are separated by a membrane permeable only to the solvent

osseous tissue (os'-ee-us tish'-yoo): bony; composed of or resembling bone

ossification (os"-eh-fi-kay'-shun): process of bone formation

osteoarthritis (os"-tee-oh-ahr-thry'-tis): degenerative joint disease

osteoblast (os'-tee-oh-blast): cells involved in formation of bony tissue

osteoclast (os'-tee-oh-klast): cells involved in resorption of bony tissue

osteocyte (os'-tee-oh-site): bone cell

osteomyelitis (os'-tee-oh-mi-e-lit'-is): inflammation of the bone

osteoporosis (os"-tee-oh-pour-oh'-sis): loss of calcium in bone, causing brittleness, occurs mainly in females after menopause

osteosarcoma (os-tee-oh-sar-koh'-mah): bone cancer

otitis media (o-teye'-tis mee'-dee-uh): an infection of the middle ear

otosclerosis (ah"-toh-skle-roh'-sis): chronic, progressive ear disorder in which the bone in the region of the oval window first becomes spongy and then hardened, causing the stirrup or stapes to become fixed or immobile.

ova (o'-va): female reproductive cell

ovary (o'-veh-ree): female reproductive organ produces ova, estrogen, and progesterone

oviduct (ov'-i-duct): *see* fallopian tube

ovulation (ah"-vyoo-lay'-shun): second stage of the menstrual cycle, when a ripe egg cell is released from an ovarian follicle cell

oxidation (oks-in-day-shun): *see* cellular respiration

oxygenate (ok"-si-ji'-nate): to saturate a substance with oxygen, either by chemical combination or by mixture

oxyhemoglobin (ok"-see-hee'-muh-gloh"-bin): hemoglobin combined with oxygen

oxytocin (ocks"-see-toh'-sin): hormone released during childbirth to cause strong contractions of the uertus

P

pacemaker (pace maker): *see* sinoatrial valve

palatine (pal'-ah-tine): tonsils located on the side of the soft palate

palpitation (pal"-pah-tay'-shun): irregular, rapid pulsation of the heart

pancreas (pan'-kree-as): organ of digestion lies behind the stomach, produces digestive juices, insulin, and glucagon

pancreatitis (pan"-kree-ah-teye'-tis): inflammation of the pancreas

Pap or **Papanicolaou** (pap or pah"-peh-nik'-oh-low) **smear:** cytological, diagnostic cancer technique that studies exfoliated cells, especially those from vagina

papillae (pa-pil'-uh): small, nipple-shaped elevations

papilloma (pap-ih-loh'-mah): a type of tumor of the epithelial tissue; also known as a wart

parasympathetic system (par'-ah-sim'-pah-thet'-ik sis'-tem): division of the autonomic nervous system inhibits or opposes the effects of the sympathetic nervous system

parathormone (par"-ah-thor'-mone): hormone that controls the concentration of calcium in the bloodstream

parathyroid gland (par"-uh-thiy'-royd gland): four small endocrine glands embedded in the thyroid gland; secretes parathormone

paresthesia (par"-es-theez'-shuh): ensation of tingling, crawling, or burning of skin

parietal (pah-ryi'-eh-tahl): bone that forms the roof and sides of the skull

parietal lobe (pah-ryi'-ah-tel lobe): division of the cerebrum lies beneath the parietal bone

parietal membrane (pah-ryi'ah-tel mem'-brayn): the lining of a body cavity

Parkinson's disease (par'-kin-senz di-zeez'): marked tremors may be due to decrease of neurotransmitter dopamine

parotid salivary gland (pah-rot'-id sal'-ah-ver-ee gland): largest of the salivary glands

passive acquired immunity (pas'-iv a-kwi'-erd i-mu'-ni-tee): borrowed immunity, has a temporary effect (i.e., gamma globulin)

passive transport ('pas-siv' trans-pōrt): the process of moving materials across a cell membrane that does not require energy such as disfussion, osmosis, and filtration.

patella (pah-tel'-uh): kneecap

pathogenic (path"-uh-jen'-ik): disease causing

pathogenicity (path"-oh-jeh-nis'-ih-tee): ability of a microorganism to produce disease

pectoral (pek'-tuh-rul): pertaining to the chest

pelvic cavity (pel'-vick kav'-ih-tee): the area of the body containing the urinary bladder, reproductive organs, rectum, remainder of the large intestine, and appendix

pelvic inflammatory disease (PID) (pel'-vick in-flam'-ah-tor-ee dih-seez'): a disease resulting from infections of the reproductive organs

pelvis (pel'-vis): any basin-shaped structure or cavity

penile shaft (pee'-nile shaft): erectile tissue that becomes rigid during intercourse

penis (pee'-nis): male reproductive organ

peptic ulcer (pep'-tick uhl'-sir): sore or lesion that forms in the lining of the stomach or duodenum

pericardial membrane (per"-ih-kahr'-dee-ahl mem'-brayn): lines the heart cavity

pericarditis (per"-ih-kahr'-deye'-tis): an inflammation of the outer membrane covering the heart

pericardium (per"-ih-kahr'-dee-um): closed membranous sac surrounding heart

perineum (per'ah-nee-um): area between the vagina and the rectum

periodontal membrane (per-ee-o-dan'-tel mem'-brayn): membrane that anchors a tooth in place

periosteum (per-ee-os'-tee-um): fibrous tissue covering the bone

perioxisome (per"-ee-ock'-sih-sohm): membranous sacs that contain oxidase enzymes

peripheral (pe-rif'-er-al): outside surface, or the area away from the center

peripheral nervous system (pe-rif'-er-al): made up of 12 pairs of cranial nerves and 31 pairs of spinal nerves

peripheral vascular disease (pe-rif'-er-al vas'-kul-ar di-zeez'): blockage of arteries usually in the legs

peristalsis (per"-ih-stal'-sis): progressive wave of contraction in tubular structures provided with longitudinal and transverse muscular fibers, as in esophagus, stomach, small and large intestines

peritoneal dialysis (per"-ih-toh-nee'-ahl dye-al'-ih-sis): filtering of the client's blood through the client's own peritoneal lining

peritoneal membrane (per"-ih-toh-nee'-ahl mem'-brayn): lines the abdominal cavity

peritoneum (per-ih-toh'-nee-um): serous membrane lining of abdominal cavity

peritonitis (per"-ih-toh'-neye-tis): inflammation of the membrane lining the abdominal cavity

pernicious anemia (per-nish'-us a-nee'-mee-a): caused by decrease of B_{12} or lack of intrinsic factor in the stomach

pertussis (per-tus'-is): severe coughing attacks and dyspnea; also known as whooping cough

pH scale The measure of the acidity or alkalinity of a solution

phagocyte (fag'-oh-sight): cell having property of engulfing and digesting foreign particles or cells harmful to body

phagocytosis (fag"-oh-si-toh'-sis): ingestion of foreign or other particles by certain cells

phalanges (fah-lan'-jez): bones of fingers and toes

pharyngitis (fair"-in-jeye'-tis): a red, inflamed throat caused by a bacteria or virus

pharynx (fair'-inks): throat

phase (faze): condition or stage of a disease or a biological, chemical, physiological, and psychological function at a given time

phenylketonuria (PKU) (fen"-il-kee-toh-new'-ree-uh): a metabolic disorder; the body cannot make an enzyme needed for normal metabolism or breakdown of the amino acid phenylalanine. Excess phenylalanine will disrupt the normal development of neurons in the brain

phlebitis (fle-bye'-tis): inflammation of a vein, with or without infection and thrombus formation

phospholipids (fos'-foh-lip'-ids): fats that contain carbon, hydrogen, oxygen, and phosphorous

phrenic nerve (fren'-ik nurv): stimulates the diaphragm

physical agent (fiz'-ih-cahl ay'-jent): factor in the environment capable of causing disease in a host

physiology (fiz"-ee-ol'-uh-jee): study of functions of living organisms and their parts

physiotherapy (fiz"-ee-oh-ther'-uh-pee): the treatment of disease and injury by physical means using light, heat, cold, water, electricity, massage, and exercise

pia mater (pee'-uh may'-tur): innermost vascular covering of brain and spinal cord

pineal gland (pin'-ee-al gland): located in the third ventricle of the brain; produces melatonin

pinna (pin'-ah): outer ear

pinocytic vessel (pin"-oh-si'-tik ves'-el): formed by having the cell membrane fold inward to form a pocket

pinocytosis (pin"-oh-sye-toh'-sis): process of engulfing large molecules in solution and taking them into the cell

pituitary gland (pi-too'-e-tayr'-ee gland): a small gland located in the sphenoid bone in the cranium, its hormones affect all other glandular activity; called the master gland

pivot joint (piv'-et joynt): joint in which an extension of one bone rotates in a second arch-shaped bone

planes (plahnz): imaginary, anatomical dividing lines useful in separating body structures

plasma (plaz'-muh): liquid part of blood containing corpuscles

pleura (ploor'-uh): or pleural membrane; serous membrane protecting the lungs and lining the internal surface of thoracic cavity

pleural fluid (ploo'-rahl floo'-id): serous fluid necessary to prevent friction between the pleural membranes

pleural membrane (ploo'-rahl mem'-brayn): lines the thoracic cavity

pleurisy (ploor'-ih-see): inflammation of pleura

plexus (plek'-sus): a network of spinal nerves

pneumonia (noo-mon'-ya): infection of the lung

pneumothorax (noo-moh-tho'-racks): a buildup of air within the pleural cavity on one side of the chest

poliomyelitis (po"-le-o-mye-lye'-tis): disease of nerve pathways of spinal cord, rarely seen because of polio vaccines

polycythemia (pol"-eh-si-thee'-mee-ah): too many red blood cells

polydipsia (pol"-eh-dip'-see-ah): excessive thirst

polyphagia (pol"-e-fay'-jah): excessive hunger

polysaccharide (pol"-ee-sak'-uh-ride): a complex sugar

polyuria (pol"-e-yoor'-ee-ah): excessive urination

pons (ponz): part of the brainstem

popliteal (pop-lit'-ee-ul): area behind knee

popliteal artery (pop-lih-tee'-al ar'-ter-ee): artery located behind the knee

portal circulation (por'-tul sir-kul-ay'-shun): brings blood from the organs of digestion through the portal vein to the liver

portal of entry (por'-tul of en'-tree): route by which an infectious agent enters the host

portal of exit (por'-tul of ecks'-it): route by which an infectious agent leaves the reservoir

portal vein (por'-tul vane): major vein leading to the liver

posterior (pos-teer'-ee-ur): located behind or at the back; opposite to anterior

posterior chamber (pos-teer'-ee-or chaym'-bur): chamber of the eye filled with vitreous humor

posterior pituitary lobe (pos-teer'-ee-or pih-too'-ih-tair"-ee lobe): stores the hormones produced by the hypothalamus

potential energy (poh-ten'-shul en'-er-jee): energy stored in cells waiting to be released

premenstrual syndrome (PMS) (pree-men'-strahl sin'-drome): a group of symptoms exhibited just prior to the menstrual cycle caused by water retention in body tissue

prepuce (pre'-poos): *see* foreskin

presbycusis (prez"-bih-kyoo'-sis): a condition that causes deafness due to the aging process

presbyopia (prez"-bee-oh'-pee-uh): farsightedness of advanced age due to loss of elasticity in lens of eye

primary repair (preye'-mair-ee ree-pair'): repair of epithelial tissue when no infection is present; new epithelial cells push themselves up toward the skin surface to repair the damage

prime mover (prime muv'-er): muscle that provides movement in a single direction

prodromal stage (proh-droh'-mahl stayj): time interval from the onset of nonspecific symptoms until specific symptoms of the infectious process begin to manifest

progesterone (pro-jes'-tur-ohn): steroid hormone secreted by ovary from corpus luteum to help maintain pregnancy

prolactin hormone (PR) (pro-lack'-tin hor'-mone): hormone that develops breast tissue and the production of milk after childbirth

pronation (pro-nay'-shun): (1) condition of being prone; (2) turning of palm of hand downward

prophase (pro'-faze): phase two in the process of mitosis

prostaglandin (pros-tah-glan'-din): hormones secreted by various tissue, their function depends on which tissue they are excreted from

prostate gland (pros'-tate gland): gland located just under the urinary bladder; secretes a thin, milky alkaline fluid that enhances sperm motility

prostatectomy (pros"-tuh-tek'-tuh-mee): surgical removal of all or part of prostate

prostatitis (pross"-tah-teye'-tis): an infection of the prostate gland

protease (pro'-tee-ace): pancreatic juice that breaks down protein into amino acids

protein synthesis (proh'-teen sin'-theh-sis): production of protein by the cells that are essential to life

prothrombin (proh-throm'-bin): a globulin that helps blood to coagulate

protozoa (proh-tah-zoh'-ah): single-celled parasitic organisms with the ability to move

proximal (prok'-sih-mul): located nearest the center of the body; point of attachment of a structure

proximal convoluted tubule (prok'-sih-mul con-voh-loo'-ted too'-byool): twisted tubular branch off the Bowman's capsule

psoriasis (so-rye'-ah-sis): chronic inflammatory skin disease with silvery patches

ptyalin (teye'-ah-lihn): found in saliva; it converts starches into simple sugars

puberty (pew'-bur-tee): age when reproductive organs become functional

pubis (pew'-bis): pubic bone, portion of hipbone forming front of pelvis

pulmonary artery (pool-'ma-ner-ee ar'-ter-ee): structure takes blood from the right ventricle to the lungs

pulmonary embolism (pool-'ma-ner-ee em'-boh-lism): a blood clot that travels to the lungs

pulmonary semilunar valve (pool-'ma-ner-ee sem"-ee-loo'-nar valv): heart valve at the opening of the pulmonary artery that allows blood to flow from the right ventricle into the pulmonary artery

pulmonary veins (pool-'ma-ner-ee vayns): structure which takes blood from the lungs to the right atrium

pulp cavity (pulp kav'-ih-tee): inside of the tooth contains blood vessels and nerve

pulse (puls): measures the number of times the heart beats per minute

pulse pressure (puls preh'-shur): the difference between systolic and diastolic blood pressure

pupil (pew'-pil): opening in iris of eye for passage of light

Purkinje fibers (per-kin'-jee fye'-burs): conduction fibers which conduct the impulses through the ventricles of the heart

pus (pus): product of inflammation; a cream-colored liquid that is a combination of dead tissue, dead and living bacteria, dead white blood cells, and blood plasma

pyelonephritis (pye-loh-nef-right'-is): inflammation of the kidneys and the pelvis of the ureter

pyloric sphincter (pye-lor'-ick sfink'-ter): valve that regulates entrance of food from the stomach to the duodenum

pyloric stenosis (pye-lor'-ik sten-oh'-sis): narrowing of the pyloric sphincter

pylorospasm (pye-lor'-oh-spazm): vomiting of undigested food due to failure of the pyloric sphincter to relax

pylorus (pye-lo'-rus): circular opening of stomach into duodenum

pyrexia (pye-rek'-see-uh): fever

R

radial artery (ray'-dee-ahl ar'-ter-ee): artery located at the wrist

radial nerve (ray'-dee-ahl nurv): found in the brachial plexus; it stimulates the wrist and hand

radioactive (ra'-dee-oh-ak'-tiv): capable of emitting energy in the form of radiation

radius (ra'-dee-us): bone on the thumb side of the forearm

rales (railz): raspy sounding breathing

receptor (ree-sep'-tur): sensory nerve that receives a stimulus and transmits it to the CNS

recombinant DNA (ree-com'-bih-nant DNA): replication and artificial manipulation of DNA

Recommended Dietary Allowances (RDA) (reh-coh-men'-ded deye-ih-tair'-ee ah-low'-en-ses): nutritional requirements established by the Food and Nutrition Board of the National Academy of Sciences

rectum (reck'-tum): portion of the colon that opens into the anus

reflex (ree'-fleks): involuntary action; automatic response

rehabilitation (ree-ha-bil-eh-tay'-shun): the process of restoring function through therapeutic exercise

renal (ree'-nul): pertaining to the kidney

renal calculi (ree'-null cal'-cu-lye): *see* kidney stones

renal column (ree'-nul col'-uhm): support structures between the renal pyramids

renal fascia (ree'-nul fa'-shah): tough fibrous tissue covering the kidney

renal papilla (ree'-null pap'-ih-lah): apex of the renal pyramid

renal pelvis (ree'-nul pel'-vis): funnel-shaped structure at the beginning of the ureter

renal pyramid (ree'-nul peer'-ah-mid): striated cones that make up the medulla of the kidney

renin (ren'-in): enzyme produced by the kidney

replication (rep"-li-kay'-shun): occurs when an exact copy of each nuclear chromosome is made during the early part of the first stage of mitosis (early interphase)

reservoir (rez'-er-vwor): place where the agent can survive

resident flora (rez'-ih-dent floor'-ah): microorganisms that are always present, usually without altering the client's health

residual volume (reh-zid'-yoo-ahl vol'-yoom): the amount of air that cannot be voluntarily expelled in the lungs

respiratory mucosa (res-pir'-ah-tor-ee myoo-coh'-sah): lines the respiratory passages

retina (ret'-in-ah): innermost layer of the eye contains the rods and cones

retroperitoneal (ret"-ro-per"-i-toh-nee'-ul): located behind the peritoneum

reverse isolation (ree-vers' eye-soh-lay'-shun): barrier protection designed to prevent infection in clients who are severely compromised and highly susceptible to infection

Rh factor (r h fak'-tor): antigen found in red blood cells

rheumatic heart disease (roo-mat'-ick hart dih-seez'): a disease of the lining of the heart thought to be caused by frequent strep throat infections

rheumatoid arthritis (roo'-mah-toyd arth-ri'-tis) chronic inflammatory disease affects connective tissue and joints

rhinitis (rih-ni'-tis): inflammation of the lining of the nose

RHO Gam (row'-gam): specific preparation of immune globulin given

ribonucleic acid (RNA) (rye'-boh-noo-kley'-ik as'-id): type of nucleic acid

ribosome (rye'-bo-sohm): submicroscopic particle attached to endoplasmic reticulum, site of protein synthesis in cytoplasm of cell

rickets (rik'-its): bones soften due to lack of vitamin D

rickettsia (rih-ket'-see-ah): intercellular parasites that need to be in living cells to reproduce

right lymphatic duct (rite lim-fat'-ick dukt): the lymphatic duct that receives lymph from the right side of the body

right ventricle (rite ven'-trick-ul): one of the lower chambers of the heart

ringworm (ring'-worm): contagious fungal infection with raised circular patches

rods (rodz): cells in the retina, sensitive to dim light

root (root): part of the tooth imbedded into the alveolar process of the jaw; part of the hair that is implanted in the skin

rotation (roh-tay'-shun): allows a bone to move around a central axis

rotator cuff disease (roh'-tay-tor cuf dih-seez'): an inflammation of a group of tendons that fuse together and surround the shoulder joint

roughage (raftage) (ruf'-aj): the coarse parts of certain foods that are undigestible and stimulate peristalses

rugae (roo'-jee): wrinkles or folds

rule of nines (rule of nines): measures the percent of the body burned

S

sacrum (sa'-krum): wedge-shaped bone below the lumbar vertebra at the end of the spinal column

sagittal plane (sadj'-ih-tul plane): longitudinal; shaped like an arrow

salivary amylase (sal'-ih-vair-ee am'-ih-lace): found in saliva; converts starches into simple sugars

salpingitis (sal"-pin-jeye'-tis): an inflammation of the fallopian tubes

salt (salt): compound formed when a negative ion of acid combines with a positive ion of a base

sarcolemma (sar-koh'-lem-mah): muscle cell membrane

sarcoplasm (sahr'-ko-plazm): the hyaline or finely granular interfibrillar material of muscle tissue

scab (skab): dried capillary fluid that seals a wound

scapula (skap'-yoo-luh): large, flat, triangular bone forming back of shoulder

sciatica (siy-at'-ik-ah): neuritis of the sciatic nerve

sciatic nerve (siy-at'-ik nurv): largest nerve in the body originates in the sacral plexus, runs through the pelvis and down the leg

sclera (skleer'-uh): tough, white covering, part of external coat of eye

scleroderma (skler"-ah-der'-mah): disease that results in the thickening of the skin and blood vessels

scoliosis (skoh"-lee-oh'-sis): lateral curvature of the spine

scrotum (skro'-tum): pouch that contains the testicles

sebaceous gland (se-bay'-shus gland): gland that secretes sebum, a fatty material

sebum (see'-bum): secretion of sebaceous glands that lubricate the skin

second degree burn *see* burn

secondary repair (seck-on-dair'-ee ree-pair'): repair of a wound with small or large tissue loss

section (seck'-shun): a cut made through the body in the direction of a certain plane

sedimentation rate (sed"-e-men-tay'-shun rate): time it takes red blood cells to settle to the bottom in an upright tube

segmented movement (seg-men'-ted moov'-ment): single segments of the intestine alternate between contraction and relaxation

selective semipermeable membrane (se-lek'-tiv sem"-ih-per'-mee-ah-bul mem'-brayn): the cell membrane regulates the passage of certain material in and out of the cell

sella turcica (sel'-uh tur'-si-kuh): saddle-shaped depression in sphenoid bone

semen (see'-mun): male reproductive fluid containing sperm

semicircular canals (sem'-ih-sir'-kuh-lar kan-als'): structures in the inner ear involved with equilibrium

semilunar (sem"-ih-lew'-nur): half-moon shaped valve of aorta and pulmonary artery

seminal vesicles (sem'-i-nul ves'-i-kuls): two highly convoluted membranous tubes that produce substances found to help nourish and protect sperm on its journey up the female reproductive system

seminiferous tubule (sem-in-if'-er-us too'-byool): highly twisted tubules within the testicle

sensory nerve (sen'-soh-ree nurv): nerve fibers carrying impulses from the brain or spinal cord to the muscles or glands; also called the afferent nerve.

sensory neuron (sen'-soh-ree neur'-on): *see* afferent neuron

septicemia (sep"-tih-see'-mee-a): presence of pathogenic organisms in the blood

septum (sep'-tum): partition; dividing wall between two spaces or cavities, such as the septum between left and right side of heart or nose

serosa (see-roh'-sa): the name given to a double-walled serous membrane beginning with the letter *p*

serous fluid (seer'-us floo'-id): (1) normal lymph fluid; (2) thin, watery body fluid

serous membrane (seer'-us mem'-brayn): a double-walled membrane that produces serous fluid

serum (seer'-um): clear, pale yellow fluid that separates from a clot of blood; plasma that contains no fibrinogen

shaft (shaft): (1) part of the hair that extends from the skin surface; (2) the diaphysis of the long bone

shin splints (shin splintz): injury to muscle tendon in front of the shins

shingles (shing'-elz): herpes zoster, a virus infection of the nerve endings

sickle cell anemia (sick'-ul sel uh-nee'-mee-uh): blood disorder; the shape of the red blood cell is a sickle shape, which makes the red blood cells clump together

sigmoid colon (sig'-moyd col'-on): distal, S-shaped part of colon

silicosis (sil'-ah-koh'sis): lung condition caused by breathing dust containing silicon dioxide; lungs become fibrotic

sinoatrial (SA) node (sigh"-no-ay'-tree-ul node): dense network of fibers of conduction at junction of superior vena cava and right atrium

sinus (sigh'-nus): recessed cavity or hollow space

sinusitis (sigh-nyoos-eye'-tis): an infection of the mucous membrane which lines the sinus cavity

skeletal muscle (skel'-e-tal mus'-ul): muscle attached to a bone or bones of skeleton and aids in body movements; also known as voluntary or striated muscle

skeletal system (skel'-e-tal sis'-tem): the bony framework of the body

skin cancer (skin kan'-sir): a tumor that develops on the skin as a result of exposure to ultraviolet light

slipped (herniated) disc (slipt her'-nee-a"-ted disk): a cartilage disc between the vertebra ruptures or protrudes out of place

smooth muscle (smooth mus'-ul): nonstriated, involuntary muscle

sneezing (sneez'ing): deep breath followed by exhalation from the nose

solute (sol'-yoot): dissolved substance in a solution

somatic cell mutation (soh-mat'-ick sell myoo-tay'-shun): alterations that occur within individual body cells

somatotropin (soh'-ma-te-troh'-fin): growth hormone

spastic quadriplegia (spas'-tik kwod'-re-plee'-ja): spastic paralysis of all four limbs

sperm (spurm): the reproductive cell of the male

spermatic cord (spur-mat'-ik kord): cord that extends from the testis to the deep inguinal ring; contains the ductus deferens, the blood vessels and nerves of the testis and epididymis, and the surrounding connective tissue

spermatogenesis (spur'-mat'-ah-jen'ah-sis): the process of the formation of sperm

spermatozoa (sper"-mat-oh-zoh'-ah): the male gametes

sphenoid (sfen'-oid): the key bone of the skull

sphincter muscle (sfink'-tur mus'ul): circular muscle, such as the anus

spinal cavity (spye'-nul kav'-ih-tee): area of the body containing the spinal cord

spinal cord (spye'-nul kord): part of the central nervous system within the spinal column; begins at foramen magnum of occipital bone and continues to the second lumbar vertebra

spinal nerve (spye'-nul nurv): thirty one pairs, originate in the spinal cord

spirometer (spy-rom'-eh-ter): a device that measures the volume and flow of air during inspiration and expiration

spleen (spleen): lymph organ situated below and behind the stomach

spongy bone (spon'-jee bone): the result of hard bone when it is broken down

spore (spoor): bacteria in a resistant stage that can withstand unfavorable environments

sprain (sprayn): wrenching of a joint, producing a stretching or laceration of ligaments

squamous cell carcinoma (skwa'-mes sel kahr"-si-noh'-muh) cancer of the epidermis

stapes (stay'-peez): stirrup-shaped bone in middle ear

steapsin (stee-ap'-sin): pancreatic lipase

sterile (ster'-el): incapable of reproducing, or free from bacteria or other microorganisms

sterilization (ster"-ill-ih-zay'-shun): total elimination of all microorganisms including spores

sternum (stur'-num): flat, narrow bone in median line in front of chest, composed of three parts: manubrium, body, and xiphoid process

steroid (ster'-oyd): lipids or fats that contain cholesterol

stethoscope (steth'-uh-skope): instrument used for detection and study of sounds arising within body

stimulus (stim'-ye-lus): any change in environment

stirrup (stir'-up): a tiny bone found in the middle ear; also known as stapes

stomach (stum'-ik): a major organ of digestion; a pouch-like structure located in the upper left quadrant of the abdominal cavity, between the esophagus and the duodenum

stomach cancer (stum'-ik kan'-sir): abnormal cell growth in the stomach

stomatitis (sto-me-tiy'-tis): inflammation of the mucous membrane of the mouth

strabismus (strah-biz'-mus): a condition in which the muscles of the eyeball do not coordinate their action; also known as crosseyes

strain (strayn): tear in a muscle or stress

stratum corneum (strat'-um kor'-nee-um): the surface layer of the skin

stratum germinativum (strat'-um jer"-min-ah-teye'-vum): the deepest epidermal layer of the skin

strength (strength): capacity to do work

stress test (stress test): test to determine how the physiological stress of vigorous exercise affects the heart

stroke volume (strohk vol'-yoom): the amount of blood ejected from the ventricles with each heart beat

stroke *see* CVA

sty (stye): infection of gland along the eyelid

sublingual gland (sub-ling'-gwal gland): salivary gland located under the sides of the tongue

submandibular gland (sub"-man-dib'-yoo-lar gland): salivary gland located near the angle of the lower jaw

sudden infant death syndrome (SIDS) (suh'-den in'-fant deth sin'-drome [SIDZ]): death of an infant due to a stoppage of breathing while the infant sleeps

sudoriferous gland (sue"-dur-if'-ur-us gland): producing perspiration

sulci (sul'-ce): fissure or grooves separating cerebral convolutions

superficial (soo"-per-fish'-al): on or near the surface of the body

superior (su-peer'-ee-ur): in anatomy, higher; denoting upper of two parts, toward vertex

supination (sue-pih-nay'-shun): turning of palm of hand upward, condition of being supine (lying on back)

surfactant (sir-fack'-tant): lipid material covering the inner surfaces of the alveoli

susceptible host (suh-sep'-tih-bl host): person who lacks resistance to an agent and is thus vulnerable to diease

suspensory ligament (sus-pen'-soh-ree lig'-ah-ment): the ligaments that hold the lens of the eye in place

suture (sue'-chur): (1) in osteology, a line of connection or closure between bones, as in a cranial suture; (2) in surgery, a fine threadlike catgut or silk used to repair or close a wound

sympathetic system (sim-pah-theh'-tik sis'-tem): division of autonomic nervous system

synapse (sin'-aps): space between adjacent neurons through which an impulse is transmitted

synaptic cleft (si-nap'-tik kleft): space between the axon of one neuron and the dendrite of another

synarthroses (sin-ar-thro'-ses): immovable joints connected by fibrous connective tissue

synergist (sin'-er-jist): muscles that help steady a joint

synovial cavity (sin-oh'-vee-ahl kav'-ih-tee): an area between the two articular cartilages

synovial fluid (si-noh'-vee-ahl floo'-id): a lubricating substance

synovial membrane (si-noh'-vee-al mem'-brayn): double layer of connective tissue that lines joint cavities and produces synovial fluid

syphilis (sif'-eh-lis): infectious disease transmitted by sexual contact

systematic anatomy (sis-teh-mat'-ick ah-nat'-oh-me): study of the structure and function of various organs or parts comprising a particular organ system

systole (sis'-tuh-lee): contraction of ventricles, forcing blood into aorta and pulmonary artery

systolic blood pressure (sis-tol'-ick blud preh'-shur): pressure measured at the moment of contraction

T

tachycardia (tak"-i-kahr'-dee-uh): abnormally rapid heartbeat

tachypnea (tak"-ip'-nee-uh): abnormally rapid rate of breathing

talus (tay'-lus): ankle bone that articulates with bones of leg

tarsals (tahr'-sals): ankle bones

tarsus (tahr'-sus): instep

taste buds (tayst budz): cells on the papillae of the tongue which can distinguish salt, bitter, sweet, and sour qualities of dissolved substances

Tay-Sachs disease (tay-saks' di-zeez'): genetic mutation caused by lack of a particular enzyme (hexosaminidase) needed for the breakdown of lipid molecules in the brain

telophase (tel'-ah-faze): final stage in the mitosis process

temporal (tem'-per-el): side of the head

temporal artery (tem'-per-al ar'-ter-ee): artery located slightly above the outer edge of the eye

temporal lobe (tem'-per-el lobe): part of the cerebral hemisphere associated with the perception and interpretation of sound

tendon (ten'-dun): cord of fibrous connective tissue that attaches a muscle to a bone or other structure

tennis elbow (ten'-is el'-boh): inflammation of the tendon that connects the arm muscles to the elbow

testes (tes'-tis): male reproductive organ produces sperm and testosterone

testosterone (tes-tos'-te-rohn): male sex hormone responsible for male secondary sex characteristics

tetanus (tet'-uh-nus): infectious disease, usually fatal, characterized by spasm of voluntary muscles and convulsions caused by toxin from tetanus bacillus (*Clostridium tetani*)

tetany (tet'-ah-nee): a condition in which severely decreased levels of calcium affect the normal function of nerves

thalamus (thal'-a-mus): part of the diencephalon, relays sensory stimuli to the cerebral cortex

thalassemia (thal-ah-see-mee-a): *see* Cooley's anemia

third degree burn *see* burn

thoracentesis (thor"-ruh-sen-tee'-sis): aspiration of chest cavity for removal of fluid, usually for empyema

thoracic cavity (thoh-rass'-ick kav'-ih-tee): area of the body divided into two cavities, the left pleural cavity containing the left lung and the right pleural cavity containing the right lung

thoracic duct (thoh-rass'-ick dukt): lymphatic duct that receives lymph from the left side of the body

thoracic vertebrae (thoh-rass'-ick ver'-teh-bray): the 12 bones of the spine located in the chest area

thorax (tho'-raks): chest; portion of trunk above diaphragm and below neck

threshold (thresh'-hold): limit of reabsorption in the urinary system

thrombin (throm'-bin): enzyme found in blood; produced from an inactive precursor, prothrombin, inducing clotting by converting fibrinogen to fibrin

thrombocyte (throm'-boh-site): platelet, part of megakaryocyte cells necessary for blood clotting

thrombocytopenia (throm"-boh-siy-toh-pen'-ee-ah): decrease in the number of platelets

thromboplastin (throm'-boh-plas-tin): substance secreted by platelets when tissue is injured; necessary for blood clotting

thrombosis (throm-boh'-sis): formation of a clot in a blood vessel

thrombus (throm'-bus): blood clot formed in a blood vessel

thymus (thiy'-mus): endocrine located under the sternum; produces T-lymphocytes

thyroid gland (thiy'-royd gland): endocrine gland located on anterior portion of the neck produces thyroxine triiodothyronine and calcitonin

thyroid-stimulating hormone (TSH) (thiy'-royd stim'-yoo-lay-ting hor'-mone): hormone that stimulates the growth and secretion of the thyroid gland

thyroxine (T_4) (thigh-rok'-seen): hormone secreted by thyroid gland or prepared synthetically

TIA (t-i-a): transient ischemic attacks, temporary interruption of the blood flow in the brain

tibia (tib'-ee-uh): larger, inner bone of the leg, below the knee

tidal volume (teye'-dal vol'-yoom): amount of air that moves in and out of the lungs with each breath

tinnitus (tin-i'-tus): ringing sensation in one or both ears

tissue (tish'-yoo): cells grouped according to size, shape, and function; epithelial, connective, muscle, and nerve tissues are examples

T-lymphocyte (tee lim'-foh-cite): cells synthesized in the thymus gland

tonsillitis (ton-sill-eye'-tis): infection and swelling of the tonsils

tonsils (ton'-silz): mass of lymph tissue in the back of the throat which produces lymphocytes

torticollis (tor-ti-kol'-is): a contracted state of the neck muscles producing an unnatural position of the head; also called wryneck

total lung capacity (toh'-tal lung cah-pa'-sih-tee): measurement that includes tidal volume, inspiratory reserve, expiratory reserve, and residual air

toxic shock syndrome (tock'-sick shock sin'-drome): a bacterial infection caused by a staphylococcus organism

trace element (trays el'-eh-ment): substances found in the body in very small amounts

trachea (tray'-kee-ah): a thin-walled tube between the larynx and the bronchi; conducts air to the lungs

transient flora (tran'-see-ent floor'-ah): microorganisms that attach to the skin for a brief time but do not continuously live on the skin

transient ischemic attack (TIA) (tran'-see-ent is-kee'-mick ah-tack'): temporary interruptions in blood flow to the brain

transmyocardial laser revascularization (TMR) (tranz'-meye-oh-car'-dee-ahl lay'-zer re-vass''-kyoo-lar-ih-zay'-shun):

transverse (trans-vurse'): crosswise; at right angles to longitudinal axis of body

transverse colon (trans-verse' koh'-lun): portion of the colon that veers left across the abdomen to just below the spleen

triceps (tri'-seps): three-headed muscle on back of upper arm

trichomoniasis (trick''-oh-moh-neye'-ah-sis): a sexually transmitted disease caused by infection with the protozoan *Trichomonas vaginalis*

tricuspid valve (tri-kus'-pid valv): three-part valve located between the right atrium and right ventricle (AV Valve)

trigeminal neuralgia (tri-jem'-i-nel noo-ral'-ja): painful condition affecting the fifth cranial nerve; also known as tic douloureux

triglyceride (try-glis'-er-ide): fat and oil in food

triiodothyronine (T$_3$) (try''-eye-oh''-doh-thigh'-roh-nen): hormone that serves to regulate body systems

trisomy 21 (try-soh-mee 21): *see* Down syndrome

true ribs (tru ribz): first seven pairs of ribs which are attached to the sternum by costal cartilage

trypsin (trip'-sin): one of four protein-digesting enzymes found in pancreatic juice

tuberculosis (too-bur''-kya-loh'-sis): infectious disease caused by tubercule bacillus, mainly affects lung

tumor (too'-mer): abnormal and uncontrolled growth of cell

tunica adventitia (too'-nih-kah ad-ven-tish'-uh): the outer layer of the arterial walls

tunica intima (too'-nih-kah in'-tim-uh): the inner arterial layer

tunica media (too'-nih-kah mee'-dee-uh): the middle arterial layer

turbinate (tur'-bin-ut): shaped like a spiral; the three bones situated on the lateral side of the nasal cavity

tympanic membrane (tim-pan'-ik mem'-brayn): membrane that separates the external ear from a middle ear

U

ulcer (ul'-sur): inflammation that occurs on the mucosal skin surface

ulna (ul'-nuh): bone on inner forearm

umbilical (um-bil'-ih-kal): area located around the naval; the right and left lumbar region

umbilicus (um-bil'-i-kus): navel

unicellular (yoo''-nih-sel'-yoo-lur): composed of one cell

universal donor (yoo''-nih-vur'-sul do'-nur): type O blood; has no A or B antigens; can be donated to all blood types

universal recipient (yoo''-nih-vur'-sul re-sip'-ee-unt): individual belonging to AB blood group

upper limit (UL) (uh'-per lih'-mit): the maximum amount of a vitamin or mineral recommended to be taken in

uremia (yoo-ree'-mee-ah): the presence of urea and excess waste products in the blood

ureter (yoor'-ah-ter): the long narrow tube that conveys urine from the kidney to the urinary bladder

urethra (yoo-re'-thra): the tube that takes urine from the bladder to the outside of the body

urinalysis (yoor-i-nal'-ah-sis): the chemical analysis of urine

urinary bladder (yoor'-i-ner-ee blad'-er): a muscular membrane-lined sac situated in the anterior part of the pelvic cavity and used to hold urine

urinary meatus (yoor'-i-ner-ee mee'-tus): the opening to the urethra

urticaria (ur''-ti-kar'-ee-a): skin condition characterized by itching wheals or welts and usually caused by an allergic reaction also known as hives

uterus (yoo'-ter-us): hollow, thick-walled, muscular organ that houses the fetus during pregnancy

uvula (yoo'-vew-luh): projection hanging from soft palate, in back of throat

V

vacuole (vak'-yoo-ole): (1) clear space in cell; (2) cavity bound by a single membrane; usually a storage area for fat, glycogen, secretions, liquid, or debris

vagina (va-jie'-nuh): sheathlike structure; tube in females, extending from the uterus to the vulva

valve (valv): structure which permits flow of a fluid in only one direction

varicose veins (var'-i-kose vayns): veins that have become abnormally dilated and tortuous, due to interference with venous drainage or weakness of their walls

vas deferens (vas deaf'-er-ens): a continuation of the epididymis

vasopressin (vay"-zo-pres'-in): hormone secreted by the posterior pituitary gland; has an antidiuretic effect; also called antidiuretic hormone (ADH)

vectorborne transmission (veck'-tor-born trans-mish'-un): transfer of an agent to a susceptible host by animate means such as mosquitoes, fleas, and ticks

vehicle transmission (vee'-hih-cahl trans-mish'-un): transfer of an agent to a susceptible host by contaminated inanimate objects such as food, milk, and drugs

vein (vane): vessel that carries blood toward the heart

vena cava (ve'-nah ka'-vah): large blood vessel that returns blood to the right atrium; there are two: superior and inferior

ventral (ven'-trul): front or anterior; opposite of posterior or dorsal

venule (ven'-yoo-ul): small vein

vermiform appendix (vur'-mi-form a-pen'-diks): small, blind gut projecting from cecum

vertigo (vur'-ti-go): sensation of dizziness

very low density lipoprotein (VLDL) (ver'-ee low den'-sih-tee lip-oh-proh'-teen): lipoprotein that carries fat to the cells

vestibule (ves'-tih-byool): a small cavity at the beginning of a canal

villi (vil'-eye): hairlike projections, as in intestinal mucous membrane

virulence (vir'-u-lens): frequency with which a pathogen causes disease

virus (veye'-rus): a disease-causing agent

visceral membrane (vis'-er-al mem'-brayn): the membrane covering each organ in a body cavity

vital lung capacity (veye'-tahl lung cah-pa'-sih-tee): total amount of air involved with tidal volume, inspiratory reserve volume, and expiratory reserve volume

vitamin (vye'-tuh-min): any of a group of organic compounds found in very small amounts in natural food; needed for the normal growth and maintenance of an organism

vitreous humor (vit'-ree-us hew'-mur): transparent, gelatinlike substance filling greater part of eyeball

vomer (vo'-mer): flat, thin bone that forms part of the nasal septum

vulva (vull'-vah): external female genitalia

W

wart (wart): a type of tumor of the epithelial tissue; also known as papilloma

wheezing (wee'-zing): sound produced by a rush of air through a narrowed passageway

whiplash injury (wip'lash in'-jer-ee): trauma to cervical vertebra

whooping cough (hoop'-ing kof): infectious disease characterized by repeated coughing attacks that end in a "whooping" sound; also called *pertussis*

wisdom tooth (wiz'-dum tooth): third molar tooth in adult mouth

Y

yawning (yawn'-ing): deep, prolonged breath that fills the lungs

yeast infection (yeest in-feck'-shun): an infection caused by the *Candida albicans* organism

Z

zygote (zye'-gote): organism produced by union of two gametes

zygomatic (zeye"-goh-mat'-ick): bone that forms the prominence of the cheek

INDEX

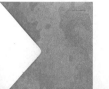

Getting Started with Delmar's Anatomy & Physiology CD-ROM

System Requirements

- 100 MHz Pentium w/24 MB of RAM
- Windows® 95 or newer
- Sound card and speakers
- SVGA 24-bit color display
- 8 megabytes of free disk space

Windows 95 ® is either registered trademarks or trademarks of Microsoft Corporation in the United States and/or other countries

Set-Up Instructions

1. Insert disk into CD ROM player

2. From the Start Menu, choose RUN

3. In the Open text box, enter ***d: setup.exe*** then click the OK button.(Substitute the letter of your CD ROM drive for ***d:***)

4. Follow the installation prompts from there.

License Agreement for Delmar Learning, a division of Thomson Learning, Inc.

Educational Software/Data

You the customer, and Delmar Learning, a division of Thomson Learning, Inc. incur certain benefits, rights, and obligations to each other when you open this package and use the software/data it contains. BE SURE YOU READ THE LICENSE AGREEMENT CAREFULLY, SINCE BY USING THE SOFTWARE/DATA YOU INDICATE YOU HAVE READ, UNDERSTOOD, AND ACCEPTED THE TERMS OF THIS AGREEMENT.

Your rights:
1. You enjoy a non-exclusive license to use the software/data on a single microcomputer in consideration for payment of the required license fee, (which may be included in the purchase price of an accompanying print component), or receipt of this software/data, and your acceptance of the terms and conditions of this agreement.
2. You acknowledge that you do not own the aforesaid software/data. You also acknowledge that the software/data is furnished "as is," and contains copyrighted and/or proprietary and confidential information of Delmar Learning, a division of Thomson Learning, Inc. or its licensors.

There are limitations on your rights:
1. You may not copy or print the software/data for any reason whatsoever, except to install it on a hard drive on a single microcomputer and to make one archival copy, unless copying or printing is expressly permitted in writing or statements recorded on the diskette(s).
2. You may not revise, translate, convert, disassemble or otherwise reverse engineer the software/data except that you may add to or rearrange any data recorded on the media as part of the normal use of the software/data.
3. You may not sell, license, lease, rent, loan or otherwise distribute or network the software/data except that you may give the software/data to a student or and instructor for use at school or, temporarily at home.

Should you fail to abide by the Copyright Law of the United States as it applies to this software/data your license to use it will become invalid. You agree to erase or otherwise destroy the software/data immediately after receiving note of termination of this agreement for violation of its provisions from Delmar Learning.

Delmar Learning, a division of Thomson Learning, Inc. gives you a LIMITED WARRANTY covering the enclosed software/data. The LIMITED WARRANTY follows this License.

This license is the entire agreement between you and Delmar Learning, a division of Thomson Learning, Inc. interpreted and enforced under New York law.

LIMITED WARRANTY

Delmar Learning, a division of Thomson Learning, Inc. warrants to the original licensee/purchaser of this copy of microcomputer software/data and the media on which it is recorded that the media will be free from defects in material and workmanship for ninety (90) days from the date of original purchase. All implied warranties are limited in duration to this ninety (90) day period. THEREAFTER, ANY IMPLIED WARRANTIES, INCLUDING IMPLIED WARRANTIES OF MERCHANTABILITY AND FITNESS FOR A PARTICULAR PURPOSE, ARE EXCLUDED. THIS WARRANTY IS IN LIEU OF ALL OTHER WARRANTIES, WHETHER ORAL OR WRITTEN, EXPRESS OR IMPLIED.

If you believe the media is defective please return it during the ninety day period to the address shown below. Defective media will be replaced without charge provided that it has not been subjected to misuse or damage.

This warranty does not extend to the software or information recorded on the media. The software and information are provided "AS IS." Any statements made about the utility of the software or information are not to be considered as express or implied warranties.

Limitation of liability: Our liability to you for any losses shall be limited to direct damages, and shall not exceed the amount you paid for the software. In no event will we be liable to you for any indirect, special, incidental, or consequential damages (including loss of profits) even if we have been advised of the possibility of such damages.

Some states do not allow the exclusion or limitation of incidental or consequential damages, or limitations on the duration of implied warranties, so the above limitation or exclusion may not apply to you. This warranty gives you specific legal rights, and you may also have other rights which vary from state to state. Address all correspondence to: Delmar Learning, a division of Thomson Learning, Inc., 5 Maxwell Drive, P.O. Box 8007, Clifton Park, NY 12065-8007. Attention: Technology Department